Health in
Elementary
Schools

HEALTH IN ELEMENTARY SCHOOLS

HAROLD J. CORNACCHIA, Ed.D.

Emeritus Professor of Health Education,
San Francisco State University,
San Francisco, California

LARRY K. OLSEN, Dr.P.H.

Professor, Health Education,
The Pennsylvania State University,
University Park, Pennsylvania

CARL J. NICKERSON, Ed.D.

School Health Consultant,
Olympia, Washington

SEVENTH EDITION
with 70 illustrations

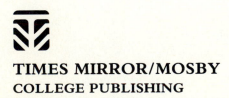

TIMES MIRROR/MOSBY
COLLEGE PUBLISHING

ST. LOUIS   TORONTO   SANTA CLARA   1988

Editor: Nancy K. Roberson
Editorial assistant: Susan Clancy
Project manager: Teri Merchant
Production editor: Deborah L. Vogel
Design: Gail Morey Hudson

SEVENTH EDITION

Copyright © 1988 by Times Mirror/Mosby College Publishing

A division of The C.V. Mosby Company
11830 Westline Industrial Drive
St. Louis, Missouri 63146

Previous editions copyrighted 1962, 1966, 1970, 1974, 1979, 1984

Printed in the United States of America

Library of Congress Cataloging-in-Publication Data

Cornacchia, Harold J.
  Health in elementary schools.

  Includes bibliographies and index.
  1. School hygiene—United States.   2. Health
education (Elementary)—United States.   I. Olsen,
Larry K.   II. Nickerson, Carl J.   III. Title.
[DNLM: 1. Health Education—United States.   2. School
Health Services—United States. QT 200 C812h]
LB3409.U5C63   1988   372.3'7   87-17996
ISBN 0-8016-1120-2

GW/VH/VH   9 8 7 6 5 4 3 2 1   02/B/245

PREFACE

Numerous health problems need attention in the United States. Communicable diseases such as smallpox, diphtheria, and poliomyelitis have been brought under control through immunization and improvements in sanitation, housing, and nutrition. However, heart disease, high blood pressure, cancer, accidents, stress, sexually transmitted diseases, AIDS, and the misuse and abuse of alcohol, tobacco (including smokeless tobacco), and other drugs (including cocaine) are common today. Elementary school-age children generally are in good health, yet there are numerous health conditions such as respiratory and gastrointestinal disturbances, vision and hearing problems, emotional difficulties, child neglect and abuse, suicide, drug abuse, dental caries, pregnancies, and obesity that need to be identified by school personnel, with information and guidance provided for pupils and parents.

Much of the illness found among children and adults can be *prevented* or at least reduced in incidence and severity through the avoidance of *risk factors* and through *lifestyle modifications*. Since many adult conditions depend on habit patterns established in the early years of life, programs in schools that provide health education, health services, and a healthful environment will aid in the establishment of practices of healthful living and contribute to pupil well-being when conducted in cooperation with the home and the community.

NEED FOR ELEMENTARY SCHOOL HEALTH EDUCATION

Awareness of the need for health education has greatly increased in recent years. It is widely recognized that individuals must assume more responsibility for their own health. Individuals now realize that health care involves not only physiological considerations but also psychological, sociological, and spiritual emphasis. Health education is needed because of the (1) high cost of medical care, (2) existence of health misconceptions, (3) millions of dollars spent on useless, unnecessary, and harmful products and services, (4) influences on behavior by peers, adults, and the media, (5) confusing and often inaccurate health information disseminated, and (6) desire of people to be healthy.

Health education programs are now supported by the American School Health Association, the Association of the Advancement of Health Education, The American Public Health Association, The American Association of School Administrators, The National Association of State Boards of Education, the American Medical Association, The American Academy of Pediatrics, and the National Congress of Parents and Teachers. The federal government has established the Center for Health Promotion and Education in the Centers for Disease Control, Public Health Service, and Department of Health and Human Services. In the private sector, the National Center for Health Education has been functioning for over 5 years. Numerous companies and foundations such as the Metropolitan Life Foundation are providing funds for demonstrations of comprehensive school health education programs. Thirty-eight states (76%) have mandated school health education, and seven more have encouraged the subject to be included in the curriculum.

Unfortunately, less than 22% of the elementary schools in the United States have health

v

education programs, and few of these programs are comprehensive. The legal provisions in states often are so loosely written that numerous programs are limited to one or more health topics such as nutrition, drugs, or safety. The term *comprehensive* has been subject to a variety of interpretations. Its meaning as defined in this text and accepted by school health experts has not been implemented to any great extent in U.S. schools. Several problems related to the lack of school finances and the public's demand for a return to teaching the basic subjects have compounded the difficulty of developing health instruction programs despite the increased awareness of need and the progress made in recent years.

GOALS FOR THIS REVISION

The authors of this text continue to firmly believe that:

1. Good health is essential to learning.
2. The prevention approach to health and the need for self-care must be initiated in the early years of life.
3. Schools play an important role in the well-being of students.
4. Despite present problems, health education can be introduced into schools.

It follows therefore that teachers, especially at the elementary level, need to understand the nature and purpose of school health programs and must learn their role in such programs. Thus the major goal of this text has not changed from that of previous editions. To this end this book has been organized to deal primarily with *health education*—curriculum, learning applied to health education, methods and techniques of teaching, instructional aids, evaluation—and with *health services*, the *healthful school environment*, and *coordination* of the program.

AUDIENCE FOR THIS BOOK

This book has been designed to be a practical guide for prospective and in-service elementary teachers and for health service personnel and school administrators. Prospective teachers will obtain a preview of their role in the school health program. In-service teachers may use the text to evaluate and develop health education programs for schools that do not have such programs. School health coordinators, curriculum coordinators, principals, school board members, and health specialists will find this volume to be helpful in the development and implementation of curricula and in the preparation of guiding principles and programs. Public health personnel will be able to clarify problems concerning organization, objectives, curriculum development, supervision, and teaching methods and material related to elementary school health programs.

ORGANIZATION OF TEXT

This text is arranged to provide an introduction to school health in Part One by identifying its nature and purpose, as well as the role of the classroom teacher.

Coverage of healthful school living and health services is found in Parts Two and Three, with some information located in the Appendixes.

Parts Four, Five, and Six, and most of the Appendixes focus on health education. The content represents about 70% of the text material.

The status of health education today, the learning process in health education, illustrations of popular and effective programs, and principles and procedures of organization are covered in Part Four.

Methods and materials in health education, including an introduction to general methods with over 1200 teacher-tested techniques categorized by subject area and grade level group, are contained in Part Five.

An understanding of evaluation with practical suggestions for teacher use in the classroom are found in Part Six.

The Appendixes include sources of programs and teaching aids, the American School Health Association statement on AIDS, evaluation information, and partial health units that may be used to develop units and curricula.

NEW IN THIS EDITION

The changes that follow are the result of a critical analysis of the sixth edition by several reviewers, a computer search for data, and author contributions:

1. Part Four "Health Education," has been changed to provide a more complete and orderly approach to health education. Chapter 9, "The Learning Process and Health Education," has been changed to focus more on the principles of learning as they apply to health education. This is followed by Chapter 10, "Health Education Approaches," and Chapter 11, "Organizing For Health Teaching."

2. Up-to-date information on AIDS as it applies to schools today can be found in Chapter 5, and the official statement on AIDS by the American School Health Association can be found in Appendix A.

3. The Surgeon General's Health Goals for 1990 and their implied challenges for school health programs have been highlighted in Chapter 1.

4. The latest research on environmental impacts as they affect a child's emotional health, such as family crises, latchkey children, and alcohol and drug abuse, have been addressed in Chapter 4, "Emotional Climate and The Teacher." How the teacher can improve the emotional climate of the child follows.

5. A variety of new photos and illustrations have been provided and the illustrations on first aid in Chapter 7 were redrawn to improve clarity.

6. Key concepts and chapter summaries have been added to assist the student in understanding the material presented.

PEDAGOGICAL FEATURES

1. A key concept opens each chapter to provide a content focus for the student.

2. Summaries end each chapter with a brief review of the material covered, assisting the student in understanding and retaining chapter content.

3. Updated references for each chapter provide students with further information about the subjects discussed within the chapters.

4. Questions for discussion are found at the end of each chapter; they may be used for classroom activities or essay test questions.

5. Table 9-2, "Principles of Learning and Their Reference to Test Information" can be used to show relations, importance, and application of principles.

INSTRUCTOR'S MANUAL

The Instructor's Manual provides specific help for teachers when planning course outlines and teacher/learning activities. The manual contains a rating utilizing the principles of learning in the selection of effective teaching techniques. It has been improved to provide additional useful material and information. It contains general and specific student objectives, new suggestions for classroom teaching/learning activities, and the latest audiovisual aids available. The objective type of true-false, multiple choice, and completion questions for examinations have been reviewed, modified where necessary, and increased in number.

IN CONCLUSION

The authors have made every effort to present the latest and best in research, practice, and thought in school health in light of what is feasible and practical for elementary schools throughout the nation. We have attempted to provide a synthesis of fundamental principles that are generally accepted by professionals and that we in our many years of experience have found to work best in elementary schools. It is necessary for teachers, administrators, and others to implement these principles and practices for health education programs to be effective.

If this volume helps to bring about favorable changes in elementary school health programs, if we lead classroom teachers to recognize the powerful potential influence they have on the health of children, if we provoke principals to take a critical look at school health, if we touch the conscience of superintendents or school board members, if we pique the curiosity of health departments or voluntary health agencies, or above all, if we in some way enrich the lives of elementary school children, we will have achieved the goal for which this book was written.

ACKNOWLEDGMENTS

Finally, we are grateful to all those people and organizations who have helped us make this seventh edition of *Health in Elementary Schools* a better book. We are especially indebted to those classroom teachers, our friends in the profession, and our students who offered stimulation and useful suggestions. We wish to thank Lynda Garitone and Sue Nickerson for their assistance in typing the manuscript.

In addition, we would like to thank the following reviewers for their valuable input, which helped in the revision of this edition:

June Gorski
University of Tennessee

Kathleen Shreve
University of Florida

Norm Eburn
Western Oregon State College

Frank Schabel
Iowa State University

Harold J. Cornacchia
Larry K. Olsen
Carl J. Nickerson

CONTENTS

PART

I

THE ELEMENTARY SCHOOL HEALTH PROGRAM

CHAPTER 1

SCHOOL HEALTH: ITS NATURE AND PURPOSE

The health of the American people has never been better. American children today are healthier than ever before.

JULIUS B. RICHMOND, M.D.

Former Surgeon General of the United States*

KEY CONCEPT: Comprehensive school health programs that include instruction, services, and environmental phases play an important role in the promotion, prevention, and maintenance of student health.

Since 1900 the death rate in America has been reduced as a result of medical control over such diseases as tuberculosis, diphtheria, poliomyelitis, and gastroenteritis. Infant, child, and maternal mortality have decreased, and the life expectancy of individuals has increased from approximately 50 years in 1900 to almost 75 years in 1985. Improvements in sanitation, housing, nutrition, and immunization have resulted in control over typhoid fever, smallpox, plague, and other diseases. Progress is evident in the control of heart disease, some cancers, and other

chronic conditions. Despite these advances, however, many health and safety problems among young people, especially the poor, still exist in the United States. Acute illnesses result in an average loss per school year of 4.9 days for each American child. Numerous children are not completely immunized. Accidents are a major cause of death. Child abuse and neglect are of major concern. Students are experiencing learning difficulties related to such problems as hyperkinesis and dyslexia. Pupils are exposed to a variety of risk factors that lead to adult diseases and conditions. Infants, school-age children, adolescents, and adults are all affected by these risk factors.

The need for preventive actions and services

---

*U.S. Department of Health, Education and Welfare, Public Health Service: Healthy People—the Surgeon General's report on health promotion and disease prevention 1979, Washington, D.C., 1979, Superintendent of Documents.

to promote and preserve the health of individuals has now been recognized by Americans who have become increasingly aware and concerned with the preventive aspects of health. The American Academy of Pediatrics* advocates that children must be healthy to learn effectively and maintains that schools have a responsibility to promote optimal health in pupils. According to the American School Health Association,† a child needs to be healthy to learn. Attention to lifestyles and behavior together with control of environmental factors can reduce the need for medical and hospital care according to Julius B. Richmond, M.D., former Surgeon General of the United States. Dr. Richmond indicated the Public Health Service reviewed its priorities for the expenditure of funds in America and decided that the improvement of the health status of citizens could be achieved predominantly through preventive actions rather than through the treatment of disease.

In 1979, the first Surgeon General's report on health promotion and disease prevention, Healthy People, was published. It stated that good health could be preserved and ill health could be prevented. The report identified 15 priority areas in which if appropriate actions were taken, further health gains could be expected between the years 1980 and 1990. Broad national goals were established that could lead to the improvement of the health of Americans. These goals were expressed as reductions in overall death rates or days of disability. In 1980, the report Promoting Health/Preventing Disease was produced. It identified 207 specific objectives necessary to achieve the broad national goals. Over 65 of these had implications for school programs. Selected objectives that have school implications for most of the areas are listed in Table 1-1. Progress toward the achievement of some of these goals is charted in Table 1-2.

Authorities agree that the best time for build-

ing the foundations for better health is early in life. It follows then that one of society's largest— and potentially most influential—organizations offers vast opportunities for raising the level of health of the individual, the family, and the community. Obviously, we speak here of the 58,000 public and private elementary schools dotting the cities, suburbs, towns, and countryside of America. We think too of the almost limitless ways in which elementary teachers and school administrators—with the help of health specialists *and* the support of parents and the community—can favorably affect the health of 45 million boys and girls in schools across the land. This is through enlightened *health teaching* and provision for *health services* and a *healthful school environment*. Fig. 1-1 outlines the main activities of the entire school health program.

But our schools are in trouble. Teachers, prospective teachers, educational administrators, legislators, parents, education faculty in colleges and universities, taxpayers, and the news media have all become increasingly concerned about our schools. As problems continue to mount, cluttering the road to quality education for all children, it is clear that bold measures must be taken if we are to give more than lip service to repeated statements of lofty objectives and high ideals for America's schools.

Our schools and our society are beset with the harsh reality of economic, political, and other social problems that affect the quality of life. The question of tax sources for the equitable and adequate support of our schools has become critical. Piled atop the money problems are the tangled issues of busing, lowered enrollments, school closings, collective negotiations between teachers and school boards, health and safety conditions for pupils and teachers, conflicts in administrative and learning theories, "accountability" procedures for both pupils and teachers, and recently, public concern over the quality of education and teachers, and the call for a return to the basic subjects in education.

However, since this is a book about elementary schools and their health programs, we cannot properly analyze all those forces that tend

---

*Committee on School Health: School health: a guide for health professionals, Evanston, Ill., 1981, American Academy of Pediatrics.

†American School Health Association, Marketing Kit, 1985.

TABLE 1-1. Selected areas and objectives from the Surgeon General's report, Promoting Health/Preventing Disease

Areas	Objectives
	By 1990:
High blood pressure	At least 50% of adults should be able to state the principal risk factors for coronary heart disease and stroke (i.e., high blood pressure, cigarette smoking, elevated blood cholesterol levels, diabetes).
Family planning	There should be no unintended births to girls 14 years old or younger.
	At least 75% of men and women over the age of 14 should be able to describe accurately the various contraceptive methods including the relative safety and effectiveness of one method versus the other.
Pregnancy and infant health	85% of women of childbearing age should be able to choose foods wisely and understand the hazards of smoking, alcohol, pharmaceutical products, and other drugs during pregnancy and lactation.
Immunization	At least 95% of children attending licensed day care facilities, and kindergarten through twelfth grade should be fully immunized.
Sexually transmitted diseases	Every junior and senior high school student in the United States should receive accurate, timely education about sexually transmitted diseases.
Toxic agent control	At least half of all people ages 15 years and older should be able to identify the major categories of environmental threats to health and note some of the health consequences of those threats.
Accident prevention and control	The motor vehicle fatality rate for children under 15 should be reduced to no greater than 5.5 per 100,000 children; the home accident fatality rate should be no greater than 5.0 per 100,000 population.
Fluoridation and dental health	At least 95% of school children and their parents should be able to identify the principal risk factors related to dental diseases and be aware of the importance of fluoridation and other measures in controlling these diseases.
	At least 65% of school children should be proficient in personal oral hygiene practices and should be receiving other needed preventive dental services in addition to fluoridation.
	No public elementary or secondary school should offer highly cariogenic foods or snacks in vending machines or in school breakfast or lunch programs.
Smoking and health	The proportion of children and youth aged 12 to 18 years old who smoke should be reduced to below 6%.
Misuse of alcohol and drugs	The proportion of adolescents 12 to 17 years old who abstain from using alcohol or other drugs should not fall below the 1977 levels (alcohol, 46%; marijuana, 89%; heroin, 99.9%).
	The proportion of adolescents 14 to 17 years old who report acute drinking-related problems during the past year should be reduced to below 17%.
	The proportion of adolescents 12 to 17 years old reporting frequent use of other drugs should not exceed 1977 levels (marijuana, 19%; other drugs, 1%).
Nutrition	All states should include nutrition education as part of required comprehensive school health education at elementary and secondary schools.
Physical fitness and exercise	The proportion of children and adolescents aged 10 to 17 participating in daily school physical education programs should be greater than 60%.
	The proportion of children and adolescents aged 10 to 17 participating regularly in appropriate physical activities, particularly cardiorespiratory fitness programs which can be carried into adulthood should be greater than 90%.
Control of stress and violent behavior	Stress identification and control should become integral components of the continuum of health services.
	Injuries and deaths to children inflicted by abusing parents should be reduced by at least 25%.
	The rate of suicide among people 15 to 24 years should be below 11 per 1,000.

U.S. Department of Health and Human Services, Public Health Service: Promoting health/preventing disease: objectives for the nation, Washington, D.C., 1980, U.S. Government Printing Office.

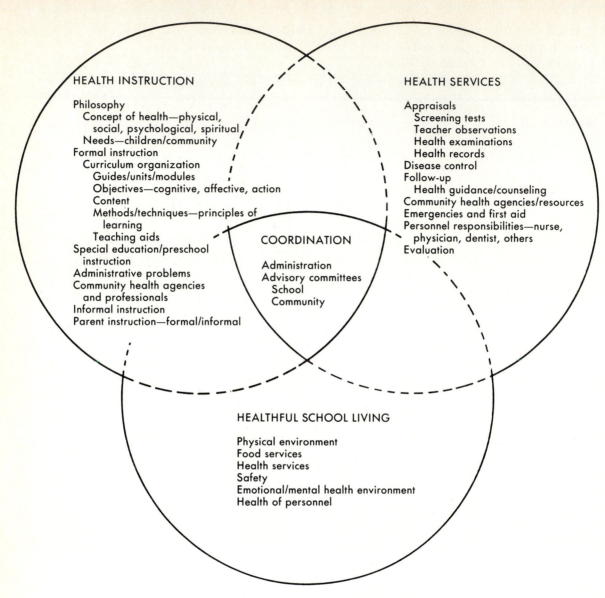

HEALTH INSTRUCTION

Philosophy
   Concept of health—physical,
     social, psychological, spiritual
   Needs—children/community
Formal instruction
   Curriculum organization
     Guides/units/modules
     Objectives—cognitive, affective, action
     Content
     Methods/techniques—principles of
      learning
     Teaching aids
Special education/preschool
   instruction
Administrative problems
Community health agencies
   and professionals
Informal instruction
Parent instruction—formal/informal

HEALTH SERVICES

Appraisals
   Screening tests
   Teacher observations
   Health examinations
   Health records
Disease control
Follow-up
   Health guidance/counseling
Community health agencies/resources
Emergencies and first aid
Personnel responsibilities—nurse,
   physician, dentist, others
Evaluation

COORDINATION

Administration
Advisory committees
   School
   Community

HEALTHFUL SCHOOL LIVING

Physical environment
Food services
Health services
Safety
Emotional/mental health environment
Health of personnel

FIG. 1-1. Elementary school health program.

to shape our culture and our schools. Nevertheless, the need for *preventive* health care has never been more critical, and its advocacy is increasing substantially each year. Authorities now realize that it is not only necessary but also economically more feasible and desirable to reduce the incidence of health problems. The schools have a vital role to play in such action.

Yet, school health does not exist in a vacuum. The school health program is part of the lifeblood of America's better schools, and like all aspects of good schools, it is sensitive to significant thinking and events in the community in which it thrives. In a very real sense the school reflects the character of its community—local, state, and national. Health instruction must be

TABLE 1-2. 1983 Progress report toward achievement of selected Surgeon General's goals for 1990

Areas	Progress
High blood pressure	24% of adults have blood pressure under control
Family planning	Slight decline in teen pregnancies; births among unmarried women on the rise
Sexually transmitted diseases	Problem is increasing and expanding in scope and complexity
Accident prevention and control	Motor vehicle fatality rate down from 23.6 in 1978 to 19.0 in 1983 per 100,000 population
	Home injury fatality rate of children under 15 dropped from 6.0 in 1978 to 5.0 in 1983 per 100,000 population
	Fatalities from residential fires were down from 5,400 in 1978 to 4,500 in 1983.
Smoking and health	Proportion of people who have smoked down from 33.5% to 30.5%
	Far greater awareness of smoking hazards
Alcohol and drugs	Rate of alcohol-related vehicle fatalities down from 11.5 to 9 per 100,000 population
	Deaths from nonmotor vehicle accidents attributable to alcohol down from 7 to 4.3 per 100,000 population
	Drug deaths on the rise
Stress and violent behavior	Homicide deaths among blacks 15 to 24 down from 70.7 in 1980 to 66.8 in 1983 per 100,000 population

Review of progress on prevention: heartening, tragic, and in between, The Nation's Health, 1, 14, 20, Feb., 1987.

closely related to day-to-day problems of health and safety; school health services depend in large measure on the community's health resources; and the healthful school environment is in itself part of the community.

It is the basic thesis of education that the thinking and the behavior of people can be changed for the better. We assume with the confidence that grows out of research and experience that good teaching in a favorable setting will raise the quality of living for pupils. By enriching the lives of millions of children, elementary education cannot help contributing to forming a better society.

This "better society" and "the good life" have challenged humans for thousands of years. Along with the family, the church and temple, and the community in general, schools have continuously sought to help people live better individually and in groups. Although there have been shifts in philosophy from time to time, the ultimate purpose of our schools has remained constant.

Teachers and elementary school personnel in the United States are in a unique position to contribute significantly to the preventive concept of health. They can help preserve and promote the well-being of students through the provision of services, programs, and activities that will have great influence on pupil behavior and lifestyles.

WHAT IS PREVENTION?

Prevention has multiple meanings. Literally, to prevent is to keep something from happening. Prevention includes the protection and promotion of health. It involves primary, secondary, and tertiary aspects. Schools generally provide for primary and secondary preventive assistance.

Primary prevention refers to action taken to interfere with something happening or a procedure to stop something before it starts. Specifically, it is an attempt through education and other procedures to help students refrain from the use of or reduce the misuse of drugs, obtain immunizations, and generally make intelligent decisions in regard to their health. This type of prevention may take place in the school or in the community. Within the school the education may be formal or informal and may be provided for students, parents, school personnel, and others.

Secondary prevention relates to procedures taken after an illness or abnormal condition has occurred so that it does not get worse or become more advanced. It includes early detection of conditions and the use of follow-up procedures to obtain the necessary treatment or adjustments. For example, a teacher who observes a student with a suspicious skin rash sends the child to the school nurse. The nurse concludes that the problem needs medical attention and telephones the child's parent, advising that the student be examined by a physician. The school health program usually provides counseling and guidance that may include referral of children to community resources.

Tertiary prevention is an extension of secondary prevention in which action is taken to interrupt the development of more serious conditions. It refers to treatment and rehabilitation services rendered by physicians, psychiatrists, and other professionals to save lives, restore pupils to high levels of wellness, and prevent serious personality damage. This service is generally not a function of schools and usually takes place outside the school setting. For example, a child with diabetes, epilepsy, heart disease, or hyperkinesis is in need of medical assistance. Communication between the school, parents, and physicians is needed for appropriate adjustments to be made in the school setting.

WHAT IS HEALTH?

Health includes multiple phenomena and therefore cannot be simply or easily defined. Comprehension of the variety of components that comprise health is essential to understanding health's nature and its importance in the school health program.

Health is a condition of the organism that may be represented on a continuum from so-called good health to so-called bad health, or from "wellness" to "illness," with many variations in between. People desire to find themselves at the positive end of the health scale and not at the negative end. Where any person fits on the continuum at any given time depends on these factors:

1. *Health is personal.* Each person is born with a specific constitution or physical body that is provided through the genetic structure inherited from parents. Individuals are the same in many ways (number of arms, legs, and eyes) and different in many ways (size, shape, and color of skin and eyes). Some children may be tall, obese, have only one kidney, have allergies, or perhaps minimal brain damage. Some pupils have susceptibilities to certain diseases and conditions. Thus health is individual and variable.

2. *Health is frequently changing.* It is the result of the interaction of the individual (genetic heredity) with many factors and experiences in the environment.

3. *Health depends on self-actualization.* It necessitates internalization by the individual. Each person must make a decision whether to promote and preserve his or her own health.

4. *Health is a means to an end.* Health is necessary for effective learning and living. A child with poor health may have difficulty learning to read, doing arithmetic, or speaking and may have trouble later in life, such as when trying to obtain a job.

Health is a complex phenomenon that includes a composite of the physiological, psychological, sociological, and spiritual interrelated components of the modified concept of health shown in Fig. 1-2. These components have special significance in helping students make *intelligent decisions* as to the environmental health factors and experiences they face in society. These components must receive greater consideration in teaching to achieve more effective health education.

The isosceles triangle in Fig. 1-2 shows that physiological aspects form the base of the triangle and are fundamental to all learning. Students need to understand the structure and function of the human organism and the nature of good and ill health and diseases and conditions. However, this is of less importance in health instruction than the psychological and sociological aspects represented by the longer, vertical sides of the triangle. The diagram also indicates that emotional and physical needs are reciprocally related to people—friends, rela-

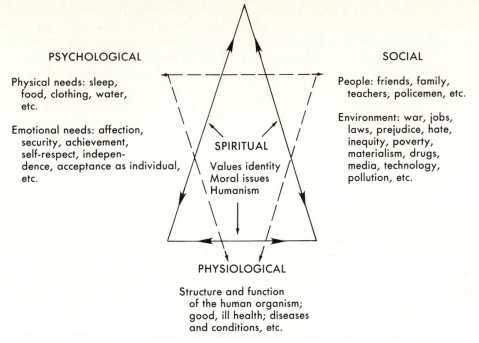

PSYCHOLOGICAL

Physical needs: sleep,
food, clothing, water,
etc.

Emotional needs: affection,
security, achievement,
self-respect, indepen-
dence, acceptance as individual,
etc.

SPIRITUAL

Values identity
Moral issues
Humanism

SOCIAL

People: friends, family,
teachers, policemen, etc.

Environment: war, jobs,
laws, prejudice, hate,
inequity, poverty,
materialism, drugs,
media, technology,
pollution, etc.

PHYSIOLOGICAL

Structure and function
of the human organism;
good, ill health; diseases
and conditions, etc.

FIG. 1-2. A modified concept of health. *(Health is a complex phenomenon. Adapted from Cornacchia, H.J., Smith, D.E., and Bentel, D.J.: Drugs in the classroom: a conceptual model for school programs, ed. 2, St. Louis, 1978, The C.V. Mosby Co.)*

tives, and others—and to the environment found in the social arena. These interrelating factors influence the structure and function of the human body (see dotted lines in Fig. 1-2). Unfortunately, these components are not often stressed in health instruction.

For example, a pupil may start to smoke cigarettes to satisfy an emotional need for acceptance or affection as well as to satisfy a desire to be part of a school peer group or to enter into adulthood. Cigarettes are readily available to the public and widely advertised as an acceptable form of social behavior. Thus the psychological need promotes the demand on the part of the manufacturers to satisfy the need and, reciprocally, the need is satisfied by the availability of the cigarettes and the encouragement of their use. There would be considerably less lung cancer, bronchitis, and emphysema if students could be directed toward alternative ways of satisfying their psychological needs. Pupils need

assistance in this regard as well as help in learning how to cope with societal pressures.

Probably the most important influence on health behavior, yet the one most frequently overlooked or omitted in the classroom, is the spiritual aspect. People's motivations toward health depend on their values, their recognition of moral issues in society, and their concern for the welfare of others. These are the driving forces of human behavior. They provide direction and establish the purposes or meanings of life, helping people determine their life goals. If individuals value their health, they will attempt to satisfy their emotional and physical needs through positive rather than negative behavior. They will learn to cope with the environmental and peer influences previously identified. They will conclude that their actions can also affect other people.

Unfortunately, few health education curricula in schools (see Chapter 10) have been designed to use the total-person concept of health described in this section. The holistic approach to health is being widely advocated and promoted. There is need to prepare instructional programs that help students understand their own health motivational factors and make them aware of the influence of the environment in which they live on these motivations. In addition, programs must help pupils with the development of values, comprehension of moral issues, and understandings of their effect. Such emphasis will enable children to *learn to make intelligent health decisions* and *learn to cope;* it will help them make adjustments to the social climate in which they live. Health instruction programs designed to include the total health concept will have more of an effect on the students' lives.

The concept of health described in this chapter, which includes the physiological, psychological, sociological, and spiritual aspects of health, has been used in the development of the illustrative units found in Appendix B. The extent to which emphasis of these components should be made at various grade levels is also identified in Appendix B.

WHAT FACTORS INFLUENCE PUPIL HEALTH?

A child's health is determined by three basic factors: *heredity, environment,* and *behavior.* Each boy and girl, as an individual personality, is a product of these fundamental forces.

As individuals, pupils differ in many ways. Differences in their facial and physical features are readily apparent, even to the casual observer. As a teacher, however, you observe other differences. You find that some learn quickly, others slowly; some show rapid rates of physical growth yet others lag behind, at least temporarily. Some learn motor skills easily and quickly; others seem never able to quite "get the hang of it" when a new physical skill is taught. All these and more are evidence of biological traits transmitted from parents to children. All these are proof of the miracle of heredity.

It is *heredity* that establishes a child's health endowment fund. What is passed on to the child by the genes and their constituent deoxyribonucleic acid (DNA) and ribonucleic acid (RNA) molecules from the parents, grandparents, and more distant ancestors has much to do with the child's capacity for good health. Heredity also plays a part in the predisposition to some mental disorders, infectious diseases, and chronic conditions such as cancer, heart disease, diabetes, hemophilia, and sickle cell anemia. All experienced teachers have seen the pupil with a strong constitution. This is the boy or girl who is alert, vigorous, seemingly indefatigable, and relatively free from illness. Similarly, teachers are familiar with the opposite—the weak, sickly child who seems always to be perched precariously on the figurative fence dividing health and illness. Often both children are exposed to essentially the same environment and follow much the same daily routine. In the absence of other explanations, such as previous illness or impairment, these health variances must be considered as being significantly influenced by heredity.

Environment has a direct bearing on the health of pupils. Boys and girls must interact with and adjust to an environment that is physical, biological, and social. *Physical* factors, such as weather and climate, housing, soil, water and food supply, medicines, radiation, clean or polluted air, recreational facilities, automobiles, hospitals, school buildings and sites, and many more physical things around us can affect health for better or worse. *Biological* influences include germs, plants, animals, and other people. These, too, may be helpful or harmful to health. For example, a pupil may catch a cold from a parent. At the same time that parent provides shelter, food, clothing, medical care, and other necessities that serve to maintain and improve the child's health. Some "friendly" germs in the intestinal tract manufacture certain vitamins that help prevent deficiencies; other germs are capable of causing disease and death. *Social* or *cultural environment* comprises all the interactions between and among people. These complex human relationships influence and are themselves influenced by patterns of culture at a given time and place. Hence, boys and girls are constantly exposed to the beliefs, attitudes, ideals, values, and customs of family, neighborhood, school, church, and the general community (local, state, national, and world) in which they live. In terms of nationwide values there remains little doubt that the thinking of both children and adults is influenced by vigorous and persuasive advertising through TV and other mass media. These cultural forces can directly or indirectly, for better or worse, affect the physical, mental, or emotional health of elementary school pupils.

To a far greater extent than either heredity or environment, *behavior*, or *lifestyle* that includes decision making, is generally the most influential factor in pupil health. Behavior is the result of the interaction of the psychological, social, and spiritual factors previously discussed. Young people in elementary schools are at impressionable ages, and teachers and schools can have a great impact on their lifestyles. With proper guidance and motivation, children can make corrections in their behavior or learn to make adjustments to hereditary limitations and environmental factors. An effective health instruction program can guide pupils toward lifestyles that will enable them to live in a healthful manner. It is the fundamental purpose of this text to help teachers and school personnel aid students in elementary schools achieve high levels of wellness.

WHAT ARE THE HEALTH PROBLEMS OF CHILDREN?

Despite the apparent good health of many children in the United States, there continues to be a variety of health and safety problems, especially among the poor, that have a draining effect on their energies, stamina, and capabilities. These problems are of such magnitude and diversity that the quality of education will be affected for students in those schools that fail to give them attention and do not provide a health program of the nature described in this text.

According to the American Academy of Pediatrics,* the most common health problems in children 3 to 5 years of age are acute infectious diseases (respiratory illnesses and gastrointestinal disorders), accidents, emotional disorders, dental caries, sensory defects (vision, hearing), and iron deficiency. Cancers are the leading cause of death in children aged 1 to 7, with 3,214 deaths occurring yearly. The American Cancer Society's data† for 1983 reveal that approximately 1,000 children ages 1 to 7 died of cancer that year, whereas 1,318 died who were between the ages of 5 and 14.

Early elementary school–age pupils have the next-to-lowest mortality and serious morbidity of any age group. Most physical illness in this age group is the result of accidental trauma and respiratory illness, usually of infectious origin. These students also have a variety of problems such as hearing, vision, and speech defects, dental caries, mental retardation, and emotional and educational problems.

What are the death rates of children and adults?

The average expected lifespan for all white Americans is 74.6 years (males, 71.7 years; females, 78.7 years), and for nonwhite Americans it is 69.5 years (males, 65.4 years; females, 73.6 years).

The 10 leading causes of death in 1986 are listed in Table 1-3. Almost 1.5 million people die annually from heart disease, cancer, and cerebrovascular diseases and accidents. These conditions may be prevented or reduced in incidence in elementary school children if the students receive attention and develop good lifestyle habits.

The death rates, estimated numbers of deaths, and percentages of deaths from selected causes for young people aged 5 to 14 years are shown

---

*American Academy of Pediatrics: School health: a guide for professionals, Evanston, Ill., 1981, The Academy.
†American Cancer Society: Personal communication, Oct. 1, 1986.

TABLE 1–3. Death rates, percent of total deaths, and estimated numbers of deaths for the 10 leading causes of death in the United States, 1986 (rates per 100,000 population)

Rank*	Cause of death	Rate	Percent of total deaths	Estimated numbers of deaths
	All causes	872.3	100.0	2,055,420
1	Diseases of heart	320.8	37.0	755,870
2	Malignant neoplasms, including neoplasms of lymphatic and hematopoietic tissues	193.2	22.0	455,524
3	Cerebrovascular diseases	62.8	7.0	147,960
4	Accidents and adverse effects	38.3	4.3	90,350
	Motor vehicle	19.6	—	43,840
	All other accidents	19.7	—	46,510
5	Chronic obstructive pulmonary diseases and allied conditions	31.0	3.5	72,930
6	Pneumonia and influenza	27.8	3.0	65,450
7	Diabetes mellitus	12.1	1.38	28,500
8	Suicide	11.3	1.29	26,660
9	Chronic liver disease and cirrhosis	9.4	1.0	22,080
10	Atherosclerosis	8.1	0.9	19,020

U.S. Department of Health and Human Services, Public Health Service: Monthly vital statistics report, vol. 35, National Center for Health Statistics, July 17, 1986, Births, marriages, divorces and deaths for April, 1986, Washington, D.C., 1986, U.S. Government Printing Office.
*Based on number of deaths.

TABLE 1–4. Death rates and estimated numbers and percentages for selected causes for children and youth 5 to 14 years of age, United States, 1983

Causes	Death rate (per 100,000 population)	Estimated number of deaths	Percentage
All	26.9	9,143	100
Accidents and adverse effects	12.7	4,321	47
Motor vehicle	6.6	2,241	
All other accidents	6.1	2,080	
Malignant neoplasms	3.9	1,318	14
Malignant neoplasms—all other and unspecific sites	1.7	563	6
Leukemia	1.5	507	5.5
Congenital anomalies	1.4	471	5
Major cardiovascular diseases	1.2	432	4.5
Homicide and legal interventions	1.0	357	4
Diseases of heart	0.9	318	3.5
Suicide	0.6	205	2
Pneumonia and influenza	0.4	130	1.5
Chronic obstructive pulmonary diseases and allied conditions	0.3	93	1.0

From U.S. Department of Health and Human Services, Public Health Service, National Center for Health Statistics: Monthly vital statistics report, 34(6):(Suppl. 2), Sept. 26, 1985, Advance report of final mortality statistics, Washington, D.C., 1983, U.S. Government Printing Office.

TABLE 1-5. Student accident* rates and school days lost for students in grades K-9 according to grades and location of activity, United States, 1983-84 school year

Location/activity	Grades				Days lost per injury
	K	1-3	4-6	7-9	
	(Accidents per 100,000 student days)				
Shops and labs	4.67	3.57	6.54	7.55	1.51
Buildings	1.67	1.05	1.49	1.97	1.40
Grounds—unorganized activities	1.23	1.30	1.98	0.31	1.42
Physical education	0.69	0.52	1.93	3.48	1.31
To and from school (motor vehicles)	0.22	0.20	0.22	0.21	2.26
To and from school (non–motor vehicles)	0.22	0.12	0.13	0.13	3.59

National Safety Council: Accident facts, Chicago, 1985, The Council.
*Accidents are those causing (1) the loss of ½ day or more of school time, (2) the loss of ½ day or more of activity during nonschool time, or (3) any property damage as a result of a school jurisdictional accident.

in Table 1-4. These rates and numbers are exceedingly low in comparison with other age groups when one considers there are over 26 million children of elementary school age in the United States.

What are the safety hazards for pupils?

Accidents are the leading cause of death and disability among children and youth. Approximately 4,300 young people aged 5 to 14 years were killed in 1983. Motor vehicle accidents accounted for almost 50% of these deaths, drownings for 16%, fire burns for 11%, and firearms for 5%. In 1984, 100 people (50 pupils) were killed in school bus accidents. There were 6,700 student injuries. Table 1-5 shows the student accident rates and school days lost per injury for 1983. Of the 8,600 school jurisdiction accidents 23% were related to playground equipment. One fourth of these were severe—concussions, crush wounds, fractures, and multiple injuries.

What are the physical illnesses and conditions?

Illnesses. Respiratory and gastrointestinal illnesses are the most common physical illnesses among young people. Allergic disease* (nasal allergy, asthma, other allergies) is the number one chronic illness of childhood. Streptococcal infection ("strep sore throat") has occurred 2 to 3 times in young people by the age of 10 years. Acute rheumatic fever, a serious complication of sore throat, may lead to permanent heart disease. Approximately 61% of school days missed by children are because of acute illnesses, primarily respiratory conditions. The common health problems contributing to short-term disability and school absenteeism of elementary pupils may be identified by rank as follows:

1. *Respiratory conditions:* including the common cold, sore throat, earache, bronchitis, influenza, asthma, and related conditions
2. *Infectious diseases:* including measles, chickenpox, German measles, and mumps; skin infections; sexually transmitted diseases among upper grade students
3. *Digestive disorders:* including viral and bacterial intestinal infections, food allergy, constipation, and appendicitis

Although the incidence of measles, rubella, mumps, pertussis, diphtheria, and poliomyelitis has dropped markedly since 1950, it is estimated that one third or more of preschool and school-age children in the U.S. are incompletely immunized.* Approximately one third of 12- to 17-year-olds have skin disorders in need of medical

*Richards, W., M.D.: Allergy, asthma, and school problems, Journal of School Health **56:**151-152, April, 1986.

*Miller, C.A., et al.: Monitoring children's health: key indicatives, Washington, D.C., 1986, American Public Health Association.

attention. About 8 out of every 1,000 children born in the United States each year have one or more congenital heart defects. Up to 1987, 498 cases of AIDS were reported in children and adolescents 18 years old or younger.

The two most common dental diseases are caries and periodontal disease. Many pupils also have gingivitis. The incidence of these increases as children get older. Decay probably affects more children than any other health problem with the exception of respiratory infections and injuries. Dental caries has been on the decline because of dietary changes and the use of fluorides in water, topical applications, and mouth washes.* It is estimated that 37% of children 5 to 17 years of age are presently caries free.

Conditions. Approximately 1 child in 20 aged 3 to 5 has a vision problem. About 20% of school-age pupils have visual acuity problems, and another 5% to 7% have some form of eye disease. Many of those in need of glasses do not have them. It is estimated that 10% of students have hearing difficulties, with 3% of these caused by middle-ear infections. Two percent of pupils are epileptic, and an additional 1% have major speech disorders.

What are the emotional problems?

It is estimated that 10% of pupils (4 to 5 million) have emotional problems requiring psychiatric help. An additional 2% to 3% have seriously psychotic or prepsychotic conditions. In a class of 30 children, a teacher may expect to recognize emotional difficulties in 3 children and possibly be able to identify 1 child in need of psychiatric assistance. Educational failure, or the "failure syndrome," is one of the underlying stress factors related to depression, acting-out in school, truancy, and maladjustments. Stress has a significant correlation to a variety of illnesses, including depression, asthma, and diabetes. It is also related to skin rashes, children's streptococcal infections, accidents, suicide, and substance abuse.

*Children's dental caries decreased dramatically, The Nation's Health Feb., 1982.

What are the social and lifestyle-related problems?

Approximately 59% of children aged 6 to 17 years have mothers in the work place. It is anticipated that by 1990 25% of all families will be headed by a single parent. The children of these families have been labeled "latchkey" children and have problems that may have implications for school health. (See Chapter 4.)

Child neglect and abuse. J. Fontana,* Medical Director of the New York Foundling Hospital, said child neglect and abuse is increasing in the United States at the yearly rate of 15%. He adds that these are the children who assault, rob, murder, and commit suicide. Although the incidence is unknown because many occurrences are never reported, the yearly estimate indicates that over 200 of the 1.4 to 1.9 million abused children die. The types of child neglect and abuse include physical and emotional neglect and physical and sexual abuse. Neglect refers to lack of adequate nutrition, clothing, and shelter, and failure of parents and caretakers to provide an emotionally stable environment. Neglect is more common than physical abuse, which causes bodily harm to children and is manifested by bruises, welts, abrasions, fractures, lacerations, and burns. Sexual abuse includes incest, sodomy, and rape.

Suicide. In 1983 over 28,000 people committed suicide and it is estimated 280,000 to 2,800,000 attempted suicide. White males generally have the highest suicide rate. The rate among teenagers has been steadily increasing. In 1985, 4,845 teenagers took their own lives, with 205 being children aged 5 to 14 years.† Girls attempt suicide 3 times more often than boys, but boys succeed more often. The young people with increased risk of committing suicide include those with a history of major psychiatric

*House of Representatives, Joint Hearing, Subcommittee on Oversight, Committee on Ways and Means and Select Committee on Children, Youth, and Families: Child abuse and day care, Sept., 1984, Washington, D.C., 1985, U.S. Government Printing Office.
†Miller, C.A., et al.: Monitoring children's health: key indicatives, Washington, D.C., 1986, American Public Health Association.

disorders, drug and alcohol abuse, recent behavioral changes such as depression or truancy, previous suicide attempts, or suicide by another family member. Also involved may be such factors as divorce or separation of parents, loss of a parent or relative, sense of failure, and recent humiliation or punishment.

Cigarette smoking. Lung cancer in 1983 caused 25% of the cancer deaths or 5% of all deaths in the United States. Over 80% of these cancer deaths (117,000) were caused by cigarette smoking.* Smokers run a higher risk than nonsmokers of cancer of the larynx, oral cavity, esophagus, and stomach. Smoking is the major cause of emphysema and chronic bronchitis. Reports of retrospective studies of high school seniors show that a small percentage started smoking in the sixth grade and as they moved upward through the grades, larger numbers began to use tobacco. By their senior year 90% had tried cigarettes and 20% to 30% smoked on a regular basis. There are 3.3 million teenagers smoking regularly with girls outnumbering the boys.†

Smokeless tobacco products, particularly chewing tobacco and snuff, have recently emerged as popular products among teenagers. Some studies reveal that 16% of teenagers 12 to 17 years of age have tried them. The dangers of their use include increased risk of oral cancer, gingival recession (receding gums leading to tooth loss), oral leukoplakia (white patches in the mouth that may become cancerous), and nicotine addiction.

Alcohol. Alcoholic beverages are the primary drug of choice in the United States and have been tried by 93% of all high school seniors, with 5% reporting daily use. Of these students, 10% claim they had their first drink by the sixth grade and 30% began drinking by the eighth grade. The National Institute on Alcohol Abuse and Alcoholism stated that 10% (3.3 million) of

14- to 17-year-olds are problem drinkers.* The American Academy of Pediatrics† stated there are 500,000 child and adolescent alcoholics. Although the extent of involvement is not known, apparently fourth-grade children are being introduced to and trying alcoholic beverages. Early drinking behavior is a predictor of drinking habits later in life.

Other drugs. Although the drug problem appears to have leveled off and is not rising in terms of extent of use, it continues as a major health problem for young people. A Gallup poll‡ has identified drugs as the biggest problem confronting schools. With the possible exception of marijuana, 40% to 50% of students have first tried illicit drugs before the tenth grade, with 1% having tried them before the sixth grade. Two thirds of all young people have tried an illegal drug before high school graduation. We live in a drug-oriented society. We take drugs to wake up, to go to sleep, to keep alert, to escape from reality, to relax, to ease pain, and for many other reasons. People use, misuse, and abuse legal as well as illegal drugs. A recent survey§ of the extent of drug use among 12- to 17-year-olds revealed the following percentages:

Legal drugs
   Opiates (cough syrups, painkillers)—2% to 10%
   Stimulants—6% to 28%
   Tranquilizers—2% to 12%
   Sedatives—2% to 13%
Illegal drugs
   Marijuana—20% to 50%
   Inhalants (glue, gasoline, etc.)—2% to 19%

---

*Miller, C.A., et al.: Monitoring children's health: key indicatives, Washington, D.C., 1986, American Public Health Association.
†Reported in Smoking and Health Reporter, National Interagency on Smoking and Health **3**:April, 1986.

*National Institute on Alcohol Abuse and Alcoholics: Focus on the Fourth Special Report to the U.S. Congress on Alcohol and Health: patterns of alcohol comsumption, Alcohol World **5**:Spring 1981.
†American Academy of Pediatrics: School health: a guide for health professionals, Evanston, Ill., 1981, Committee on School Health.
‡18th annual Gallup poll for the Phi Delta Kappan **67**:Sept., 1986.
§U.S. Department of Health and Human Services, Public Health Service, Alcohol, Drug Use and Mental Health Administration, National Institute of Drug Abuse: Use of licit and illicit drugs by American high school students 1975-1984, Washington, D.C., 1985, U.S. Government Printing Office.

Hallucinogens (LSD)—3% to 13%
Cocaine—4% to 16%
Heroin—1%

Nutrition. Nutrition is generally good among school-age children but the most prevalent problems are overeating causing obesity and overweight, anorexia nervosa (willful self-starvation) and bulemia (vomiting) in teenage girls, and poor food choices. The obese 1- to 11-year olds apparently are more sedentary than the thin children. The problem may be one of adjustment and is a precursor to adolescent and adult obesity. Poor food choices result in low intakes of the minerals calcium and copper and the vitamins A, C, and B_2 (riboflavin).

Exercise and fitness. It is estimated that 50% or more of school-age children do not participate in daily physical education programs. Sedentary living is one of the factors that increase the probability of cardiovascular disease. Although there are no substantial data available that clearly identify the effect of exercise and fitness in reducing the risks of recurring illness, exercise can help in the control of weight and in stress reduction through relaxation. It can help to increase the efficiency of the heart and blood vessels and may aid digestion.

Sexual activity. About 12 million of the 29 million young people between the ages of 13 and 19 years have had sexual intercourse (18% of boys and 6% of girls 13 to 14 years old). Eight in 10 males and 7 in 10 females report having had sexual intercourse in their teens.* Sexually transmitted diseases appear to be on the increase.

In 1984 the National Center for Health Statistics† reported that 9,965 children were born to mothers under 15 years of age. Almost 42% (4,276) did not begin pregnancy and prenatal care until the fourth to sixth month.

A variety of problems complicate pregnancies in young mothers and they include toxemia, anemia, lack of prenatal care, resulting in such problems as low birth rate, increased infant mortality, and mental retardation of the child.

Teenage pregnancy is widely viewed as related to poverty. Young black women in the United States are almost 7 times more likely than young white women to give birth before the age of 15 years.*

What factors are related to school underachievement?

The American Academy of Pediatrics identified a variety of external and internal factors that affect school underachievement of students.

External factors. External factors include (1) improper educational management—curriculum, motivation, resources, class size, and school design; (2) family problems—marital discord, anxiety, and depression; (3) unrealistic parental expectations; and (4) lack of motivation—lack of home support, socially and financially successful parents, and peer pressure.

Internal factors. Internal factors include (1) chronic and recurring physical problems—cerebral palsy and heart problems; (2) sensory defects—defects in vision or hearing; (3) handicapping neurologic and neuromuscular problems—defects of brain, epilepsy, and dysphasia; (4) psychiatric and psychosocial problems; and (5) mental retardation.

Who are the children with special educational needs?

There are approximately 4 million children with special educational needs, as indicated in Table 1-6. The largest group is the learning disabled, including children with such conditions as minimal brain dysfunction, dyslexia, and hyperkinesis.

*The Alan Guttmacher Institute: Teenage pregnancy: the problem hasn't gone away, New York, 1981, The Institute.
†U.S. Department of Health and Human Services, Public Health Services, Monthly Vital Statistics Report, National Center for Health Statistics, **35**(4)(Suppl.): July 18, 1986; Advance report of final natality statistics, Washington, D.C., 1984, U.S. Government Printing Office.

*Miller, C.A., et al.: Monitoring children's health: key indicators, Washington, D.C., 1986, American Public Health Association.

TABLE 1-6. Number and percentage of school enrollment of children and youth aged 3 to 21 years served under P.L. 89-313 and P.L. 94-142 by handicapping condition, 1983-1984

Handicapping condition	Number	Percentage of total school enrollment
Learning disabled	1,811,489	4.57
Speech impaired	1,130,569	2.86
Mentally retarded	750,534	1.84
Emotionally disturbed	362,073	0.91
Other health impaired	54,621	0.13
Multihandicapped	67,537	0.07
Hard of hearing/deaf	74,279	0.18
Orthopedically impaired	56,209	0.14
Visually handicapped	31,576	0.07
Deaf-blind	2,512	0.01
TOTAL	4,341,399	10.89

U.S. Department of Education, Office of Special Education and Rehabilitative Services: 7th annual report to Congress on the implementation of the handicapped act, Washington, D.C., 1985, U.S. Government Printing Office.

What are the special problems of the poor?

Children from low-income families, especially those families with only one parent, are generally in poorer health than children from high-income families. Of families living below the poverty level, 50% are headed by a woman. Nearly 50% of black children live in poverty. A study completed several years ago revealed that of young people under 17 years of age, 70% from high-income families were in excellent health whereas only 41% of children from low-income families were in excellent health.

In recent years increasing attention has been accorded the unusually high rate of illness among the poor and minority groups such as black Americans, Mexican Americans, and native Americans. Poverty and ignorance are the common contributory causes of these higher disease rates. Poor diet, inadequate medical and dental care, unhealthful housing, health misconceptions and superstitions, high incidence of child abuse and neglect, and lack of adequate childhood immunizations are major reasons for the generally subpar health of low-income families.

Some of the health problems of minority groups are based on genetic variances (such as sickle cell anemia in blacks and Tay-Sachs dis-

ease in Jewish and other groups of Middle East origin), whereas others appear to be related to lifestyle and environment (such as alcoholism among Irish Americans, accidents among native Americans, and high blood pressure among black Americans). Migrant and seasonal farmworkers and their children, most of whom are black or Hispanic, suffer severaly under the burden of poverty, poor housing, inadequate diets, discrimination, occupational accidents, emotional problems, and exposure to agricultural pesticides. Among native Americans these conditions are prevalent: tuberculosis, dental decay, alcoholism, drug abuse, diabetes, and a variety of emotional problems.

WHAT IS SCHOOL HEALTH?

A multiphasic differential health program as illustrated in Fig. 1-1 is needed to adequately care for the variety of students and health and safety problems found in schools. The comprehensive school health program is one that includes *health instruction, health services, healthful school living*, and *coordination*. The instructional component should be both formal and informal and for students and parents. The health service phase attempts to identify pupils with problems and provide counseling and guidance to obtain corrections where possible and to make adjustments in school programs where necessary. It provides policies and procedures to prevent the spread of communicable diseases and to take care of children who may be injured or become ill while at school. The environmental phase includes a physical plant that is healthful and safe, is staffed by well-adjusted employees, and offers an atmosphere of friendliness and comfort conducive to learning. No program of this nature can function effectively without co-ordination.

An understanding of school health is more easily gained through familiarity with the terminology that follows:

school health The physiological, psychological, sociological, and spiritual aspects of health as they relate to the school setting.

school health program The procedures and activities designed to protect and promote the well-being of students and school personnel. It has four categorical phases: health education/instruction, health services, healthful school living/healthful school environment, and coordination.

health education A broad term referring to both formal and informal learning about health that will enable individuals to make intelligent, informed decisions affecting their personal, family, and community well-being. It may take place in school, outside school, and through the media.

health instruction The formal program that takes place in the school. It includes a program of planned activities in a classroom setting that offers understandings and attempts to develop attitudes and practices of healthful living that will enable children to reach high levels of wellness. The formal program is one that is planned, is sequential, and includes all grades in a school or school district. It is now considered to be a *comprehensive school health education* program. It should be based on sound principles of curriculum development and include all subject areas necessary to satisfy student health needs and interests. The subject areas must (1) be repeated at several grade levels to ensure reinforcement of learning, and (2) increase in depth of content, progressing from simple to complex concepts as pupils move upward in grade.

health services Those activities that involve nurses and other health professionals in the identification and follow-up of pupil health problems with students and parents, the control of disease, and pupil emergencies and first aid.

healthful school environment The phase sometimes referred to as healthful school living and relates to those activities that provide a safe and healthful school atmosphere. It includes the physical plant—lighting, heating, ventilation, food services, health services unit, and health of school personnel—as well as the emotional climate in the school.

coordination Those activities usually carried out by a school administrator in cooperation with school and community health committees or councils. They include the administration and supervision of the school health program with specific responsibilities to integrate the various phases with health instruction, to develop curriculum, to provide in-service teacher and staff training, and to prepare policies and procedures.

WHY SCHOOL HEALTH?

The health of children and their learning are reciprocally related. Young people must be healthy to obtain optimal benefit from their elementary school experiences. Educational experiences must be provided that will enable pupils to live in a healthful manner.

The curriculum in America's elementary schools must include substantially more than the three Rs despite the present trend to return to so-called basic education. Reading, writing, spelling, arithmetic, social studies, and science need not be neglected with the inclusion of health education. Although health should be included as a separate subject area, it can also be integrated easily into all instructional areas. Teachers, with the help of parents, family members, and the community, must aid students to learn how to live and make adjustments to the society in which they find themselves. Health is basic to the basics. Without good health, pupils will have difficulty learning to read, write, add, and perform the necessary activities for learning.

Students who are frequently absent because of illness, uncorrected vision problems, emotional disturbances, malnourishment or under-nourishment, or fatigue or other health problems are simply not able to learn most efficiently and effectively even with the best teaching. The American Academy of Pediatrics* identifies these factors that contribute to underachievement in pupils: chronic and frequently recurring physical problems; specific sensory defects (vision, hearing, speech); neurologic and neuro-muscular problems (brain defects, epilepsy); psychological problems (passive-aggressive behavior, fears, anxieties); and mental retardation.

Although parents have the primary responsibility for the health of their children, schools must offer supportive and complementary programs to help counsel pupils and parents. The role of the school is primarily to educate. Schools are expected to provide education to help students live in and adjust to society. Since society places high value on human life and health, schools have a responsibility and an opportunity to help protect and promote the health of pupils and to aid in the prevention of ill health.

WHAT IS THE ROLE OF THE SCHOOL AND THE TEACHER IN PREVENTION?

The role of the school in preventive health is identified in the total school health program (Fig. 1-1).

Schools have both a legal and a moral responsibility to provide a safe, sanitary, and healthful environment for pupils and school personnel. An atmosphere conducive to learning is one that is friendly and comfortable, offers a curriculum that motivates and meets the needs of students, minimizes stress situations, and includes well-adjusted, competent teachers.

The central purpose of the school health program is to help children learn to be responsible for their own health. Students should be able to acquire scientific understandings and attitudes

---

*American Academy of Pediatrics: School health: a guide for health professionals, Evanston, Ill., 1981, The Academy.

through the health instruction program that will enable them to act intelligently. The health habits established in these formative years greatly influence the quality of life that emerges in adulthood. Young people in elementary schools can be exposed to many useful health experiences and activities, since they legally must attend school for approximately 6 hours daily, 180 days yearly, for 8 or more years.

Children attend school with a variety of illnesses and conditions such as communicable diseases, speech impediments, and dental problems that are in need of identification, or possible correction, or both. The school health services program should provide nurses, physicians, dentists, and other professionals who can assist with these problems to protect other students, to counsel and guide pupils and parents, and to recommend adjustments in school programs for more effective learning.

Teachers are expected to protect and try to improve the health of the children in their charge. Generally they are to be active participants in the comprehensive school health program (Fig. 1-1). Specifically they need to understand the concept of health previously discussed, to be aware of the factors that influence pupil health (p. 10), to enthusiastically be involved in the instructional program, and to know how to tell if pupils are in good health. The basic competencies needed for teachers to take part in the school health program are identified in Chapter 2.

HOW CAN YOU TELL IF PUPILS ARE IN GOOD HEALTH?

The classroom teacher is not qualified to diagnose illness or make a clinical assessment of pupil health. However, some specific characteristics distinguish healthy children from those who are not healthy. (Refer to Appendix K for details.) Actually, these attributes help spell out a definition of good health. To be able to enumerate, albeit roughly and incompletely, the more basic telltale clues of good health is to be better prepared to recognize and promote buoy-

FIG. 1-3. The healthy child. *(Courtesy of the San Jose Nutrition Project.)*

ant health among your pupils (Fig. 1-3). Generally these behaviors should be looked for in the healthy child:

1. Carries out routine learning activities in school and in homework assignments without undue fatigue or emotional upset
2. Participates regularly in physical education and other physical activities in the school curriculum
3. Demonstrates skill in games and basic body movements appropriate to age, sex, body type, and motor learning experiences
4. Shows progressive gains in weight and heights without unusually wide deviations
5. Has enough energy to do the things that most children of this age and sex want to do
6. Has smooth and clear skin, without discoloration, eruptions, or excessive dryness or oiliness
7. Has a good appetite
8. Has no more frequent illnesses or accidents than are typical of his or her age and sex group
9. Is interested in and enthusiastic about most activities that are popular with classmates
10. Has confidence in own abilities yet enjoys working and playing with others
11. Controls emotions about as well as most of the other children in class

WHERE DO WE STAND NOW?

A great deal of progress has been made in the development and expansion of health instruction programs. Little or no progress has been made to improve health services programs, and the growth of the environmental and coordination of the school health program has remained static or regressed somewhat.

Some of the numerous professional and other organizations that have helped nurture the growth of school health in the United States include the American School Health Association, the American Public Health Association, and the Association for the Advancement of Health Education. The American Medical Association, the

American Academy of Pediatricians, the American Heart Association, the American Lung Association, and the National Congress of Parents and Teachers are among other groups that have been supportive over the years.

It should be noted that at the federal level there is the Center for Health Promotion and Education in the Centers for Disease Control, in the Public Health Service, within the Department of Health and Human Services. The Center for Health Promotion and Education, formerly the Bureau of Health, has supported school health education and provided funds for the development of demonstration and model programs. Until it was eliminated by budget cuts, there was also an Office of Comprehensive School Health within the Department of Education. There is also the Office of Disease Prevention and Health Promotion, (ODPHP), Public Health Service, Department of Health and Human Services. These offices have all cooperated in efforts to advance school health.

In the private sector, the National Center for Health Education is an organization supported by funds from industry and other sources that promote health education. The National Congress of Parents and Teachers has for many years conducted a program of support for health education, especially comprehensive health education. Several other major curriculum projects are now under way. They have received financial support from several foundations and other sources.

Health education in schools has perhaps made its greatest progress in the last 25 years. The following list of advances in school health was compiled by Kolbe and others* (with the help of the staff of the Center for Health Promotion Research and Development at the University of Health Science Center in Houston) in a report prepared for the American School Health Association. It said:

---

*Kolbe, L.J., et al.: School health in America: an assessment of state policies to protect and improve the health of students, ed. 4, July 18, 1986, Kent, Ohio, 1986, American School Health Assocation (draft of material to be published).

1. School health education is mandated in 38 states (76%); 7 states (14%) encourage the subject; 25 states (50%) have policies by state boards of education or departments of education supporting health education; and 23 states (46%) have resolutions, bylaws, or formal endorsements.

2. In 15 states (30%) there are education officials whose sole responsibility is for health education; 9 states (18%) also include health services, and 15 states (30%) have people with dual responsibilities for health education and physical education. Only 16% of these officials have degrees in health education or health science, whereas 8% have degrees in health and physical education.

3. Elementary teachers are required in 22 states (44%) to take coursework in health education while preparing to become teachers. In addition to state mandates, many colleges and universities require or offer health education coursework.

4. A curriculum or planning guide for health education is available to school districts in 39 states (78%).

5. In 29 states (58%) persons responsible for school health services are employed by the state department of education, and 18 states (36%) have persons employed by departments of health. In 8 (16%) states these individuals also have responsibilities for health education.

6. There is a state-level school health advisory council in 24 states (48%). In 38 states (76%) there is no policy in regard to a local-level school health advisory council.

Despite the tremendous efforts in support of school health education programs in recent years, they are not universally found in elementary schools in the United States. It is estimated that fewer than 22% of the nation's schools provide health instruction programs. Many of these are not comprehensive, and often are not evaluated in terms of their impact on students. State laws requiring health programs, despite their apparent prevalence, are often written in such general terms that schools can comply with the requirements without providing instructional programs such as those outlined in this text.

With the exception of some large districts, the health services programs found in schools may not be recognizable as such because they are fragmented, uncoordinated, and poorly planned; in many instances, there may be little or no administrative leadership. In a number of schools and school districts, some of the services may be provided by local health departments. At best a nurse or some administrator may have the responsibility for the supervision and conduct of such programs. In many districts there may be no nurses or only part-time nurses in schools. Large districts may have specific departments with physicians, nurses, and other health professionals.

In recent years federal legislation has helped to provide some measure of improvement in health services programs. In 1967 Congress approved a program that required states to provide early and periodic screening, diagnosis, and treatment (EPSDT) as a mandatory Medicaid service to improve the health of children from low-income families through preventive health services. It included identification and preventive care for vision, hearing, and dental problems, among others. The program has been under the supervision of local and state health departments but it necessitated school involvement and coordination. In 1975 Congress passed the Education for All Handicapped Children Act, which required that "free appropriate public education" be available to all handicapped children from ages 3 to 21 years regardless of their disabilities and their ability to pay for services. The law requires that provision be made for school health services, speech therapy, medical services, psychological and parent counseling, and other types of programs.

The patterns of organization for health services vary widely in America's schools. Many schools hire their own nurses and other professionals to conduct programs, some have all services provided by local health departments, and a few schools and school districts coordinate their own activities.

School districts in general are attentive to the physical plant including food services, health services, and to a lesser extent, the health of school personnel. The emotional climate may receive consideration to a greater or lesser degree but this depends on the nature of the school services rendered and the individual efforts of teachers and personnel.

Coordination of the phases of the school health program outlined here does not exist except in some large school districts. In those few districts that have administrative personnel to oversee programs, these individuals may be called supervisors, coordinators, consultants, or directors. In some districts, physicians or other health professionals may serve in this capacity. School health advisory committees can render useful and important aid but such committees are few in number except possibly in large districts. The same probably holds true for community health committees. It should be noted that without administrative supervision, health services or health instruction programs will be hard pressed to develop, and if in operation, will slowly disappear.

Despite the progress and advances that have been made in school health, health education continues to receive low priority for curriculum inclusion by school superintendents and school board members. Additional awareness programs for such individuals with pressures exerted by parents and community health organizations and professionals must be initiated. Finances and resources for health instruction are greatly limited.

Perhaps the state of school health programs is best described by these remarks of former Secretary of Health, Education, and Welfare, Joseph A. Califano, when he addressed the American School Health Association annual meeting in Minneapolis several years ago:

Improved school health programs will be a key element in the comprehensive national child health policy which I will ask the Public Health Serivce to develop for the Department . . . I believe that the time has come again to forge ahead in expanding and improving these programs.

The school health program outlined in this text may be considered as a conceptual model of the ideal program. It illustrates the pattern for school health that should exist in America's schools and has been advocated by the American School Health Association and other professional health organizations. This program identifies the specific components and their organization that if implemented will enable children to achieve high levels of wellness. It will contribute to quality education and aid young people to grow into worthwhile and productive adults.

The health program described here has emerged as a result of a thorough review of the scientific literature and numerous school health programs, consultation with many school health authorities, discussions with a variety of health professionals, and the authors' years of experience with schools. We have served in numerous capacities in elementary schools at local and state levels as teachers and administrators. We have participated in professional organizations, conducted many in-service teacher-training activities, and been active in health education projects at local, state, and national levels.

IN SUMMARY WE BELIEVE

Comprehensive school health programs that include health instruction and health services and provide a healthful environment are necessary to protect and promote the health of America's elementary school children.

Comprehensive school health programs will continue to expand and become more readily available in elementary schools despite present difficulties.

Comprehensive school health programs will emerge because people have become aware of their need and will take action to provide for this need.

Comprehensive school health with emphasis on health instruction in elementary schools requires that teachers, administrators, and the community be more assertive in the promotion of their need.

Comprehensive school health programs need the involvement of parents, professional health personnel, and other community representatives in development, implementation, and financial support.

Comprehensive school health and health instruction programs for classrooms, schools, and school districts can be prepared by teachers and administrators through the use of the information found in this textbook.

QUESTIONS FOR DISCUSSION

1. In the Surgeon General's report, Promoting Health/ Preventing Disease, what are five areas and their objectives for achievement by 1990 that have school implications?
2. What is the nature of a comprehensive school health program? Identify its components and interrelations.
3. What is the meaning of the preventive health concept? Provide illustrations. What is the role of the school and teachers?
4. What are the components of health as described in the text? Briefly describe their significance to individuals.
5. What is the modified concept of health as illustrated in the text? Give examples of its application to health education.
6. What factors influence the health of pupils? Provide illustrations.
7. What are 10 important health problems of children? Identify the extent to which they exist in elementary school pupils.
8. What are five of the social and lifestyle-related health problems of elementary pupils, and what can teachers do about such problems?
9. What are five student health problems in need of special education? What can teachers do to help these children socially and psychologically?
10. Name the special health problems of the poor, and indicate their significance for health education.
11. Why do schools have a responsibility to provide for a comprehensive school health program?
12. How can a teacher tell whether children are in good health?
13. What is the status of school health programs in the United States today?

SELECTED REFERENCES

American Academy of Pediatrics, School health: a guide for health professionals, Evanston, Ill., 1981, The Academy.

Black, J.L.: AIDS: preschool and school issues, Journal of School Health **56**:151-152 April, 1986.

Comprehensive school health education, Journal of School Health **54**:312-315 Sept., 1984.

Cornacchia, H.J., Smith, D.E., and Bentel, D.J.: Drugs in the classroom: a conceptual model for school programs, ed. 2, St. Louis, 1978, The C.V. Mosby Co.

DiAngelis, A.T., et al.: Dental needs in children of Mexican-American migrant workers, Journal of School Health **51:**312-315 Aug., 1981.

Education Commission of States: Recommendations for school health education: a handbook for state policymakers, Report No. 130, Denver, 1981, The Commission.

Gephart, J., et al.: Perspectives on health of school-age children: expectations for the future, Journal of School Health **54:**11-17 Jan., 1984.

Health education: practical application of research, Newsletter of Phi Delta Kappa's Center on Evaluation, Development and Research **5:**1-4 June, 1983.

Health interview survey, United States, 1976, Vital Health Statistics **119** (10): Nov., 1977.

Miller, C.A., et al.: Monitoring children's health: key indicators, Washington, D.C., 1986, American Public Health Association.

National Safety Council: Accident facts, Chicago, 1985, The Council.

Prevention of Child Abuse, The Nation's Health ISSN 0028-0496: 12-13 Aug., 1986.

Richards, W., M.D., Allergy, asthma and school problems, Journal of School Health **56:**151-152 April, 1986.

The Robert Wood Johnson Foundation, Special Report, No. 1, National school health services program 1985, Princeton, N.J., 1985, The Foundation.

U.S. Department of Health and Human Services, Public Health Service, Alcohol, Drug Abuse and Mental Health, National Institute on Alcohol Abuse and Alcoholism: Fifth Special Report to the U.S. Congress on alcohol and health, Washington, D.C., 1983, U.S. Government Printing Office.

U.S. Department of Health and Human Services, Public Health Service, Office of Secretary for Health and Surgeon General: Healthy people: the Surgeon General's report on health promotion and disease prevention, Washington, D.C., 1979, U.S. Government Printing Office.

U.S. Department of Health and Human Services, Public Health Service, Health Resources and Services Administration: Health status of minorities and low income groups, Bureau of Health Professions, Division of Disadvantaged Assistance, Washington, D.C., 1985, U.S. Government Printing Office.

U.S. Department of Health and Human Services, Public Health Service, National Center for Health Statistics: Health United States 1985, Washington, D.C., 1985, U.S. Government Printing Office.

CHAPTER 2

THE TEACHER'S ROLE IN SCHOOL HEALTH

Today there is a real sense of urgency about our need to convey to young people of this country the kinds of information they can use to protect and promote their own health and the health of their families.

EDWARD N. BRANDT, JR., M.D., Ph.D.
Assistant Secretary for Health, U.S. Department of Health and Human Services

KEY CONCEPT: Teachers with appropriate competencies in the comprehensive school health program have a positive effect on student health.

The elementary classroom teacher has a unique and vital role in the protection and improvement of the health of students through the development of positive health attitudes and behavior. The teacher, one of the most influential factors in the life of young persons, has contact with children during their most formative and sensitive years—a precious time when what they know, what they think, and what they do can be significantly affected. Often the teacher sees and communicates with a child for more hours each day than do the parents. This reality becomes increasingly important in light of Department of Labor reports showing that over half of the mothers of school-age children hold regular jobs.

What teachers do with this combined opportunity and responsibility depends on whether they are ready, willing, and competent to assume a prominent role in school health, especially classroom health instruction.

To better understand the ways teachers can contribute to children's health and safety, let us briefly reexamine the interrelationship of the three phases (health education, health services, and healthful school environment) of the comprehensive school health program (Fig. 1-1).

Health instruction, through formally planned and sequentially arranged activities (see Chapters 9 and 11 through 13) and informal counseling and guidance, is designed to promote health knowledge (cognitive), attitudes (affective), and practices (action) that contribute to the highest levels of individual, family, and community health. There are opportunities for both formal and informal instruction through health services as well as through the environmental phase. The formal health instruction program provides the greatest responsibility and opportunity for the teacher. Yet, informally, individual health problems can often be given attention through counseling and guidance.

Health services (see Chapters 5, 6, 7) include activities that identify the health problems of children and seek corrections and adjustments of school programs to ensure the greatest learning. The purpose of the school health services program is to protect, maintain, and improve the health of children. This involves nurses, physicians, dentists, and others. Teachers must be prepared to deal with common childhood problems such as colds, stomachaches, fevers, sore throats, toothaches, headaches, and allergies. Teachers must be able to recognize signs and symptoms of student health problems, refer pupils to health personnel, and assist with screening programs. The teacher may also use service activities as teachable moments (see Chapter 12) to provide formal and informal instruction.

A healthful school environment includes the physical aspects (see Chapter 3) and the emotional climate (see Chapter 4) of the school setting. The school must be free of hazards and offer a safe, comfortable, warm atmosphere with stable teachers to enable children to learn most effectively. Teachers must assume some responsibility for the proper lighting, heating, and ventilation of the classroom and offer assurance that pupils are free of exposure to hazardous conditions through the provision of safe environment and practices. The emotional climate is a part of the school environment that includes teacher health, fairness in dealing with pupils, consideration for individual differences, creation of a friendly classroom setting, and avoidance of bias and prejudice.

The elementary classroom teacher has often been called a "specialized generalist," "a jack-of-all trades," in recognition of the diversity of talents necessary to be a good teacher. Few people in the entire field of education, or in any of the other professions for that matter, need the diversity of competencies required of the good elementary school teacher. Summarily, that person must be a grammarian, mathematician, psychologist, space-age scientist, nutritionist, editor, art and drama critic, geographer, health educator, sociologist, physical educator, agriculture expert, historian, recreation leader, zoologist, anthropologist, safety specialist, chemist, economist, nurse, counselor, and more.

WHAT COMPETENCIES DOES THE ELEMENTARY TEACHER NEED?

It would be unrealistic to expect each classroom teacher to be a health education specialist. However, the teacher must have an understanding of the nature and process of health education as well as the total school health program for an effective instructional program. The specific competencies that will enable the teacher to participate in a comprehensive program are identified on pp. 27, 28.

In addition to these specific competencies the teacher as a health educator should (1) realize that health education requires the use of a different approach, (2) understand the controversial nature of some health topics, (3) appreciate the special need for the consideration of individual pupil differences, (4) be familiar with a variety of sources of current scientific health information (see Chapter 13 and Appendixes F and G), (5) be able to identify health problems to include in the instructional program (see Chapters 1, 5, and 11), and (6) plan for the orderly conduct of formal educational experiences and use teachable moments for health instruction (see Chapters 8 through 13).

Health teaching is different

Although in many ways health teaching is much like all other teaching, it does differ in certain crucial respects.

COMPETENCIES

General

The teacher understands and appreciates:

1. The meaning of health as a multidimensional state of well-being that includes physical, psychological, social, and spiritual aspects
2. That health of individuals is influenced by the reciprocal interaction of the growing and developing organism and environmental factors and is necessary for optimal functioning as productive members of society
3. The significance of children's and youth's health problems on learning
4. The importance and the need for the school health program in today's society
5. The nature of the total school health program
6. The role of the teacher in each of the school health program components—services, environment, and instruction
7. The influence on students of teacher health and teacher health habits
8. The need for basic scientific information about a variety of health content areas, including dental health; drugs (alcohol, tobacco, and other drugs); care of eyes, ears, and feet; exercise, fitness, rest, and fatigue; prevention and control of diseases and disorders (communicable and chronic); safety and first aid; family health; consumer health; community health; environmental health; nutrition; mental health; anatomy; and physiology

Health instruction

The teacher:

1. Can identify and use a variety of techniques and procedures to determine the health needs and interests of pupils
2. Is able to organize the health instruction program around the needs and interests of students and can develop effective teaching units for the grade being taught
3. Is able to stress the development of attitudes and behaviors for healthful living based on scientific health information
4. Can distinguish between the various patterns of health instruction and attempts to use the direct approach in teaching whenever possible
5. Realizes that health education must receive time in the school program along with other subject areas
6. Possesses current scientific information about a variety of health content areas
7. Can use a variety of stimulating and motivating teaching techniques derived from fundamental principles of learning
8. Is able to identify and use "teachable moments" or incidents that occur in the classroom, in the school, or in the community
9. Uses a variety of teaching aids in the instructional program and is familiar with their sources
10. Is familiar with the sources of scientific information and the procedures necessary to keep up to date with current health information
11. Is able to provide a variety of alternative solutions to health problems to enable students to make wiser decisions
12. Can integrate health into other phases of the curriculum, such as social science, science, and language arts
13. Uses a variety of evaluative procedures periodically to (a) assess the effectiveness of the program on students and (b) determine the quality and usefulness of teaching aids and materials

Continued.

COMPETENCIES—cont'd

Health services

The teacher:

1. Is familiar with the characteristics of the healthy child and can recognize signs and symptoms of unhealthy conditions; refers problems to the school nurse or other appropriate school personnel
2. Is familiar with the variety of health appraisal procedures used in schools and uses them to enrich the health instruction program
3. Acquires limited skill in counseling and guiding students and parents regarding student health problems
4. Understands the value and purposes of teacher-nurse conferences
5. Is familiar with the variety of health personnel found in schools, their functions, responsibilities, and usefulness to the teacher
6. Is able to use information contained on health records
7. Can identify and follow the policies and procedures in schools in regard to such matters as emergency care, accidents, disease control, and referrals, exclusions, and readmittance of pupils
8. Can administer immediate care when accidents or illnesses to pupils occur or can act promptly to obtain sources of help within the school
9. Is able to adjust the school program to the individual health needs of students
10. Is able to relate the health services program to the health instruction program

Healthful school living

The teacher:

1. Is familiar with the standards for hygiene, sanitation, and safety needed in schools to provide a safe and healthful environment
2. Is familiar with the physical and emotional needs of students and adjusts classroom activities to help students satisfy these needs whenever possible
3. Understands the nature and importance of the food services program and is able to relate it to the instructional program
4. Is able to recognize hazardous conditions on the playground, in the classroom, and elsewhere in the school and takes appropriate action to eliminate or correct such conditions
5. Is cognizant of the effect of teacher health, personality, biases, and prejudices on student health and learning and is concerned with the humane treatment of pupils
6. Integrates healthful environmental aspects into the health instruction program

Coordination

The teacher:

1. Understands the need for school and community health councils or committees and is willing to participate as a member if requested to do so
2. Realizes the importance of and need for a coordinator, consultant, or a person with administrative responsibility being in charge of the school health program

In the first place, although much of the content of health education is basic to the complete physical, psychological, social, and spiritual development of the child, motivation is often difficult. The normal, healthy child is largely unconcerned about his or her health and safety. In fact, if public apathy toward the value of auto seat belts and the serious danger of cigarette smoking is any criterion, one may conclude that many youths and adults demonstrate a rather perverse antagonism toward established facts of safe and healthful living. Quite possibly this is because the essential knowledge and favorable attitudes and practices needed to combat this apathy were not developed a decade or more ago when these people were student's in elementary school. In any event, the classroom teacher faces special challenges in the influential motivation of pupils in health education. At the same time, fear psychology, vague exhortation, and the possibility of developing an unhealthy overconcern for health among pupils must be avoided. The balance is often a most delicate one.

Second, health teaching is inextricably bound up in our cultural and social patterns of thinking and doing. Perhaps no other area of learning in the elementary school depends so heavily on positively influencing attitudes and behavior. A person's actions are rooted in feelings, and feelings are colored by experiences and understandings. Even though children may come to school without any preconceived notions regarding reading or arithmetic, they often already have begun to develop some false ideas, poor attitudes, and harmful practices in health and safety. Altering these unsound patterns of thinking and behaving is often difficult because of the rigidity of family and community culture and its powerful influence on the child.

Third, health information is constantly changing. What was unknown yesterday will be commonplace tomorrow; what was true last year is false this year; what was an apparently insurmountable problem a decade ago is now relegated to the museum of scientific antiques. Moreover, health science is not a simple listing of pure "blacks and whites." Whereas some concepts are clearly and unalterably established by research, others are supported in varying degrees of authenticity given current scientific evidence. The classroom teacher, therefore, must prepare pupils for scientific change without developing a negative skepticism. The teacher must lead children to understand the scientific method so that, using this understanding, they may weigh the facts at hand and make choices and decisions that will favorably affect health. This idea of decision making is critical, for unlike most other subject matter areas, health and safety demand that children be participants, not merely spectators.

Health teaching can be controversial

Some of the topics in health education may occasionally provoke emotional reactions among pupils, parents, and other concerned persons or groups in the community. Such areas of instruction include sex education, sexually transmitted disease, fluoridation, tobacco, alcohol and other drugs, the choice of a health advisor, and medical care plans.

Of course, sex education and tobacco and alcohol instruction have certain moral and religious implications. Yet the evidence clearly indicates that despite the hue and cry of small vocal groups, the majority of parents and religious leaders generally favor school instruction in these areas. Fluoridation of public water supplies has been associated with emotionally tinged publicity in some communities. Despite the fact that every responsible scientific organization has endorsed fluoridation as safe and effective in reducing tooth decay, there is still occasional criticism of this topic. Members of some healing professions may take exception to the generalization that medical diagnosis and treatment are best performed by licensed doctors of medicine and osteopathy. Some persons may urge that an ultraliberal view of medical care—barely short of socialized medicine—be presented in class. Those who oppose this tend to question any approach to medical care that suggests anything other than the traditional fee-for-service agreement between patient and physician.

Because health education is so intimately related to the cultural patterns of any community, teachers can expect that now and then some objections will arise. Neither teachers nor administrators should be intimidated by sporadic criticism of this kind. However, to be sure of standing on firm ground in these provocative areas, the classroom teacher should do the following:

1. Maintain a scientific, unbiased approach
2. Follow course and unit outlines recommended or approved by local school officials
3. Seek the help of resource people and groups in the community (for example, local medical and dental societies, the PTA representative, religious leaders, and public health officials) in preparing units of study
4. Wherever possible, use materials that have been prepared by such reputable groups and organizations as the American Alliance for Health, Physical Education, Recreation, and Dance; American Medical Association; American School Health Association; U.S. Public Health Service; National Education Asssociation; National Council on Alcoholism; American Red Cross; local or state health departments; American Social Health Association; and other recognized scientific groups
5. Use resources that are up to date and scientifically sound (detailed criteria are discussed in Chapter 13)
6. Maintain adequate records of pupil activities, questions, interests, and problems
7. Allow for cultural differences and student exemptions when subjects or topics interfere with religious or parental beliefs
8. Inform parents of the program's intent and methods (this might be a function of the school administrator)
9. Permit parents to attend classes and review outlines of subject matter and teaching materials to be used

A variety of teaching techniques should be effectively used in a well-planned health instruction program. However, there are numerous pitfalls to avoid if the program is to be a positive learning experience for children. Some of the pitfalls to avoid include the following:

1. Using extrinsic rewards—especially "unhealthy" rewards (e.g., candy) for a child who demonstrates positive health behavior
2. Inserting personal bias into instruction
3. Using students as examples of poor health practices or of health problems
4. Creating a "clean plate" club
5. Overuse of fear tactics or overly graphic portrayals of disease entities or health problems
6. Conducting competition between students on health practices such as grooming or posture
7. Overly emphasizing perfect attendance at school
8. Pushing personal values or interests as fact
9. Setting forth unrealistic standards in terms of health knowledge and practices for children
10. Ridiculing a child's home situation or using it as an example of a poor health practice or environment

Teacher-pupil planning of units and participation by parents and other citizens in curriculum study and development are procedures that help assure public understanding and acceptance of what is taught in the schools. Increasingly closer ties among school, home, and community tend to lessen substantially the possibility of any misunderstandings regarding teaching concepts in controversial areas.

Ethical issues

Teachers and all personnel must be aware that a variety of ethical questions regarding student health related to health services and health education need consideration. Health records will often contain information from a variety of sources including health appraisals, physicians' reports, and parental notes. Such information entrusted to school personnel by nurses and others is for educational purposes and must be considered confidential and not subject to discussion (except possibly with the specific children, parents, physicians, or school nurses). When such information is shared with teachers it is for the purpose of enhancing learning or aiding children to make adjustments. Teachers must value and respect the dignity, worth, and right to privacy of all individuals regardless of their age, sex, socioeconomic or health status, race, creed, or ethnic origin. It is an infringement on student rights for teachers and other school personnel to openly discuss with friends or teachers specific children's conditions or illnesses such as diabetes, epilepsy, mental retardation, or emotional disturbances unless they have specific bearing on the student's educational experiences.

When teaching about health, especially as it applies to the controversial areas previously mentioned, teachers must be aware that students have the right to freely choose their own styles of living if fully aware of the risks (informed consent). Since elementary school–age children may not be able to do this, the wishes of parents or guardians must be honored. However, all individuals have the right to be protected against other individuals if their rights, health, or welfare are endangered. The school, therefore, has the right to prevent illness or injury by imposing restrictions wherever communicable disease or safety is concerned.

Sources of current scientific information

Elementary education programs in the teacher-training institutions have varying school health requirements—from no coursework to one or more courses in personal health, first aid, and school health. This inadequacy of training was recently illustrated in a limited study of Michigan elementary school teachers,* in which the need for in-service training to carry out

school health responsibilities was evident. This lack of preparation together with the constant flow of changing health knowledge uncovered by new research, stresses the importance of teachers keeping up to date and seeking reliable sources of health information.

Unfortunately, the sources of reliable and new information and the methods used to assess such information present problems not readily or easily resolved. There are no simple or definitive ways to discover with certainty whether material contained in publications is truthful and accurate. There are several reasons for this difficulty: (1) data are limited or inconclusive regarding the cause, treatment, or cure of many conditions such as arthritis, cancer, and obesity; (2) published research data are frequently in conflict; and (3) a number of so-called authorities, including scientists, nutritionists, physicians, and others who may disseminate health information may have been motivated to disseminate inaccurate information for purely profit-related reasons—information clearly not in the best interest of the health consumer. Further, the elementary teacher does not usually have access to basic medical literature for the purpose of double-checking the information contained in varied publications. Therefore it is important that teachers attempt to determine the validity of health information they read. These guidelines should be helpful in the evaluation of publications and other printed materials*:

1. What is the purpose of the printed material; is it produced to sell products, make money, or present factual information to the reader?

2. Is it presented in an educational or scientific manner, or does it use exaggerated claims and make misleading and inaccurate statements?

3. Is the author qualified by way of educational background and professional experience? It must be kept in mind that even though the author may be qualified, the information may be inaccurate.

---

*Davis, C., et al.: Health concerns of teacher training of selected elementary teachers in Michigan, Journal of School Health **55:**151-153 April, 1985.

*Adapted from Cornacchia, H., and Barrett S.: Consumer health, ed. 3, St. Louis, 1985, Times Mirror/Mosby College Publishing.

4. Are the data based on appropriate research and experience of experts in the health field or on the opinions of a few individuals?

5. Are the research data acceptable by medical, dental, public health, and other authorities and organizations?

6. What evidence exists to support or refute conflicting claims about health information? Has the claimant generalized from a particular incident or from broad research?

Sources of reliable current information and ways for teachers to keep up to date may be found in Chapter 13 and Appendixes F and G.

Providing for individual differences

Providing for individual differences, including cultural and ethnic differences, is something we talk about a great deal in education. Doing much about it becomes increasingly difficult. Overcrowded schools and oversized classes make individual guidance of pupil learning more a theoretical goal than an accomplished fact.

There are numerous ways teachers can learn more about their pupils. Of course, school records furnish significant information on a child's intellectual capacity, status, and progress. Often these records also contain data on a pupil's social and emotional development. Well-kept cumulative health records should provide information on illnesses, injuries, major surgical operations, allergies, health examination findings, dental health, physical growth, and teacher observations from previous years. These, combined with notes and recommendations of the school nurse and physician, can be most helpful to the teacher in understanding the health status of each child and the implications such status may have for learning (see Chapter 5).

Intellectually, one must realize that it is not physically possible for a teacher to meet every need of every student within a given classroom. When a teacher must deal with anywhere from 20 to 30 or more students in a classroom and considerably more than that throughout the school day, the chance is quite good that the teacher will come into contact with one or more students with whom it will be difficult to establish rapport. When this occurs, the teacher would be well advised to examine his or her personal biases to determine if they might be a barrier to the rapport. In like manner, the teacher will have a profound effect on the lives of many other students with whom rapport has been established.

Beyond the variances in the health and growth of pupils (see Chapter 5 and Appendix L), there are important differences that relate to each child's environment. Most important of these is the home background. Economic conditions, cultural level, parental attitude toward the school, social position, marital status, value systems, leisure time activities, parents' occupations, and racial or ethnic origins of parents—all these, and more tend to leave their mark on the child. Children's purposes, interests, and values will tend to align themselves with those of their parents. Thus whereas one child comes from a home where meals are carefully planned and medical and dental care readily available, another may leave a home where a full stomach is the only measure of good nutrition, where breakfast is not served, or where the physician or dentist is seen only for the most extreme conditions, if at all. Surely the needs and interests of these two pupils are different in many respects.

In the same classroom there are pupils whose neighborhoods vary widely. Whereas some live in the town or city, others may be transported to school from outlying rural areas; some enjoy a pleasant suburban neighborhood, and yet others live in the shadow of factories, railroad yards, commercial sections, or in the ghettos. Home, family, and neighborhood influences will shape the kinds of out-of-school experiences a pupil has. Travel, work, and recreation also play a part in contributing to differences among children.

Attempting to adapt teaching-learning situations and experiences to fit the needs, concerns, and abilities of children, the teacher must also bear in mind that children mature at different rates. What is appealing and important to one fifth grader is, at the moment, beyond the understanding and interest of a classmate. Children grow and mature according to a general pattern, yet each child sets his or her own unique schedule. This is a most important concept for teachers to recognize.

Finally, teachers should remember that effective learning also takes place in many situations. A balance must be maintained between individual guidance and small and large group learning activities. The very nature of these human differences often provides the raw materials with which a good teacher can actually mold a superior setting for health education. Although there are many more similarities than differences among children of the same age and sex, the areas of variance constitute both a stimulating challenge and a rich opportunity for alert teachers to achieve effectiveness in two fundamental functions of good teaching: (1) providing learning experiences suited to individual purposes, needs, concerns, and interests, and (2) providing opportunities for pupil sharing of diversified experiences relating to safe and healthful living.

Teachers must choose

Perhaps the most significant function of the classroom teacher is deciding how much time and emphasis to give to various health and safety topics. In general, the teacher designs the curriculum in those districts where none exists. Even with textbooks, courses of study, teaching units, and lesson plans as guides, the classroom teacher ususlly has considerable latitude in selecting course content at a given grade level. Moreover, the teacher may have to decide just how much emphasis to place on subtopics within a broad unit. More detailed information is provided in Chapter 11 and Appendix B.

It is important that teachers remember that their primary responsibility and function is to teach, but they also have a role in the elementary school's health services and environment programs.

THE TEACHER AS COUNSELOR AND GUIDANCE PERSON

The classroom teacher assumes the role of counselor and guidance person mainly in connection with the health services program. The teacher is in a unique position to observe deviances within the student population. The teacher spends a great deal of time with the child and thus is able to see patterns develop within each child. When a deviation from the normal pattern for a given child occurs, the teacher can refer the child to appropriate sources of care.

Once the child has been referred, the conscientious teacher will follow the progress of the child to be sure that the condition for which the child was referred is alleviated. In some cases, all that will be needed is to move the child's desk to enable that student to see or hear more easily. In other cases, major alterations may be required. Regardless of what needs to be done, the teacher must maintain contact with the school nurse, the parents, and often the referral source if the school health services component is to reach its full potential.

Another way the teacher serves as counselor and guidance person is through the *informal education approach*. Information, counseling, and guidance that is nondirective, voluntary, and of little if any structure can be provided to children and parents. The teacher must be constantly alert for the child who expresses a need for help.

Naturally, any informal counseling is intended to supplement and complement the formal program. If the school health services program is to be effective, both formal and informal opportunities for counseling must be available to the student. An excellent means of informal counseling involves the use of peer groups that can serve as referral sources for students. By informally discussing the various problems that come to the teacher's attention within the classroom setting, the teacher is enhancing the total school health services program.

HEALTH OF SCHOOL PERSONNEL

The health of school personnel is important when one considers the many daily contact hours these persons have with school-age children. It is important to know whether they are emotionally well adjusted, have communicable diseases, or are physically able to perform the multitude of required duties.

School districts over the years, however, have not given adequate consideration to personnel health. Varied attention has been given mainly to health insurance, counseling by health professionals, and provisions for sick leave, maternity leave, and leave of absence. In recent years the focus on preventive aspects of health and the need to reduce skyrocketing health care costs have caused districts and insurance programs to provide monetary rewards at the end of the school year to personnel who stay well. Some companies provide reduced premiums to nonsmokers. A prevention-oriented educational program recently conducted in Texas schools* gives promise of greater attention and participation. The program focused on areas of self-management, coping and adapting, exercise and fitness, and nutrition.

Teachers and all school personnel not only have a responsibility to protect children's health, but they have a responsibility for their own health as well. Expected to provide the best physical and emotional climate (see Chapters 3 and 4) for pupils in the classroom, school personnel need to periodically assess their own health needs and problems to maintain a high level of wellness, and they also need to utilize school and community health personnel and services.

*Falck, V.T., and Kilcoyne, M.E., Jr.: A health promotion program for school personnel, Journal of School Health 54:239-242 Aug., 1984.

Teachers have little opportunity to be completely alone during the school day. Teaching is demanding and time consuming. It is common for teachers to have inadequate sleep, not find the time for proper exercise or relaxation, and feel great stress associated with their responsibilities.

The teacher is a role model for the child. As stated in the beginning of this chapter, the teacher exerts a great influence over the child. Thus if the teacher is ill, many additional untoward features may manifest themselves. If the teacher does not feel well, it is quite likely this will show in his or her disposition or in the way classroom problems are handled. How can students gain from the teacher who is chronically tired, is obese, has poor personal hygiene, or constantly complains about one or more physical, psychological, social, or spiritual problems?

Health standards for school personnel

When a child is legally mandated to attend school for at least 10 years, it is only right that parents would expect that their child not be exposed to undue health hazards. Thus having health standards for school personnel benefits children, the school personnel themselves, and the community at large.

The School Health Education and Services Section (formerly the School Health Section) of the American Public Health Association summarized the varied benefits to be derived from having health standards for school personnel. These benefits are presented in the box on p. 35.

COORDINATION OF THE SCHOOL HEALTH PROGRAM

For a school health program to be effective, coordination of all three major aspects of the program is necessary. In some cases, one individual is given primary responsibility for this administrative function. Thus the likelihood of efficient use of various school resources and fa-

BENEFITS DERIVED FROM HEALTH STANDARDS FOR SCHOOL PERSONNEL

Benefits for children

1. Increased quality of learning experiences when the staff is well
2. Lessening of stress in classrooms and other school areas
3. Greater continuity in the learning experience resulting from fewer absences of teachers and other school staff
4. Lessened exposure to communicable disease
5. Decreased risk of accidents (as from fitness of bus drivers)
6. Increased awareness and value of health when employees are good role models

Benefits for school employees

1. Early detection of conditions that can be corrected or minimized
2. Assistance in locating health resources when needed
3. Financial assistance (for health leaves, sickness disability insurance)
4. Placement in positions or assigned tasks based on consideration of the individual's health status
5. Realization that one's health behavior does relate to his/her fitness and job competency
6. Assistance in coping with stressful situations

Benefits for the community

1. Increased cost-effectiveness when staff members have fewer absences
2. Greater competence of personnel when they are well
3. Improved emotional climate in the schools
4. Increased understanding of how teacher and labor negotiations relate to health issues
5. Established and written health policies are available
6. Reduced incidence of communicable diseases
7. Assured compliance with federal regulations for hiring and placement of handicapped persons

From Doster, M., et al.: Health of school personnel: report of the American Public Health Association, Education and Services School Health Section, Washington, D.C., 1980, The Association.

cilities is enhanced since the linkage between the instructional, service, and environmental aspects of the program can be brought more clearly into focus.

The teacher and the health coordinator

In an ideal situation, each school district or system should have a coordinator or supervisor for the district's school health program. Unfortunately, few districts have employed such a person. In those instances where employment of a health coordinator is possible, the person employed should be a professionally trained school health educator who works with all of the professional and ancillary school staff, including administrators, to assure that a well-developed school health program is operating within the district. In those cases where a coordinator is not hired, the classroom teacher may have to assume the role of coordinator for a given building.

Numerous functions have been attributed to

the health coordinator, but a summary of those most commonly found include the following*:

Organize and supervise the school health program

Coordinate the activities of such a program with those in the community—health departments, civic and professional organizations, parents, police safety programs, physicians, dentists, private and voluntary health agencies, and school and community health councils

Help teach in the instructional program

Maintain a continuous evaluation program

Plan for in-service education

Help develop an articulated health and safety curriculum

Counsel individual students following referral

Serve on the community health council

Chair the school health council

Establish procedures for purchasing and distributing instructional material

Furnish the staff with information about the total school health program

Help prepare policies and procedures for school health services

Develop a plan for keeping health records

Provide procedures for student referral

Prepare and interpret emergency care procedures for faculty and staff

Provide leadership in the promotion of healthful school living

In-service education. The provision of in-service education programs for teachers is a responsibility of central administration but is often coordinated by the health coordinator. The in-service program provides one way teachers can keep up to date on health matters that affect the school-age child. A good program of in-service education can help boost teacher morale and keep the school health program dynamic.

Individual guidance. Through planned conferences and informal talks the supervisor can help teachers analyze and solve the problems that relate to their own classroom situations and teaching. Much of this is concerned with evaluation of the teaching-learning process. The conference may be based on classroom observation by the coordinator. Such observation is concerned with helping the teacher do a better job, *not* with personal criticism of the teacher.

Refer to Chapter 6 for detailed information on health guidance and informal education.

Communication. To bring helpful information and ideas to teachers is one of the chief functions of the school health coordinator. Elementary classroom teachers cannot possibly keep up with all the important literature in school health, thus the coordinator has a major function to keep the staff aware of new developments in the field.

Research and curriculum development. An important but often overlooked function of the health coordinator is that of stimulating and guiding teachers in research projects. Of course, most teachers cannot be expected to carry out extensive investigations in addition to their normal teaching load. Yet with help and guidance from the supervisor, significant problems can be selected and delineated for worthwhile study in an elementary school. Important data can often be collected within the framework of routine classroom activities. Policy and procedures based on objective evidence offer far more likelihood of success than those predicated on empirical opinion. By having teachers directly involved in policy making, it is more likely that the policy will be understood and accepted than if the policy were externally developed.

The teacher and the administrator

Administrators and school board members who understand the problems and appreciate the values of school health and health education are essential to an effective program. Experience with health programs in elementary schools has shown with vivid clarity that the success of any such program basically depends on the attitude of school administrators and school board mem-

---

*Adapted from Schaller, W.: The school health program, ed. 5, New York, 1981, W.B. Saunders Co., and Creswell, W., Newman, I., and Anderson, C.: School health practice, ed. 8, St. Louis, 1985, Times Mirror/Mosby College Publishing.

bers. When administrators favor and support a sound health program, it is more likely to be initiated and carried out successfully. Fortunately, in recent years the leading professional societies of administrators have recommended that school health programs be established for all schools. However, teachers may need to encourage administrators to take active leadership in providing effective school health programs. Teachers may encourage the formation of a school health council and indicate their willingness to serve on such a committee.

At the superintendent level this leadership often takes shape through stimulation of school evaluations by professional groups and citizens' advisory committees. Specific criteria for evaluation of the school health program are presented in some detail in Appendix H.

As the official leader in an individual elementary school, the principal has much influence on the health program. Through concern for a sound program, provision of released time for conferences, establishment of in-service programs on health-related topics, encouragement of teachers, efforts to secure textbooks and other learning materials, and consistent interest in the many activities of the school health program, the principal helps classroom teachers assume their responsible roles in school health.

The teacher and the school nurse

With the lack of coordinators in the schools, the school nurse may commonly be the individual who promotes and coordinates the health program. The classroom teacher should make every effort to work closely with the school nurse in matters of student health. Although some school nurses are employed directly by the school and others are employed by local or state health departments, it is a fundamental school staff function of the teacher to offer full cooperation to the nurse serving the school.

There are numerous areas in which the teacher and nurse can be of great help to each other. The nurse can help the teacher by letting the teacher know the signs and symptoms of various health problems, establishing referral mechanisms, assisting with the instructional program through securing speakers and material aids, working with the teacher in terms of health guidance (see Chapter 6), and aiding the returning student to readjust to the classroom. The teacher can help the nurse by observing the children daily, assisting in screening, and referring suspected health problems, including child abuse or neglect. Child abuse is not always physically manifested. In fact, mental abuse may be more devastating to the child in the long run. A child who is "beaten" mentally may become disconsolate, dispirited, and withdrawn. In any case, the basic procedure for reporting any suspected health problem should be part of the written policies and procedures of the school district. The administration should acquaint all employees with these materials.

Once a child has been referred, the teacher is not free of responsibility. It is important that the teacher follow up the referral to see that something is done. Naturally this could and should be done in conjunction with other school personnel. It is usually rather easy to determine if something has been done, since the teacher will have daily contact with the referred child. Further, the teacher can exert some control over the situation through rearrangement of the classroom environment, including seating, and through altering the daily classroom schedule.

The teacher can aid the school nurse through assisting with screening procedures (see Chapter 5). The most common measures include growth and development, vision, hearing, and possibly postural defects (primarily scoliosis). Some schools may offer mental health screening. It must be remembered that these procedures are not diagnostic tools. They are used merely to determine whether a potential problem exists. The teacher should be familiar with various mental health screening measures and know how to explain the results to the parents.

The teacher will be able to do some health counseling using the screening procedures as objective evidence. This should be coordinated with the school nurse. Often this counseling occurs on a less formal basis throughout the progress of the average school day.

Screening tests also afford the opportunity for incidental instruction. As the tests are being administered, the teacher has an opportunity to do incidental health teaching on topics directly related to the screening process. Such questions as "Why should this screening be done?" "What might be detected?" and "Will this hurt?" all provide excellent instructional potential.

To assure close rapport between the teacher and the nurse, teacher-nurse conferences are necessary. Unfortunately, it is often difficult to find the time in the already crowded school day to schedule such meetings, but with the help of the school principal, this problem should not be difficult to resolve. These conferences may be formal or informal, depending on the topics to be considered. Further information concerning the nature of teacher-nurse conferences is presented in Chapter 5.

THE TEACHER AS A LINK WITH THE COMMUNITY IN SCHOOL HEALTH

As the school and the community join more closely in their efforts to improve education, many reciprocal advantages accrue. Opportunities that will benefit the school health program are abundantly evident. The teacher has many occasions to work with resource people in the community and should capitalize on these opportunities.

Community organizations and people who are capable of providing cooperative assistance include the following:

Medical societies and individual physicians
Dental societies, individual dentists, and dental hygienists
Local and state health departments
Local and state voluntary health agencies
Parent-teacher associations
Police and fire departments
Community health and safety councils
Child guidance clinics, individual psychiatrists and clinical psychologists
Red Cross

Service clubs
Departments of education
Departments of welfare
Youth councils
Boy Scouts and Girl Scouts
YMCA, YWCA, CYO, 4-H Clubs, Future Farmers of America, and other youth organizations

These organizations often have speakers' bureaus, among other services, or will provide resource materials to the classroom teacher. For example, the fire department may be willing to present demonstrations of home fire safety hazards or assist the teacher in teaching children techniques of artificial resuscitation. Voluntary, government, and professional organizations and agencies may provide pamphlets, posters, slides, cassettes or films for classroom use. All the teacher has to do is ask for the material.

The new teacher would be well advised to consult with the school nurse, the school administrator or coordinator, and other teachers in the school to learn the resources available in a given area.

SCHOOL HEALTH COUNCILS

One of the best ways to fully coordinate the personnel resources of the community is through the school health council. Membership of the school health council can include representatives from the following groups:

Teachers
Pupils
Parents
Medical society
Dental society
Health department
Voluntary health agencies
Food service and custodial staffs
School administrators (principal and school health coordinator)
School nurses and physicians

Membership of the council will vary depending on the size of the school and the nature of the community. However, even in small rural elementary schools, council membership can include the principal or a delegated representative, parents, pupils, classroom teachers, and custodians. In some communities an advisory health council is established for all schools in the area; in others each school has its own council. Regardless of the size or makeup of the school health council, it has three basic functions: (1) to identify health and safety problems of pupils and school personnel, (2) to study these problems, and (3) to make recommendations to the school administration for solution of the problems. It is important to understand that the council is an advisory body to the superintendent and school baord; it is not responsible for taking direct action. The council may, however, conduct evaluation studies, propose changes in the policies for the instructional, service, or environmental aspects of the program, or propose the need for a total curriculum revision. The school health council is also a good forum to receive input from parents and interested citizens on matters related to school health policies and practices.

Councils have not been found in many schools or school districts in recent years. However, they are still needed to develop interest in, support, initiate, and assess school health programs.

COMMUNITY HEALTH COUNCILS

The community health council is the community counterpart to the school health council. It has the potential of linking the school health program and the community health program. This council becomes a community voice for the airing of health problems seen by the various groups within the community. By having a close, cooperative link with the community, the school health program can become more responsive to the needs of that community. Membership of the community health council may include representatives from the following:

School health council
Voluntary health agencies
Medical and dental organizations
Private industry
Civic or community service clubs
Religious organizations
Educational organizations
Parent-teacher groups
Youth organizations
Police and fire departments

In cities where the community health council has been successfully established, the school health program has been used as a focal point for community health services. Such things as sickle cell screening, school safety (especially crosswalks in the vicinity of the school), drug education referral centers, and many other health problems can be coordinated between the school and the community health programs.

THE TEACHER AS A MEMBER OF THE SCHOOL STAFF IN HEALTH MATTERS

As has been discussed, teachers do many things with and for pupils beyond the routine classroom learning activities. The teacher's role as counselor in the various health services, and several ways in which a teacher provides a link between school and community has been presented. In many of these activities the teacher also serves as a member of the school staff.

However, in the role of staff member, the elementary classroom teacher also has the responsibility for taking part in committee work and other organized efforts aimed at improvement of the school health program. The teacher may also serve on committees concerned with textbook selection, curriculum development, civil defense, special events planning, safety patrol, school clubs, building and grounds, audiovisual aids, and food service. The work of certain committees, particularly the health council, and the proper concern of all teachers commonly relates to the safety and health of the school environment.

THE TEACHER AS A MEMBER OF THE PROFESSION IN SCHOOL HEALTH

A good teacher tries constantly to improve health instruction by using better methods and keeping abreast of new developments in a variety of fields, including school health. As has been suggested earlier, many teachers will conduct surveys and experiments in connection with their health teaching or other school health work. This, too, is the mark of a professional person. Objective conferences with the health coordinator about teaching methods and materials also help the teacher improve approaches in the classroom.

Through membership in national and state educational associations the elementary teacher takes part in the profession to a fuller extent. National and state societies generally make provision for school health concerns through member associations, divisions, or sections. Organizations specifically concerned with school health include the American Alliance for Health, Physical Education, Recreation, and Dance; the American School Health Association; the American Public Health Association (School Health Education and Services Section); and regional and state branches of such groups.

All in all, the life of elementary school classroom teachers is a diversified one in regard to school health. As has been discussed, they must live up to a reputation as "specialized generalists" if they are to make contributions in the three basic phases of the health program. Although many teachers-to-be approach their first positions with some trepidation, all the evidence and experience indicate that the majority of classroom teachers can and do make substantial contributions to school health and health education. All they need is a bit of confidence and an understanding of the fundamental concepts of health instruction, health services, and healthful school living. The raw material is America's richest resource; the product is a healthier nation.

SUMMARY

Elementary school teachers have the opportunity to greatly influence the health of students through the instruction, services, and environmental aspects of the school health program. To be effective, these teachers need to acquire the competencies outlined in this chapter. They must be aware that in teaching about health: (1) the approach requires a different emphasis than other subject areas in the curriculum, (2) the inclusion of controversial topics is involved, (3) current scientific information must be imparted without bias, (4) ethical issues need consideration, and (5) provision for individual pupil health differences must be made. Teachers must realize that the status of their own health has a considerable effect on student health. They must be ready and willing to coordinate their health efforts with a variety of school and community personnel, organizations, and agencies.

QUESTIONS FOR DISCUSSION

1. Identify the five basic areas of competency for the elementary teacher and list one competency for each area. Do you feel it is realistic to expect elementary teachers to possess all these qualities? Why or why not?
2. Why does the teaching of health require a different approach than other subject areas in the school curriculum?
3. What are some of the areas when teaching health that may be considered to be controversial and why is this true? How might teachers deal with these areas in the classroom?
4. What are two ethical issues related to the school health program and indicate what teachers can do about them?
5. Why must teachers keep up to date with current scientific information? What evaluation procedures may be used to assess the reliability of sources of health information?
6. What are three ways teachers may provide for individual differences in the classroom?
7. What are two ways teachers may provide health counseling and guidance?
8. How can the health of teachers affect students? What may teachers do to protect student health in this regard?
9. Identify three ways the school health coordinator may provide services to schools and three ways this person may assist teachers.
10. Identify three ways teachers can assist the school nurse and three ways the nurse can assist teachers in regard to the health of students.
11. What might comprise the membership of a school health council and identify the council's functions? Might teachers play a role in starting a council if none exists in a school or school district?

SELECTED REFERENCES

American Public Health Association: Health of school personnel, report of the School Health Education and Services Section, Washington, D.C., 1980, The Association.

Barnes, S.E.: Ethical issues in health education, Health Education **11:**7-9 March/April, 1980.

Charles, C.M.: Individualizing instruction, ed. 2, St. Louis, 1980, The C.V. Mosby Co.

Cornacchia, H. and Barrett, S.: Consumer health, ed. 3, St. Louis, 1985, Times Mirror/Mosby College Publishing.

Creswell, W., Newman, I., and Anderson, C.: School health practice, ed. 8, St. Louis, 1985, Times Mirror/Mosby College Publishing.

Davis, C., et al.: Health concerns and teacher training of selected elementary teachers in Michigan, Journal of School Health **55:**151-153 April, 1985.

Falck, V.T. and Kilcoyne, M.E., Jr.: A health promotion program for school personnel, Journal of School Health **54:**239-242 Aug., 1984.

Hochbaum, G.M.: Ethical dilemmas in health education, Health Education **11:**4-6 March/April, 1980.

Hosokowa, M.C.: Insurance incentives for health promotion, Health Education **17:**9-12 Oct./Nov., 1984.

Levy, M.R., Greene, W.H., and Jenne, F.H.: Competency-based professional preparation, School Health Review July/Aug., 1972.

Ludwig, D.J.: Teacher preparation in health education, School Health Review Sept./Oct., 1972.

Proceedings of the National Conference on School Health Education Research in the Heart, Lungs and Blood Area, Bethesda, Md., 1983 National Institutes of Health.

Richardson, G.E.: Ethical issues in school health: a survey, Health Education **14:**5-9, 1983.

Russo, R.M., et al.: The use of community health aids in a school health program, Journal of School Health **52:**425-427 Sept., 1982.

Schaller, W.: The school health program, ed. 5, New York, 1981, W.B. Saunders Co.

Valente, C., and Lumb, K.: Organization and function of a school health council, Journal of School Health **51:**466-468 Sept., 1981.

PART

II

HEALTHFUL SCHOOL LIVING

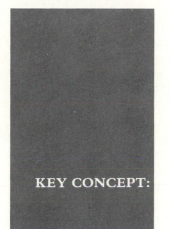

HEALTHFUL SCHOOL ENVIRONMENT: PHYSICAL ASPECTS

The physical environment of the school can affect the health of pupils and school personnel.

AMERICAN ACADEMY OF PEDIATRICS

KEY CONCEPT: A safe and healthful school environment enhances the quality of student life and learning.

When we by law require children to spend so many of their formative years in our schools, we assume a legal and ethical responsibility to provide safe and healthful buildings, equipment, facilities, and services.

Even though this obligation is accepted and the concept understood in our educational literature and professional pronouncements, tens of thousands of American schools fail to meet minimal health and safety standards for students. Many schools are considered by experts to be firetraps; others maintain overcrowded classrooms; some are hotbeds of violence; still others carry tenured teachers who are emotionally unstable; many are not meeting the emotional needs of students; many have question-

able water and sewerage systems; most are operating unsafe school buses; and few provide a sanitary, nutritious food service.

A physically and emotionally healthful school environment is essential to the highest quality of education in our schools. The quality of life cannot be enriched for students who are forced to strive to learn and grow in schools that fail to provide a pleasant, conducive atmosphere.

WHAT IS A HEALTHFUL SCHOOL ENVIRONMENT?

Healthful school living is "the promotion, maintenance, and utilization of safe and wholesome surroundings (Fig. 3-1), organization of

FIG. 3-1. Safe playgrounds contribute to a positive school environment.

day-to-day experiences and planned learning procedures to influence favorable emotional, physical, and social health."*

Clearly this definition dispels the idea that healthful school living is confined to the mere provisions of a safe and sanitary environment in which learning can occur. The overriding purpose for providing a healthful school environment is to establish a climate for children and staff that is supportive of their health and quality of life, enables them to feel good about being in school, and enhances opportunities for student learning.

HOW DO SCHOOL SITE AND BUILDINGS AFFECT STUDENT HEALTH?

Some specific physical components of healthful school living include site and building construction, internal organization such as thermal

*Green, L.: New definitions: report of the 1972-73 joint committee on health education terminology, Health Education Monographs 33:33-37, 1973.

control, lighting and acoustics, water supply, sanitation, food services, school bus safety, and fire prevention and protection.

School site and construction

The construction of facilities in which learning is to occur has been a major concern for many decades. In 1829 Alcott wrote an "Essay on the Construction of Schoolhouses,"* which emphasized the impact of the environment on the education process. Ever since that time, many rules, regulations, and standards have been promulgated to help assure that the school physical plant promotes safety and is sanitary, free of unnecessary hazards, and conducive to maximizing the potential for learning. The critical factor is to plan ahead and not operate on a crisis basis. The mere construction of a new building is no assurance that it contributes favorably to the educational experience of the child. A facility poorly planned in terms of location, internal space, color, internal and external traffic patterns, and many other environmental considerations too numerous to mention here may in fact detract from overall learning. The school environment should support the holistic nature of the student.

The selection of a site involves such considerations as the following:
Accessibility for local traffic
Distance from busy or noisy streets
External odor and noise factors (airports, railway stations, dumps, industrial areas)
Adequate space (playgrounds, athletic fields)
Freedom from unnecessary hazards (open holes, water hazards)
Adequate drainage
Hookups to community water and sewage lines
Amenability to esthetic landscaping
Adequate pupil population within a rather limited radius (often considered one-half mile or less in large cities)
Numerous innovations in school construction

*Means, R.: A history of health education in the United States, Philadelphia, 1962, Lea & Febiger.

occurred in the early 1960s. Too often, however, these new facilities were based on an architectural idea rather than the effective use of the facility as an institution of learning. Frequently, these new ideas in construction did not adequately facilitate learning. Unfortunately, little research that demonstrates what would be best in school facilities has taken place. Now, however, much more consideration than before has been given the interiors of the building. Modular construction, open classrooms, learning wings, and central resource libraries, as well as the more traditional single-level or multilevel self-contained classroom may be found in new school building construction.

Recently another problem associated with school construction has surfaced—that of asbestos removal. Before 1973, asbestos was often used in school construction, primarily as a fire retardant. The Environmental Protection Agency estimates that as many as 33,000 school buildings involving 15 million children and 1.3 million teachers, administrators, and other staff have deteriorating walls and ceilings containing asbestos fibers. When this deterioration occurs, the asbestos fibers are allowed to float free in the buildings. Since exposure to asbestos fibers has been linked with several debilitating lung diseases, schools containing asbestos can cause a health hazard for the occupants.

In April, 1987, the Environmental Protection Agency proposed new rules that will require school systems that find dangerous asbestos in their buildings to use certified contractors to remove the asbestos. This will require school districts to submit a plan for the removal of the asbestos and to begin the work by mid-October, 1988. It is estimated that the cost of this removal will exceed $3.2 billion over the next 30 years. To help school districts pay for the removal, Congress has voted to provide $50 million this year to assist in the process. Although there is a great deal of controversy whether the problem of asbestos removal should be a federal, state, or local issue, the fact remains that it is a hazard that cannot be allowed to remain in the school environment.

Internal organization. It is important when designing a new or refurbishing an existent school building that the architect give consideration to the needs of children and provide lowered and recessed drinking fountains, as well as lowered toilets, sinks, light switches, chalkboards, and storage space for coats, hats, lunches, and other items. Of special concern are the needs of the handicapped who might attend the school. Additionally, classrooms large enough to permit physical activities of children, areas that can be used in quiet study or activity, and overall internal classroom flexibility such as mobile walls must be planned. The well-being of the faculty and staff must also be provided for with a teacher's lounge and separate restroom facilities that are both functional and appealing in appearance. Some new constructions contain two teacher/staff lounges, one for smokers and one for nonsmokers.

THERMAL CONTROL. The teacher often neglects to make adequate provisions for heating, ventilation, and air-conditioning. Elementary school children have a higher metabolic rate than adult teachers and tend to be able to stay warm in seemingly cold conditions; thus making the room temperature comfortable for the teacher may make it too warm for the students. Since the human body radiates heat, the teacher can avoid adjusting the room temperature upward by wearing a sweater or long-sleeve shirt, blouse, or jacket in the classroom.

A classroom that is too cold for children can have an impact on their learning. The general recommendation for classroom temperature is between 65° to 70° Fahrenheit, depending on the age of the students and the type of activity that will occur in the classroom.

The flow of air in a classroom must receive primary attention. If the school is not equipped with air-conditioning, the teacher should open windows or doors or secure a fan to assure adequate air movement.

LIGHTING. Footcandles of illumination at the work surface and in halls were commonly the determining factor for number, location, and intensity of lights located in schools. Today the role of color, the use of natural as opposed to artificial lighting, the reflection and glare of light, and the type of activity to be performed in the room are factors of greater importance.

The teacher should be aware that glare is an annoying problem in the classroom setting. Speaking to the class while standing in front of unshaded windows so that the sun is shining brightly into the eyes of students is certainly not in their best interests. Further, if there is a great deal of activity outside the window where the teacher is standing, the child's attention will be more easily distracted. The prudent and judicious use of window shades as well as teacher movement can greatly reduce the problem of glare and outside movement. Glare can be further reduced by the proper use of color and placement of student desks or tables. Children should not directly face windows or other sources of illumination. Teachers should use bulletin board materials that have a dull, nonreflecting surface rather than a shiny or highly reflective finish. If the bulletin boards are portable, they should be placed in an area of the classroom where the glare is at a minimum.

ACOUSTICS. For the most part, the teacher will not have much control over the classroom acoustics. In newer schools this matter has received attention. However, by keeping doors and windows closed except when ventilation is needed, the teacher can begin to reduce the amount of outside noise that filters into the classroom. Also, noise control can be maintained by (1) keeping the noise level within the classroom to a minimum, (2) remembering to alert children to keep noise down in the halls by not shouting or conducting other rowdy activities therein, (3) careful planning of the location of the school facility, (4) careful placement of areas that have the potential for a high level of noise (such as shops, playgrounds, and music rooms), and (5) using carpeting and acoustic tile in the construction or remodeling of school facilities.

Water supply. School authorities have a legal and moral responsibility to provide a safe and sanitary water supply for the schools. Availability of a clean and sufficient water supply is a primary consideration when selecting the site for new school construction.

The best way to assure a safe water supply is to receive it from the local municipality, which has a civil responsibility to ensure that the water is safe for consumption for its constituents. In those areas where it is not possible to connect to the municipal water supply, wells can be drilled. Wells must conform to local sanitary standards available from the various city, county, and state health departments. The water supply should be tested monthly by experienced personnel to assure that it is free of contamination. Since water is a daily essential, whatever the water supply, it must be adequate for all of the daily school activities that require water. Automatic toilet flushing devices used in the school restrooms greatly increase the demand for water. Thus careful planning is needed to ensure an adequate water supply if these devices are to be used in either new or remodeled facilities.

FOUNTAINS. Drinking fountains should be recessed in the wall, located in accessible positions, and operable by those who must remain in a wheelchair. Use of "arc stream" fountains is preferable to using the "bubbler" type fountain because the arc stream keeps the person who is drinking away from the direct source of the water. If the individual has a communicable disease, the likelihood of contaminating the bubbler fountain is much greater than that of the arc stream fountain. It is also important that the pressure of the water emitted from the fountain be powerful enough that children will not have to put their mouths too close to the outlet jet to drink.

TOILET ROOMS. It is preferable that toilet facilities have an outside exposure to direct, natural lighting because of the effect of sunlight on select disease-causing organisms. It is important that the toilet facilities be accessible and not located in the basement; there are supervisory reasons for this as well as considerations of distance from the various classrooms in the school. There should be easy access to toilets for the handicapped, which is yet another reason for lavatories to be located on the ground level.

Both washbasins and commodes should be accessible to the handicapped. At least one commode that has a closable door for privacy should be provided for the handicapped.

Washbasins in the restrooms (or in classrooms for that matter) should be equipped with hot and cold running water. They should have liquid soap dispensers rather than solid soap. The major problem with bar soap is the possibility of it causing an accident should someone step on it, slip, and be injured.

Sanitation. Students should not be subjected to an unsanitary environment. Provisions must be made for the safe and effective removal of waste from the school. Where daily pick up of garbage is not possible, refuse should be kept in a secure place where it will not attract animals or vermin that will scatter it around the school site. The use of sturdy disposal cans with tight lids for sanitary storage of waste is advisable.

SEWAGE DISPOSAL. Connection with the municipal sewage system is the best way to dispose of sewage. If this is not possible, septic tanks must be installed. Where running water is not available, chemical holding tanks will have to be used. Regular disposal of the contents of the holding tanks can be accomplished through a professional sanitary disposal firm.

It is important that school officials consult with sewage experts before installing a septic or chemical tank. The septic tank should be located below the source of water in schools that use wells to avoid the possibility of contaminating the water supply. The tank should be accessible for annual cleaning to ensure that there are no disease-causing organisms contained in the tank.

SCHOOL FOOD SERVICES: ARE THEY ADEQUATE?

With over 4.2 billion lunches and 630 million breakfasts served in 1985, the feeding of children in schools obviously has become big business. It is also big politics, and it certainly is "no small potatoes" when it comes to the nutrition and health of millions of American children.

Yet for millions of America's students the school breakfast, school lunch, or both is their only chance for a nutritious meal during the day. Repeated surveys show that many school-age children and youth, from *all* socioeconomic levels, are subsisting on diets that are nutritionally marginal if not deficient. There is a pressing need for better school lunches and expansion of the school breakfast program. In 1985, over 85,500 schools participated in one or both of these programs.

School lunch program

Originating in 1935 under Section 32 of Public Law 74-320 (the Agricultural Adjustment Act) under which the federal government bought farm commodities for distribution to schools as a way to absorb farm surplus and support agricultural incomes, the National School Lunch Act (PL 79-396) was authorized in 1946. The goals of the program were to (1) distribute surplus farm commodities and support farm income, and (2) safeguard the health of school children.

In 1954 the Agricultural Act (PL 83-690), which encouraged fluid milk consumption along with the lunch program, was passed. Since both the National School Lunch Program and the Agricultural Act were basically temporary programs, Congress passed the Child Nutrition Act (PL 89-642) in 1966, giving both prior acts permanent authorization. The programs are administered by the U.S. Department of Agriculture.

Participation in the National School Lunch Program has grown from 6.6 million children in 1946 (approximately 24% of eligible school children) to 23.6 million children (60.5% of eligible school children) in 1985. At present it is estimated that over 94% of all schools in the United States participate in the National School Lunch Program.

The cost of school lunches is over $6.8 billion a year. Although the amounts expended in each state differ, about half of the cost is divided between federal and state governments, and the other half comes from "lunch money" from parents. In 1985 the federal government paid over $3.4 billion for school lunches. Half of the federal contribution is in the form of food commodities. The federal government contributes to each school meal based on the percentage of students who get free or reduced-price meals. The amount of this reimbursement fluctuates each year.

School breakfast program

Because of recognition of the urgent need for many elementary and secondary children to have the opportunity to eat a well-balanced breakfast, breakfast programs have been initiated with the support of the U.S. Department of Agriculture. As in the school lunch program, all public and nonprofit private schools may participate in the breakfast program. In 1985 over 3.5 million children participated. The federal government paid over $385 million in cash and commodities for the school breakfast program in 1985. In addition, over $15.9 million was spent for the special milk program available in schools.

Study and experience have shown that, as with the lunch program, when students participate in a school breakfast program, they learn better, have fewer complaints of headache and stomachache, and have fewer behavior problems.

The problems

A number of problems have become painfully apparent since the National School Lunch Act was passed during the Truman Administration over 4 decades ago. The program has made substantial contribution to the health of millions of American students, but critics from the field of nutritional science and the congressional arena continue to point up these problems:

1. The *quantity* of food, affected by the changing availability of farm surplus commodities, does not necessarily assure a *quality* diet for growing children and youth.

2. Increasing financial burden has fallen on parents, since, by implicit Congressional sanction, states can count students' lunch payments as part of the matching formula.

3. Economic eligibility guidelines—who pays how much for what students—have contributed to administrative, political, social, and (for the student) psychological problems.

4. Early in the program, studies showed that many school lunches were deficient in complete proteins and in vitamins A, B_1 (thiamine), B_6 (pyridoxine), C (ascorbic acid), and D, and contained excess fats, salt, and sugar. This led to the National Evaluation of School Nutrition Programs published in 1983.

5. U.S. Department of Agriculture regulations now permit competitive foods to be sold in vending machines in school lunchrooms but they can't operate at the time of the regular lunch program. Sharp criticism has been leveled at this modification of the national school lunch program since it opens the door for students to pass up the school lunch for more appealing, but less nutritious, "junk" foods. However, an increasing number of school systems are limiting vending machine sales to milk, fruit juices, and nutritious foods.

6. Food and labor costs are causing a financial crisis for schools and parents in providing nutritious school lunches and breakfasts. A U.S. Department of Agriculture study revealed that for every 1-cent increase in cost to the student, there was a 1% drop in participation in the program.

Too much too soon?

A growing body of evidence indicates that high serum cholesterol levels are a major risk factor in the development of coronary heart disease and premature fatal heart attack. It has also been clearly established that this buildup of blood cholesterol accelerates during adolescence, especially among boys.

In a classic, carefully controlled study at Saint Paul's School in New Hampshire,* researchers were able to substantially lower the serum cholesterol of approximately 500 boys by substituting polyunsaturated foods for those high in saturated fats. These Harvard School of Public Health investigators modified students' dining

---

*Stare, F.J., editor: Atherosclerosis, New York, 1974, Medcom, Inc.

hall diets by substituting low-fat milk for whole milk, using polyunsaturated vegetable oil in baked products and for frying doughnuts, replacing butter and regular margarine with a soft margarine, and serving whole eggs just once a week and a low-cholesterol egg mix twice a week. Other dietary modifications were made with the same purpose in mind—reduction of cholesterol and other hard fats. At present the Galveston, Texas Public Schools are engaged in a large nutrition education project that involves the application of social learning theory across the entire food service program.

Compounding the problem of high cholesterol and coronary heart disease is the hard fact that obesity continues to be a serious threat to health and a high quality of life for millions of American parents and their children. Obesity and malnutrition often go hand in hand—too many calories with too few essential nutrients.

We also have learned that most cases of adult obesity have their beginnings in childhood and adolescence. Yet we continue to serve school lunches and breakfasts that are high in fats, salts, sugars, and additives. Surveys of large samples of school foods throughout the nation confirm this. Under current standards such hard-fat foods as regular peanut butter, whole-fat milk, processed cheese, fatty meats, frankfurters, and regular margarine or butter qualify for federal reimbursement under the national school lunch program.

Too little too late

As previously mentioned, studies show that many school lunches are deficient in complete proteins, iron, and vitamins A and C. More than a few schools also fail to provide adequate amounts of such important nutrients as thiamine, pyridoxine, vitamin D, and magnesium. All of these are needed for optimal growth and development during childhood and adolescence.

Further, the American Heart Association recommends that not over 30% to 35% of the recommended daily allowance of calories be fat. Too often U.S. Department of Agriculture meals exceed this recommendation.

Dispelling the myths

Although there are still problems with the various school feeding programs, it is important to dispel some of the myths and misconceptions that surround them. Only 20% of the food used in school lunch or breakfast programs is provided by the U.S. Department of Agriculture. The remainder is purchased by local school districts from the same vendors who supply restaurants. Thus the problem of less-than-optimal nutritional value attributed the government may well be a local problem instead. Improper preparation and storage of the food that is made available through government sources or through local vendors may be responsible for less-than-optimal nutritional value in the school feeding program.

Often teachers grumble about having to pay a higher price for their meals than the students, even though they get the same meal as the students. Federal regulations stipulate that reimbursement, or commodities for the nutrition programs in schools, exclude meals served to adults. As such, no money collected from students, commodities that are either provided or purchased, or money that is reimbursed to the school may be utilized in serving meals to adults. Thus schools must charge adults an amount for each meal that would pay for the foods that are included in that meal.

Finally, the National Evaluation of School Nutrition Programs* showed that the diets of all students were low in vitamins A, and B_6, and the minerals calcium and magnesium, but if the children ate breakfast or lunch at school, they generally showed a higher energy level and a better overall nutrient intake than they would if no school feeding program were available. Further, it was shown that when a school breakfast program existed, more children ate breakfast than would have eaten breakfast if that particular program did not exist and the student was expected to eat breakfast at home before arriving at school.

---

*Wellish, J., et al.: National evaluation of school nutrition programs, Final Report, vols. 1 and 2, Santa Monica, Cal., 1983, System Development Corporation.

Streamlining school food services

Perhaps like America's railroad dining car—a nostalgic financial failure—our school lunchrooms need to move into the jet age of airline-type central food service. The day of the haphazardly run kitchen must now give way to a more businesslike organization.

Evidence is mounting that the planning and operation of school food services is best done by organizations experienced in large-scale meal delivery systems. Studies show that for the same worker cost, centrally located kitchens can provide 3 times the number of meals that can be served under the existing unit kitchen system where meals are prepared in each individual school. However, plate wastage (food served but not eaten) may offset any of the advantages that might be attained. Thus careful planning is critical.

The chief drawback to a central kitchen system is the high initial cost. Although such systems usually become economically stable in 1 or 2 years, many school districts cannot afford the initial financial outlay.

Improving school food services

Regardless of the merits or limitations of new school food program legislation, teachers, school board members, administrators, and others concerned with student health can get information and assistance from the Child Nutrition Division of the U.S. Department of Agriculture (Washington, D.C. 20250), and the American School Food Services Association (5600 S. Quebec, Suite 300B, Englewood, Colo., 80110). In addition, teachers and those directly concerned with providing school food services can write or call their state office for specific information.

At local and state levels there is continuing need for studies to determine the most efficient methods—lowest cost and highest nutrient meals—for raising the important contribution of the school feeding program to the health of elementary and secondary school children and youth.

School feeding and nutrition education

Certainly one of the chief advantages of the school lunch or breakfast is the opportunity it provides for relating classroom information on healthful diets to school feeding programs. Teachers can have students keep daily records of what they eat, including school meals, and discussions can be a significant part of a unit on nutrition. Of course, any diary records from students must be anonymous if reliable responses are to be obtained.

A news story told about an elementary school principal who was distressed at the food wastage in the lunchroom and had pupils take inventory of what had been thrown in trash cans in 1 day. A pupil-prepared report disclosed that students had discarded the following items: 41 sandwiches, 2 cartons of milk, 2 whole pieces of chicken, 3 bags of potato chips, 19 apples, 13 oranges, 1 piece of cake, an untouched carton of chocolate pudding, 4 whole carrots, 2 boxes of raisins, 19 pieces of candy, and 14 cookies! Obviously, simply offering food to children does not ensure that they will eat it.

Without sound nutrition education students may discard nutritious foods from the school lunch or breakfast, buy calorie-rich nutritionally poor foods from vending machines, or patronize one of the quick-food commercial establishments in the neighborhood. Again, health education appears as the crucial influence in choices and decisions of students whatever the environmental situation.

WHAT ABOUT SCHOOL BUS SAFETY?

School buses are part of the school environment because once the child steps aboard the bus he or she is under the jurisdiction and responsibility of the schools. The child's health and safety on the bus are just as important as they are when that child is in any other school facility or activity (Fig. 3-2).

Between 1984 and 1985, 50 students lost their lives in school bus accidents—20 as passengers

FIG. 3-2. School buses must be safe and can be equipped to meet the needs of the physically challenged individual. *(Courtesy of Wichita Public Schools.)*

and 30 while getting on or off the bus. An additional 6,700 students were injured. Every day more than 390,000 school buses carry over 21.5 million boys and girls to and from school.

Schwartz and Klenetsky* stated that school buses are the safest vehicles on the road and that they are 37 times safer than an automobile. Even so, there is substantial room for improvement. At present, there is a growing movement across the nation to improve the safety of school buses, including the installation of seat belts in them.

In May, 1984, the National Coalition for Seat Belts on School Buses was formed to help coordinate seat belt installation efforts nationwide. Through the efforts of this national coalition, more and more school districts are not only equipping their existing buses with seat belts, but also are purchasing buses with seat belts

factory installed. The estimated cost of these safety devices runs $1,200 to $3,000 for each bus, for an average cost of about 75 cents for each child per year, based on a 66-passenger bus that lasts 13 years and transports more than one "set" of passengers each day. Over 70 school districts nationwide require seat belts for their school buses. The problem is that use of the seat belt by a student is generally made optional. Unfortunately, parents and the general public usually are apathetic except for brief transient periods of emotional concern following a tragic accident killing large numbers of students.

Many of America's school buses are unsafe for one reason or another. The National Highway Traffic Safety Administration has proposed new, tough requirements for all public transport buses, including school buses. Chief among these is the provision for padded, high-backed seats and safety belts for all passengers. The National Conference on School Transportation has developed a code that contains minimum standards for school buses. This code is available from the National Education Association.

Congressional legislation, in the face of powerful lobbying and bureaucratic inertia, offers the promise of safer school buses. One of the better recent proposals in the U.S. House of Representatives includes these new national standards:

1. Seating systems including proper padding, firm anchoring to the floor, approved passenger belts, and higher seat backs
2. Improved emergency exits
3. Interior protection for passengers
4. Greater floor strength
5. More crash-resistant bodies and frames
6. Safer vehicle operating systems
7. Improved safety glass for windshields and passenger windows

Safety experts also believe that school bus transportation can be made safer by careful selection and training of drivers, skilled mechanical maintenance, nationwide uniformity of exterior color and bus stopping requirements, and avoidance of overcrowding and unruly pupil behavior.

*Schwartz, L.G., and Klenetsky, F.: Seat belts in school buses, Journal of School Health **55**(3):119, 1985.

ARE OUR SCHOOLS FIRETRAPS?*

Not too many years ago some fire safety experts estimated that approximately 30,000 schools in America could be classified as firetraps. Many magazine articles, continued public education by the National Safety Council and local and national fire officials, such popular films as *Towering Inferno*, and the Kentucky nightclub fire in 1977 have tended to increase public concern for fire prevention and protection. In the years 1980 to 1984, the National Fire Protection Association estimates that an average of 12,200 fires per year occurred in the nation's schools. The average annual cost of these fires exceeded $80.9 million.

Still, many schools lack automatic fire alarm systems, and few have automatic sprinkler systems. Such systems should, at least, be installed in shops, chemistry laboratories, boiler rooms, supply rooms, and other fire-hazard areas. Local fire inspectors should be consulted by school administrators for regular inspections and recommendations for eliminating any existing dangerous conditions. The cost of alarm and sprinkler systems is a small price to pay for protecting the lives of children and youth in our schools.

The American Insurance Association urges that the following school fire-hazard conditions be checked and, when necessary, immediately corrected†:

1. Buildings where the walls or ceilings of exit corridors are surfaced with highly combustible finishes
2. Buildings with wood floors and masonry walls, especially if the pupils in the upper floors have no means of exit other than through stairs open to lower stories
3. Buildings of wood construction with pupils housed above the second story
4. Buildings with unventilated space below them where gas may collect and explode
5. Buildings with exit doors to the outside that cannot be readily opened from the inside
6. Buildings in which pupils on upper floors have no means of exit except down stairs that are open to lower stories having combustible walls and finishes or contents in storage that are combustible

With the increasing use of electrical current for audiovisual and other equipment in schools, careful periodic inspection by professionals should be made for faulty or overloaded wiring systems—a major fire hazard.

Monthly fire and disaster drills should be held for students and school personnel, and evacuation plans should be posted in every room. Fire extinguishers should be approved by local fire officials, inspected regularly, and their location and operation understood by teachers and other school personnel. All school personnel and students should be aware of the location of fire extinguishers and manually operated fire alarms in the school and of regular fire alarm boxes near the school.

As with other aspects of a safe and healthful school environment, instruction is essential for optimal fire prevention and protection.

RESPONSIBILITIES FOR HEALTHFUL SCHOOL LIVING

Healthful school living implies a joint responsibility among all persons who come into contact with the school. This would extend to those responsible for developing the physical plant (the board of education and the architect), school administrators, students, parents, custodians, and all ancillary staff.

Board of education

Probably the most critical role in healthful school living falls on the board of education. This group decides if, when, and where a school will be built or if existing facilities will be renovated to meet new standards. The group's authority for these decisions is derived from the voters of the community as their elected representatives. These same voters must ultimately provide the

---

*See the fire safety unit in Appendix B for use in educational programs.
†American Insurance Association: Safe schools, New York, 1968, The Association.

funds for any building or renovation programs suggested by the board.

A responsible board will consider carefully any recommendations for the construction of new or the renovation of existing facilities. It will hold meetings with school administrators, teachers, architects, and community representatives before it makes its decision. The decision to construct a new school is not just a board project but also a project of the community. The community will ultimately benefit from a well-planned and well-constructed school building that contributes positively to the students who attend the facility, or will suffer as the result of a facility that does not meet the needs of the students and the community.

It is the responsibility of the board to retain an architect who is reputable and has experience in school design. Before accepting a school design, the board should consult with school administrators and teachers to be sure that those persons are satisfied with the basic design, that it meets their needs as professional educators, and that it contributes to the learning of students. By taking this extra step, the board can add a great deal to the overall efficacy of any school planning. By consulting school officials the board develops within those individuals a greater sense of dedication and appreciation of the role they play in maintaining a healthful school environment.

Architect

Once the decision to construct or renovate has been made, the role of the architect becomes formidable. The construction of schools has, in fact, become a specialty within the architectural profession.

Working closely with school personnel and the board of health (which issues the building permits and does construction approval inspections), the architect has the primary responsibility to present a school plant design that embodies the considerations discussed earlier in this chapter. Too often the initial appearance of a school is appealing but on closer examination the school is not as functional as it might be.

To help overcome potential problems, the special needs of not only students but also school personnel should be considered. It is also quite important that the design be compatible with accessibility for handicapped and in compliance with Public Law 94-142, the Education for All Handicapped Children Act of 1975.

Administrators

School administrators have the major responsibility for keeping the board of education informed of needed changes within the educational system. They direct and control the daily operation of the school and must be informed of the needed changes in the physical plant that affect the overall quality of education. School population increases or decreases, deterioration of facilities, and other changes must be reported by school personnel to the superintendent, who then must relay this information with proposals for action to the board of education.

Teachers

The teachers are "on the firing line." They must make administrators aware of any special needs they may have. This far surpasses the mere physical component of the classroom and extends into all facets of school operation.

It is important that the teacher understand the unique features of a particular building so that those features can become an enhancement to the educational experience of the students. The teacher can also instill a sense of "ownership" of the school into students through the regular instructional program. By keeping the custodial staff informed of needed repairs and the administrators aware of any special needs, the teacher can contribute positively to the overall environment of the school.

Students

The students stand to benefit most from having a healthful school environment. Teachers must help them learn how to assume responsibility for keeping the school safe, sanitary, and clean. Students will greatly assist in keeping a healthful school environment by, among other things, using trash cans rather than throwing paper on the ground or floor; refraining from writing graffiti on the restroom walls; not defacing desks, chairs, and tables; keeping their feet off the walls; and wiping their shoes on doormats before entering the building.

Custodians

In today's modern school facility, the custodian must possess a broad range of mechanical and carpentry skills, knowledge of safety and sanitation principles, and general concepts of disease control. The custodian must also possess the ability to work with both students and staff.

The custodian must constantly be aware of the advantages and disadvantages of the wide range of cleaning and painting products on today's market and the new equipment available for use in the schools. In many cases the custodian will be called on to repair equipment. This person should periodically attend training workshops designed to update custodial knowledge and skills.

Lunchroom personnel

General sanitation as well as the serving of nutritious, low-fat, and attractive food should be of primary concern to lunchroom personnel. By being aware of and practicing good sanitation and food handling techniques, the lunchroom staff can help control possible food-borne disease outbreaks.

Most states require all persons who deal with feeding the public to undergo a food handler's sanitation course and a medical examination to show that they are free of any type of communicable disease. The food handler's course generally consists of learning about the need for refrigeration and heating, storage of foods, dishwashing, simple equipment maintenance, and various sanitation standards. Personal health habits and their potential for disease causation are also included.

It is important for teachers to keep the lunchroom personnel informed of various nutrition-related projects being conducted in the classroom; thus the lunchroom can become an extension of the classroom. In addition, lunchroom personnel can act in an advisory capacity for the teachers or can assist in the various classroom projects being undertaken. It is also important for parents to keep school officials informed of any possible food allergies of their children. This information must be passed to teachers, school nurses, and the lunchroom staff so that they might be alert for a potential food allergy problem.

SUMMARY

Of course, teachers have no choice in school site or construction unless they are among the few who have the opportunity to serve on a school planning committee for a new school. Hence, they must make the very best of what they inherit. Whatever the age or other problems of school site, buildings, and facilities, improvements can be affected by concerned administrators, teachers, school nurses, and others involved with the health and safety of students. School health councils are especially effective as instruments in bringing about favorable change.

Every school building in America should be maintained in accordance with state and local standards of safety, sanitation, and educational utility. Regular inspections of school buildings and facilities should be made by school administrators, local building inspectors, fire inspectors, health department sanitarians and safety experts, and other qualified personnel. Principals, teachers, custodial staff, food service personnel, school nurses, and others in the school should be alert each day for unhealthful or dangerous conditions in the building and on the school grounds.

School bus drivers should be specifically trained to deal with large numbers of students. They should be particularly safety conscious because the safety of students in their bus is their responsibility. The bus drivers should also be trained in basic first aid and emergency care.

Preventable fire hazards should never be allowed to exist in the school environment. All fire safety equipment such as alarms, fire extinguishers, hoses, and sprinkler systems should be tested regularly and maintained in good working condition. Regular fire drills should be conducted so that all students and school personnel know how to evacuate the school in a safe and orderly fashion. Finally, all school personnel should know how to use the fire-fighting equipment that is available in the schools.

A healthful school environment contributes to overall student learning and is the responsibility of all persons (who have reason to be) associated with the school. By working together, the health and safety of students and school personnel alike is enhanced.

QUESTIONS FOR DISCUSSION

1. What are the aims of a healthful school environment?
2. What considerations are included in a good program for healthful school living?
3. How can teachers and other school personnel help make improvements in old school buildings and poor school sites?
4. Why are school food service programs important to student health?
5. What are some of the major problems still existing in developing better school lunch and breakfast programs?
6. Why are central food service facilities considered to be better than individual school food preparation facilities?
7. What nutrients are often found lacking in many school lunch programs? What nutrients may be served in excess and too often?
8. What organizations can help start a new school feeding program or improve an existing one?
9. Why are so many school buses considered by safety experts to be dangerous?
10. What changes need to be made in the construction of school buses to make them safer?
11. What changes need to be made in the operation of school buses to make student transportation safer?
12. Do you think seat belts should be made mandatory for all school buses? Why or why not?
13. Should use of seat belts be made mandatory for both students and adults who ride school buses? Justify your response and include how you would suggest implementing any programs to accomplish your ideas.
14. What are the chief fire dangers in today's schools?
15. How can school administrators and teachers improve programs of fire prevention and protection?
16. Why should the school be obligated to provide a healthful environment for students?
17. What factors have contributed to the school lunch program becoming a national controversy?
18. Discuss how the school physical environment might enhance or detract from the health services program and the health instruction program.

SELECTED REFERENCES

American Academy of Pediatrics: School health: a guide for health professionals, Evanston, Ill., 1978, The Academy.

Commission on School Buildings of the American Association of School Administrators, Schools for America, Washington, D.C., 1967, The Association.

Fire Analysis Division of the National Fire Protection Association: U.S. school fire trends and patterns, Quincy, Mass., 1986, The Association.

Gilbert, G.G., and Scatarige, C.S.: Update on asbestos in schools, Journal of School Health 53(3):212-213, 1983.

Green, L.: New definitions: report of the 1972-73 joint committee on health education terminology, Health Education Monographs 33:33-37, 1973.

Joint Committee of Health Problems in Education; Healthful school environment, Washington, D.C., 1969, National Education Association and the American Medical Association.

Knotts, G., and McGovern, J.: School health problems, Springfield, Ill., 1975, Charles C Thomas, Publisher.

Means, R.: A history of health education in the United States, Philadelphia, 1962, Lea & Febiger.

Means, R.: Historical perspectives on school health, Thorofare, N.J., 1975, Charles B. Slack, Inc.

National Dairy Council: Child nutrition programs update, Dairy Council Digest 53(6):31-36, 1982.

National Safety Council: Accident facts, Chicago, 1986, The Council.

Nelson, K., et al., editors: The national evaluation of school nutrition programs: review of research, vol. 2, Santa Monica, Cal., 1981, System Development Corporation.

Riggs, S., and Woodman, K.: It's back to basics for school foodservice: refining menus, renovating kitchens, Restaurants and Institutions 95(2):148-157 Jan., 1985.

Schwartz, L.G., and Klenetsky, F.: Seatbelts in school buses, Journal of School Health 55(3):119, 1985.

Spital, M., Spital, A., and Spital, R.: The compelling case for seat belts on school buses, Pediatrics 78(5):928-932, 1986.

Wellish, J., et al.: National evaluation of school nutrition programs, final report vols. 1 and 2, Santa Monica, Cal., 1983, System Development Corporation.

CHAPTER 4

EMOTIONAL CLIMATE AND THE TEACHER

Some teachers are great. . . . They put bandages on my hurts—on my heart, on my mind, on my spirit. Those teachers cared about me, and let me know it. They gave me wings.

Thoughts from a drop-out★

KEY CONCEPT: A positive emotional climate in the classroom is dependent on adequate provision for the physical and psychological needs of children.

When John Locke used the phrase, "mens sana in corpore sano"—a sound mind in a sound body—he expressed the interrelationships that exist between physical and mental health. He envisioned mental health as a condition of the whole personality, not as an entity separate from physical health. He stressed the importance of the total health of children. Current concepts of health also include reference to social and spiritual aspects introduced in Chapter 1.

The mental phase of health today has never had greater meaning. The tremendous anxieties, pressures, and concerns in the world have their effect on children and youth. The young people living in poverty and among bias and prejudice are especially subjected to extensive biological, psychological, sociological, and economic stress. The cultural, ethnic, racial, and economic inequalities, the tensions over world peace, the dichotomy of moral and social values, the stress on materialism, the need for good grades, the conformities to outmoded and antiquated practices and traditions in schools, and the inadequacies of educational opportunities create a social climate conducive to mental illness. The Joint Commission on Mental Health of Children stated★:

---

*McLeod, A.: Growing up in America: a background to contemporary drug abuse, Rockville, Md., 1973, National Institute of Mental Health.

---

*Report of Task Force VI and excerpts from the Report of the Committee on Children of Minority Groups by the Joint Commission on Mental Health of Children, New York, 1973, Harper & Row, Publishers, Inc.

The major crisis of our time is a crisis of human relations . . . we have lost our capacity for mutual trust, love and responsibility. . . . Social changes on a major scale are required if all our children and youth are to . . . enjoy optimal mental health.

It is imperative that schools recognize these conditions and that teachers become aware of their roles in the promotion and maintenance of good mental health.

In Chapter 3 the physical components of the environment as they relate to healthful school living received consideration. However, healthful school living includes the sum of the internal as well as external factors that act on the individual. Therefore the emotional climate in the school is a critical component affecting the mental health of both students and teachers. The *emotional climate* may be defined as a setting that gives consideration to students—their feelings, their beliefs, their physiological and psychological needs—as well as subject matter. It is a setting that treats pupils with kindness and humaneness. The following poem illustrates its meaning:

If a child lives with criticism, he learns to condemn.
If a child lives with hostility, he learns to fight.
If a child lives with fear, he learns to be apprehensive.
If a child lives with pity, he learns to feel sorry for himself.
If a child lives with jealousy, he learns to feel guilty.
If a child lives with encouragement, he learns to be confident.
If a child lives with tolerance, he learns to be patient.
If a child lives with praise, he learns to be appreciative.
If a child lives with acceptance, he learns to love.
If a child lives with approval, he learns to like himself.
If a child lives with recognition, he learns to have a goal.
If a child lives with fairness, he learns what justice is.
If a child lives with honesty, he learns what truth is.
If a child lives with security, he learns to have faith in himself and those about him.
If a child lives with friendliness, he learns the world is a nice place in which to live.

DOROTHY LAW NOLTE

Observations of pupil behaviors may indicate mental health difficulties that may be the result of a poor school atmosphere. They may cause teachers to ask:

"Why is Bill always boisterous and rude?"
"Why does Ann cry easily?"
"Why is Susan so hard to reach?"
"Why is Jack so nervous?"
"Why does Sam use drugs?"
"What can I do to help Bob whose parents are alcoholics?"
"Why is Nancy frequently truant?"
"Why is Mary always so quiet and withdrawn?"
"Why does Bill become frightened so easily?"
"Why is Jane always sullen and unhappy?"
"Why is Ed constantly picking on other children?"
"Why is Marion having trouble getting along with her classmates?"
"How can I help, and what should I do to best understand children with behavior problems?"

Architects, builders, and school administrators to a large extent control the physical aspects of the school, whereas teachers exert tremendous influence over the emotional climate in the classroom and in the school. The classroom is the teacher's domain. The atmosphere provided there contributes significantly to student learning. The perceptions pupils have of their physical surroundings, their teachers, and their peers all have an impact on learning.

This chapter is designed to provide (1) understanding about mental/emotional health, (2) information about some of the factors that have an impact on mental/emotional health of children, (3) the reasons schools need to be concerned, and (4) ways schools and teachers can improve the emotional atmosphere so children will make worthwhile contributions to the society in which they live by growing into happy, productive, and useful individuals.

WHAT IS MENTAL/EMOTIONAL HEALTH?

Teachers need to understand the nature of mental/emotional health to be able to have an effect on emotional atmosphere in schools. Although it is difficult to define mental health to the satisfaction of everyone, for the purpose of this chapter it refers to the adjustment of the individual to self and to society so that the realities of life can be faced and the individual can function most effectively with the greatest satisfaction, cheerfulness, and socially acceptable behavior. Mentally healthy persons are able to control their emotions and adequately meet situations that occur in their environment; they possess positive self-esteem, insight, and self-acceptance. The observable features of this adjustment may be identified in what is called *personality* or the *individual's personality*—the sum of the traits and characteristics that make each person unique. Just as children have numerous combinations of traits and characteristics, many types and varieties of personalities exist.

Mental health is affected by the environment in which a person lives and by that person's experiences (Fig. 4-1). It is an outgrowth of one's total life. Teachers and schools can contribute to the mental health of pupils by helping with the satisfactory fulfillment of their physiological and psychological or emotional needs. The physiological needs include food, air, water, warmth, rest and sleep, clothing, and freedom from disease and other health hazards. The psychological or emotional needs include the following:

1. Affection—love
2. Security—to belong, to have roots, to have protection
3. Acceptance as an individual—free of prejudice or bias, concern for the individual differences
4. Achievement—success experiences, recognition
5. Independence—create and develop things, be on one's own, do things under one's own guidance and direction
6. Authority—guidance and direction by adults
7. Self-respect—courteous, fair, and just treatment

Mentally healthy individuals exhibit these characteristics:

FIG. 4–1. Fun activities contribute to positive mental health. *(Courtesy of San Jose Nutrition Project.)*

1. Pursue reasonable goals using their talents and abilities
2. Have a sense of self-respect, self-reliance, and achievement; feel worthwhile; have a high level of self-esteem
3. Know they are liked, loved, and wanted
4. Have a sense of security and are reasonably at peace with themselves and their environment; enjoy life
5. Can think and act rationally and realistically when seeking solutions to problems; are able to withstand frustration and anxiety, to persevere despite difficulty, and to ask for help without loss of self-esteem
6. Can distinguish between feelings and facts
7. Can maintain integrity in work and play; exhibit confidence and orderliness

FIG. 4-2. Self-concept identification. *(Courtesy of Miss Betty Jane Mobley, teacher, Tacoma Public Schools, Tacoma, Wash.)*

8. Are able to work in groups; are interested in others
9. Respect the rights of others
10. Face the realities of life and are able to accept responsibilities; are self-disciplined

The mentally healthy individual has a positive self-concept (Fig. 4-2) and a realistic view of the culture in which that person lives. The individual can accept bigness or smallness of size, good or poor looks, artistic talent or lack of it, and intellectual capacities or limitations. The individual can get along with children and adults in school, at home, in the neighborhood, and elsewhere. Normal individuals can function in the world about them by being able to adjust to its rules and conformities, express their feelings by behaving in personally gratifying ways that the social order will accept, and contribute to a changing and challenging society.

Mental health is usually considered a positive aspect of health. If it were placed on a continuum, it would be located at the extreme end and would represent the highest level of health

to be achieved. However, it may also be considered to be negative and then would be found at the lowest level of health, representing mental illness. There are varying degrees of positive mental health just as there are varying degrees and kinds of mental illness. Often these variations are difficult to define or identify.

When basic physical and emotional needs are not met or are threatened, a variety of deviate behaviors may result*:

1. Overtimidity—withdrawing, crying easily
2. Overaggressiveness—bullying, quarreling, boisterousness
3. Excessive daydreaming—persistent inattentiveness
4. Excessive boasting or showing off
5. Poor sportsmanship
6. Undue restlessness—habit tics, stammering, nail-biting

---

*Adapted from Cornacchia, H., Smith, D., and Bentel, D.: Drugs in the classroom: a conceptual model for school programs, ed. 2, St. Louis, 1978, The C.V. Mosby Co.

7. Frequent accidents or near-accidents
8. Abnormal sex behavior
9. Difficulty in reading or reciting
10. Failure to advance in school at normal rate
11. Stuttering or other forms of speech difficulty
12. Lying, stealing, cheating
13. Resistance to authority, constant complaints of unfairness
14. Unhappiness and depression
15. Gradual deterioration and marked sudden drop in educational achievement
16. Lack of interest or motivation
17. Constantly seeking attention or popularity
18. Emotional outburst such as temper tantrums or antisocial behavior
19. Overuse of various adjustment mechanisms such as rationalization, compensation, or projection

ENVIRONMENTAL IMPACTS ON MENTAL HEALTH

Teachers and students affect and are affected by the overall environment of the school. Thus the emotional climate of the school is a reflection of the various attitudes and behaviors students and staff bring to the school. Teachers and administrators have an ethical responsibility to provide a positive atmosphere for the most effective learning. School personnel should be alert for signs that may lead to the deterioration of the school emotional atmosphere.

This chapter focuses on children of divorced or separated parents, latchkey children, child abuse and neglect, and student misuse and abuse of alcohol and other drugs and its relation to suicide. However there are many other factors including nutrition, child growth and development, fear and uncertainty, peer pressure, and family standards among others that have an impact on the mental health of students.

Child abuse

A conservative estimate is that over 1 million children per year are abused or neglected, with as many as 2,000 children dying as a result. Al-
though it is generally easier to identify a physically abused child than a neglected child, child neglect is 4 to 5 times more common than physical abuse. The teacher is in a good position to observe deviations in normal childhood behavior that may be an indication of abuse or neglect. What is generally termed *child abuse* may be physical or sexual in nature, whereas neglect often assumes a more complex nature.

Physical abuse. Physical abuse of the child is often disguised as discipline or punishment of the child. The teacher needs to realize, however, that the distinction between discipline and abuse can be difficult to make. The U.S. Department of Health and Human Services has defined physical abuse as "any abuse that results in physical injury, including fractures, burns, welts, cuts and or internal injuries."* Whenever the teacher sees any of these outward physical signs of injury, the child should be questioned as to how the injury occurred. Children will often deny that their parents, guardians, or other adults have caused the injury because they fear additional retaliation. The teacher should refer a child to the school nurse, counselor, or administrator if it is suspected that the child is a victim of abuse. State laws and school district procedures may *require* the reporting of these children.

The outward signs of possible child abuse include bruises, welts, burns, abrasions and contusions, wounds of any type, and fractures. Marks on the torso, legs, or arms can be difficult to discern because they are covered by clothing. Other abuse indicators that are difficult to assess include burns on the palms of hands or the soles of feet; bruises on the ears that are covered by long hair; ruptured eardrums caused by blows to the head; loosened or missing teeth; and internal injuries resulting in blood being passed in the urine or stool. If the child complains that walking, writing, moving, using the toilet, or eating causes pain, the teacher should refer the

---

*U.S. Department of Health and Human Services: Child abuse and neglect: curriculum in the schools, Washington, D.C., 1981, PHS Pub. #0 81-30312, The Department.

child. Additionally, if the child seems to complain of earaches or appears with missing teeth, especially if there are bruises around the mouth, abuse should be suspected.

Sexual abuse. Sexual abuse is one of the most difficult forms of child abuse to identify and has been defined as "any contact or interaction between child and adult in which the child is being used *for the sexual* stimulation of the perpetrator or of another person."* Almost all states indicate that any sexual involvement between a child and a parent, guardian, other adult, or an older child is sexual abuse. The majority of sexual abuse cases involve incest between a father and daughter, but cases involving mothers and sons, fathers and sons, and mothers and daughters have also been seen by the nation's courts. The teacher might suspect that a child is being sexually abused if there is a sudden behavior change, especially if the behavior is of a regressive or totally aggressive nature. Sexually abused children often flee to a fantasy world or direct their hostility for a parent or guardian toward other children or adults. Clearly something must be done if a child confides in the teacher. Rather than a direct revealing of the abusive situation, the confidential statement is often rather subtle, "I would like to come and live with you."

Children who refuse to participate in physical education or playground activities, turn to drugs and alcohol, become sexually promiscuous, or even attempt to run away from home may be sending out a plea that they are being sexually abused at home. The teacher who observes these signs should refer the child for additional help and guidance.

Neglect. Neglect is the failure of a parent or guardian to care for the basic needs of the child. This may take the form of denigrating the child to such an extent that the child feels whatever he or she does, it is not good enough for the parent and may result in the withholding of suitable clothing, food, or shelter from the child.

*U.S. Department of Health and Human Services: Child abuse and neglect: curriculum in the schools, Washington, D.C., 1981, PHS Pub. #0 81-30312, The Department.

Mental neglect of a child is much more difficult to identify than physical neglect. If the child begins to come to school with dirty or torn clothing on, appears haggard, emaciated, or lethargic, the teacher should suspect something might be occurring in the home situation that might be in need of remediation. Often a great deal of professional counseling and interpretation of the observations is needed.

The teacher's role. Teachers are in a unique position to notice whenever a student begins to behave or appear markedly different than usual. Teachers also have a responsibility to report these deviations to the proper authorities according to school procedure. This is especially true if abuse or neglect is suspected so immediate action can be taken to help the child and those who are abusing the child. Those who make these reports are generally immune from legal prosecution as long as the report was made in the interest of the child. Most states mandate that suspected cases of child abuse or neglect be reported to the proper authorities and a failure to do so may result in criminal action being taken against those who fail to make such a report.

Alcohol and other drug misuse and abuse

Alcohol and other drug misuse and abuse can be a personal, as well as family problem for a child. Statistical evidence indicates that a teacher will have children in class who come from families where one or more members abuse drugs. Over 7 million children face fear, uncertainty, or other problems daily as a result of parental alcohol abuse. Researchers have shown that children who come from families where alcohol is abused enter school with emotional burdens in addition to the general problems faced by all children as a result of growing and maturing. Children from these homes often lack self-confidence, spontaneity, or autonomy in their dealings with others. These children may withdraw and refuse to discuss anything about home or family and sometimes are viewed by teachers as problem children. This is compounded by the fact that these children often exhibit poor academic and verbal skills. This may be the result of not being able to study at home, talk with their parents, or get assistance with studying.

In 1973 a special drug warning network (DAWN) was formed combining a network of hospital emergency rooms and medical examiner/coroner offices in 26 major metropolitan areas. In 1985 over 900 facilities were linked by this system. The purpose of this network is to identify trends in drug and alcohol use among children and adults. Between 1974 and 1980 there was a significant increase seen in the use of alcohol in combination with other drugs—most notably methaqualone and marijuana. It was further determined that in half of the cases seen, the use of alcohol and some other substance resulted in an attempt at suicide or a suicide gesture. For every 100,000 hospital emergency room visits, 29 were students who ingested drugs in a suicide attempt. With 76 million emergency room visits per year, it is estimated that 22,000 students per year attempt suicide or make a suicidal gesture as a result of the abuse of alcohol and other drugs.*

Evidence indicates that 60% of those who enter an emergency room for an alcohol or drug emergency have their medical symptoms treated and then are released. School officials should be informed when children have been admitted to emergency rooms for drug-related problems. If these children are to be given the opportunity to benefit from their educational experience, community and school personnel must help them solve the problems that predisposed them to substance abuse. The teacher must be alert for the signs and symptoms (see Appendix J) that children may be using drugs in order to cope with personal problems. Young people who may be at high risk include:

1. Children of parents with alcohol and drug abuse problems
2. Children seen by health care providers be-

*Ryser, P.E.: Students and drug abuse, 1974 and 1980, Journal of School Health **53**(7):435-436, 1983.

cause of abuse, numerous accidents, or psychosomatic disorders
3. Children seen by various school personnel because of high levels of absenteeism, poor academic motivation, signs of depression, shyness or withdrawal, or acting-out behaviors
4. Children seen by social service workers because of abuse, neglect, depression, running away, and other home problems
5. Children seen by juvenile justice workers for lying, stealing, or other delinquent behaviors
6. Military dependents
7. Youths in institutionalized settings

Children who may be troubled are those who:
1. Miss a lot of school
2. Run away from home
3. Appear extremely apathetic or bored
4. Are careless and accident prone
5. Lose their appetite or eat a lot
6. Don't talk a great deal
7. Withdraw from peer activities; lack self-confidence
8. Smoke cigarettes or consume alcoholic beverages
9. Experience nightmares, insomnia, or early morning waking
10. Have a prolonged reaction following a loss
11. Engage in lying and stealing

Telltale evidence such as syringes, pills, solvents, special cigarette papers, and other items found in student possession and around school are additional clues.

Children of separated or divorced families

The number of children attending schools from separated and divorced families is growing. Over 1 million divorces occur annually in the United States with 49% of all second marriages ending in divorce. Over 12.5 million children are in families where divorce has occurred, and it is estimated that one third of all children born in this country will live with only one parent before the age of 18. Within a 5-year period after a divorce, one third of the children will be severely emotionally damaged, one third will be muddling through, and one third will adjust fairly well.

Children who are from families going through divorce experience unique problems. These children are preoccupied with the family situation, thus school work and other activities become secondary. They face an inconsistent family life, may spend weekends with the noncustodial parent, and may miss being with friends, thus impairing their socialization process. These children may also face increased responsibilities at home, especially if there are younger children and the custodial parent must work.

Often these children feel alone or betrayed by parents who no longer are in the household. As a result they may direct their energies at trying to get the parents back together again. Children may feel the need to choose between the parents and also may feel that "unchosen" parents will either be hurt or will not love them as much as before. Children of divorced parents may begin to request more nurse office visits, as well as need attention and become discipline problems. They may also begin to skip school or look for ways to get suspended from school because they feel they have additional home responsibilities or do not want to be confronted by other children who might ask them about their family situation.

In divorce or separation situations the school may be the only stable element in the life of the child, and these children need a great deal of support, both moral and social. They need to know that divorce is an adult problem, not a child problem, and that even though they live with only one parent, they are still a family unit.

Helping children of divorce. Often the teacher does not know that a child is in a family crisis. However, if the teacher remains alert for behavior changes such as over-aggressiveness or over-helpfulness; refusal or reticence to discuss anything related to parents or family; lack of classroom concentration; failure to do homework; constantly seeking adult attention; becoming a "loner;" dropping out of school activities; showing excessive tardiness or absence at the beginning of the school day; or even listlessness, nervousness, or sleepiness; the teacher should certainly suspect that something is awry and may want to refer the child to the school nurse or counselor. The teacher should also discuss the situation with the proper school authorities.

In addition to referring the child, the teacher should be aware of the problems and express a genuine concern to the child that the child was not to blame for an adult decision. The teacher should watch carefully for falling grades, be ready to assist the child whenever possible, and help the child maintain friendships and relationships with other children in the class. The child will eventually realize that the situation is not unique—that there are other children in the same position. Teachers should make sure that when discussions of family arise in the classroom, one-parent families, guardianships, stepfamilies, adoptive families, and foster parents are all included in the discussion.*

Latchkey children

Latchkey children is a term used to describe over 7 million children under the age of 13 whose parent or parents are working, therefore the children must go to school or return home from school without direct adult supervision. They are the result of economics rather than divorce. This is another factor that can have an impact on the mental/emotional health of the school-age child. Often these children come to school without breakfast, and many of them are afraid to return home at the end of the day.†

Several school districts have developed special curricula designed to teach these children survival skills that enable them to take care of themselves in the absence of parents. Other districts have developed after-school supervised recreational activities. However, a controversy

---

*Additional information can be obtained by contacting: Children Facing Divorce, 5136 East Karen, Scottsdale, Ariz., 85254.

†Seligson, M., et al.: School-age child care: a policy report, Wellesley, Mass., 1983, School Age Child Care Project, Wellesley College Center for Research on Women.

still exists as to the nature of the school's responsibility to aid these children and their parents.

Should programs be provided for those children whose parents cannot supervise them? Should these programs involve the use of empty classrooms? Such action may help to reduce school vandalism and ensure children's safety. However, the additional teacher workloads, school costs, and increased facility use create problems in need of attention.

Researchers have shown that latchkey children, especially those in urban areas, face risks. These children must face loneliness and the fear of being alone. Faced with general boredom, they may get into trouble just "horsing around," or they may face academic problems because they do not do their homework after school, or feel rejected because they have no place to go and cannot invite friends to the house as long as their parents are not there. These children also may experience fear for personal safety either from someone breaking into their homes, or from older siblings. Taking all of this into consideration, it is clear that latchkey children are expected to assume a great deal of responsibility at an unusually young age.

Some communities have developed telephone hotlines for latchkey children. One such program is located in State College, Pennsylvania. This project, called *Project PhoneFriend*, is run by the American Association of University Women. This free hotline is open from 2:30 to 5:30 PM on weekdays and is staffed by adult volunteers who offer advice, comfort, and general conversation to the school children who contact them. Other communites have developed recreational programs in cooperation with the parks and recreation departments of the local communities. Increasing emphasis is also being placed on self-reliance activities and programs such as scouting.

The teacher and latchkey children. The teacher should be aware that latchkey children will be present in the school setting. Strother*

*Strother, D.B.: Latchkey children: the fastest growing special interest group in the schools: The Journal of School Health, **56**(1):13-16, 1986.

has suggested several ways teachers can help latchkey children:

1. Carefully structure homework assignments since these children do not have adults around to help them complete assignments correctly
2. Consider the possibility of establishing a telephone hotline to help students with homework (such a system is currently available in Mesa, Arizona)
3. During the school day, allow time for children to discuss their personal concerns with the teacher
4. Establish streamlined, workable procedures for contacting the parents when emergency situations involving the child arise
5. Develop both before-school and after-school day-care programs for these children

WHY SHOULD SCHOOLS BE CONCERNED WITH THE MENTAL/EMOTIONAL HEALTH OF STUDENTS?

The school is usually thought to rank second to the family as the most important unit in society affecting the mental health of children and must be concerned for these reasons:

1. The effectiveness of the educative process will be seriously hampered, since approximately 10% of pupils (5 million) are afflicted with emotional disturbances.

2. Educational failure, or the "failure syndrome," is one of the underlying factors that triggers acting-out in schools, depression, drug abuse, truancy, and other maladjustments. Children who exhibit such behavior have a lower self-concept, or self-identity.

3. The experiences to which a child is exposed can help prevent serious difficulties or hasten mental problems. Hence, schools play a role in both primary and secondary prevention—before conditions occur and in the control of existing conditions. Early identification of children with emotional difficulties is important because remedial help can hopefully be provided at a time when intervention is maximally effective. The increase of problems and the great shortage of

community mental health services and facilities add to the need for emphasis on prevention.

4. Behavior is more readily modified at the elementary level than later in life.

5. It is important for children to experience success in school with special attention given to their physical and psychological needs. Many children who enter school are educationally handicapped in terms of readiness to enter school. This has led some to suggest that children should not enter school until they are 11 or 12 years of age.*

6. The school is the only agency outside the home that reaches practically all children and youths.

Schools and teachers should promote positive mental health in all students, thus helping prevent mental illness and emotional disturbances and assisting children with mental health problems.

WHAT IS THE TEACHER'S ROLE IN IMPROVING THE EMOTIONAL CLIMATE?

There is much being said and written about the effect of schools and school personnel on the emotional health and mental development of children. It has been estimated by some psychologists that the average child is exposed to two emotionally unstable teachers during his school years. This estimate might be considered too conservative.

In any case, the teacher is the person children see day after day during the school year. Next to the parent the teacher probably has more influence on most students than any other person in their young lives. What a challenge this is; yet what an opportunity!

Practically all certified teachers have had at least some background of study in the field of mental health. Still, teachers find it difficult to deal effectively with the emotional problems presented from time to time in the classroom

and in extracurricular settings. The reason for this in most instances is that we know so little about mental health and emotional development. One of the things we do know reasonably well is that people need to be motivated, to have perceivable goals if they are to learn, perform, and develop as individual personalities capable of coping with and contributing to their world.

The single most important contribution to student mental health is the development of a wholesome emotional climate in the classroom. This atmosphere affects students' personal goals, their gaiety and depression; in fact, the moods of the different pupils in the room have great influence on all the students. What teachers say, do, and think has great significance on the patterns of behavior that are exhibited by students. Teachers have profound and lasting influences on children. The extent to which teachers can develop good human relationships with their pupils largely determines the extent to which a wholesome classroom atmosphere will exist. The setting in which children work together and are secure in the knowledge and feeling that they are accepted by the group and the teacher is what teachers should strive to achieve. This environment is influenced by teachers' preconceptions of pupils, concern with self, fear of witnessing emotion, values, biases, prejudices, and feelings of social class barriers.

The learning that takes place in school is affected by how people feel and believe, and what they value as well as how people treat each other. Teachers must be concerned with individuals and not just subject matter. There is a need to focus on the learner in the classroom. It is important not only to be concerned with what takes place in school, but also more importantly, to be concerned with what happens to students. An emphasis on humaneness must take place. Teachers must be concerned with justice, equality, friendship, tolerance, respect for the individual, self-expression, and decision making. These few suggestions should help to provide ways to achieve such a climate:

1. Maximize individual learning through the recognition of individual differences (Fig. 4-3)

*Moore, R.S., and Moore, D.: When education becomes abuse: a different look at the mental health of children, The Journal of School Health, **56**(2):73-75, 1986.

FIG. 4-3. It is important that schools provide for individual differences. *(Courtesy of Wichita Public Schools.)*

2. Encourage and increase student involvement in the education process
3. Provide a meaningful curriculum that satisfies the needs of students
4. Provide opportunities for success experiences for all students
5. Permit freedom of expression in the classroom
6. Listen to students in a nonjudgmental fashion
7. Help students to assess their own value systems
8. Make grades and grading procedures noncompetitive

9. Aid young people to improve their abilities to cope with the complex world
10. Aid young people to assume responsibility for their own behavior

The teacher who is interested in developing the best atmosphere must do the following:

1. Want to help children; establish a classroom environment free from fear and tensions; include an atmosphere of warmth and friendliness; aid in improvement of self-concept
2. Believe that children are trying to do the best work possible
3. Get acquainted with children and attempt to develop friendly relations; know their health and guidance records; be cheerful; let children talk; call students by name; talk with pupils; do not be shocked easily; provide warmth to the room by color and displays, using children to help
4. Avoid ridicule, sarcasm, and belittling remarks and help pupils to do likewise
5. Accept the emotional outbursts of children and not condemn or reproach hostility—everyone gets angry sometimes
6. Understand the many factors that affect the mental health of children, including the family and the home, peer group relations, socioeconomic class, communications media, and the tensions of the times
7. Be alert for indications of latent skills and interests and encourage pupils in their development
8. Arouse interest in cultures and religions of all groups and accept pupils regardless of race, creed, or color
9. Develop trust in students as individuals
10. Practice tolerance and humanity in dealing with all people in the school—students, teachers, administrators, and staff
11. Avoid punitive disciplinary action
12. Provide for individual guidance to help students understand their strengths and weaknesses and how to enhance strengths and overcome weaknesses
13. Show concern for each student
14. Make the classroom a friendly place
15. Make learning fun

16. Treat all students with kindness and respect
17. Encourage students to help plan class activities such as field trips or PTA presentations

Additional factors affecting the emotional climate in the classroom include the following:

1. Clarity and meaning of school activity
2. Excessive competition
3. Curriculum not adjusted to the needs of pupils
4. Uneven and unfair distribution of rewards and punishments (Is the teacher always negative to some students?)
5. Biases regarding students in terms of race, creed, color, or ability
6. Authoritarianism or permissive environment
7. Grades and their uniformity
8. Liberal use of praise and encouragement
9. Attainable goals within pupils' abilities

Anxieties and tensions are acquired and can quickly and easily become evident in class. The teacher can help to ease these conditions by being cognizant of the factors previously mentioned and also by providing relaxation outlets through music, art, drama, play, dance, exercise, or creative reading or writing.

Teachers who are self-confident and able to motivate their students will generally realize a greater degree of teaching success by providing a positive emotional climate. The ability of the teacher to handle the daily demands of teaching, as well as the teacher's self-concept, personal appearance, and health status can positively influence the emotional climate of the school.

How does teacher health affect the school climate?

Well-adjusted teachers are needed if the most wholesome emotional climate is to be found in the classroom. The teacher who suffers from anxiety and lack of self-confidence will communicate this to children. The teacher's personality is extremely important since a maladjusted teacher is in a strategic position to do great harm to young people. It is estimated that the percentage of mentally ill or maladjusted teachers is about the same as in the general population—approximately 10%. Teachers therefore need to give attention to their personal needs and make adequate provision for sleep, rest, exercise, appropriate diet, and relaxation, as well as maintain the highest level of health possible.

The teacher's physical health status, diet, sexual activities, and personal health practices, including the use of alcoholic beverages and mood-altering drugs may have an impact on the emotional climate within the classroom. It is important for teachers to realize that they become role models for students. As such, the way the teacher reacts to varying stressful situations within the school day will have an impact on the students exposed to that teacher. If the teacher cannot handle the daily stresses of the school day, as well as stresses outside of school, how will that teacher be able to transfer good coping skills to students?

Teachers must realize that stress is experienced by everyone. It is a part of living. Individuals vary widely in their ability to adapt to stress. How a person responds to stressful conditions, therefore, is important; it has both positive and negative effects. In the classroom stress may stimulate and motivate students positively to increase learning, whereas repeated negative reactions may result in adverse behaviors previously identified as occurring when needs remained unmet. When this occurs, a repetitive cycle is initiated wherein the negative behavior evokes negative responses from others, causing more stress.

Stress in the classroom setting, however, is part of the process of education. Any teacher requirement or demand will create differing degrees of stress among pupils. It is important that teachers help children learn how to deal with these as well as other stresses that must be faced as the child grows and matures.

Health instruction and mental health

The need for health education as part of the curriculum has been mentioned often as a means of promoting positive mental health. Education can help pupils to understand themselves, their drives, their prejudices, their emotions, their ambitions, their growth and personality development, and their values, as well as help them learn how to get along with others, live in society, and be socially acceptable members of the world in which they live. Satisfaction that comes with self-esteem and self-concept leads to feelings of confidence, worth, strength, capability, and adequacy. Children who attain such attitudes are able to learn with increased interest, enthusiasm, and efficiency.

Instruction should include both formal and informal programs (see Chapter 1 and Appendix B). The suggested outline of content for mental health, the concepts that should receive consideration, and the objectives to be achieved through grade level groups in the formal phase may be found in Appendix B. They can be integrated into all phases of the curriculum, or specific units can be prepared and taught as part of health education using a variety of techniques (see Chapter 12).

Informally, mental health concepts and understandings of self can be learned and modified indirectly through interpersonal relations between teachers and pupils. The wholesome classroom atmosphere provides numerous opportunities for incidental teaching through informal discussion, counseling and guidance, and working with children in many ways. In addition, awareness groups can be convened voluntarily to permit students to express opinions and feelings on a variety of topics through verbal and other forms of communication.

Parent education programs need consideration for inclusion in schools. Family understanding of children's needs and the need for communication are extremely important for positive mental health.

SUMMARY

The teacher plays a primary role in establishing the emotional atmosphere in the school. Teachers therefore must understand the nature of mental/emotional health and its effect on learning. To aid pupils in their development, teachers must help provide for their physical and psychological needs. They must be alert in their observations of changes in students' attitudes and behaviors and understand which ones are in need of attention.

A variety of environmental impacts affect the mental/emotional health of children. These include child abuse, alcohol and other drug use, parental separation or divorce, and economics (latchkey children).

The teacher must be aware of the various stresses that face both student and staff each day. The teacher must also understand that the reaction to these stresses varies for each individual. Knowing how children react to stress, however, is not enough. The teacher must also be aware of how he or she reacts to stress, since the teacher becomes a role model for students. If the teacher constantly reacts in a negative way to stress, it is quite likely that the teacher's students will react in the same way.

Personal health practices are important. If the teacher is constantly slovenly in appearance, or lets mood-altering substances provide substitutes for good judgment and professional pride, then that teacher is not doing much to contribute to the total emotional climate of the school. As Plato stated, "Know thyself." By knowing oneself, the teacher is in a better position to positively influence the emotional climate created in the classroom and the total school environment.

Formal and informal instructional programs aid children in the development of positive mental health.

QUESTIONS FOR DISCUSSION

1. How would you summarize the poem by Dorothy Law Nolte?
2. What is the meaning of the term, *mental health*?
3. Why do you think child neglect is 4 to 5 times more prevalent than physical child abuse?
4. Some people feel alcohol and substance abuse should not be discussed in schools. State and justify your position on this issue.
5. Why is it important for teachers to know if a child has gone to a hospital emergency room as the result of a drug or alcohol emergency?
6. What special problems might confront the child who comes from a family where the parents are separated or divorced?

7. What do you think the role of the school should be in caring for latchkey children?
8. Why should teachers be concerned with the mental/emotional health of students?
9. What can the teacher do to provide an emotional climate in the classroom that promotes good mental health?
10. What might teachers do to be more humane in their dealings with pupils?
11. How can health instruction help the mental health of pupils?
12. What impact does the health of the teacher have on the emotional climate of the classroom?

SELECTED REFERENCES

Belcastro, P.A., and Gold, R.S.: Teacher stress and burnout: implications for school health personnel, Journal of School Health **54**(7):404-407, 1983.

Cornacchia, H.J., Smith, D.E., and Bentel, D.J.: Drugs in the classroom; a conceptual model for school programs, ed. 2, St. Louis, 1978, The C.V. Mosby Co.

Epstein, M.H., and Cullinan, D.: Depression in children, Journal of School Health **56**(1):10-12, 1986.

Frick, S.B.: Diagnosing boredom, confusion and adaptation in school children, Journal of School Health **55**(7):254-257, 1985.

Gray, B.J., and Pippin, G.D.: Stepfamilies: a concern health education should address, Journal of School Health **54**(8):292-295, 1984.

McCleod, A.: Growing up in America: a background to contemporary drug abuse, Rockville, Md., 1973, National Institute of Mental Health.

Moore, R.S., and Moore, D.: When education becomes abuse: a different look at the mental health of children, Journal of School Health **56**(2):73-75, 1986.

Patten-Seward, P.: Assessing student emotional behavior after parental separation or divorce, Journal of School Health **54**(4):152-153, 1986.

Redican, K.J., Olsen, L.K., and Baffi, C.R.: Organization of school health programs, New York, 1986, Macmillan Inc.

Report of Task Forces IV and V and the Report of the Committee on Clinical Issues by the Joint Commission on Mental Health of Children: The mental health of children: services, research, and manpower, New York, 1973, Harper & Row, Publishers, Inc.

Ryser, P.E.: Students and drug abuse, 1974 and 1984, Journal of School Health **53**(7):435-436, 1985.

Seligson, M., et al.: School-age child care: a policy report, Wellesley, Mass., 1983, School Age Child Care Project, Wellesley College Center for Research on Women.

Strother, D.B.: Latchkey children: the fastest growing special interest group in the schools, Journal of School Health **56**(1):13-16, 1986.

Swan, H.L., and Houston, V.: Alone after school: a self-care guide for latchkey children and their parents, Englewood Cliffs, N.J., 1985, Prentice-Hall, Inc.

PART
III

HEALTH SERVICES

CHAPTER 5

HEALTH APPRAISALS OF SCHOOL CHILDREN

. . . early identification of problems can alert school personnel to potential barriers to learning.

SUSAN FRINK AND PHILIP NADER

Journal of School Health, 1984

KEY CONCEPT: Teachers and other school personnel are involved in a variety of appraisals used to identify children with health problems.

Teachers often ask such questions as the following:

"Why must I be concerned with the health of boys and girls in my class?"

"How can I find out about the health status of children in my room?"

"Is the failure of children to learn related to their health problems?"

"Can the nurse help me to know more about the health of my pupils?"

"Why must children have periodic vision and hearing tests?"

"What is the teacher's responsibility in preparing children for vision testing, hearing testing, dental inspections, health examinations, and other appraisals?"

"Should I be concerned about a child with a runny nose or a skin infection or one who is always extremely fatigued?"

"What can I do about the overly active, fidgety, aggressive child in class?"

"Why are health records used in schools?"

"What should I do about children in my class who are diabetic or epileptic or who have heart problems?"

Although educators and medical specialists generally believe the home has the primary responsibility for the health of children, schools need to maintan strong supportive programs (1) because of the relationship of good health to effective learning, (2) because there are hazards associated with communicable diseases, and (3) because numerous parents fail to, or do not know how to, accept their responsibilities for maintaining high levels of health in their children. Students with communicable diseases may transmit these conditions to others. Children who cannot see or hear well may have difficulty in acquiring an education. Students with emotional problems may have trouble learning. Pupils who fail to eat breakfast or who are malnourished may not have sufficient stamina to endure the daily classroom activities. Dental health problems may be of sufficient severity or degree to cause young people constant pain or emotional upset, which adversely affects their concentration and attention to learning. Children who are asthmatic, diabetic, epileptic, or hyperkinetic need to be identified as such to arrange adjustments of their educational programs.

Unfortunately, the home has not always satisfactorily or completely assumed its health role. In some instances this responsibility has been ignored or has not been recognized. With about 50% of mothers working away from the home, communication with parents has become difficult. Children continue to be sent to school with physical and emotional conditions that are unknown to parents or considered unimportant. The school therefore has found it necessary to locate those boys and girls with health problems. The procedures used to identify these children with health problems are called health appraisals.

Health appraisals are part of the comprehensive health services program that should be found in all schools (see Fig. 1-1). Health services are those actions taken to help children with problems. They also include follow-up and guidance (Chapter 6), emergencies and first aid (Chapter 7), health personnel such as nurses, nurse practitioners, physicians, and others, and communications with community health agencies and organizations. National, state, and local laws mandate the availability of various service components. However, those services found in schools are uneven in quality and quantity and often barely comply with the letter of the law. Except in large school districts, very little money is appropriated for these services, and therefore they are generally inadequate. In most schools, nurses or nurse practitioners are responsible for segments of the program. The amount of nursing services provided varies widely and is greatly limited in many school districts.

PROBLEMS OF THE POOR

It was pointed out in Chapter 1 that low-income families generally have more health problems than those children and youth whose families are at higher socioeconomic levels. The American Academy of Pediatrics* has advocated that where school children do not receive adequate health care, school programs may be necessary to provide screening, preventive, and some treatment services. Since 1967, states have been required by Congress to provide early and periodic health screening, diagnosis, and treatment (EPSDT) for eligible poor children as part of Medicaid. These procedures have included screening tests (vision, hearing, blood pressure, and others), immunizations, dental care, and well-care supervision. Unfortunately, this program has not met the needs of poor children and youth not covered by Medicaid.

This failure to take care of the needs of poor children and youth prompted four school districts (Cambridge, Massachusetts; Hartford, Connecticut; Galveston, Texas; and Chicago, Illinois) in the 1970s to attempt to provide primary health care.† Such an attempt was made possible by the emergence of school nurse practitioners who receive special medical school training in diagnosing (not merely screening) and performing limited treatment under physician supervision. The Robert Wood Johnson Foundation‡ funded a 5-year demonstration project in medically underserved areas in a total of 18 school districts in New York, Colorado, Utah, and North Dakota. The purpose of this project was to establish primary health care and determine

*Committee on School Health: School health; a guide for health professionals, Evanston, Ill., 1981, American Academy of Pediatrics.

†Cronin, G.E., and Young, W.: 400 navels, the future of school health in America, Bloomington, Ind., 1970, Phi Delta Kappa.

‡Robert Wood Johnson Foundation, National school health services program, Spec. Rep. No. 1, Princeton, N.J., 1985.

whether school nurse practitioners supported by community physicians could improve student health.* The findings revealed that nurse practitioners could correctly diagnose and treat many health problems of the school-age child.

Comprehensive school-based health clinics are becoming prevalent throughout the United States. Kirby† reveals that 71 clinics in 17 states have been recognized by the Support Center for School Based Clinics in Washington, D.C., with more being established every week. The majority of the clinics service high school students, but at least 10 are located in junior high schools.‡

The school-based clinic concept is controversial for some of these reasons: (1) parental responsibility for primary health care is invaded, (2) private treatment services are generally considered the responsibility of private physicians, not schools, and (3) lack of school funds.

WHAT ARE HEALTH APPRAISALS?

Health appraisals refer to a series of procedures designed to assess the health status of children. Although the nature and frequency of appraisals vary in school districts throughout the United States, they generally include teacher observations, screening tests (vision, hearing, and others), health histories or inventories, dental inspections, medical examinations, and psychological tests. (See box, p. 78.)

Appraisals exist for the following reasons:

1. To locate pupils needing medical or dental treatment
2. To locate pupils who are poorly adjusted and in need of special attention at school or treatment by a psychiatrist or child guidance clinic

(for example, concerning behavior problems and emotional disturbances)

3. To locate pupils who need modified educational programs (for example, those who are hard of hearing, partially sighted, blind, or mentally retarded)
4. To locate pupils who need more thorough examinations than provided in school (for example, x-ray examinations, laboratory examinations, or examinations by specialists)
5. To inform school personnel and parents about the health status of children and to encourage parents to recognize and accept the responsibility for seeking necessary corrections
6. To make adjustments or compensations in school for pupils with health problems
7. To serve as learning experiences for children, teachers, and parents

The nature of health appraisals and the responsibilities of the teachers are discussed in the pages that follow. The degree to which the teacher participates differs in every school district and is dependent on the extent of the school program as well as on the availability of special school health personnel.

Three important points related to the teacher's role must be recognized:

1. Teachers, nurses, and non-medically trained people should not attempt to make diagnoses. However, nurses are able to make preliminary diagnoses because of their training and experience. Observations of runny noses, flushed faces, and elevations of temperatures do not permit untrained individuals to identify these conditions as colds, influenza, or other diseases. Signs and symptoms that are noted in young people should result in the referral of these children to the school personnel capable of making diagnoses or of determining necessary action.

2. Ordinarily schools and school personnel should not render medical care, and employees in general should not attempt to provide treatment services; this is the function of physicians, dentists, and other qualified specialists. Some school districts try to make provision for treatment services for poor children.

*Kort, M.: The delivery of primary health care in American public schools, 1890-1980, Journal of School Health **54**(11):453-457, 1984.
†Kirby, D.: Comprehensive school-based clinics: a growing movement to improve adolescent health and reduce teenage pregnancy, Journal of School Health **56**(7):289-291, 1986.
‡Lovick, S.R., and Wesson, W.F.: School-based clinics: update, Washington, D.C., 1986, Center for Population Options.

SCHOOL HEALTH SCREENING PROGRAMS BY GRADE LEVEL AND FREQUENCY, DENVER PUBLIC SCHOOLS, 1980

Type of service	Grade													
	ECE*	K	1	2	3	4	5	6	7	8	9	10	11	12
Vision screening tests†	X	X	X	X	X		X		X		X			
Hearing screening tests†	X	X	X	X	X		X		X		X			
Dental inspections		X			X		X		X					
Weight and growth measurements on all new and referred pupils (often done cooperatively with P.E. fitness program)	X	X	X	X	X	X	X	X						
Nurse interviews with parents of new children	X	X	X	X	X	X	X	X	X	X	X	X	X	X
Medical and/or school nurse practitioner — All pupils with suspected health or learning problems without current or complete reports from family or clinic physicians		X	X	X	X	X	X	X	X	X	X	X	X	X
All pupils being considered for placement in special education without current or complete reports		X	X	X	X	X	X	X	X	X	X	X	X	X
Pupils who participate in swimming classes when private or clinic physician reports are not obtained									X	X	X	X	X	X
Special services — Mandatory tuberculin skin tests for those who have not had one within 9 months	No longer mandatory, so not being done at this time. X													
Scoliosis screening							X	X	X	X				
Inspections for nuisance diseases	(as needed)													
Color vision tests										X	(new pupils)			

Permission to publish granted by the Department of Health and Social Services, Denver Public Schools, Denver, Colorado, 1980. Revised 1986 according to telephone information.
*Early Childhood Education.
†At certain grades; all new pupils at other grades and referrals.

3. Health information about pupils should remain confidential. Teachers and others in schools who need this knowledge should have access to school health records.

WHAT ARE TEACHER OBSERVATIONS?

Teachers are in an excellent position to observe the appearance and behavior of children because they are with pupils for many hours each school day and many weeks each year. They see children perform a variety of activities under different environmental circumstances. They note pupils with headaches, frequent respiratory infections, and recurrent earaches, or those suffering from overfatigue, skin infections, and emotional disturbances. They are capable of becoming skilled observers of the signs and symptoms of ill health. The constant attention that they give to observing boys and girls throughout the day often results in the identification of pupils who are in the early stages of communicable diseases or who are suffering from physical defects or emotional disturbances needing care. Prompt attention to symptomatic behavior greatly helps in the maintenance and improvement of the children's health.

The responsibility of observing children for illness indications does not carry with it the responsibility of diagnosing specific conditions. Diagnosis is a matter that rests with individuals with special professional ability. However, the more detailed and accurate the teacher's noting of pertinent symptoms, the more valuable the information can be for those responsible for diagnosis. A comment such as "George does not seem to feel well today" gives the physician little specific aid; but a brief account of the signs and symptoms (such as a runny nose, frequent fatigue, and constant cough) that led the teacher to believe George was not feeling well is likely to be much more helpful.

Health observation by the teacher is a continuous procedure that takes place daily and throughout the entire day. A pupil's health may change suddenly, and the teacher therefore must constantly be on the alert for such changes. The Colorado Department of Health has prepared a brief list of observations (Table 5-1) that can serve as a guide for referring students to the school nurse or other designated school official. More detailed signs and symptoms of health defects and illnesses may be found in Appendix J.

The teacher must also be aware of the good health characteristics (Appendix K) of children not only so deviant behavior may be more easily identified, but also so the teacher's competency in making student referrals will improve.

Understanding and observing student growth and development characteristics (Appendix L) can have implications for health education, serve as teachable moments, and can be used in the development of curriculum for the instructional program.

Allergies

Allergies are one of the complex health problems that may confront the teacher. Allergic conditions account for an estimated one third of the chronic conditions seen in children. This means that approximately one in five children suffers from some sort of allergy. Over 4.5 million children suffer from asthma, an allergic condition that accounts for nearly 20% of the school days lost in elementary and secondary schools each year. When children miss school as a result of any illness, their overall school performance can be affected. However, children who suffer from asthma and other allergic conditions may have to face additional problems even though they remain in school.* Some of these problems include fatigue from lack of sleep, discomfort from the various symptoms, episodic hearing loss, sleepiness, and other side effects from medications they must take to control their condition. Additionally, these children affect the concentration of other children in the classroom because they often wheeze, cough, sniff, clear their

---

*U.S. Department of Health, Education, and Welfare: Asthma and the other allergic diseases, NIAID, Pub. No. 79-387, Washington, D.C., 1979, National Institutes of Health.

TABLE 5-1. Guide for teacher's referral to nurse

It is recommended that the following observations be referred to the nurse:

EYES:

a. Sties or crusted eyelids
b. Inflamed eyelids
c. Crossed eyes
d. Repeated headaches
e. Squinting, frowning, or scowling
f. Protruding eyes
g. Watery eyes
h. Rubbing of eyes
i. Twitching of the lids
j. Excessive blinking
k. Holding head to one side
l. Complaints of blurry vision

TEETH AND MOUTH

a. State of uncleanliness
b. Gross caries
c. Irregular teeth
d. Stained teeth
e. Gum boils
f. Offensive breath
g. Mouth habits such as thumb sucking
h. Complaints of toothache
i. Swollen jaw

HEART:

a. Excessive breathlessness
b. Tires easily
c. Any history of "growing pains"
d. Bluish lips or fingernails
e. Excessive pallor

GROWTH:

a. Failure to gain regularly over 6-month period
b. Unexplained loss in weight
c. Unexplained rapid gain in weight.

EARS:

a. Discharge from ears
b. Earache
c. Failure to hear questions
d. Picking at the ears
e. Turning head to hear
f. Talking in a monotone
g. Inattention
h. Anxious expression
i. Excessive noisiness of child
j. Ringing in ears
k. Dizziness

GLANDS:

a. Enlarged glands at side of neck
b. Enlarged thyroid

GENERAL APPEARANCE AND CONDITION

a. Underweight—very thin
b. Overweight—very obese
c. Does not appear well
d. Tires easily
e. Chronic fatigue
f. Nausea or vomiting
g. Faintness or dizziness
h. Chronic menstrual discomfort

POSTURE AND MUSCULATURE:

a. Alignment of shoulders
b. Peculiarity of gait
c. Obvious deformities of any type
d. Alignment of spine on "standing tall"
e. Muscular development
f. Coordination
g. Muscle tone
h. Use of feet in standing and walking

NOSE AND THROAT:

a. Persistent mouth breathing
b. Frequent sore throats
c. Recurrent colds
d. Chronic nasal discharge
e. Frequent nose bleeding
f. Nasal speech
g. Frequent tonsilitis
h. Chronic coughing

ANY CHRONIC ILLNESS (known or suspected diagnosis)

a. Diabetes
b. Epilepsy
c. Rheumatic Fever
d. Cystic Fibrosis
e. Orthopedic condition
f. Severe hearing loss
g. Unremedial visual loss or handicap
h. Other special conditions

OTHER:

a. Students who lack medical care due to financial stress or religious views
b. Known or suspected social, family, financial situations affecting the health of the student
c. Prolonged absenteeism due to illness
d. Homebound students
e. Suspected or known pregnancies
f. Children subjected to physical abuse
g. Children receiving medications for a prolonged time and for chronic conditions
h. Students new to school district

SKIN AND SCALP:

a. Unusual pallor of face
b. Eruptions or rashes
c. Habitual scratching of scalp or skin
d. Nits on the hair
e. State of uncleanliness
f. Excessive redness of face

BEHAVIOR:

a. Over studious, docile, withdrawing
b. Bullying, overaggressiveness, domineering
c. Unhappy and depressed
d. Overexcitable, uncontrollable emotions
e. Stuttering or other forms of speech difficulty
f. Poor accomplishment in comparison with ability
g. Lying (imaginative or defensive)
h. Lack of appreciation of property rights
i. Abnormal sex behavior
j. Antagonistic, negativistic, continual quarreling
k. Excessive use of toilet
l. Enuresis (involuntary urination at night and during sleep)

Reprinted by permission: Colorado Department of Education and Colorado Department of Health: Colorado School Health Guidelines, ed. 2, Denver, 1986, The Departments.

throats, blow their noses, or display other disruptive mannerisms.

Students with allergic rhinitis, or hay fever, may suffer a great deal from eye irritation, itching, congestion, and sneezing. This condition may also create headaches and cause numerous ear infections. Obviously, when vision and hearing are impaired, learning may be affected.

The teacher should be aware of children who have allergies, asthma, or other respiratory conditions that may adversely affect school performance. Engagement in vigorous physical activity can cause the symptoms of asthma to appear, with running and swimming likely to evoke problems.

In most instances, however, the presence of asthma should not completely preclude the child's participation in regularly scheduled physical activities. However, since several studies have shown that asthmatic students miss significantly more school than their nonasthmatic peers, participation in activities that require a great deal of exertion should be carefully evaluated.*

Reye's syndrome

Health officials are becoming increasingly concerned with the relationship of aspirin and the development of Reye's syndrome in children. Although no direct cause of the syndrome has been discovered it has appeared in children given aspirin when they have chickenpox or influenza.

Reye's syndrome is a serious disease that causes rapid brain and liver deterioration. It is known to produce permanent brain damage, and the mortality is as high as 30%.† Fortunately, the disease is rare, affecting approximately 3 per 100,000 individuals annually.

Although teachers and school personnel should not be giving aspirin to children for any

reason, they need to be aware of this condition and may be able to counsel parents in this regard.

Learning disabilities or perceptual problems

Approximately 7% of all school-age children suffer from one or more learning disabilities. Learning disabilities may be characterized as problems in understanding or using spoken or written language. The use of language involves complex psychological processes, and failure of these processes to function properly may result in a learning problem.

Teachers may also observe a variety of children's problems that have been characterized as minimal brain dysfunction (MBD), minimal brain damage, or minimal cerebral function. They include such conditions as dyslexia (inability to read more than a few lines with understanding), hyperkinesis, hyperkinetic impulsive disorders or hyperactivity, autism (disturbances of language, cognition, and human relations—self-centeredness), and developmental aphasia (inability to transmit ideas by language, including writing and speaking, and through reading). These central nervous system disabilities are not clearly defined but generally refer to those pupils with near average, average, or above average general intelligence with learning or behavioral abnormalities ranging from mild to severe that are associated with subtle deviant functions of the central nervous system. They are characterized by difficulties in listening, thinking, talking, reading, writing, spelling, and arithmetic. They involve memory and control of attention, impulse, or motor function. There is a significant difference between children's achievement level and their functioning capabilities based on their mental abilities. These conditions are independent of errors of refraction, muscle imbalance, and imperfect binocular vision, including problems caused primarily by hearing or motor handicaps, mental retardation, emotional disturbance, or environmental disadvantage.

*Richards, W.: Allergy, asthma, and school problems, Journal of School Health **56**(4):4-6, 1986.
†Food and Drug Administration: Labeling for salicylate-containing drug products, Federal Register **47**:57886-57901, Dec., 1982.

Children with specific learning disabilities may exhibit the following behavior:

1. Hyperactivity—constantly moving, poor concentration, short attention span, talkativeness
2. Impulsiveness—easily distracted by stimuli; speaks out of turn
3. Variability and unpredictability—may cry or laugh easily; explosive irritability
4. Emotional instability—overreacts to trips, parties, and such activities; delay and failure may produce tears and temper tantrums; not accepted by peers; gullible and trusting; low tolerance for failure and frustration
5. Perseveration—continuous repetition of an action or response after a successful performance; may write a letter over and over, or talk incessantly about a subject for months
6. Poor sleep habits—easily awakened; difficulty falling asleep
7. Poor muscle coordination—cannot function in sports; exceptionally clumsy; difficulty with buttoning, writing, speaking, reading (dyslexia)

Since the causes for these conditions are not known, the diagnosis of students with perceptual problems is difficult and complex. It is a medical matter. It may involve a team of individuals including school personnel. The procedure involves obtaining a complete medical history, conducting a thorough physical examination, including a neurological survey, as well as a psychiatric and psychological examination and an electroencephalogram (EEG). There is question by some authorities regarding the use of the EEG because they claim so-called normal children may exhibit abnormal brain wave patterns.

Treatment for learning disabilities is not easily rendered. It may include helping students recognize sensory information (perception), improve memory, understand oral and written language, or increase cognitive skills—conceptualize rational, psychological, and social factors. It may also include the use of such drugs as stimulants (Ritalin, Dexedrine, Mellaril), tranquilizers, sedatives, antidepressants, antihistamines, and anticonvulsants, which have been beneficial to many children. If drugs are to be administered at school, the role of the teacher should be clearly defined (see Prescribed medications at school, Chapter 6).

A number of unproved therapies are also being promoted. The Feingold diet (removal of additives, especially artificial colors and flavors from foods and beverages) for hyperkinesis has been recommended by some allergists and endorsed by some parents. Adherence to this program requires a drastic change in lifestyle and eating patterns, but good evidence for this treatment has not yet been provided.* According to the American Academy of Pediatrics,† motor patterning therapy for brain-damaged or mentally retarded children (review with child of various motor development stages) is not effective. Eye-tracking exercises for reading disability (dyslexia) do not help because the brain learns to read, not the eyes.

Control of communicable diseases

Although local health departments generally have the legal responsibility for the prevention and control of disease, teachers and school personnel need to be concerned with the control of communicable diseases because of the hazards they present to students. A variety of microorganisms including bacteria, viruses, protozoa, and fungi can enter the body and cause infectious disease. If they are transmissible from person to person, they are considered to be communicable.

Teachers must be alert for symptoms (Table 5-1 and Appendix J) that will identify suspected disease conditions in pupils. They are expected to isolate those children discovered and send them to the nurse, principal, or appropriate school authority for possible exclusion from school. Schools generally have written policies

---

*Johnson, G.J., M.D., and Goldfinger, S.G., M.D., editors: The Harvard Medical School health letter book, Cambridge, Mass., 1981, Harvard University Press.
†Cardwell, M.A., Jr.: The pitfall of unproven therapies, Journal of School Health **49:**421, Sept., 1979.

FIG. 5-1. Control of communicable disease is part of the school health services program.

in this regard that have been developed with the help of health departments. Should no such policies exist, however, school nurses or administrators can provide information when needed, and local or state health departments can render school assistance when necessary. When such pupils return to school, teachers should be familiar with the readmission procedures to be certain that the pupils have sufficiently recovered to permit their return.

It is possible to prevent and control many diseases through immunizations for diphtheria, whooping cough, tetanus, poliomyelitis, measles, mumps, and German measles (Fig. 5-1). Some school districts make available these immunizations.

Acquired immunodeficiency syndrome (AIDS). AIDS* was first reported in the United States in May, 1981.† It is estimated that 2 million Americans may be infected with the virus

and that by the mid-1990s, the disease will kill more Americans than were killed in World War II. As of 1987, 498 cases of AIDS have been reported in youth 18 years or younger. No disease since the Bubonic plague has evoked as much fear, anguish, and emotion as AIDS.

AIDS is caused by a virus (HTLV-III) that invades many cells of the body but particularly those vital to the immune defense system. It reproduces rapidly and eliminates all of the T-helper cells that are crucial to resisting some kinds of disease. Thus many germs that ordinarily would not be harmful with a normal immune system can produce devastating and ultimately lethal diseases in persons with AIDS. There are no screening tests to identify the disease in its early stages. The tests used to identify people with antibodies cannot be administered with certainty. Once the infection is established, it is probably a lifelong infection and those people who carry the virus are potentially infectious to others. No cure has been found and little can be done by way of treatment.

The people especially susceptible are intravenous drug users who share needles, homo-

---

*For a more detailed discussion of AIDS, see Appendix A.
†Toolief, M.S., et al.: Pneumocystic carinii pneumonia and mucosal candidiasis in previously healthy homosexual men: evidence of a new acquired cellular immunodeficiency, New England Journal of Medicine **305**:1425-1431, 1981.

sexually active men, persons with hemophilia, and Haitian immigrants; although others are being identified. Heterosexual contact and contact with blood or blood products through transfusions may also result in the disease being transmitted. For children, receiving blood transfusions or being from a mother who has the disease is another way to acquire AIDS.

Treatment is limited to the use of antimicrobial agents and drugs (interferon) to bolster the immune system. The result at best may be prolonged life.

Whereas the best prevention for AIDS would be a vaccine, one unfortunately has not been discovered. In the meantime, although the disease *is not easily transmitted*, education in preventive procedures, including the need to reduce or eliminate sex contacts and to sterilize needles used by drug users, seems advisable.

Despite the fact the AIDS virus has been found in body fluids such as blood, semen, saliva, and tears, there are no documented cases showing that anyone has become infected with AIDS as a result of contact with saliva or tears. Also, there is no documented evidence that AIDS is transmitted person-to-person through the air or by casual contact.

Schools and parents have been concerned because children infected with the disease are coming to school and possibly exposing school personnel and other students to the disease. Teachers and other personnel therefore must be aware of the factual data, establish policies to deal with this disease, and be prepared to inform pupils and parents about the disease.

When establishing policies on the exclusion of students with AIDS, teachers and school personnel should keep in mind "no scientific reason exists for school personnel to be excused from education involvement with otherwise normal children with AIDS."* They should also keep in mind that "no identified U.S. cases of HTLV-III infections are known to have been transmitted

in school, day-care, or other casual person-to-person contact."*

Professional associations suggest that school attendance should not be precluded except for children who are neurologically handicapped to the extent that they lack control of their body secretions or for young preschool children infected with AIDS.

Regardless of the policy of the school, according to Philip Nader, M.D., Professor of Pediatrics at the University of California, San Diego, and former President of the American School Health Association:

No greater public health urgency exists today than to inform students frankly and explicitly how to avoid AIDS infection. The education needs to be directed to all students, regardless of their developing sexual preferences and behaviors. To fail to do so may sentence unknown numbers of children and adolescents to contract not just a sexually transmitted disease (STD) but one with potential mortality.*

Pediculosis (head lice). Every year school districts contact health departments to inform them of outbreaks of pediculosis. To combat these outbreaks, a variety of treatment methods have been used, including using special shampoos, soaking the head in carbolic acid and totally shaving the hair on the head. Regardless of these efforts, however, infestation rates seem to be climbing.†

Itching seems to be the major complaint of students infested with head lice. Infections can be caused from the open wounds that may result from the scratching that accompanies the itching.

It is important for teachers to stress with children that they should not share combs, brushes, hats, or other headgear or clothing since this type of direct contact is the major way head lice are transmitted. Since elementary students sometimes invite friends to spend the night,

---

*Black, J.: AIDS: preschool and school issues, Journal of School Health **56**(3):93-95, 1986.

*Nader, P.: AIDS: a commentary, Journal of School Health **56**(3):107-108, 1986.
†Monheit, B.M., and Norris, M.M.: Is combing the answer to headlice? Journal of School Health **56**(4):158-159, 1986.

contact with the bed linen of an infested individual also might result in spread of the lice.

When teachers observe a student continually scratching his head, or if children complain of an itchy scalp, pediculosis might be suspected. If the teacher notes whitish specks attached to the hair shafts, the child should be referred to the school nurse or other school authority.

Scabies. Like head lice, scabies is highly contagious. Scabies is caused by a mite that burrows under the skin, and the individual who has scabies will appear to scratch a lot or will complain of severe itching, especially at the finger webs, wrists, elbows, beltline, armpits, thighs, or buttocks. Once the mite has burrowed into the skin, small lesions will appear. Because of the intense itching and subsequent scratching, secondary infections are common.

The major means of transmission of scabies is through direct person-to-person contact. However, contact with undergarments or bed linens of an infected person can also result in disease transmission. Once the mite has moved to a new individual, it can burrow beneath the skin in less than 3 minutes.

As with pediculosis, any student suspected of having scabies should be referred to the school nurse. Once a child has been referred, the teacher should take care to watch the class closely for other children who may have become infected.

Tuberculosis. The prevalence of tuberculosis in the United States has been on the decline for many years, and its incidence generally is not high except in some communities. A procedure used to detect the disease through the identification of positive reactors is tuberculin testing. In the Mantoux test, a fluid containing proteins extracted from tubercle bacilli called tuberculin is injected intradermally (between the layers of the skin) or into the skin through multiple punctures (tine, Heaf, Mono-Vac, or Sterneedle test). If the test is positive, a reaction, an inflamed or red area, appears in about 48 hours on the skin where the injection was made.

A positive reaction to the test (inflammation, redness) does not necessarily mean that a person has active tuberculosis. It is an indication that the person has tubercle bacilli within his or her body and there has been an allergic reaction to these germs. In areas of high socioeconomic conditions less than 2% of elementary children have positive reactions, whereas in low socioeconomic areas this percentage may be as high as 10%. Children with positive reactions to tuberculin tests should receive thorough medical examinations, including chest x-ray films, to determine whether active tuberculosis exists.

The American Lung Association* recommends that tuberculin testing should be concentrated in areas where the prevalence of infection is constantly high over a period of time. Therefore routine or periodic testing of school children and young adolescents should be stressed in those schools where the reactor rate is 1% or more and should take place in other schools on a selective basis only. The American Academy of Pediatrics† agrees with this procedure. They also state that schools can determine whether the incidence of tuberculin sensitivity exceeds 1% by testing all those starting school for the first time and children in grades 8 and 9 at intervals of 3 years or by testing randomly selected subsamples annually.

WHAT ARE SCREENING TESTS?

Screening tests are those preliminary health evaluations used in schools to assess the health status of pupils. They are not diagnostic tests. The primary goal of conducting these screenings is to identify those health conditions among students that may adversely affect the child's ability to learn. Secondary goals include serving as a referral and resource mechanism and making

---

*Your patient's risk of tuberculosis, New York, 1975, American Lung Association.
†Committee on School Health: School health: a guide for health professionals, Evanston, Ill., 1981, American Academy of Pediatrics.

recommendations for adjustments in the school program to accommodate children found to have educationally limiting health problems. Screening may include tests for vision and hearing problems, growth and development, tuberculosis, dental problems, posture, nutrition, sickle cell anemia, and others. They should be low cost so they can be available to all students. They are likely to be administered by teachers, nurses, technologists, and other school personnel. They serve as rough measuring devices that supplement and complement teacher observations as well as other procedures used to determine the health of students. If children are found to be in need, they should be referred to health specialists for diagnostic tests.

Vision

Vision screening is usually concerned with problems of central visual acuity, direct vision of near and far objects, and ability to perceive the shape and form of objects in the direct line of vision. However, constant alertness for signs of eye diseases and other abnormalities must also be maintained. Children with acuity defects cannot perceive and discriminate the details of objects or printed symbols. Thus they are likely to encounter learning difficulties.

School vision screening usually attempts to reveal the following eye problems:

1. Errors of refraction—eye defects in which images are focused improperly on the retina.
   a. Hyperopia—farsightedness; light rays focus behind the retina, common in those under 10 to 12 years and usually corrects itself as the eye matures.
   b. Myopia—nearsightedness; light rays focus in front of the retina.
   c. Astigmatism—irregular curvature of the cornea or lens.
2. Strabismus—crossed eyes caused by muscle imbalance; the muscles of the two eyes do not work in coordination, resulting in failure of the alignment of the eyes. It is estimated that 1.5% of children are so af-

flicted. The afflicted eye may not be used and may bring about deterioration of visual acuity, a condition known as amblyopia, which can usually be prevented if treated early; some schools are advising preschool examinations, and others are trying to identify children in Head Start programs.

3. Color blindness—inability to perceive colors; this condition may be congenital or acquired, with the congenital form being more prevalent. Congenital defects may be either total or partial; total color blindness is rare and when it occurs, all colors appear as grays. The partial type is more common and is primarily inherited through the mother who carries the recessive gene and is generally not affected. Red and green colors are usually confused in most cases, but blue-yellow defects also occur; acquired defects of color may often develop in the course of ocular, mainly retinal, disease. Approximately 3.8%* of children 6 to 11 years of age have color vision deficiencies; by sex 6.95% of boys and 0.53% of girls are affected; the problem among white boys is about twice as great as among black boys.

The American Academy of Pediatrics states that every child should have a test for visual acuity by the age of 4 years, before entry into school.

Basic minimum recommended procedure. The minimum recommended vision screening program varies in schools throughout the United States. The National Society to Prevent Blindness† claims that where a professional eye examination is not possible a child should have an *annual* test for distance visual acuity. However, realizing that time and personnel may not permit such screenings, the basic minimum using the Snellen charts (Fig. 5-2) should be:

---

*U.S. Department of Health, Education, and Welfare, Public Health Service, National Center for Health Statistics: Color vision deficiencies in children, United States, Washington, D.C., 1972, U.S. Government Printing Office.
†National Society to Prevent Blindness: Vision screening for children, New York, 1980, The Society.

FIG. 5–2. Snellen charts. *(Courtesy National Society to Prevent Blindness, New York, N.Y.)*

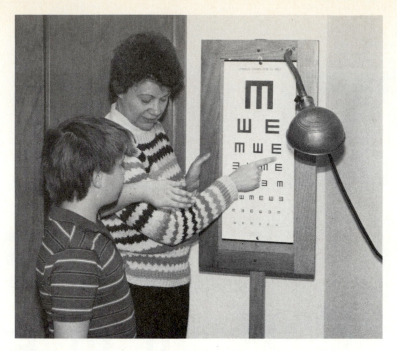

FIG. 5-3. Students must be taught how to respond to vision screening charts. *(Courtesy of Wichita Public Schools.)*

1. Kindergarten or first grade (5 to 6 years)—use symbol "E"chart (Fig. 5-3)
2. Second grade (7 years), fifth grade (10 to 11 years), eighth grade (13 years), tenth or eleventh grade (15 to 17 years)
3. All new students and teacher referrals
4. All children who exhibit a change in behavior or learning disability

Continuous observation by the teacher and the tester for symptoms related to eye problems should be correlated with the screening procedure. Several research studies have indicated high correlation of this action with clinical findings by ophthalmologists.

Preschool vision screening is now being recommended. Identification of such defects as cross-eye and amblyopia or so-called lazy eye is important. These conditions can lead to unnecessary loss of vision unless detected and treated before the age of 6 years. Screening with isolated symbols is recommended because a "crowding effect" results when more than one letter is used.

Teacher involvement. Who conducts the screening differs among schools and school districts. Common practice indicates that teachers, nurses, technicians, and volunteers are assigned to perform this service. Some state laws require teachers to administer the tests. Reasons often advanced for teacher involvement in vision testing are the following:

1. They understand better the children with vision problems in their classes.
2. They become more sensitive to and concerned with opportunities for continually observing children with vision problems.
3. They can make the vision screening program a part of the health instruction program.

Snellen test. Probably the most commonly used vision screening device, the Snellen test is designed to discover those children with myopia, although other difficulties may also be found. It has been widely used in schools because it is simple, economical, and practical. It has been considered by the National Society to Prevent Blindness as well as other authoritative groups as the best single measurement for vision screening.

The test makes use of a chart that has square-shaped letters or symbols resembling the letter E (Fig. 5-2). These are in specified sizes and in printed rows. The symbol at the top line of the chart is of such a size that a person with normal vision is able to see it from a distance of 200 feet, whereas the person with a vision problem can view it only from 20 feet. In each succeeding row, from the top downward, the size of the symbols is reduced to a point that a person with normal vision can see them at distances of 100, 70, 50, 30, and 20 feet, respectively.

To determine visual acuity, the student stands at a distance of 20 feet from the chart and with one eye covered reads the smallest letter that can be seen. The student's acuity is recorded by stating the distance at which the test has been completed and the line the student reads. These numbers are recorded as fractions: 20/20, 20/40, 20/70. They are not actually fractions, but represent a simple method of reporting facts. Thus an acuity of 20/70 means that the student was tested at 20 feet and could read only the letters on line 70. The vision of each eye is tested separately.

Criteria for recommending students for a retest may be the following:

1. Four-year-olds through grade 3—20/40 visual acuity or less in one or both eyes; inability to read the 30-foot line
2. Grade 4 and up—20/30 visual acuity or less in one or both eyes; inability to read the 20-foot line

After being retested, children for whom the second findings are the same as those recorded after the first test, provided that the teacher's observations indicate an abnormality, should be referred for examination by a professionally qualified person.

Additional tests. The National Society to Prevent Blindness indicates there are several other tests that may be added to the basic minimum procedure. These include the plus sphere lens, muscle imbalance, and color vision tests.

PLUS SPHERE LENS. The plus sphere lens is used to detect students with hyperopia. The test is administered by having children wear a pair of glasses with convex (hyperopic) lenses of specified strength (+2.25 diopters* for the first three grades and +1.75 diopters from fourth grade on) and requiring them to read the 20-foot line of the Snellen chart. Each eye is tested separately. If they read the line, they have failed the test. The convex lens blurs the vision of the children with no refractive error and makes correction for the hyperopic youngsters enabling them to read the chart. Pupils who fail the test should be retested. If the results are the same and there are other signs noted through teacher observations, these children should be referred for professional diagnosis. The plus sphere test should be given only to those pupils who do not wear glasses and who satisfactorily pass the Snellen test.

MUSCLE IMBALANCE. Muscle imbalance refers to the inability of the two eyes to work together. There are a number of instruments, such as Maddox's rod, to measure this condition, but there is no satisfactory screening procedure. A rough, and not very accurate, method still in use is the cover test. It is a simple way to detect latent strabismus (crossed eye not readily noticed). In some children this condition reveals itself only when they are very tired or under emotional stress. Latent strabismus may manifest itself in only one eye, or it may alternate between the eyes.

The cover test determines whether eye alignment is maintained when one eye is covered while the other is fixed on an object. The alignment of each eye should be determined for both distant and near points.

The procedure for testing should be as follows:

1. Have the pupil look at a small light or object 20 feet away.

---

*Diopter, unit of measurement of strength or refractive power of lenses.

2. Place a cover card in front of one of the pupil's eyes in a manner so that the light or object cannot be seen with that eye. Watch to see if the alignment of the covered eye is maintained; note whether the eye turns in, out, up, or down or holds its fixed position.

3. After a few seconds, move the cover card to the other eye. The previously covered eye is watched for a shift in the direction of its fixation.

4. Repeat the test, having the pupil look at a small light or object 8 to 10 inches in front of the nose. If the muscle balance of the eye is essentially normal, there should be no marked change in its fixation on covering or when the cover is removed.

Pupils who show marked deviation from normal should be retested, and if the same results are discovered, they should be referred for professional diagnosis.

COLOR VISION TEST. The color vision test is a procedure to determine whether a person is color blind, or unable to discriminate between certain colors, usually red and green and sometimes blue and yellow. Two satisfactory tests for school use are the Hardy-Rand-Ritter test and the Ishihara test.

Color blindness is inherited and cannot be corrected. Adjustments to the abnormality are important, and students should be aware of this limitation, especially when making vocational choices, when learning to drive automobiles, or when crossing streets. It is desirable to test young people before they enter junior high school.

Other devices and procedures. Numerous other instruments, devices, and procedures are available for vision screening and testing. A variety of opinions (including that they cause over-referral of pupils) regarding their value exist. They include Maddox's rod test (for muscle imbalance), the Telebinocular (a stereoscopic instrument to measure muscle imbalance, visual acuity, and color vision), the Ortho-Rater (similar to the Telebinocular), the Titmus vision tester (for near- and far-sightedness), and the Massachusetts vision kit (visual acuity, plus sphere, and Maddox's rod test). Several modi-

fied clinic techniques (MCT) have been used. One involves the cooperative use of optometrists and ophthalmologists; a second uses only ophthalmologists. The procedures used to test vision include visual acuity (Snellen "E" Chart), binocular coordination (cover test for muscle imbalance), refractive error (retinoscope for myopia, hyperopia, and astigmatism), and ocular health (use of ophthalmoscope to inspect the internal and external eye structures). It is claimed the MCT procedures reduce the numbers of children in need of eye attention who were missed (underreferrals).

Hearing

The procedure generally used to test the hearing of children is performed with the puretone audiometer. It requires technical training to administer and interpret.

Puretone audiometer. The puretone audiometer (Fig. 5-4) is an individual testing device that measures the ability to hear sounds of vary-

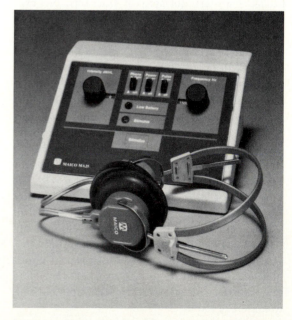

FIG. 5-4. Puretone audiometer. *(Courtesy Maico Hearing Instruments, Inc.)*

ing frequencies* or hertz (Hz) at different intensities of sound called decibels.†

A procedure known as the sweep-check test method has been used in schools to expedite the hearing screening process. Testing each ear separately, the intensity dial is set at 10 decibels. The tone dial is changed rather quickly through the 1,000, 2,000, 4,000, and 6,000 frequencies and reset at 20 decibels for 4,000 frequencies. The extremely low and high tones may be omitted. Some sweep-check methods involve the 500, 1,000, 2,000, and 4,000 frequencies at 20

*Frequencies, qualities of sound caused by the number of vibrations per second of an object resulting in high and low tones, for example, strings on a piano.
†Decibels, units of sound intensity.

decibels. It is estimated that from 5% to 10% of the students will fail this test. Those students who fail to hear one tone or more in either ear in this sweep-check method should be given a second screening test. Failure to pass the repeated screening should be followed by a threshold test. In this test, pupils listen to all the intensities of sound of each frequency, with the results plotted on audiograms (Fig. 5-5). The findings are then interpreted by technologists administering the test, and decisions are made whether to refer these children for specialized examinations. The criteria for referral generally include hearing losses of 20 decibels or more at any two frequencies in either ear, or a loss of 30 decibels or more at any single frequency in ei-

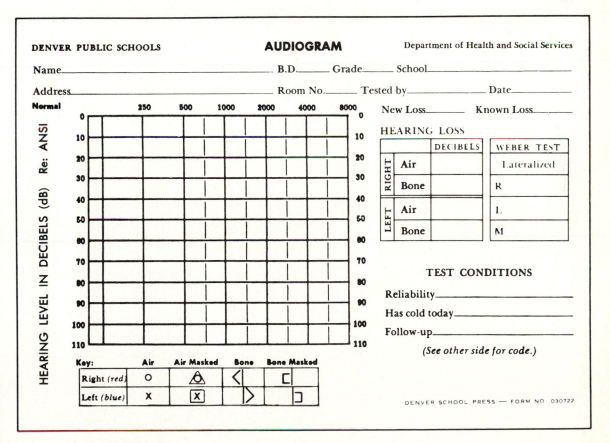

FIG. 5-5. Audiogram. *(Courtesy Department of Health and Social Services, Denver Public Schools, 1981.)*

ther ear. The degrees of hearing disability may be categorized as mild, moderate, moderately severe, and severe.

Audiometers are usually calibrated in round-numbered frequencies such as 125, 250, 500, 1,000, 2,000, on up to 8,000; the range of sounds that are normally heard by human beings. The machines are also calibrated by sound intensities with the step intervals being from 5 or 10 decibels to a maximum of 100 decibels.

The American Academy of Pediatrics* recommends that every child have a hearing test

---

*Committee on School Health: School health: a guide for health professionals, Evanston, Ill., 1981, American Academy of Pediatrics.

by the age of 4 years (Fig. 5-6). Children with ear disease, language or speech problems, or other indications of possible hearing abnormality should be tested when conditions are first recognized regardless of age. Hearing testing in schools should be done annually in preschool, kindergarten, and grade 1 and then in grades 3, 6, 9, and 12. Children with persistent hearing impairments should be tested annually.

Growth and development

Periodic measurements of the heights and weights of children will aid in understanding the growth and development (see Appendix L) of boys and girls in terms of (1) normal progression,

CODE: 1. RETEST
2A "HOME REPORT"—*To recommend medical care.*
2B "HOME REPORT"—*With no medical care recommended at present.*
3. REPORT OF HIGH FREQUENCY LOSS
4. EDUCATION AUDIOMETRY

Significant medical history:_____

_____

Significant educational history:_____

Recommendations:_____
Special seating, etc.:_____

_____

General:_____

_____

FIG. 5-5, cont'd. For legend see p. 91.

(2) extent of overweight, and (3) extent of underweight. However, Eisner and others* state that routine growth measurements have not proved their general usefulness in health service programs and are not of sufficient educational value to justify a large investment of nurse time. Mere observation of weight and height increases, or the failure of children to gain weight, may not in themselves be of much significance in the growth process. Children's growth patterns are individual, and unless an instrument is used to show this, school personnel may be led to erroneous conclusions about overweight, underweight, or abnormal growth conditions. Weighing and measuring can be valuable in the appraisal process if the information is recorded

---

*Eisner, V., Oglesby, A., and Peck, E.B.: Health assessment of school children, VI. height and weight, Journal of School Health **42:**March, 1972.

and plotted on growth charts for interpretation, as illustrated in the height-weight records shown in Figs. 5-7 and 5-8.

The taking of heights and weights should be done at the beginning, middle, and end of the school year. It is important that measurements be accurately taken and recorded (Fig. 5-9).

Children in grade 3 and upward can be taught to take these measurements. Teachers, nurses, or nurse assistants can aid by recording these data on the growth charts. This activity provides an excellent teachable moment for health instruction about growth and development.

Dental inspections

Dental inspections refer to procedures generally performed by dentists or dental hygienists using mouth mirrors and explorers to locate decayed teeth, as well as to check for diseases of

FIG. 5-6. Hearing screening is an important component of the school health services program. *(Courtesy of Wichita Public Schools.)*

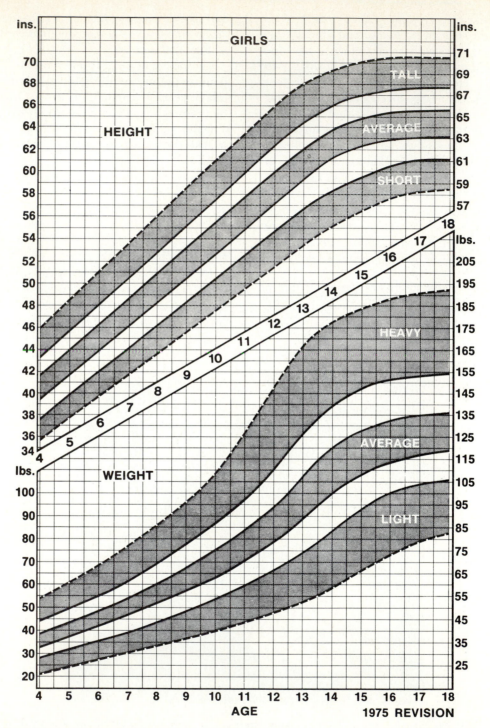

FIG. 5-7. Growth of girls. *(Copyright 1975, 1978, American Medical Association. Publication of A.M.A. Medicine/Education Committee. Material produced by John H. Spurgeon and Howard V. Meredith, University of Southern California.)*

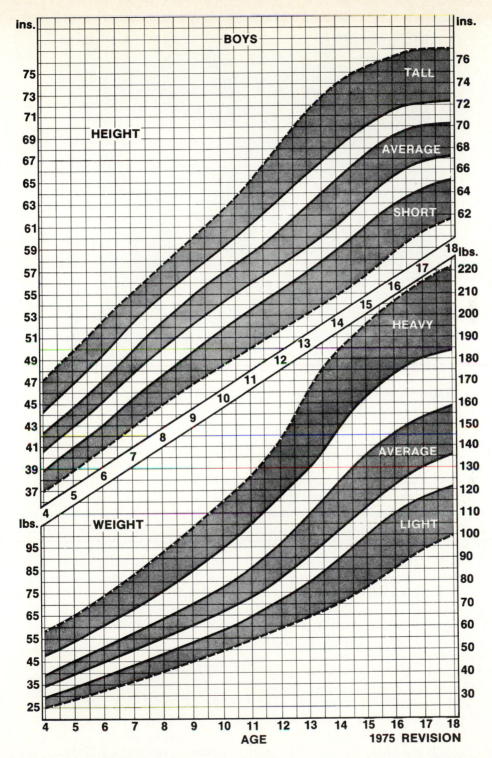

FIG. 5–8. Growth of boys. (*Copyright 1975, 1978, American Medical Association. Publication of A.M.A. Medicine/Education Committee. Material produced by John H. Spurgeon and Howard V. Meredith, University of Southern California.*)

FIG. 5-9. Height and weight screening. *(Courtesy of Wichita Public Schools.)*

tissue surrounding the teeth and for malocclusion. These inspections are not complete examinations since they do not include x-ray examinations.

Ideally, children should visit their family dentists twice yearly for appraisal and necessary treatment. There is evidence to indicate only 20% of the population is following this practice.

Opinions differ regarding whether periodic dental inspections should be conducted in schools. Several reasons causing this dilemma include the following:

1. Since dental decay is the most common health defect found in school-age children, there is little need to locate problem cases.

2. There may be a poor geographic distribution of dentists and dental hygienists. Therefore increased pressure on parents by the schools to obtain corrections may make it impossible for dentists to provide the needed services. The schools would be criticized for not being aware of this difficulty.

3. Most school districts do not employ dentists or dental hygienists.

Dental inspections in schools vary widely as to their inclusion and frequency. In Pennsylvania, dental examinations by a dentist must be conducted by schools on the original entry of children as well as in the third and seventh grades. In elementary schools, however, substitution is permitted by service from dental hygienists provided it includes a screening process, prophylactic care, and an educational program. In Denver, all pupils are inspected at selected grades by dental hygienists.

Sickle cell disease

Sickle cell disease is a disorder of red blood cells caused by abnormal hemoglobin and affects the cells' ability to carry oxygen. The normal red blood cells that usually appear disc shaped are crescent or sickle shaped. The condition is found among the black population and to a lesser degree in individuals with Mediterranean ancestry (Greek, Italian), in Caribbean islanders, and in people in South and Central America. The sickle cell trait is a genetic factor estimated to be found in 10% of the black population, whereas the disease itself, sickle cell anemia, is found in approximately 1 in 400 to 500 blacks. The condition results in the swelling of joints, pain in the abdomen, legs, and arms, and fatigue. The anemia cannot be cured, but the "crisis" situation when cells are deprived of oxygen can be treated. The crisis condition can be prevented or ameliorated.

One valid procedure used to identify this condition among junior and senior high school students is to draw venous blood and test it by direct hemoglobin electrophoresis to determine if the blood cells differ from normal ones. Only one test is needed to determine an individual's status. The American Academy of Pediatrics* states that routine screening of well school-aged children is not desirable.

Diabetes

Approximately 13 million people in the United States have diabetes. Diabetes is not an infectious disease. It can be detected by urinalysis to determine the level of sugar in the blood. Although schools generally do not conduct such tests, every effort should be made to identify those afflicted children to be able to provide needed help. When students first enter school, parent interviews, completion of health histories, physician contacts, and other means should be used to locate diabetic pupils.

Diabetes results from failure of the pancreas to make a sufficient amount of insulin. Without insulin, food cannot be used properly. Diabetes currently cannot be cured but can be controlled by daily injections of insulin and a prescribed food plan.

There are two types of diabetes: type I and

type II. Type II, or non-insulin-dependent diabetes usually develops in individuals over 40 years of age. Thus the teacher will generally see the child who has type I, or insulin-dependent diabetes. In general, students with type I diabetes will already be under the care of a physician, but the teacher should be aware of which children in class have this disorder in case one of them begins to show symptoms of insulin shock or diabetic acidosis. If a child with diabetes seems to show uncharacteristic sleepiness, or complains of stomach pain and begins vomiting, immediately refer the child to appropriate school personnel.

Afflicted children can participate in all school activities but should be carefully observed in class. Physical education should not be scheduled just before lunch nor should a child be assigned a late lunch period. These young people may need midmorning or midafternoon snacks. Teachers should have sugar readily available in the event of insulin shock (a condition in which too much insulin is circulating in the bloodstream).

Epilepsy

Epilepsy is a disruption of the electrical impulses to the brain that causes nerves to send out erratic impulses through the body resulting in a seizure, or sudden onset of symptoms, such as convulsions. It occurs in approximately 1 child in 50, with 75% of the cases beginning before the eighteenth birthday. Four out of five cases of epilepsy, where known, can be controlled with medication; 50% can be totally controlled, and 30% partially. Teachers should be aware that excessive fatigue, overexposure to heat or sunlight, and situations that cause emotional disturbances can affect the seizure threshold in children and increase the incidence of attacks.

Schools must identify students with epilepsy to be able to best provide for their safety and to enable classmates to help these pupils. Screening to locate such children can take place when they first enter school through parent interviews and the completion of health histories, through

---

*Committee on School Health: School health: a guide for health professionals, Evanston, Ill., 1981, American Academy of Pediatrics.

a review of health records and physician contacts, and by other means. (See Chapter 7 for ways to handle seizures at school.)

Scoliosis

Scoliosis is a condition in which there is a lateral curvature and rotation of the spine. It is found in 0.5% to 2.0% of young people. It is most commonly observed in children aged 12 through 16 years and progresses until skeletal maturity is attained. It occurs more often in girls than boys and is generally the result of poor muscle tone and fatigue and sometimes may reflect depression and lack of self-esteem.

The procedure used in screening for scoliosis should be done with pupils stripped to the waist. Girls may wear brassieres. Pupils should be observed from the back and should stand erect with the shoulders back, head up and looking forward, hands hanging at sides, knees straight, and feet together. The screener should note whether the shoulders, scapulae, arm hang, and hips are in a level plane; one should not be higher or lower than the other. Also, the straightness of the spine should be checked; it should not bend right or left. The pupil should then bend forward at the waist, head hanging relaxed, arms dangling from the shoulders, and knees straight (Fig. 5-10). The screener should observe the surface of the back at eye level to detect prominence of the thoracic ribs and the area around the vertebral column. The chest should be symmetrical, and an imaginary line drawn from scapula to scapula should be parallel to the floor. As the student resumes an upright position, the back movement should be checked to note prominences or spinal curvatures. Abnormalities detected should be referred to a physician for examination and treatment.

The purpose of scoliosis screening is to detect abnormal curvature of the spine at an early stage so that corrective procedures can be instituted. It should take place when skeletal growth is rapid—in girls at 9 to 14 years of age and boys at 11 to 15 years of age. Schools commonly conduct the screening in grades 5 through 9 or 10. The number and frequency of these procedures

FIG. 5-10. Correct procedure should be followed in scoliosis screening. *(Courtesy of Wichita Public Schools.)*

are dependent on the resources available and local school district policy. The procedure can be completed by nurses and others with special training.

Scoliosis screening may be controversial because the testing procedure (the bending test) produces a large number of false-positives and marginal cases that may not need assistance. Since the best method of diagnosis is through the use of x-ray examinations,* it has been suggested that this screening should remain a part of the family physician's routine examination.†

---

*Edwards, D.D.: Toward safer scoliosis screening, Science News **128**:262 October 26, 1985.

†Morais, T., Bernier, M., and Turcotte, F.: Age- and sex-specific prevalence of scoliosis and the value of school screening programs, American Journal of Public Health **75**(12):1377-1380, 1985.

DENVER PUBLIC SCHOOLS   **SCHOOL NURSE INTERVIEW WITH PARENT**   DEPARTMENT OF HEALTH AND SOCIAL SERVICES

Pupil's name_____ Birth date_____ Date of interview_____

I. BIRTH AND DEVELOPMENT

Pregnancy - Delivery

Gravida_____ Para_____

Birthweight_____

Birthplace_____

Baby's condition at birth_____

Days in hospital_____

Age - sat up_____ crawled_____
    walked_____
    talked_____ words_____ sentences_____
    Any speech problems_____

Weaned at age_____

Toilet training_____ age_____

Constipation_____ Diarrhea_____

Enuresis_____ Encopresis_____

Handedness: Right_____ Left_____ Both_____

Are you satisfied with child's progress and development?

Do you have any particular concerns about your child?

DENVER SCHOOL PRESS — STOCK NO. 01-030025

II. BEHAVIORAL DEVELOPMENT

How does child get along with
    peers?_____
    siblings?_____
    parents?_____

Assumes responsibility_____

Expresses anger by_____

Expresses insecurity by_____

Method of discipline_____

Habits:
    Eating_____
    Sleeping_____ Nightmares_____
    Thumbsucking_____ Nail biting_____
    Masturbation_____ Other_____

Reading and early listening experiences_____

TV and recreation_____

Attention span_____

School experience_____

III. PAST ILLNESSES (include age of child or date)

Allergies_____

Contagious diseases_____

Serious illnesses or chronic diseases_____

High fever_____

History of convulsions_____

Accidents_____

Head injury or unconsciousness_____

Fractures_____

Surgery_____ Hospitalization_____

Emotional problems_____

Significant family episodes (include dates)
    for example:
        death_____
        severe accident_____
        loss of job_____
        divorce/separation_____
        remarriage_____
        other_____
                                    (OVER)

IV. FAMILY MEDICAL HISTORY

Mother_____

_____

Father_____

_____

Siblings_____

_____

Maternal grandparents_____

_____

Paternal grandparents_____

_____

Others_____

Previous tests or screening of child:
    Sickle cell_____ Speech_____
    DDST_____ Hearing_____ Vision_____
    Dental_____
Medical care resource_____

V. FAMILY HISTORY

Father's age_____ Occupation_____
                        Work hours_____

Last grade in school_____

Glasses?_____

Mother's age_____ Occupation_____
                        Work hours_____

Last grade in school_____

Glasses?_____

Language (s) spoken in home_____

School experience of siblings_____

_____

_____

_____

_____

VI. CONCLUSIONS

How do you think your child will do or does in school?

How would you describe your child?

School nurse and/or family plans, following this interview:

_____
Name of person interviewed and relationship to child

_____, RN

FIG. 5-11. School nurse interview with parent. *(Courtesy Department of Health and Social Services, Denver Public Schools, 1981.)*

Other screening procedures

A variety of additional types of screening appraisals such as teacher observations of nutritional deficiencies (Appendix J), speech difficulties, hypertension, and assessment for conditions such as anemia, hemophilia, and muscular dystrophy occur in schools. Their frequency and extent show wide variation throughout the United States.

WHAT ARE HEALTH HISTORIES AND INVENTORIES?

Histories and inventories (Fig. 5-11) are informational accounts of the health practices and behavior of children that take the form of written questionnaires or checklists. They are often neglected, yet they are one of the most important parts of periodic health appraisals. The basic content should include information about major past health problems (physical and emotional) and their treatment, an orderly review of body systems, information about current and past special problems of other members of the family, and information about the student's academic achievement and school adjustments. This information provides background data about the health of children not usually revealed by other procedures but are useful in the health appraisals of pupils. The teacher needs to know that a child with diabetes is taking insulin. A periodic health examination may not reveal that a student has asthma or occasional epileptic attacks. These inventories help in understanding the health status of boys and girls and may be particularly useful when school medical examinations are conducted. The forms may be sent to parents of young children for completion or may be finished at school when the child is brought in for enrollment. The data obtained become a part of the child's health record.

WHAT ARE MEDICAL EXAMINATIONS?

Medical, health, or physical examinations refer to those appraisals usually completed by qualified physicians. Accurate evaluations of health require medical examinations.

The health examination usually includes the following conditions and parts of the body:

Nutrition
Skin and hair
Head and neck
Lungs
Muscle tone
Nose, throat, and tonsils
Feet
Eyes
Genitalia
Heart
Nervous system
Posture
Thyroid gland
Teeth and gums
Bones and joints
Ears
Pulse—resting and after exercise
Blood pressure
Abdomen
Lymph nodes
Inguinal and umbilical region for hernia
Laboratory tests such as urinalysis and blood tests

The American Academy of Pediatrics believes the child's health care provider or family physician is the most desirable source for a health appraisal. Therefore it generally should be performed outside the school setting. However circumstances such as legal requirements, poverty, and lack of health care resources may necessitate such examinations being conducted in some schools.

The Academy states that routine, periodic, health examinations in schools have proved to have low effectiveness in the identification of serious, uncared for medical problems. They indicate that the continuance of such appraisals is inadvisable.

The frequency of health examinations for children in school is set by law in some states. Where there are no legal directives, local school and medical officials must make these decisions. Appraisals probably should be performed when pupils start school, again in grades 6 or 7, and before leaving school in grades 11 or 12. In addition, they should be conducted for those who have been identified as having particular problems. The Academy states that priority for school examinations should be given to high-risk children, who may be those with low socioeconomic status, poor school performance, existing handicaps, frequent absence, and disciplinary problems.

WHAT ARE PSYCHOLOGICAL EXAMINATIONS AND TESTS?

Psychological examinations and tests include a variety of procedures to test personality, behavior, and social acceptance of pupils as well as intelligence, achievements, and aptitudes. They are usually administered by psychologists and psychometrists who are members of a child guidance or pupil personnel services program. School districts occasionally employ consulting psychiatrists to help with emotionally disturbed students. Mental health specialists and mental health counselors are beginning to be trained and used in some schools. The findings from these appraisals, together with teacher observations, help determine the necessary action. Pupils with suspected emotional difficulties who are located through these evaluations may need to be referred for medical or psychiatric consultation. The American Academy of Pediatrics states that children with emotional problems are difficult to identify. It also claims that the management of children with emotional problems is the most common unmet health need of school children.

Teacher feelings, emotions, and expressions affect pupil emotions. Teacher attitudes are reflected in the attitudes of pupils. The teacher who is kind but firm, sympathetic but exacting, and friendly but reserved exerts a beneficial influence on emotional health. The nagging, scolding, domineering, sarcastic, or emotionally unstable teacher may lead to serious emotional difficulties in pupils.

Locating children with emotional problems

Children who are emotionally disturbed or who exhibit behavior that causes one to suspect mental illness need to be identified and located early if they are to receive the greatest help. The teacher is the main contact person with pupils and is in a strategic position to render valuable service. The importance of teacher observations was previously stressed; however, the specific signs of maladjustment that the teacher must know and recognize are found in Table 5-1 and Appendix J. It has been estimated that teachers can identify 70% of the emotionally disturbed children, and with a clinic team, 90% of their problems can be discovered. The deviant behaviors observed are generally the result of pupil needs not being fulfilled. Teachers must be alert throughout the entire school day and be observant in their informal contacts, conferences, and interviews with pupils and parents for clues that will help to identify the problems of their pupils.

Some procedures teachers may use with discretion to help identify indicators that children may have problems include the following:

1. Sociometric technique—the teacher may ask pupils to list the three classmates they would like to have sit next to them in order of preference. This information can then be plotted on paper, and those pupils with few, if any friends, can be readily identified. The isolates are easily located through the use of this method.

2. Examination of school records including health records—these contain chronological reports of children's performances and health status.

3. Written assignments—the teacher may have pupils write compositions on such topics as the following:

> "What I criticize about myself"
> "What others criticize about me"
> "What makes me mad"
> "The person I would like to be"
> "My life 10 years from now"

Finding problem children is not easy and is also the responsibility of other school personnel, including nurses and psychologists. Their specific responsibilities vary in schools, but they should be observant of pupil behavior, assess pupil records, and use a variety of formal procedures.

Numerous intelligence, personality, and adjustment inventories and tests used by school or private psychologists can be employed to help identify emotionally disturbed children.*

Counselors, physicians, nurses, psychiatric social workers, psychologists, and psychiatrists may individually or collectively be involved in case studies of pupils. Teachers and other personnel may also be requested to report their observations. This is a technique whereby the

---

*For a discussion of various tests that may be used in mental health evaluation of children, see Reinert, H.R.: Children in conflict, ed. 2, St. Louis, 1980, The C.V. Mosby Co.; and Johnson, R.B., and Magrab, P.: Developmental disorders, Austin, Tex., 1978, Proed, Inc.

conclusions of a variety of people are brought together to help identify and understand deviant children, determine needed action to help children, and suggest school adjustments.

The assessment of the mental health status of pupils is both difficult and complex. Accurate, objective observations of behavior together with the pooling of information obtained from many sources are necessary.

WHAT ARE HEALTH RECORDS?

Health records (Fig. 5-12) refer to those materials that contain all pertinent data about the health status of pupils. Cumulative records should be maintained for all pupils in school and not merely for those with known health problems. They should be accessible to those persons who need to use them and should follow students from grade to grade, from school to school, and from school district to school district.

There is no common type of health record used in schools. However, records information should be kept confidential and should not be available without permission of school health personnel. They should not contain personal observations by the teacher that label children as slow learners, mentally retarded, and the like. Parents or guardians should have access to the contents.

Records usually contain the following information:
1. Teacher observations
2. Results of screening tests
3. Findings of medical, dental, and psychological examinations
4. Notes on health counseling and follow-up procedures

Despite the amount of information found in health records, the records are not used with any degree of consistency by teachers and others. This is probably because of any, or all, of the following reasons: (1) there is no central, master file on every student, and retrieval of information is difficult; (2) it takes a great deal of time to transcribe the data by hand; (3) information is often lost or misinterpreted, and

records may be incomplete; (4) little anecdotal information can be included; (5) if a record is lost, a completely new one must be reconstructed; and (6) an adequate study of the total student population is virtually impossible.

In an effort to solve problems related to health records, including recording and having access to data, school districts are beginning to computerize these records. The technology exists today to do this on a wide scale.* Ontario, Canada has been successful with this procedure since the early 1970s.

Teachers can better understand the health status of students by reviewing health records at the beginning of the semester as well as at other times. They may be expected to enter notations of observations and other essential information about the health of children in their classes on the health records.

THE NURSE AND APPRAISALS

The more than 35,000 employed professional nurses who work as school nurses have an important role in school health appraisals. They are an integral part of the professional health team within the school and community. Their responsibilites vary depending on the size of the school district, whether physician services are available, and the amount of time they serve in schools. Generally, they are expected to (1) supervise and conduct screening procedures, (2) prepare schedules and logistical arrangements for tests, (3) help teachers conduct certain appraisal procedures, (4) assist with examinations conducted by physicians and other health professionals, (5) aid teachers with pupil observations and referrals, (6) interpret appraisal findings to pupils, teachers, and parents, (7) counsel pupils and parents, and (8) maintain health records.

Referral of students to community resources for the remediation of health problems is an important part of the school health service pro-

---

*Shea, S., and Marguiles, D.: The paperless medical record, Social Science and Medicine **21**:741-746, 1985.

NAME _____ Last, _____ First, _____ Middle _____

Father's Name _____ **Mother's Name** _____ **Birthdate** _____ **Sex** _____

GROWTH AND SCREENING RECORD

SCHOOL															
YEAR															
LEVEL															
Height															
Weight															
Vision- With glasses R.	20	20	20	20	20	20	20	20							
Vision- With glasses L.	20	20	20	20	20	20	20	20							
Vision- Without glasses R.	20	20	20	20	20	20	20	20							
Vision- Without glasses L.	20	20	20	20	20	20	20	20							
Vision referral															
Near vision															
Stereo test															
Color vision															
Hearing, R.															
Hearing, L.															
Hearing referral															
Dental screening															
Dental referral															
Scoliosis															
Scoliosis referral															
Physical Examination															
Health Assessment															
Special ed Staffing															

HISTORY OF IMMUNIZATION
Code: Date of immunization   D for disease

	DATE	DATE	DATE	BOOSTERS			
DPT							
DT							
Tetanus							
Polio (Trivalent)							
Measles (Rubeola)							
Measles (Rubella)							
Mumps							
Other							

MAJOR HEALTH CONCERNS

KINDS	DATE	KINDS	DATE
Allergies:		Hospitalizations	
Animal		Operations	
Drug		Serious injury	
Food		Seizures	
Insect stings		Skin infections	
Chickenpox		Prone to colds	
Dental		Prone to strep	
Diabetes		Pneumonia	
Ear infections		On medications	
Eye concerns		Other:	
If yes to any of these, please remark:			

FIG. 5-12. Cumulative school health record. *(Reprinted by permission: Colorado Department of Education and Colorado Department of Health, Colorado school health guidelines, ed. 2, Denver, 1986, The Department.)*

ACTIVE PROBLEM LIST

MO/YR	ACTIVE PROBLEM LIST (Include Special Instructions Concerning Student's Health)	DATE RESOLVED

ACTIVE PROBLEMS

MO/YR	ACTIVE PROBLEMS	DATE RESOLVED
1		
2		
3		
4		
5		
6		
7		
8		
9		
10		
11		

PHYSICAL ASSESSMENT

Date					
Eyes					
Nose					
Teeth					
Gums					
Throat					
Tonsils					
Ears					
Glands					
Heart					
Lungs					
Abdomen					
Hernia					
Orthopedic					
Skin					
Posture					
Nutrition					
Blood pressure					
Speech					
Phys. ed. rec.					

FIG. 5-12, cont'd. For legend see p. 103.

FIG. 5–13. Nurse takes blood pressure. *(Courtesy of Wisconsin Department of Public Instruction, Madison, Wis.)*

gram. However, unless follow-up activities including telephone calls, health counseling, and health education are conducted, the full impact of the referral may be lost.*

In recent years nurses have assumed expanded duties in the assessment of school-age children. Some have acquired additional special training in schools of medicine and have become *nurse practitioners*. There are now thousands of nurse practitioners licensed to practice in most states. They are especially useful in schools with limited or no physician services. In addition, they provide a close relationship with physicians and community health professionals. They are competent to conduct a complete patient assessment including neurological examinations to screen for learning difficulties. Their functions include completing health histories, performing developmental and physical examinations (Fig. 5-13), conducting laboratory tests, managing minor illnesses and accidents, and health teaching and counseling.

The expanded role of the school nurse has met with a great deal of controversy. A recent 5-year study supported by the Robert Wood Johnson Foundation found that use of nurse practitioners in schools could improve the health care for children. However, not only is the cost considerably greater than is generally spent by school districts for nursing services,* but also questions have been raised as to whether schools should provide such services.

---

*Oda, D.: Cost documentation of school nursing follow-up services, Journal of School Health **56**:20-23, 1986; and Oda, D., Fine, J.T., and Heilbran, D.C.: Impact and cost of public health nurse telephone follow-up of school dental referrals, American Journal of Public Health **76**:1348-1349, 1986.

---

*American Public Health Association: School nurse practitioners: effective, but expensive, The Nation's Health July, 1985.

TEACHER-NURSE CONFERENCES

A recommended practice in elementary schools is for teachers and nurses to hold periodic meetings during the school year to share their observations and information about the health status of pupils. This helps in coordinating the health and educational needs of the student. A general session at the start of the school year followed by individual teacher meetings could be productive. Despite the significance and wide recognition of their need, they are not often held in many schools because of limited nurse service, time constraints, and other reasons. In general, the following are some reasons for these conferences:

1. To discuss the nature of teacher observations
2. To provide understanding of known health problems, such as diabetes, epilepsy, and heart conditions, and to make provisions for individual pupil needs
3. To help teachers know what action to take in emergencies to help pupils with known health problems, such as epilepsy and diabetes
4. To help teachers make appropriate adjustments in their classrooms and in school, such as having children sit in the front of the room or having them participate in limited activities
5. To make decisions about referral cases to parents for diagnosis, information, or other action
6. To help teachers with the techniques of discussing health problems with parents
7. To inform teachers about future examinations and screening tests
8. To help teachers identify ways to integrate health instruction into the health services program

Teacher observations serve as supplementary measures to the various screening procedures and examinations that take place in schools. They help identify pupils with health problems in the interval between medical examinations and identify children with problems who need special examinations. In schools that do not conduct periodic medical and dental examinations or expect parents to have children examined, teacher observations combined with screening tests and health inventories or histories, together with teacher-nurse conferences, may have to be used in substitution.

SUMMARY

A review of the various procedures for assessing the health of pupils indicates that the teacher should:

1. Become aware of the characteristics of good health and growth and development of students
2. Observe children for signs and symptoms of health deviations and be familiar with the school's procedures for handling pupils with problems
3. Understand the meaning and importance of medical and psychological examinations and observations, dental inspections, and other assessment procedures
4. Be familiar with a variety of screening tests and be prepared to help conduct several, such as growth and development tests and the Snellen test
5. Know the importance of health records in helping to understand the pupil better and realize it may be necessary to make periodic notations on these records
6. Be prepared on occasions, when appropriate or where nurse services may be limited or nonexistent, to discuss or counsel students and parents in regard to pupil health problems
7. Periodically meet with the school nurse to exchange information about pupils, learn about school adjustments for students, and obtain help with the health instruction program

The teacher should also realize that health appraisals offer numerous opportunities for health education:

1. Teaching about care of the eyes and ears

is appropriate when pupils are taking vision and hearing tests.

2. Health examinations and dental inspections can have their greatest impact when the instruction period coincides with the examinations or the inspections.

3. The control of communicable disease should be discussed when tuberculin tests are being administered.

4. Understanding about growth and development can be achieved more easily by relating this process to the periodic taking of heights and weights.

It should be apparent that the more the teacher knows about the health status of pupils the better qualified that teacher will be to understand them, to make necessary classroom and school adjustments, to provide functional health teaching, and to increase the effectiveness of the total educational program.

QUESTIONS FOR DISCUSSION

1. Why must schools be concerned with the health status of students?
2. What is the meaning of the term *health appraisals?*
3. What are the purposes of health appraisals?
4. What is the role of the teacher when observing the health status of children?
5. What are some of the signs and symptoms of pupils' health problems that teachers can observe?
6. What is the meaning of the term *learning disabilities*, how can a teacher identify such conditions, and what can be done to help children with these problems?
7. What are several of the communicable diseases that children may bring to school, and how may teachers recognize them?
8. Why are teacher-nurse conferences necessary and important?
9. What are the general categories of health screening tests used in schools, and why are they necessary?
10. What types of vision screening tests may be used in schools?
11. How is hearing tested, and who does it in schools?
12. What are the values, problems, and frequency of periodic height and weight measurements?
13. What is meant by tuberculin testing, and under what conditions should it be completed in schools?
14. What are dental inspections, and why are they valuable?
15. What is sickle cell disease, what are its signs and symptoms, and how can it be clinically identified?
16. What is diabetes, how can it clinically be identified, and what can schools and teachers do to help such children?

17. Who should administer medical examinations to pupils, and why should they take place?
18. How frequently and why should pupil medical examinations be conducted?
19. What are psychologic examinations and tests, and what can schools and teachers do to help discovered problem children?
20. What is the procedure used in screening for scoliosis and why is it important?
21. Why is scoliosis screening controversial?
22. What is the meaning of the term *nurse practitioners*, and how may they help children with health problems?
23. What is the role of the nurse in health appraisals?
24. How would you characterize the role of the teacher in health appraisals?

SELECTED REFERENCES

American Academy of Pediatrics, Committee on School Health: School health, a guide for health professionals, Evanston, Ill., 1981, The Academy.

American Lung Association: Your patient's risk of tuberculosis, New York, 1975, The Association.

Black, J.: AIDS, preschool and school issues, Journal of School Health **56**(3):93-95, 1986.

Cronin, G.E., and Young, W.: 400 navels, the future of school health in America, Bloomington, Ind., 1970, Phi Delta Kappa.

Edwards, D.D.: Toward safer scoliosis screening, Science News **128**:262 Oct., 1985.

Eisner, V., Oglesby, A., and Peck, E.B.: Health assessment of school children, VI. height and weight, Journal of School Health **42**(3):1972.

Food and Drug Administration: Labeling for salicylate-containing drug products, Federal Register **47**:57886-57901 Dec., 1982.

Freudenberg, N., et al.: The impact of bronchial asthma on school attendance and performance, Paper presented at the 1979 annual meeting of the American Public Health Association, New York, 1979.

Gortmaker, S.L., and Sappenfield, W.: Chronic childhood disorders: prevalence and impact, Pediatric Clinics of North America **31**:3-18, 1984.

Hertel, V., and Doyen, H.: Colorado school health guidelines, ed. 2, Denver, 1986, Colorado Department of Education and Colorado Department of Education.

Holtzhauer, F.J., et al.: Reye's syndrome, American Journal of Diseases of Children **140**(12):1231-1236, 1986.

Johnson, R.B., and Magrab, P.: Developmental disorders, Austin, Tex., 1978, Proed, Inc.

Kirby, D.: Comprehensive school-based health clinics; a growing movement to improve adolescent health and reduce teen-age pregnancy, Journal of School Health **56**(7):289-291, 1986.

Kort, M.: The delivery of primary health care in American public schools, 1890-1980, Journal of School Health **54**(1):453-457, 1984.

Lovick, S.R., and Wesson, W.F.: School-based clinics: update, 1986, Washington, D.C., 1986, Center for Population Options.

Monheit, B.M., and Norris, M.M.: Is combing the answer to headlice? Journal of School Health **56**(9)158-159, 1986.

Morais, T., Bernier, M., and Turcotte, F.: Age- and sex-specific prevalence of scoliosis and the value of school screening programs, American Journal of Public Health **75**(12):1377-1380, 1985.

Nadar, P.: AIDS: a commentary, Journal of School Health **56**(3):107-108, 1986.

National Education Association: Recommended guidelines for dealing with AIDS in the schools, Journal of School Health **56**(4):129-130, 1986.

National Society to Prevent Blindness: Vision screening for children, New York, 1980, The Society.

Oda, D.: Cost documentation of school nursing follow-up services, Journal of School Health **56**(1):20-23, 1986.

Oda, D., Fine, J.T., and Heilbran, D.C.: Impact and cost of public health nurse telephone follow-up of school dental referrals, American Journal of Public Health **76**(11):1348-1349, 1986.

Parcel, G.S., Silman, S., Nader, P., et al.: A comparison of absenteeism rates of elementary school children with asthma and nonasthmatic schoolmates, Pediatrics **64**:878-881, 1979.

Pine, P.: Promoting health education in schools: problems and solutions, Arlington, Va., 1985, American Association of School Administrators Critical Issues Report.

Price, J.: AIDS, the schools and policy issues, Journal of School Health **56**(4):137-140, 1986.

Reinert, H.R.: Children in conflict, ed. 2, St. Louis, 1980, The C.V. Mosby Co.

Richards, W.: Allergy, asthma, and school problems, Journal of School Health **56**(4):4-6, 1986.

Robert Wood Johnson Foundation: National school health services program, Spec. Rep. No. 1, Princeton, N.J., 1985, The Foundation.

Shea, S., and Marguiles, D.: The paperless medical record, Social Science and Medicine **21**:741-746, 1985.

Toolief, M.S., et al.: Pneumocystic carinii pneumonia and mucosal candidiais in previously healthy homosexual men, evidence of a new acquired cellular immunodeficiency, New England Journal of Medicine **305**:1425-1431, 1981.

U.S. Department of Health, Education, and Welfare: Asthma and other allergic diseases, Pub. No. 79-387, Washington, D.C., 1979, National Institutes of Health.

U.S. Department of Health, Education, and Welfare, Public Health Service, National Center for Health Statistics: Color vision deficiencies in children, United States, Washington, D.C., 1972, U.S. Government Printing Office.

Wilson, C.E.: School health services, Washington, D.C., 1964, Joint Committee on Health Problems in Schools of the NEA and the AMA.

Wood, S.P., Walker, D.K., Gardher, J.: School health practices for children with complex medical needs, Journal of School Health **56**(6):215-217, 1986.

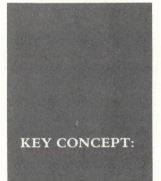

CHAPTER

6

HEALTH GUIDANCE

Parents or guardians have primary responsibility for the health care of their children.

AMERICAN ACADEMY OF PEDIATRICS

KEY CONCEPT: Helping students resolve health problems and make adjustments in school involves guidance in which teachers, other school personnel, and community resources are utilized.

The health problems of school-age children involve a broad spectrum of social, emotional, behavioral, and technological issues that requires a complex range of services delivered by various individuals and systems in a flexible, coordinated manner.* Identification of children with health problems such as vision and hearing deficiencies, undernourishment, malnutrition, overeating, dental decay, emotional disturbances, skin infections, and heart disease, all of which have an impact on student learning, clearly indicates that schools should become involved in providing assistance for children with these problems. The decision by schools

whether to aid in the improvement of students' levels of wellness should be obvious since many parents are not aware of or do not give adequate attention to their children's health problems. Failure to give attention to discovered pupil conditions may interfere with educational experiences and adversely affect learning. Many schools therefore have assumed the responsibility of providing help to students and parents. The methods used are part of the school health services program and are referred to as *follow-up* or *guidance procedures*. They include guidance and counseling, use of community health resources, and adjustment of school programs. The emphasis in this chapter is on the guidance and counseling aspects.

The most important part of the health services program, and the one given least attention, is

*U.S. Department of Health and Human Services, Division of Maternal and Child Health: Perspectives on the health of school-age children: expectations for the future, staff paper, Washington, D.C., 1982.

the follow-up phase. Schools on the whole do not provide enough nurse time and effort to obtain the needed corrective action by students and parents. By way of illustration, Griffith and Whicker* in a study of one school district in North Carolina reemphasized the need for more attention to follow-up activities. They found that over a 6-year period the school district was able to obtain corrections for its problem children at an average rate of 43%. However, when additional nurse time, nurse aides, and teacher cooperation were tried in an experimental year, the district was able to increase this rate to 66%.

WHAT IS HEALTH GUIDANCE?

Health guidance in schools is a broad term that refers to a variety of processes involving the interaction of school and community health personnel, students, and parents who aid in the discovery, understanding, and resolution of health matters through self-effort and self-direction. Health guidance includes those activities in which individuals participate voluntarily in incidental, individual, or small-group counseling or in "rap" sessions to obtain information regarding health concerns or to seek solutions to health problems. It involves communication with parents to encourage and persuade them to take action. The general aim of health guidance is to enable pupils to acquire the highest levels of wellness in accordance with their individual needs. The goal of health guidance is self-understanding and self-direction. Guidance plays an important role in *primary prevention* (before a condition arises) and in *secondary prevention* (after a condition has been discovered). (See Chapter 1.)

Health guidance involves the use of health appraisals and health records; more specifically, it involves counseling to provide information and aid in regard to health problems, immunizations, reports of health examinations, program adjustments, identification of community health resources, relations between pupils and parents with medical, dental, and other health specialists, and numerous other matters. Its objective is not to give advice but to encourage, motivate, and help individuals achieve good health through their own efforts. It is purposeful action and organized effort directed toward intelligent decision making regarding corrections, care, service, treatment, and assistance. It is educational in nature.

Opportunities for health guidance exist in the *formal school health education program*. However, they are not discussed in this chapter. The procedures used in the formal program may be considered to be group guidance methods. Pupils' requests for informal assistance often arise from the formal program. Chapters 9 to 13 and Appendix B on organizing, learning, and teaching techniques provide numerous suggestions for helping students in the classroom in a group or formal setting.

Following health appraisals, the educational procedures used in guidance are frequently referred to as *health counseling*. Health counseling focuses on helping a given individual promote his or her own well-being. This counseling is the direct personal contact between students or parents and counselors (nurses, teachers, physicians, and others) for the purpose of interpreting the nature and significance of a student's health problem. The focus of the discussion should be to provide information and understanding so that the student or the parents can formulate a plan of action that will lead to a solution of the problem.

The results of screening procedures or medical examinations are often reported to parents on cold, impersonal preprinted forms that may read somthing like:

Dear parent: On February 14, your child, John, was screened for possible visual problems. This screening revealed a visual problem that could interfere with John's health and school work. We recommend that you take John to an ophthalmologist for further diagnosis and whatever treatment is recommended.

---

*Griffith, B.B., and Whicker, P.H.: Teacher—observer of student health problems, Journal of School Health **51**:428-432 Aug., 1981.

Clearly this message has several major short-comings:

1. It may not be given to the parents by the student.

2. If it is given to the parents, they may not read it.

3. If it is read, it may be misunderstood.

4. There is no explanation or interpretation of what was found during the screening.

5. The importance of the message may not be clear and thus may not motivate the parents to take additional action.

6. There is no provision for knowing if additional action was taken by the parents.

Whereas making referrals is an important aspect of a school nurse's role, it is also one of the areas more often neglected. However, referral alone is not enough. It is important that the nurse counsel and consult with teachers, parents, and pupils, both in groups and individually. Nurses, teachers, or other school personnel should always use the appropriate moment to aid any student facing a health problem or emotional crisis. This process may be identified as the *informal school health education program*.

Informal health education

Informal health education must receive greater emphasis in schools if educational programs are to meet adequately the differing health needs of children and youth. It is a phase of the school health education program that has been neglected and has generally been thought to be the responsibility of the nurse. A great deal of such education has occurred accidentally.

Although the nurse is an important contact person, the nurse's time in school is often limited. Also, there are others who can provide assistance. On occasion, students require special, individual attention that cannot be obtained from a formal health education program. These young people need and often desire someone, some group, or some way in schools to be able to discuss concerns and interests about sex, drugs, personality development, stress and pressure, self-care, parent problems, and other

health matters. Some young people may wish to talk to their peers about their problems or about where to obtain help in solving problems. The school nurse, a teacher, a counselor, the school psychologist, or someone who will listen in a nonjudgmental fashion and have empathy for student concerns might also help. Informal health education needs to be recognized and established in schools. It would be helpful in secondary prevention of health problems and also could serve a useful purpose in primary prevention.

Informal education is learning that takes place without structure and without much planning. It may occur in the classroom, in the nurse's office, or in other school locations. It may take place in a meeting with a parent or pupil, or by telephone, note, letter sent home, or other procedure. It may take place outside the school, in the home, watching TV, talking with a parent, friend, or neighbor, reading a magazine or newspaper, or through a variety of activities. It usually occurs on a one-to-one basis or in small groups. It is a communication procedure that provides information, counseling, and guidance that is nondirective and nonthreatening to students and voluntary in terms of participation.

Implementation of informal health education may occur in a variety of ways. A student may ask a teacher a question about health or about what action to be taken because of the sudden appearance of a skin rash. A pupil visits the nurse for information and guidance in terms of excess weight, a severe cold, or fear of one or more aggressive students. The nurse, counselor, or other person encourages children and youth to make visitations to discuss health problems or concerns whenever they are free, at the noon hour, or in after-school rap sessions. The school newspaper prints articles written by students on student health problems. The nurse makes pamphlets and publications available to students. Special voluntary educational programs on drugs, sexually transmitted diseases, teenage pregnancies, and emotional problems may be held as needs arise. Parent-teacher-nurse conferences are planned.

What are the purposes of health guidance?

Health guidance seeks to achieve the following:

1. Provide information about and interpretations of pupils' health status, concerns, or problems
2. Provide information to parents of the nature of the health conditions that exist in their children and to encourage needed care (Fig. 6-1)
3. Promote pupils' acceptance of the responsibility for the promotion and preservation of their own health
4. Motivate parents and pupils to seek care and treatment when needed for existing health conditions and to accept modifications in the school program where desirable
5. Encourage and promote where necessary the establishment or expansion of school and community health service and facilities especially for needy children and families
6. Encourage pupils and parents to use available medical, dental, and other health resources to the best advantage
7. Contribute to the health education of pupils and parents in both formal and informal settings
8. Assist in the adaptation of school programs to the individual needs and abilities of students with health problems; to keep teachers informed
9. Inform teachers of pupils' health problems and concerns and to identify responsibilities
10. Work with community groups to assure availability of treatment facilities for all children

What are the general problems for which children need health guidance?

Children's health problems requiring guidance may be categorized in the following manner:

In some situations *more detailed examination* of the child is needed to establish a diagnosis. Observations of signs and symptoms might ne-

FIG. 6-1. Follow-up is part of health service.

cessitate a tuberculin test or a chest x-ray examination for tuberculosis, special tests for a heart murmur, a blood count for anemia; a urinalysis for diabetes; a medical examination when chronic fatigue, overweight, frequent colds, and blackouts are noted; or a dental examination for decay or periodontal disease.

There are some conditions for which the child needs *treatment services*, such as undernourishment, malnutrition, overfeeding, epilepsy, dental decay, vision and hearing difficulties, skin infections, diseased tonsils, or allergies.

There are conditions that need *home care improvement*. These may include the need for breakfast or help with balanced lunches, cleanliness, dental care, proper clothing, or better sleeping facilities.

Problems of emotional and social adjustment may make *special counseling* mandatory. Opportunities to talk with understanding people may be most helpful to students. Teachers who have success communicating with pupils may be able to assist them with their problems regarding the abuse and use of drugs. It also may be necessary to interpret the emotional problem to parents to encourage their seeking additional help. These problems often are difficult and delicate to present to parents.

For some problems, *assistance regarding health practices and behavior* is advisable. This might call for individual discussions with students regarding covering noses and mouths when coughing and sneezing, the importance of washing the hands before eating and after using the lavatory, the abuse of drugs, using the drinking fountains properly, remaining at home when ill, eating breakfast, and what to do about sexually transmitted diseases. Some of these matters may also involve parental communication and should be handled discreetly.

ORGANIZATION FOR SCHOOL HEALTH GUIDANCE

Although practically all schools provide some health guidance, in most cases it is done on an incidental basis. Schools in general do not have well-organized and well-developed health guidance programs, as identified in this chapter. In elementary schools the nurse is usually the key person in the counseling program. Where health guidance does exist on an organized basis, it has been found that best results accrue when the program is carried out cooperatively; all departments and personnel of a school concerned with any phase of mental, emotional, and physical health of children should cooperate and participate in the formulation of health guidance policies. Objectives and responsibilities need clear definition.

Organized health guidance programs may be considered a relatively new development; therefore it may be well to consider some of the fundamental factors that are basic to sound organization. In this respect, it seems essential that recognition be given to such factors as (1) desirable principles of operation, (2) role of the in-

dividual who counsels, (3) responsibilities of various school personnel, (4) nurse-teacher/nurse-teacher-parent conferences, (5) techniques for counseling, and (6) use of prescribed medications at school.

Desirable principles of operation

As in other functions of the school, health guidance should be based on certain fundamental principles for effective operation. The following generalized list may serve as a guide for the establishment of such principles in local school situations:

1. The health guidance program should complement and supplement the total educational program within the school.

2. The health program should be such that it serves individual pupil needs.

3. The health guidance program should have the wholehearted support of the school administrators.

4. Policies and procedures in written form identifying purposes and responsibilities of personnel should be provided.

5. School staff members responsible for health guidance programs should be knowledgeable about community agencies and specialists available for referral purposes.

6. The objectives of the health guidance program should be communicated to parents, teachers, and others.

7. Some means of in-service training in health guidance should be provided for teachers, administrators, and other members of the school personnel whenever necessary or advisable.

8. There should be full cooperation and coordination of all school departments concerned with the health of pupils.

9. The purposes and scope of each school department concerned with child health should be clearly defined to assure the most efficient service to pupils.

10. Responsibility for leadership in the health guidance program should be centered in individuals who possess, insofar as possible, interest, ability, and preparation for such service.

11. The best possible procedures for effective school and community coordination in health guidance should be provided.

12. The health guidance program should be subjected to constant and continuous evaluation so that constructive improvements may be effected (see Appendix H).

13. All health guidance personnel should be encouraged to keep abreast of the latest research and changing conditions as they relate to their specific health area.

Role of the individual who counsels

The responsibility for counseling involves a variety of school personnel including teachers, nurses, physicians, psychologists, principals, counselors, and students. Although there is no single correct philosophy or way to counsel, the person who participates as a counselor and is involved in human relations should know how to identify an individual in need of assistance and be competent to interpret findings to pupils and parents and to encourage and motivate them to action. Since parents have the primary responsibility for the health of their children, school personnel should not try to tell them how their children should be raised. School personnel should attempt to acquaint parents with the health conditions of pupils that require attention, interpret the importance of care especially as it relates to learning, and inform parents regarding the nature of community health services and the necessary adjustments of the school program.

School personnel should understand the cultural heritage and customs of blacks, native Americans, Mexican Americans, and those of other ethnic backgrounds, and some personnel should be conversant in the different languages for effective communication.

Responsibilities of various school personnel

One of the principles previously mentioned suggested that the responsibilities of all concerned with the health of pupils should be clearly defined and designated. This statement should perhaps be amplified to the extent that *every* person in the school system should accept responsibility for the health guidance of the school population. In other words, every person associated with the school should have the physical, spiritual, mental, and social well-being of pupils as a major concern. The fact that pupils' academic and nonacademic interests relate to their physical and mental health cannot be overstressed. For example, the child who is fatigued, hungry, or unable to understand why people do not want him or her around may have difficulty concentrating on learning.

Although all school personnel rightfully should take an interest in health guidance of pupils, the extent of responsibilities naturally must vary. Someone should be available in schools with whom students are able to communicate when necessary about health matters, but especially regarding sexually transmitted diseases, drugs, human sexuality, pregnancies, and home and school problems. This might be the nurse or a teacher or some other knowledgeable, capable individual. The following discussion indicates some of the more or less specific responsibilities of various school personnel depending somewhat on the size and existing conditions within the individual school system.

School administrators and officers. The responsibilities of the school board member, superintendent, and principal of the school within the community center on the leadership necessary to carry out a successful health guidance program. These individuals actually have the final vote of approval concerning the budgetary needs, the acquisition of new equipment, and the hiring of personnel. It should be strongly emphasized that these health services will entail a cooperative kind of leadership in which the administrator plans with the school staff on matters pertaining to the broad scope of the program. It is obvious that continued pooling of the competencies of mental health professionals and educators will be needed to achieve the related goals of better mental health and effective learning for more school children.

School administrators need to have adequate

knowledge of the objectives of the program, because they are usually the liaison persons between the school and the community and are expected to interpret program objectives. In addition, administrators should initiate plans for the coordination of school and community relationships and strive to maintain the highest standards for total school health. They may also need to initiate community action to help with the provision of comprehensive health care services, especially for children in poverty areas.

Health service personnel. One of the main responsibilities of the school physician, school nurse, school dentist, and others in health service is concerned with helping youths who exhibit health needs. Regular follow-up is necessary. For example, certain pertinent information derived from examinations by the school physician can be relayed to teachers and guidance counselors through the proper channels. More and more use is being made of the case study method whereby those people directly working with a child meet and discuss their findings. The various reports add to the separate impressions, and the goal of assisting in the development of the whole child is more fully realized. In other cases either the school nurse or school social worker serves as a direct link between the home and school. The nurse or social worker is in a desirable position to refer information to guidance counselors and teachers that may reveal physical, mental, and emotional health problems that arise out of home situations.

School physician. The practice of medicine in schools is a specialized area requiring expertise in identifying, observing, managing, and preventing health problems in the school setting.* School physicians must be familiar with the total school health program, not just the services component. Unlike clinical practice wherein the physician-patient relationship is the focus, the school physician is a member of a total team and often must work in a physician-group relationship.

---

*American School Health Association, Physician Study Committee: Today's school physician: a horse of a different color, Journal of School Health **52**(10):619-620, 1982.

A physician has more latitude in health matters than other school personnel and is a valuable member of the total school health team. Although a variety of job descriptions may exist, in general, the school physician may become involved in any or all of the following:
1. Administrative activities including development of health policies, procedures, and forms
2. Liaison activities between the school and the medical community, parents, and other child- or health-oriented groups
3. Consultation with school nurses regarding their health service activities
4. Consultation with teachers regarding health concerns and health education activities
5. Involvement in special education programs, including diagnostic assessment of students and interpretation of the findings for other staff professionals regarding school placement; in-service training of staff
6. Involvement in employee health programs such as mental health, physical examinations, control of communicable disease, and employee assistance
7. Attention to environmental health in the school setting for both students and employees
8. Participation in school programs such as drug and alcohol use and abuse and student behavior

School nurse. The work of the school nurse continues to gain importance in the school health program. The committee on School Health Service of the World Health Organization states that nurses, like physicians, have a different type of task when they work within the framework of the school, for it is not the clinical situation to which they have been accustomed in their hospital experiences. It is a new kind of experience, one with children to whom these nurses must bring warmth, acceptance, and understanding. Nurses must direct their energies to the educational goals of the school and remember they are not in a hospital setting. To the teacher the nurse must be a source of information and guidance. To the parent the nurse must be a friendly counselor cognizant of com-

FIG. 6-2. Nurse/parent/student conference—part of health guidance.

munity resources, sympathetic with family problems, and an interpreter par excellence of the child's needs as revealed by medical examination and school behavior.

Although the responsibilities and duties of school nurses are numerous and varied, special emphasis should be placed on their part in health guidance. The following list summarizes some of the ways the school nurse contributes to the health guidance program:

1. Keeping individual health records up to date for general use and for specific use when health counseling is indicated
2. Assisting with examinations and inspections that may reveal a need for guidance and counseling
3. Interpreting the results of health appraisals to pupils, teachers, and parents (Fig. 6-2)
4. Providing information and direction concerning community resources available for the care of physical, mental, and emotional problems of children
5. Helping motivate pupils to develop and maintain optimum health
6. Helping children to find solutions to their personal problems, particularly those involving or likely to involve physical, mental, and emotional health
7. Assisting in the identification of pupils needing modified education programs
8. Counseling pupils with health problems
9. Counseling parents concerning the health problems of children
10. Serving as a liaison between home, school, and community organizations and agencies
11. Providing care in emergencies and accidents
12. Participating in formal and informal health education

The role of the school nurse is changing. As early as 1974, Oda identified expanding school nurse duties that include the following*:

1. Greater stress on health education, counseling, and consultation
2. Emergence as a school nurse practitioner in which special training is providing competency to conduct in-depth assessment of physical, psychomedical, and psychoeducational behavior and learning disorders of children
3. Involvement in the development, implementation, and evaluation of health care plans and programs

---

*Oda, D.S.: Increasing role effectiveness of school nurses, American Journal of Public Health 64:June, 1974.

4. Use of increased technological health assessment skills

The expectations expressed by Oda are now a central part of the school nurse's duties. In studying the current activities of school nurse practice, White* identified five basic clusters of nursing activity: physical care, facilitation, instruction, administration, and clerical.

The number of nurses including school nurse practitioners found in schools varies because standards are not uniform or consistent throughout the United States. Ideally it is advisable to have a full-time nurse in every elementary school, but at the present time districts cannot afford this action. It is generally believed there should be one nurse for every 800 to 1,200 pupils. However, common practices differ widely. Many schools have no nurse services, and in others nurses are limited to one-half day weekly. Because there are so few school nurse practitioners and their usage and experience is so limited, no standard has been established regarding how many should be found in schools. In recent years nurse services have been eliminated in some districts because of budget limitations. The quality of the health services programs in these districts undoubtedly has been lowered because of this action.

Some school districts are using nonprofessional *health aides* to assist school nurses. These individuals may perform a variety of clerical responsibilities such as answering the telephone, entering data in health records, and arranging schedules. These individuals may be volunteers and occasionally are paid employees. Health aides free nurses from certain routine procedures, allowing them to devote more time to professional duties.

Health coordinator. The person assuming the responsibilities of school health coordinator should be professionally trained in health and should direct, supervise, and coordinate all activities concerning the health of students. The success or failure of health guidance programs may depend on the extent to which proper use

*White, D.H.: A study of current school nurse practice activities, Journal of School Health 55(2):52-56, 1985.

of information is made. For example, many schools have an excellent program of health appraisal, yet they do not have adequate organization or ways or means of following up the findings of the appraisals. The school health coordinator should fill any gaps that may exist by coordinating all information that might be used to guide the pupil in health matters. This person should be well informed about the total school health program as presented in Chapter 1.

Another important function of the school health coordinator is that of conducting needed research. All too often records are kept and up-to-date entries made so that the pupils' growth and development are charted, but little if any attempt made to use the data for study purposes. The analysis of records could certainly aid in pointing out trends; changes in physical, social, and emotional patterns of both boys and girls; and the limitations of the school's health program.

Unfortunately, health coordinators per se are not commonly employed in school districts. Where they are found, these individuals may be nurses, physicians, health educators, or others.

Guidance personnel. Guidance directors, psychometrists, and other guidance personnel have the responsibility of helping pupils in their efforts to handle their health problems. If counselors and others expect to have pupils referred to them for individual help, then a knowledge of the objectives of the health guidance program is essential. They should have not only sufficient background in the psychodynamics of behavior, but also an understanding of health education, since most of the problems found among children involve, either directly or indirectly, physical, mental, social, or emotional health. Counselors may also contribute to the health guidance program by offering in-service education to teachers and other school personnel with respect to the counseling methods that would be most effective for those pupils needing counseling and guidance.

Because guidance personnel are generally involved in a helping relationship, children, parents, teachers, and others often share with them various types of personal concerns, some of which may relate to the school environment. It is possible, without breaking confidence, for guidance personnel to assist in calling attention to health problems that are not receiving care.

School psychologist. In school systems in which the services of a psychologist are available, many contributions can be made to the health guidance program by the person serving in this capacity. At the present time one of the major functions of the school psychologist is more like that of a psychometrist—administering group and individual psychological tests. In addition to this primary function, many school psychologists confer with parents and teachers about individual pupils with problems that particularly concern emotional health. The school psychologist should be in close contact with the school administrators, school physician, school nurse, school social worker, teachers, and family physicians and psychiatrists who may be in a position to act on his or her recommendations regarding children who are in need of adjustment to problems that concern their health. Although most school personnel have taken course work in the area of the behavioral sciences, the school psychologist can be most helpful in aiding in the understanding of unusual behavioral patterns. Often the school psychologist will administer various types of tests and submit a report of these findings for the school to keep on record. Since these reports are more often than not psychologically descriptive, care must be taken in their use and circulation.

Elementary school teachers. Classroom teachers are actually the heart of a successful health guidance program at the elementary school level. As mentioned previously, in the majority of cases elementary school teachers are in a position to observe pupils daily. It becomes their responsibility to detect physical, social, and emotional behavior patterns that are unusual and refer them to the nurses, physicians, and administrators. Elementary teachers probably are the most important people, outside of the family, in providing for the cultivation of health attitudes and values through the health instruction program. The student will seek out the teacher for information if communication has been established in incidental and informal settings.

The elementary teacher contributes to the health guidance program by*:

1. Participating in school health appraisals, orienting students about the appraisals, and using the findings to discuss health with children
2. Providing educational information to medical and other guidance personnel
3. Listening to students and trying to assist them in clarifying and understanding any health problems they may face
4. Observing for sudden or gradual changes in child appearance or behavior and referring children suspected of having health problems (see Table 5-1 and Appendix J).
5. Contributing to the child's school records
6. Developing a good emotional climate for learning
7. Respecting students' needs and helping them develop a sense of their own well-being
8. Aiding in adapting the school program to meet the needs of the physically challenged student
9. Aiding in follow-up and referring of students
10. Assisting in interpreting for parents the significance and results of health appraisals

As a counselor, these things should be avoided:

1. Trying to diagnose or prescribe treatment
2. Taking the decision making away from the students and parents relative to what to do about a health problem
3. Suggesting only one way to resolve a health problem
4. Embarassing the child, especially in front of others
5. Ridiculing the child or the child's parents
6. Arguing basic value systems such as religion and culture as they relate to health problem resolution

---

*King, L.S., and Dodd, N.: The health educator as counselor; what does it take? Health Education **17**(2):17-22, 1986.

7. Conveying a judgmental or condescending attitude

Special teachers. Teachers dealing with special groups, as in rehabilitation, special education, and the various special subjects (physical education, home economics, and health education), definitely have considerable responsibility in all matters of pupil health, including health guidance, since they ordinarily come in close contact with situations that deal with health status. For instance, the physical education teacher has an opportunity to observe the growth and development of pupils as well as peer acceptance of the group members. Whether physical educators are aware of their responsibility for health guidance has been questioned, but it is the feeling that physical development should not be their only concern.

Drug counselor. A person known as a drug counselor has been available to students in some upper elementary and junior and senior high schools in recent years. This person may be considered to be a counselor with responsibilities related to drugs and drug use. The duties of the drug counselor may include communication with drug users, misusers, and abusers; student and parent guidance; liaison with community resources, including the police and the courts; and the preparation of policies and procedures for the school or school district. This individual should be one who is approachable by students, readily available and accessible, willing to talk and not preach, honest and trustful in approach, willing to discuss any topic of interest to pupils, and knowledgeable about the drug scene.

Students. There have been a variety of attempts by schools to use student peers to try to help pupils with drug problems. Upper elementary school youths have made formal presentations to sixth graders and other students in their own schools. They have also been available for indirect, informal individual and group meetings. Students who are familiar with drugs have been able on occasion to establish rapport with drug abusers. The value of such activities has not been clearly defined, but indications reveal they create interest and enthusiasm on the part of both the participants and the performers. The use of students in a variety of health counseling situations therefore should receive greater consideration and experimentation in schools. The problem of communication of misinformation, however, must be recognized and avoided. Success with this type of program depends on extensive training of peer educators and careful planning by program developers.*

Nurse-teacher/nurse-teacher-parent conferences

Casefinding and follow-up in the interest of the child requires a three-cornered arrangement—nurse or medical professional, teacher and parent. The absence of participation of any one of these members makes effective action on behalf of the child much less likely.

George A. Silver, M.D.†
Professor of Public Health,
Yale University School
of Medicine

The need for communication within as well as between the school and the home is clearly identified in Dr. Silver's remarks. He adds that nurse-teacher conferences are the exception rather than the general practice. He states that nurse-parent-teacher conferences rarely, if ever, occur. Unquestionably, limitations of nurse services in many schools, extensive teacher responsibilities, and the fact that more than 50% of mothers are working are factors that make the problem more complicated (see Chapter 4). In any event, it should be evident that effective guidance of pupils is not going to take place without improved communication procedures. Perhaps teachers will need to take more initiative in attempting to overcome the problems that interfere with this communication by assuming greater responsibility if the health needs of their pupils are to receive adequate attention.

Conferences may be planned or unplanned.

---

*Steinhause, G.W.: Peer education programs; a look nationally, Health Education **14**:7-8,10, 1983.
†Silver, G.A.: Redefining school work health services: comprehensive child health care as the framework, Journal of School Health **51**:157-162 March, 1981.

In planned nurse-teacher conferences, the nurse should:

1. Review each student's record in conjunction with teacher observations, and interpret recommendations and adjustments as indicated for each student
2. Plan for those students needing follow-up care; the teacher can be a valuable ally in contact with parents, especially through observation of the students and knowledge of each student's behavior in the class situation
3. Stimulate interest in health teaching utilizing screening procedures or the apparent needs of the student as educational experiences.
4. Help the teacher plan and evaluate classroom health programs and discuss availability of health education material
5. Adopt a plan for notifying the teacher of nurse follow-up on individual cases*

These basic procedures for planned teacher conferences also apply to parent meetings, but the focus must be on the individual student. The nurse or teacher should also be prepared to deal with the student or parent who just drops in to chat about various health-related matters.

Techniques for counseling

Although there is no best way to counsel, the specific procedures for communicating with students and parents include informal and formal talks, notes home, home and school visits with parents, and telephone calls.

These are the basic principles to be followed when counseling†:

1. Start where counselees are and accept them as they are
2. Treat each individual with respect and recognize the individual's potential for growth
3. Do not moralize, preach, or impose on counselees personal values, the values of the institution, or those of society

4. The key to successful or effective counseling is nonevaluative listening

When teachers counsel parents or students, or both, the following suggestions should receive consideration:

1. Try to develop rapport and thereby improve the effectiveness of the communication. Attempt to be friendly and nonofficious in approach. Demonstrate sincerity in wanting to be helpful. Create the feeling that information and aid, if desired, is the intent of the meeting. Refrain from telling the parent or student what action to take; ideally a request for help will be forthcoming. Be familiar with differences in values and cultural conflicts without becoming judgmental. Permit cultural identification to emerge in the development of a source of pride.

2. Help parents and pupils analyze or recognize the problem. A child's heart murmur may be threatening to the parents and frightening to the child. Although this condition is abnormal and may be serious, it may not be serious for that particular child. Only medical help can determine the extent of the problem.

3. Help parents and pupils understand the nature and significance of the problem by encouraging questions and by supplying information as requested. Be certain understanding and clarity occur.

4. Help parents and pupils determine the various courses of action to be taken and discuss the consequences. The solution may be relatively simple if parents have a family physician. However, if parents do not know where to go or do not have a physician or the funds, resolution of the problem may be more complex.

5. Encourage parents and students to choose a particular course of action, but indicate that the decision will rest with them.

Cormier and others* suggest these behaviors

1. Speak in a soft, soothing voice
2. Smile and look interested

---

*From: Colorado School Health Guidelines, ed. 2, Denver, 1986, Colorado Department of Education and Colorado Department of Health.
†Litwack, L., Litwack, J., and Ballou, M.: Health counseling, New York, 1980, Appleton-Century-Crofts.

---

*Cormier, L., Cormier, W., and Weisser, R.: Interviewing and helping skills for health professionals, Monterey, Cal., 1984, Wadsworth Publishing Co.

3. Lean toward the student keeping a relaxed posture
4. Look directly into the student's eyes
5. Make sure gestures are open and welcoming
6. Keep a close physical proximity

When contacting parents about student health problems that are not unusual, such as vision or hearing difficulties, the school nurse may send home a form notice because it is the quickest and easiest way to communicate with a large number of parents. The limitations of this procedure have been previously discussed and suggest that the procedures used to get in touch with parents must receive careful consideration, especially if the health problem is other than a routine matter (see pp. 110-111).

From recent studies on effective ways of communicating with parents to get action, it has been found that children of parents at high socioeconomic levels are more likely to receive attention than those at low socioeconomic levels; children whose parents give defects a high urgency rating are more likely to receive attention; notification about a child's defect by more than one contact technique (written notice, telephone call, home or school visit, and others) is more likely to secure attention than if parents are notified by one contact only. Those contacts involving personal interaction by telephone or visitation are significantly more productive than those using a written medium. Also, parents who receive two notifications of children's defects are more likely to pay attention than parents who receive only one notification. Three notifications do not appear to be worth the effort.

Research findings conclude the most effective techniques of communication for parent action are notices written by a physician and telephone calls by school nurses. However, a study in San Diego* of sixth grade pupils revealed that the face-to-face contact by a home call or a nurse-parent conference at school or at the parent's place of work resulted in over 70% of defects

identified through health appraisals receiving attention.

Prescribed medications at school

Many students with chronic health problems and others attending school are expected or required to take physician-prescribed or nonprescription medications during school hours. Because school personnel must oversee the administration of medication to students, the problems of liability arise. Errors in judgment, including use of a wrong drug, a wrong dosage or not keeping an exact schedule and record of the administration of the medications to various students contribute to the problem. It is therefore necessary for schools to establish written policies and procedures.

A study completed by Kinnison and Nimmer* revealed that fewer than 32% of the school districts reporting (48 of 159) had developed policies that dealt with the administration of medication at school. In 1974 Appleman† surveyed all 50 states. Of the 43 states that responded to the survey, only 3 had laws, 4 had regulations, and 6 had guidelines related to this issue. As recent as 1982 only 16 states had legislatively dealt with this problem.‡ According to the American Academy of Pediatrics:

Opportunities should be provided for communication between the parent, school personnel and physician regarding the efficacy of the medication administered during school hours.§

The purposes of having a written policy concerning prescription or nonprescription medications include: (1) to assure that exact instruc-

---

*Brophy, H.E.: Project pursuit: a health defect follow-up activity, Journal of School Health **40**:April, 1970.

*Kinnison, L.R., and Nimmer, D.N.: An analysis of policies regulating medication in the schools, Journal of School Health **49**:280-283, 1979.

†Appleman, M.A.: The legal issues involved in the use of stimulants on hyperactive school children, doctoral dissertation, University of Minnesota, 1974.

‡Courtnage, L.: Managing medication in the schools; a survey of state policies, Exceptional Child **49**:75, 1982.

§American Academy of Pediatrics: School health, a guide for health professions, Evanston, Ill. 1981, The Academy.

STATE COLLEGE AREA SCHOOL DISTRICT

Pupil Personnel Services
Health Services

PARENTAL REQUEST AND PHYSICIAN'S ORDER FOR MEDICATION

(For students who require medication during school hours)

Parents have the primary responsibility for the health of their child. Prescribed medication, for a specific illness and time period as indicated on a written order by the family physician, is required during school hours. If parents wish to delegate some part of their responsibility to the school, the following will apply:

Principal or designee stores medication, with the prescription label, in a secure place for the period indicated on the physician's order.

Children in kindergarten and first grade are taken to the office by their teacher or an aide or are sent to the office to get the medication from the designated person, but they take it themselves *whenever possible.* Any child *who is able* should be responsible for going to the office, obtaining the medication, taking the medication, and returning it to the designated person.

At the end of the school year, the parent is expected to pick up unused medication. Medication not picked up by the last day of school will be destroyed.

As a general rule, and if at all possible, medication should be taken at home. All reasonable precautions will be taken in storing the student's medication. Non-prescription medication, self-administered by a child during school hours, is totally the parent's responsibility.

TO BE COMPLETED BY PARENT/GUARDIAN:

Child's Name _____ Birthdate _____ School_____

I request that medication for my child (named above) be stored or administered as indicated in the physician's order below. I am aware that non-medical personnel may be administering this medication to my child. We hereby release the State College Area School District and all of its employees of and from any and all liability in law for damages either we or our child may suffer as a result of this request.

_____ Home: _____ Work: _____ Date _____
Parent/Guardian Signature   Telephone

TO BE COMPLETED BY PHYSICIAN:

IT IS NECESSARY THAT THE NAMED CHILD RECEIVE THE FOLLOWING MEDICATION AT THE TIMES STATED BELOW. PLEASE STORE OR ADMINISTER THE FOLLOWING AS DIRECTED BELOW:

_____ _____ _____
Name and Form of Medication   Dosage   Times to be Given

Route of Administration _____

Other Specific Directions _____

Purpose of Medication and/or Diagnosis _____

Side Effects to Watch For _____

Duration of Order _____

_____ _____ _____
Telephone   Physician's Name (please type)   Physician's Signature   Date

FIG. 6-3. Parental request and physician's order for medication. *(From State College Area School District, State College, Pa.)*

SCHOOL PROGRESS REPORT

Doctor _____

Child's Name _____   Teacher's Name _____

Original   Follow-up

Date of Report _____/_____   School _____

Please check only the appropriate spaces below. This will help us
to understand the situation and to adjust his medication.

	PRESENT*				AFTER† _____ Period of time		
	No Problem	A Little	Quite a Bit	Excessive	Better	Same	Worse
Rowdiness							
Wiggliness							
Out of seat							
Not attentive: to teacher							
to own desk work							
Talks to self							
Talks out of turn							
Irritable							
Crying							
Quiet and withdrawn							
Stubborn							
Belligerent							

	Good	Fair	Poor	Better	Same	Worse
Interest in work						
Follows directions						
Seems content						
Gets along with others						
Reading						
Spelling						
Writing						
Arithmetic						
Concentration						
Large muscle Coordination						
Small muscle Coordination						
Verbal communication						

OTHER COMMENTS:

*Complete and return to doctor immediately.
†Complete after stipulated time and return copy #2 to designee.

FIG. 6-4. Medication monitor. *(From Colorado School Health Guidelines, ed. 2, Denver, 1986, Colorado Department of Education and Colorado Department of Health.)*

tions are followed (right drug, right student, correct amount, and proper time), (2) to keep from embarrassing students who may have to take the medication, and (3) to minimize the amount of disruption in the school day for the student who must take the medication. In developing a set of regulations, The American Academy of Pediatrics* recommends that the following should be included:

1. A physician should provide written orders with the name of the drug, dose, time interval when the medication is to be taken, and diagnosis or reason the medicine is needed. (Fig. 6-3.)

2. The parent or guardian should provide a written request that the school district comply with the physician's order. (Fig. 6-3.)

3. Medication should be brought to school in a container appropriately labeled by the pharmacist or the physician.

4. When the student does not regularly take his or her own medication, or if the parent or physician requests that school personnel administer the medication, provision should be made for the medication to be kept in a locked cabinet. Designated personnel must be available to administer the medication at agreed-upon times, and arrangements should be made for alternate personnel to perform the task in case of absence. The person administering the medication must keep a written record. (Fig. 6-4.)

5. When the child is usually responsible for taking his/her own medication, he/she may do so in school without supervision by school personnel, provided the physician and parent have provided the required authorizations. The school administration should cooperate with the physician, parent, and child. In such instances, it is understood that the school bears no responsibility for safeguarding the medication or assuring that it is taken, and the parent should provide a written statement relieving the school of such responsibility.

6. Individual school districts should seek the advice of counsel as they assume the responsibility for giving medication during school hours. Liability coverage should be provided for the staff including nurses, teachers, athletic staff, principals, superintendents, and members of the school board.

WHICH COMMUNITY HEALTH RESOURCES ARE ESSENTIAL?

School personnel should be familiar with and use all local community health resources that can help meet the health guidance needs of pupils. Schools must take the initiative to learn about the services available and establish communications with the various physicians, dentists, psychiatrists, and other health specialists in private practice, health clinics and hospitals, as well as the voluntary health agencies, health departments, child guidance clinics, social service agencies, family service agencies, civic and service organizations, welfare agencies, and religious services located in the community.

For example, resources in the community for emotionally disturbed children may include privately practicing psychologists and psychiatrists, child guidance clinics, general and mental hospitals with inpatient and outpatient care, youth agencies, associations for the physically handicapped, special schools, family service agencies, welfare agencies, and a variety of professional and voluntary organizations.* They offer services including diagnosis, treatment, transition, rehabilitation, education, information, and consultation. In several states, public health departments make available some or many of these

---

*American Academy of Pediatrics, Committee on School Health: Administration of medication in school, Pediatrics **74**(3):433, 1984.

*Professional organizations include American Academy of Child Psychiatry, American Association for Mental Deficiency, American Association of Psychiatry Services for Children, American Orthopsychiatric Association, American Psychiatric Association, American Psychological Association. Voluntary organizations include National Association for Mental Health, Child Study Association of America, Council for Exceptional Children, National Society for Autistic Children, Inc., Al-Anon Family Group Headquarters, and Alateen.

services. The extent of community mental health services differs in school districts, with many of them being in short supply. Services for the poor are frequently inadequate. The cost for help may be partial or full payment, depending on the need of the patient. Some organizations provide free services.

It will be necessary for at least one person in the school to be familiar with the kinds and variety of resources available so the best guidance can be provided to students and parents. The school nurse often assumes this responsibility and is the best-informed person. Where nurses are not available, teachers may have to (1) try to locate someone in the school or school district who knows the resources or (2) contact the local health department for assistance.

HOW DO SCHOOLS ADJUST PROGRAMS?

Teachers who recognize symptoms of physical, mental, emotional, or social disturbances in children should initially examine their own activities in class or their relationship with the pupil to determine whether they may be the cause of, or a factor contributing to, the behavior exhibited. It is conceivable that student maladjustments may be prevented by teachers modifying their activities or pupil relationships. The teacher may find it advisable to provide additional help to a child who is having difficulty in reading or to motivate the gifted student with additional responsibility. They may have to help pupils who have trouble controlling their emotions. Teachers may have to provide success experiences for a boy or girl. They may need to be friendlier with a pupil. They may have to try to gain acceptance of a child rejected by his or her peers. These are some of the considerations that teachers must make before determining that the problem is one needing referral to others.

After appropriate care or treatment has been received by a student, it may not always mean that the child has been cured or that the child's health problem has been corrected. A child with a severe vision problem may have to wear corrective lenses but still may not be able to read the type in a textbook. A pupil with a heart problem may be under treatment and need controlled activities or all classes on one floor. A student with epilepsy may be receiving medication to control seizures but have to take the drug while at school. It therefore becomes necessary for schools to adjust programs to fit the needs of students with health problems.

Among the numerous ways schools have modified and adjusted educational programs are the following:

1. Special consideration for students in the regular classroom. The visually handicapped or hard-of-hearing child may need to be placed near the front of the room. Special rest periods during the day may have to be provided for some pupils. For others, midmorning snacks may be necessary.

2. Special teachers provided for certain handicapped children in the regular classroom. The partially sighted child may need to have special large-print textbooks and other materials provided. The pupil with speech difficulties may need special attention. Children with learning disabilities may need special guidance.

3. Special classes in the regular school. Those who are mentally handicapped, blind, or deaf may be grouped into special classes with specially prepared teachers. Greater attention to a curriculum to satisfy the needs of these children may therefore take place.

4. Special day schools. Cerebral palsied children, those who are emotionally disturbed, and those who are severely mentally retarded may be housed in a facility entirely separate from the regular school.

5. Special residential schools. Blind and deaf students may need to remain overnight for extended periods of time in these schools to receive the best education.

6. Home teachers. Those children who are ill or injured and who must remain at home for long periods of time may need to have teachers go directly to their homes.

7. Hospital teachers. Those students who must remain in hospitals for extensive periods

of time may need service of teachers while confined.

Schools differ in the nature and extent of the educational services provided for handicapped pupils. The larger school districts and those with more funds are usually able to provide greater services. Federal and state funds are often available to subsidize local programs.

With the passage of Public Law 94-142, the Education for All Handicapped Children Act of 1975, more students who previously would have been in special schools are being mainstreamed into the public schools. Unfortunately, few guidelines exist concerning placement of mainstreamed children. As a result, students might be placed in classes not consistent with their particular needs and abilities.

It is important to realize that the problem is not mainstreaming per se, but rather mainstreaming effectively. Teachers must realize that traditional methods may not be effective with these students. By law, individualized educational programs (IEPs) must be developed by an established guidance committee so that each student can benefit from the educational experience. Some districts have reacted well, whereas others have approached the concept with a negative attitude. Clearly these students face problems beyond those of the regular student, and all school personnel should be alert for any additional problems that may emerge: positive adjustments must be made.

SUMMARY

It is essential to understand that health guidance is an important and essential part of the school health services program. It should receive adequate consideration in schools. Without follow-up procedures to obtain corrections, treatment, and care including the adjustment of school programs, health appraisals by themselves are not important to the educational process. Assistance in guidance should be forthcoming from a variety of school personnel. School nurses spend a considerable portion of their time in health guidance and are important resources not only for teachers, but also for parents, students, and others. Teachers should clearly understand their responsibilities in health guidance.

For effective results when counseling, it is necessary to follow fundamental principles and techniques. School personnel should be familiar with the community resources available to help children with health problems. Schools need to use a variety of procedures when adjustments of programs for children with problems are necessary.

QUESTIONS FOR DISCUSSION

1. What procedures are necessary when children with health problems have been discovered in schools?
2. What is meant by the term *health guidance*, and what is its relationship to informal health education?
3. In your own words, define health counseling.
4. Why is informal health education an important part of the total school health program?
5. What are some of the pupil health problems needing health guidance?
6. What are the major purposes of health guidance in schools?
7. How can the health problems of children needing health guidance be generally categorized?
8. What organizational factors must receive consideration when a school health guidance program is being introduced?
9. What are the guiding principles necessary for an effective school health guidance program?
10. What should be the role of the individual who counsels in the health guidance program?
11. How would you characterize the role of the physician in the school health program?
12. What are the responsibilities of a school drug counselor, and how can such a position be justified?
13. What are some of the duties of the school nurse as the nurse's responsibilities expand?
14. What are the responsibilities of the various school personnel in health guidance?
15. What are some effective techniques for health counseling?
16. What guidelines should be used when students or parents are being counseled?
17. What health resources may be available in the community to help with student health problems?
18. What ways have schools tried to adjust programs to help pupils with health problems?
19. What policy regulations should be established in schools in regard to the use of physician-prescribed medications?

SELECTED REFERENCES

American Academy of Pediatrics: School health: a guide for health professions, Evanston, Ill., 1981, The Academy.

American Academy of Pediatrics, Committee on School Health: Administration of medication in school, Pediatrics **74**(3):433, 1984.

American School Health Association, Physician Study Committee: Today's school physician; a horse of a different color, Journal of School Health **52**(10):619-620, 1982.

Appleman, M.A.: The legal issues involved in the use of stimulants on hyperactive school children, doctoral dissertation, University of Minnesota, 1974.

Cormier, L., Cormier, W., and Weisser, R.: Interviewing and helping skills for health professionals, Monterey, Cal., 1984, Wadsworth Publishing Co.

Courtnage, L.: Managing medication in the schools; a survey of state policies, Exceptional Child **49**:75, 1982.

Griffith, B.B., and Whicker, P.H.: Teacher—observer of student health problems, Journal of School Health **51**(6):428-432 Aug., 1981.

Healthy People: The Surgeon General's report on health promotion and disease prevention, Washington, D.C., 1979, U.S. Government Printing Office.

Hertel, V., and Doyen, M.: Colorado school health guidelines, ed. 2, Denver, Colorado Department of Education and Colorado Department of Health.

King, L.S., and Dodd, N.: The health educator as counselor; what does it take? Health Education **17**(2):17-22, 1986.

Kinnison, L.R., and Nimmer, D.N.: An analysis of policies regulating medication in the schools, Journal of School Health **49**:280-283, 1979.

Litwack, L., Litwack, J., and Ballou, M.: Health counseling, New York, 1980, Appleton-Century-Crofts.

Nelson, S.: How healthy is your school: guidelines for evaluating school health promotion, New York, 1986, National Center for Health Education Press.

Oda, D.S.: Increasing role effectiveness of school nurses, American Journal of Public Health **64**:1974.

Silver, G.A.: Redefining school work health services: comprehensive child health care as the framework, Journal of School Health **51**(3):157-162, 1981.

Steinhause, G.W.: Peer education programs: a look nationally, Health Education **14**(7):7-8,10, 1983.

U.S. Department of Health and Human Services, Division of Maternal and Child Health: Perspectives on the health of school-age children: expectations for the future, staff paper, Washington, D.C., 1982.

White, D.H.: A study of current school nurse practice activities, Journal of School Health **55**(2):52-56, 1985.

Wilson, C.C., editor: School health services, Washington, D.C. 1964, National Education Association and the American Medical Association.

CHAPTER

7

EMERGENCY CARE

Every school administrator should develop a systematic procedure for handling any accident or emergency illness that occurs while children are under the school's jurisdiction.

A.E. FLORIO AND WES ALLES*

KEY CONCEPT: Teachers who are prepared to care for school emergencies enhance pupil safety.

Since children are required to attend school, all school personnel have an ethical and legal responsibility to assure that pupils have a safe and hazard-free environment and are provided care in emergencies when accidents or illnesses occur.

Accidents and illnesses are unplanned occurrences at school that all employees should be prepared to handle with promptness and efficiency in the course of the elementary school day. Regardless of the care with which a school facility is constructed, and regardless of the diligent care rendered to prevent accidents it is not possible to provide a completely safe environment.

This chapter contains basic elements of emergency care including first-aid procedures that will enable both the teacher and the staff of schools to assist children. However, all teachers are encouraged to take a course in emergency care and first aid, as well as cardiopulmonary resuscitation (CPR). It is preferable that at least one person trained in emergency care procedures be present at all times when children are in the school facility. We believe that all school personnel should be adequately trained in current emergency care procedures and CPR whether provided by the American National Red Cross or through a program provided by a college or university that certifies the individual is qualified to render first aid to the ill or injured.

For all age-groups, accidents consistently rank among the top five causes of death and are the

*Florio, A.E., and Alles, W.: Safety education, ed. 4, 1979, McGraw-Hill Book Co.

leading cause of death and disability for all persons aged 1 to 44. In 1985, accidents cost $107.3 billion in lost wages, medical expenses, insurance costs, fire losses, property damage, and indirect work loss.*

By and large elementary teachers have apparently been doing a good job in safety education. Over the past half century the accident death rate for children in the 5- to 14-year age range has continued to drop. Yet there is still room for improvement when we lose some 4,000 elementary school children each year through accidents. More tragic is the fact that approximately half of these accidents could have been prevented.

WHAT CAN TEACHERS DO?

Because health and safety are so closely related to the optimum welfare of the school child, it is important that teachers have a clear understanding of the relationship of health and safety in the school program.

Teachers, parents, and others interested in and responsible for the optimum growth and development of children should be cognizant not only of the problems in health education, but of those in safety education as well. For many years the schools have accepted responsibility in health education in attempting to help each child develop to his or her greatest possible capacity not only academically, but also emotionally and physically. Naturally, teachers and others have attempted to do everything possible to educate children concerning health as well as to try to help them maintain good health and to protect them from ill health and disabling diseases and disorders. It is recognized that safety ranks in the same category in the attempt to assure optimum growth and development of children. If teachers think in terms of protecting and providing for the optimum health and growth of children, then they must assume responsibility for safety at school.

*Data from National Safety Council.: Accident facts, Chicago, 1986, The Council.

WHAT PROVISIONS SHOULD BE MADE FOR EMERGENCY CARE OF INJURED AND ILL PUPILS?

When illnesses or injuries occur, school personnel often are not prepared to handle them properly. Every school regardless of size should have carefully organized written plans and procedures for the proper care of injured and ill pupils. These plans should be made for emergency care of both mass and individual injuries and illnesses.

Organization and administration of the school emergency care program are the responsibility of the board of education. This responsibility, however, is usually delegated to the superintendent, principal, and other school administrators.

A school district should establish a uniform policy for the emergency care of the injured and ill. The policy established by a particular school will depend on a number of factors, including the size of the community and school; availability of nurses, physicians, hospitals, and ambulances, effective communications; and trained first-aid personnel. In formulating the emergency care policy, school administrators should seek the aid, advice, and cooperation of local emergency medical services, school and community safety councils, parents, local medical and public health groups, and any of the community organizations or agencies, such as the police department, fire department, and ambulance and auxiliary services that may be able to lend aid and assistance when necessary.

The main responsibilities of the school in emergency care are to (1) *give immediate and proper first aid*, (2) *notify the parents*, (3) *not increase the severity of the injury*, and (4) *be certain that the injured or ill are placed under the care of parents or a physician designated by the parents*. The school policy including plans, procedures, and responsibility assignments should be made available *in writing* to all teachers and other school personnel who may be involved in any way in emergency care. Also, it is advisable to make the *parents* acquainted with the policy for emergency care.

Since new teachers usually join the school faculty beginning with the fall term, it is advisable for school administrators to make them familar with the emergency care program at the beginning of the term or before the school term begins. Also, the beginning of the fall semester is a good time to review the emergency care program with all teachers and acquaint them with any changes in policy, plans, or procedures. When teachers join the faculty at times other than at the beginning of the fall season, it is the duty of school administrators to familiarize these new teachers with the policy concerning school emergency care.

In the final analysis, a school district's emergency care program depends on (1) availability of *trained first-aid personnel* at the scene; (2) quick and effective *communication;* (3) a prompt, safe, well-equipped community emergency medical services system; and (4) access to *hospitals with specialized emergency care equipment and medical and nursing personnel*.

Plans for emergency care

It is important that every school district develop detailed written plans and procedures that cover all emergency situations. Although it is practically impossible to list the detailed plans that may be necessary for every district, there are a number of common procedures that should be present in all schools.

Emergency transportation. Every school should have plans for transporting injured or ill children to their homes, hospital, or physicians' or dentists' offices. Previous arrangements should be made with the community emergency medical service system. School buses, ambulances, or other suitable transportation should also be made available. Often it may be advisable for the school nurse or other school personnel to transport the children in private vehicles, but this should be done only in the absence of other alternatives. When injured children are transported in private vehicles, proper insurance coverage should be carried on those vehicles. Regardless of the means, some acceptable type of emergency transportation should be available to

the school at all times when children are in attendance. However, it is important to remember that it is always best not to move seriously injured persons unless the individual is in immediate peril from another source. Competent medical assistance should be brought to a victim at the scene of the event.

Facilities and equipment. Proper first aid and emergency care imply that there will be sufficient facilities and equipment in every school. There should be emergency lounges containing cots, blankets, lavatories, towels, chairs, and a table. Separate lounges should be provided for boys and girls. The emergency room should be equipped with adequate first-aid supplies for any type of injury or sudden illness. The first-aid supplies should be maintained in accordance with the best standards for first-aid care. The kinds and amounts of first-aid material will depend on the size of the school and the availability of community resources for assisting with emergency care. In addition to the first-aid supplies found in the emergency room, classroom teachers should have on hand such things as soap and small dressings for minor wounds. A suggested list of first-aid supplies is found on pp. 149-150.

Reports and records. An accurate report of each emergency injury or illness arising in the school should be made. The National Safety Council standard accident report form is shown in Fig. 7-1. Ordinarily the principal delegates the responsibility of making this report to the school nurse, teacher, or some other member of the school personnel. In any case, teachers are likely to have a part in making reports, particularly when children under their supervision are injured or become ill. The report should contain such information as the name of the pupil; time, location, and nature of the accident or illness; witnesses, teachers, or other persons present; possible causes of the illness or injury; description of the illness or injury including the part of the body seemingly injured; first aid given; notification of parents; and disposition of the case.

School policy on emergency care. Minor injuries and illnesses happen frequently among school children. At such times, the classroom

STANDARD STUDENT ACCIDENT REPORT FORM
Part A. Information on ALL Accidents

1. Name: _____ Home Address: _____
2. School: _____ Sex: M ☐; F ☐. Age: _____ Grade or classification: _____
3. Time accident occurred: Hour _____ A.M.; _____ P.M. Date: _____
4. Place of Accident: School Building ☐ School Grounds ☐ To or from School ☐ Home ☐ Elsewhere ☐

5. **NATURE OF INJURY**

Abrasion _____	Fracture _____
Amputation _____	Laceration _____
Asphyxiation _____	Poisoning _____
Bite _____	Puncture _____
Bruise _____	Scalds _____
Burn _____	Scratches _____
Concussion _____	Shock (el.) _____
Cut _____	Sprain _____
Dislocation _____	
Other (specify) _____	

DESCRIPTION OF THE ACCIDENT

How did accident happen? What was student doing? Where was student? List specifically unsafe acts and unsafe conditions existing. Specify any tool, machine or equipment involved. _____

PART OF BODY INJURED

Abdomen _____	Foot _____
Ankle _____	Hand _____
Arm _____	Head _____
Back _____	Knee _____
Chest _____	Leg _____
Ear _____	Mouth _____
Elbow _____	Nose _____
Eye _____	Scalp _____
Face _____	Tooth _____
Finger _____	Wrist _____
Other (specify) _____	

6. Degree of Injury: Death ☐ Permanent Impairment ☐ Temporary Disability ☐ Nondisabling ☐
7. Total number of days lost from school: _____ (To be filled in when student returns to school)

Part B. Additional Information on School Jurisdiction Accidents

8. Teacher in charge when accident occurred (Enter name): _____
   Present at scene of accident: No: _____ Yes: _____

9. **IMMEDIATE ACTION TAKEN**

First aid treatment _____ By (Name): _____
Sent to school nurse _____ By (Name): _____
Sent home _____ By (Name): _____
Sent to physician _____ By (Name): _____
Physician's Name: _____
Sent to hospital _____ By (Name): _____
Name of hospital: _____

10. Was a parent or other individual notified? No: __ Yes: __ When: _____ How: _____
    Name of individual notified: _____
    By whom? (Enter name): _____

11. Witnesses: 1. Name: _____ Address: _____
              2. Name: _____ Address: _____

12. **LOCATION**

Specify Activity	Specify Activity	Remarks
Athletic field _____	Locker _____	What recommendations do you have for preventing other accidents of this type? _____
Auditorium _____	Pool _____	
Cafeteria _____	Sch. grounds _____	
Classroom _____	_____ shop _____	
Corridor _____	Showers _____	
Dressing room _____	Stairs _____	
Gymnasium _____	Toilets and	
Home Econ. _____	washrooms _____	
Laboratories _____	Other (specify) _____	

Signed: Principal: _____ Teacher: _____

(National Safety Council—Form School 1)
Rep. 100M106002

Printed in U.S.A.

Stock No. 429.21

FIG. 7-1. National Safety Council accident report form. *(Courtesy National Safety Council, Inc., Chicago, Ill.)*

teacher should follow the policy of the school in caring for the pupil. If an illness is mild, the child should be kept warm and on a cot and be under constant or regular supervision. If the illness seems to be progressive, the parent should be called and the usual procedure invoked for caring for more serious illness. The teacher should remember that no medication of any kind should be given. First aid for such injuries as minor cuts and scratches usually can be safely cared for by the teacher. The teacher should permit limited bleeding and stress the importance of cleanliness by washing the wound with soap and water and applying a sterile dressing.

For certain seemingly major illnesses, the school policy concerning the notifying of parents and taking whatever steps necessary should be put into operation immediately. The child should rest on a cot, and body temperature should be maintained. Someone should be in constant attendance with the child until the school has fulfilled its responsibility of carrying out the parents' instructions or, in case the parents cannot be contacted, in getting the services of the family physician or taking the child to a hospital. In cases of major injuries the school policy for rendering first aid under such circumstances should be put into effect.

Information for emergencies

It is imperative that certain kinds of information be readily available to facilitate the rapid and proper handling of emergency cases. The following kinds of information should be carefully listed, organized, and placed near a telephone in the principal's office where it is accessible to all teachers or other school personnel who may be expected to assist in any way with emergency care of injured and ill children:

1. A list of all pupils with full and correct names
2. The names of both parents or guardians
3. Home address
4. Home telephone number
5. Business address of both parents or guardians
6. Business telephone numbers of parents
7. Name of family physician
8. Business telephone number of family physician
9. Home telephone number of family physician
10. Physician of choice, in case family physician cannot be reached
11. Telephone number of physician of choice if family physician cannot be reached
12. Relatives to be called in case the parents cannot be reached
13. Telephone number of relatives to be called in case parents cannot be reached
14. Hospital of choice
15. Hospital telephone number
16. Any special directions from parents concerning the handling of emergency injury or illness
17. List of homeroom teachers
18. List of pupil's daily class schedule
19. Telephone number of local ambulance services
20. Telephone number of fire department
21. Telephone number of police department

An increasing number of communities are centralizing their emergency communication systems. Through the efforts and cooperation of the telephone companies a growing number of towns and cities are using 911 as the all-purpose number to dial. School administrators and teachers as well as other school personnel should be aware of the local emergency communication system.

Notification of parents

Schools often request parents to sign a permit authorizing the proper emergency care of their children in case of injury and certain illnesses. This is particularly helpful in situations in which parents or guardians cannot be immediately contacted. The school is then free to call the designated family physician or hospital or take any other action it thinks necessary for the best welfare of the child.

Parents or guardians should be notified immediately in case of serious injury or illness. When notifying parents by telephone, the person making the call should speak in a calm, reassuring voice to allay any fear or anxiety the parent may suddenly develop. A full description of the child's injury or illness should be given so far as it is evident and possible. Parents should be told whether immediate medical attention seems needed. Sometimes emergency room hospital care may be advised and stressed to the parent. The person making the call should learn from the parents whether they will come to school for the child or whether they wish the pupil to be brought home. Parents should be encouraged to call for children whenever possible. Occasionally, it may be the desire of the parents that the family physician call at school if it seems necessary. If an ambulance is needed, parents should give permission to summon one before the school takes this action.

Sometimes it may be necessary for the child to go directly to the hospital emergency section or the family physician's office. In some cases the parents may wish someone from the school to accompany the child. Usually the nurse or principal will provide transportation and provide any other assistance necessary.

Since most physicians are not well prepared to provide emergency care in their offices in critical life-death situations, it is usually most advisable to call 911 or another emergency phone number and have the child quickly transported to the emergency unit of the nearest hospital. It is important to call the hospital and inform them of the nature of the injury or illness while the child is en route to the emergency room. This gives hospital personnel time to set up whatever equipment and medicines may be required for a specific case. It also alerts them to possible need for a surgeon or other specialists whom they may need to call to the emergency area.

Sick or injured children should never be sent home unless accompanied by a responsible adult and unless the parents or some responsible person designated by the parents is there to care for them. In cases in which parents or guardians cannot be immediately contacted, school authorities must proceed according to their best judgment. It may seem necessary to call a physician or dentist directly, or in some cases it may be necessary to call an ambulance and take the child to a hospital. In every case school personnel should give the parents every possible aid in caring for a sick or injured child. Often if specialized medical attention is indicated, the parents may be at a loss concerning the selection of a physician. In this case the school authorities should be prepared with the names of various available medical specialists such as pediatricians, otorhinolaryngologists, orthopedists, ophthalmologists, surgeons, and dentists from which parents can make a selection.

It is advisable that the school follow up emergency cases. Parents or guardians should be called within 24 to 36 hours to learn the condition of the injured or ill child. If the condition is serious, periodic telephone calls from the school might be made until the child is well on the way to full recovery. The follow-up of emergency cases costs little and usually brings a great deal of goodwill to the school. It is also important that school officials know the recovery period needed for any injury or illness so that the child's schedule can be altered appropriately. All follow-up procedures should be noted in the student's records.

TEACHER'S ROLE IN EMERGENCY CARE

Every teacher should be prepared to assume some responsibility for the school emergency and first-aid care program. Even though physicians, nurses, and others highly skilled in emergency and first-aid care may be available at practically all times, the teacher must be prepared to accept certain responsibilities, such as the following:

1. Assist with any emergency in which large numbers of pupils are injured or become suddenly ill
2. Render first aid or contact those who are officially designated to give first aid when a pupil under the teacher's direction is injured or becomes ill
3. Assist those who are officially designated to give first aid when necessary by doing such things as calling parents or physician

4. Give first aid for minor injuries such as small and insignificant wounds that do not require the attention of a physician, nurse, or others officially designated to give first aid

The legal duty of school personnel falls into four categories:

1. To foresee possible hazards and take reasonable steps to correct the hazard
2. To provide warnings about hazards that are not immediately remediable
3. To render proper first aid to the injured
4. Not to increase the severity of the injury

Although the situations are likely to be relatively few in which the teacher does not have assistance with first aid, the teacher should be prepared to assume full responsibility for those few times when there is no immediate help. The teacher should keep in mind that providing first aid does not involve medication of any kind. The teacher should never use antiseptics on a wound unless it is an established policy of the school to use them; and then *only* those that are indicated in the written policy of the school should be used. The teacher should not give the child any type of medication, including such a seemingly harmless thing as aspirin, unless directed to do so by a physician. All first-aid supplies in the schools should have the approval of those responsible for formulating the policy for emergency and first-aid care.

WHO IS LIABLE AND RESPONSIBLE FOR SCHOOL ACCIDENTS?

Although teachers have always been concerned about accidents involving school children, a study of the accident situation in the schools shows that in the past there has been a lack of proper understanding on the part of some teachers as to their full responsibility in such circumstances.

In recent years people have become suit-conscious, and the fear of being sued often dissuades teachers from rendering first aid to students. State policies differ in regard to teacher responsibilities and although in some states there may be no legal obligation, *there is a moral obligation* for teachers to provide care for students in need. Teachers who act in a reasonable and prudent manner when providing emergency care are generally protected from tort liabilities (monetary compensation).

Legal responsibility

The question is often asked, "Why is there a greater tendency today to attempt to hold the teacher financially liable for injuries to pupils?" The answer to this question in part is that today most people have come to expect accidents to be paid for. When an accident results in injury to an individual, usually the first question asked is, "Who is to pay for the accident?"

Since the teacher is supposed to be acting in loco parentis (in the place of a parent), any time a student is injured at achool, the teacher runs the risk of being sued for negligence. Negligence is generally based on failure to act as a reasonably prudent and careful individual would act given the same or similar circumstances. In general, negligence may take three forms: (1) failing to perform an expected duty (nonfeasance or an act of omission), (2) performing a duty incorrectly (misfeasance or an act of commission), or (3) performing an illegal procedure or performing a procedure without consent (malfeasance or an act of commission).

It is now commonly understood that a teacher or a school board, or both, in case of *negligence*, can be held responsible and financially liable for accidental injury to a pupil. Increasing numbers of court procedures and damage suits for accidental injuries to school children are being recorded. Each year thousands of schools are involved in lawsuits resulting in payments of millions of dollars.

The teacher would be well advised to carry a personal liability insurance policy. This policy may be purchased through private insurance companies, or may be purchased, often at less cost, through the various professional organizations to which the teacher belongs.

Teachers should familiarize themselves with

the school law in their own state regarding negligence and liability to civil suit.

The law of negligence is partly based on the theory that everyone has the right to live safely and must be protected from the negligence of others in this right. In the school situation the teacher owes a duty to the school child. In many cases the failure to act to prevent an accident to a school child would be considered negligence on the part of the teacher.

The law of negligence implies, so far as the duty of the teacher to the pupil is concerned, that there must be *foreseeability*. The teacher acting as a reasonably careful and prudent person should anticipate danger or an accident.

For negligence to be established, the court must determine that*:

1. The student was injured as a result of a school-related incident
2. The action or inaction of the school official resulted in additional injury or caused the severity of the injury to increase
3. The school official acted in a manner different from the way a reasonable and prudent person would have acted under the same or similar circumstances
4. The school official did, in fact, have a duty to act

Some conditions that may make teachers liable to legal action include:

1. Permitting pupils to play unsafe, unorganized games
2. Maintaining attractive nuisances (conditions of school environment, apparatus, equipment, machinery, and the like)
3. Permitting pupils to use dangerous devices
4. Planning and organizing inadequately for field trips
5. Permitting use of defective equipment
6. Failing to provide adequate supervision or instruction for pupil activities

Although these six points may seem rather obvious, the basic laws associated with liability were developed to protect and compensate in-

nocent victims of accidents that might have been prevented through prudent action on the part of school officials. The laws were also enacted to protect the school official from frivolous lawsuits, which are often leveled at teachers.

In some cases the injured student may be partially or wholly at fault. If the teacher gives specific directions or warnings and the student ignores them, depending on the age of the student, it is possible that the student, not the teacher, could be held liable for the injury. This is called "contributory negligence," and means that the child failed to exercise care, follow directions, or heed specific warnings. In comparative or shared negligence, both the teacher and the student contribute to the situation that results in an accident and injury. In this case, damage recovery is proportional to the amount of negligence contributed by each party to the circumstances that led to the injury.

In addition to the possibility of the teacher's being held financially liable for the injury of a child, especially in a case of negligence, there is another factor that should be taken into consideration. In many cases the teacher may not be vulnerable from the viewpoint of financial liability. However, the teacher may be quite vulnerable from the viewpoint of failing to take proper responsibility in case of an accident to a child. That is, although the teacher could not be held financially liable for the accident, the superintendent of schools or the board of education could hold the teacher negligent, perhaps resulting in discipline or even discharge for failing to use reasonable care in providing safe conditions for the child.

Legal defense

Fortunately, teachers generally exercise a great deal of caution in their dealings with students. Further, the courts have realized the difficulty of controlling or keeping under close supervision as many as 35 to 40 students who are all full of energy. Also, there has not been a successful prosecution for negligence against any person who has followed established first-aid

---

*Adapted from Hafen, B.: First aid for health emergencies, ed. 3, St. Paul, 1985, West Publishing Co.

procedures when providing aid to an injured individual. The low cost of personal liability insurance is also mute testimony to this low incidence of successful prosecutions.

Several defenses are generally used in lawsuits against teachers. These are as follows:

assumption of risk the person injured failed to heed warnings or voluntarily and with full knowledge of the possible consequences entered a hazardous situation (e.g., climbed over a fence surrounding a hazard)

contributory negligence the failure of the injured person to use due care for his or her own personal safety

proximate cause the injury was not the result of teacher negligence and would have occurred regardless of safety precautions that were taken

vis major a natural cause that could not be guarded against or anticipated by a person acting in a reasonable and prudent fashion (e.g., an earthquake or other act of God)

Obviously the best defense is not to become involved in litigation initially. This means that a well-planned safety program should be functioning within the school and that the teacher and other school staff should be prepared to handle emergency situations as they arise.

WHAT FIRST-AID PROCEDURES SHOULD TEACHERS USE?*

The emergency care given at the time a person is injured or becomes suddenly ill is known as first aid. It is the care given before medical

*Adapted in part from Airhihenbuwa, C.O.: First aid and emergency care: procedure and practice, Dubuque, Iowa, 1986, Kendall/Hunt; American National Red Cross: Advanced first aid and personal safety, ed. 2, Garden City, N.Y., 1979, Doubleday and Co., Inc.; American National Red Cross: Standard first aid and personal safety, ed. 2, Garden City, N.Y., 1979, Doubleday and Co., Inc.; Hafen, B.Q.: First aid for health emergencies, ed. 3, St. Paul, 1985, West Publishing Co.; Heimlich, H.J., and Uhley, M.H.: The Heimlich maneuver, Clinical Symposium, CIBA 31(3): 1979; Rinke, C.M., editor: Standards and guidelines for cardiopulmonary resuscitation (CPR) and emergency cardiac care (ECC), Journal of the American Medical Association 255(21):2905-2984, 1986; and Parcel, G.S.: Basic emergency care of the sick and injured, ed. 3, St. Louis, 1986, Times Mirror/Mosby College Publishing.

aid is available. Under most circumstances, medical aid is readily available. The duties of the person giving first aid end immediately when medical assistance is obtained.

It should be kept in mind by teachers that *first aid is the emergency care given at the time an injury or sudden illness first occurs*. It does not mean attempting to care for injuries or illnesses after medical aid has been obtained. Therefore such actions as repeated bandaging of wounds or attempting to care for extended illnesses is not a responsibility of the teacher and should not, under any circumstances, be attempted.

Every elementary school classroom teacher should have a knowledge of first aid. Some states now require elementary teachers to complete a university credit course in first aid or have comparable Red Cross instruction. Every person employed by the school district, every parent, and every boy and girl should have some understanding of first aid.

The following basic points should be kept in mind when giving first aid:

1. First aid is given to an injured person for the purpose of preventing further harm.
2. First aid is given for the purpose of reducing suffering and discomfort.
3. A call for emergency medical services (ambulance) should be placed for serious cases.
4. Many children injured in accidents receive further injury through improper emergency care.
5. Sometimes the failure to receive proper first aid may result in permanent injury or even death.
6. The first-aider should know what *not* to do, as well as what *to* do.
7. Hurry is seldom necessary, especially if it is likely to cause further damage to the injured person, except in cases of severe bleeding, stoppage of breathing, and poisoning.
8. If the injury is serious, a check should be made for severe bleeding, stoppage of breathing, shock, obstructions to breathing caused by a foreign body in the mouth

or throat, back and neck injuries, and broken bones.

9. If the child is vomiting, the head and body should be turned to one side to facilitate breathing.
10. Clothing should be loosened about the neck and chest, particularly if breathing is difficult.
11. The child's body temperature should be maintained by covering with blankets or coats to reduce or prevent shock (take care not to overheat).
12. An injured person should not be moved, unless it is absolutely necessary, until the exact nature of the injury is known and provisions have been made to prevent further damage.
13. An unconscious person must not be given liquid, food, or medication of any type because of the danger of obstructing breathing passages.

The teacher or person responsible for giving first aid should remember that there are three emergency situations requiring immediate and instant action to save life (hurry cases): serious bleeding, suspended breathing, and poisoning. Although shock may be extremely serious, the first-aider usually has more time to act.

Artificial respiration

A person cannot live more than 4 to 6 minutes without breathing. It is extremely important therefore when administering first aid to begin artificial respiration immediately after the cessation of breathing because the heart continues to beat only a short time after breathing has stopped.

Some of the causes of complete or partial cessation of breathing or serious interference with the oxygen supply of the body are electric shock, drowning, inhaling certain gases, choking, strangling, inhaling certain chemical fumes, and consuming drugs such as morphine, barbiturates, and alcohol. From the viewpoint of the school situation, however, mechanical obstruction is likely to be the most common cause of suspended breathing or serious interference with

breathing. The mechanical causes include foreign bodies in the throat and windpipe, drowning, and strangulation.

There are many ways of administering artificial respiration. However, the mouth-to-mouth or mouth-to-nose method is recommended as the most efficient and usually the most practical. The following directions briefly explain how to give mouth-to-mouth and mouth-to-nose artificial respiration.

First, shake the person gently and ask if he/she is all right. If you get no response, call out for help, and place your ear near the mouth to see if you detect breathing. Simultaneously, check to see if you can feel a carotid pulse (in the neck, near the Adam's apple). If you feel a pulse but detect no breathing, place the person on the back with arms at sides (see Fig. 7-2). Recheck for breathing. If you hear nothing, blow twice into the victims mouth and recheck the pulse. Place one hand on the victim's chin and your other hand on the forehead. Move the head so that the chin is pointed upward with the lower jaw in a jutting position as shown in Fig. 7-3, A. In this position the base of the tongue tends to move away from the back of the throat to give clear passage to the air.

In the mouth-to-mouth technique close the person's nostrils with your fingers or cheek. Place your mouth tightly over the person's mouth as shown in Fig. 7-3, B. Some do not wish to come in contact with the person, so they place a pocket mask over the nose and mouth of the victim. If you use the mouth-to-nose technique, close the person's mouth and place your mouth over his nose as shown in Fig. 7-3, C. Blow into the person's mouth or nose. Remove your mouth and turn your head to one side while you inhale. Repeat the blowing of air into the person's nose or mouth and remove your mouth to inhale. The rate of breathing in this way should be about *1 breath every 5 seconds*. Blow vigorously in giving artificial respiration to an adult or older child; use your diaphragm muscles, not your cheeks.

If at any time obstruction to breathing develops making it difficult to get air into and out of the person's lungs, quickly straddle the victim and administer 6 to 10 abdominal thrusts to expel any foreign object that may be blocking the airway. Then quickly resume artificial respiration.

There are a few differences in using the mouth-to-mouth method of artificial respiration on small children and on grown people.

FIG. 7-2. Initial steps of cardiopulmonary resuscitation. Top, Determining unresponsiveness; center, call for help; bottom, position the victim for resuscitation.

Place a small child on his/her back with chin pointed upward and lower jaw in a jutting position. Place your mouth over *both* the child's nose and mouth tightly enough so that air cannot escape as shown in Fig. 7-3, *C.* Hold the child's lower jaw in position with one hand and then place your other hand on the child's forehead to keep the head tilted. Puff gently and smoothly into the child's nose and mouth until the chest rises. While breathing into the nose and mouth, with your hand apply a little pressure to the child's stomach to keep if from filling with air. When you have breathed enough air into the child's lungs, as indicated by the rising of the chest, raise your head and allow the air to pass from the child's lungs. Keep one hand under the jaw and the other on the forehead and *repeat this cycle about once every 3 seconds.*

If there is any obstruction to getting air into the child's lungs, quickly bend the child over with the head down and administer three or four quick pats between the shoulders and four quick chest thrusts. Then continue artificial respiration immediately.

If no pulse can be felt in the carotid artery on the neck under the angle of the lower jaw, the *CPR technique* should be used as described next.

ABC of life support

ABC of life support* is a first-aid procedure that consists of recognizing stoppage of breathing and heartbeat and then applying cardiopulmonary resuscitation (CPR), which involves (A) opening and maintaining victim's *Airway,* (B) giving rescue *Breathing,* and (C) providing artificial *Circulation* by external cardiac compression (heart massage). CPR should be performed by people with special training. For more information contact your local Heart Association or Red Cross. These are the essential points of ABC:

A *Airway open.* Turn victim on back and quickly remove any foreign matter from the

---

*From the Metropolitan Life Insurance Co., New York, 1974

mouth. Place your hand on person's chin and lift, tilting head back as far as possible with other hand. This provides an airway.

B *Breathing restored.* If person is not breathing, place your mouth tightly over his mouth, pinch nostrils, and blow into airway until you see chest rise. Remove your mouth. Give two breaths and check for neck pulse. If pulse is present, continue rescue breathing at 12 times a minute. For a small child or infant, cover nose and mouth tightly with your mouth. Blow gently 20 times a minute.

C *Circulation maintained.* Quickly feel for neck pulse; keeping victim's head tilted with one hand, use middle and index fingers of other hand to feel for carotid pulse, in neck artery, under side angle of lower jaw. For infants, check the pulse in the upper arm artery. If no pulse, start rescue breathing and external cardiac compression.

Victim's back should be on firm surface. Place heel of your hand on center of lower breastbone with fingers off chest and other hand on top. Apply downward pressure with your hand to

FIG. 7-3. Administering artificial respiration. A, Move the head so that the chin is pointing upward. B, Close the child's nostrils and place your mouth tightly over the child's mouth. C, If the mouth-to-nose method is used, close the mouth and place your mouth over the nose.

FIG. 7-4. The ABC of life support (Cardio-Pulmonary Resuscitation, CPR).

force blood out of the heart. Be sure your shoulder is directly over the victim. Release pressure. Alternate (B) Breathing with (C) Circulation.

Two rescuers: Give 80 to 100 chest compressions a minute—one breath after each five compressions (Fig. 7-4). *One rescuer:* Perform both artificial circulation and rescue breathing giving 80 to 100 chest compressions a minute—two full breaths after each 15 compressions.

FOR SMALL CHILDREN AND INFANTS: Use only the heel of one hand and, for infants, only the tips of index and middle fingers. Give 100 compressions per minute with two breaths after each five compressions.

REMEMBER: These basic ABCs only briefly outline what to do for a person unconscious from drowning, electrocution, suffocation, accident, heart disease, or stroke. Time is crucial. Rescue

efforts must begin at once and continue until professional help arrives. To be fully effective, special training and periodic refreshers are vital.

There are a few other measures that should be followed in suspended breathing:

1. The body temperature of the person should be maintained.

2. Artificial respiration should be continued without interruption.

3. The person should not be moved until normal voluntary breathing returns.

4. If it is necessary to move the person, resuscitation should be carried on during the time the victim is being moved.

5. When the person is revived, body temperature should be maintained. The victim should remain quiet for a while and should be treated for shock by a physician.

6. Since in some cases of suspended breathing recovery is unusually slow, artificial respiration should be continued for at least 3 hours, or longer, or until rescue squad or hospital emergency personnel and equipment are available.

Choking

Occasionally students, infants, and adults will experience severe choking episodes. A total of 3,200 people died (50 in the 5 to 14 year age group) in 1985 as a result of a foreign body obstructing the airway of the individual. This represents an increase of 3% over 1984 totals.* In 1974 Dr. Henry Heimlich developed a technique to deal with foreign-body airway obstruction. Dr. Heimlich's technique consists of external compression of the air in the lungs in order to create an "artificial cough" strong enough to dislodge a foreign body blocking the airway. In 1985 a National Conference on Cardiopulmonary Resuscitation (CPR) and Emergency Cardiac Care (ECC) was convened to update standards developed in 1980. It was the recommendation of the conference participants that the Heimlich maneuver be the procedure for dealing with victims of an obstructed airway unless the victim is younger than 1 year of age. For that age group, a combination of back blows and chest thrusts was recommended.

Identifying a choking victim. In more than 90% of the instances of choking, the victim is seen to choke on food or another object. The choking victim cannot breathe or speak, becomes cyanotic, and collapses. There is obviously a life-threatening danger to the choking victim if the Heimlich maneuver is not applied.

When an individual is choking, there is a universal signal that has come to be known as the "Heimlich sign," which indicates, "I am choking." Victims grasp their neck between their thumb and index finger to indicate the choking situation (Fig. 7-5). It should be noted, however, that not every victim of choking will show

*National Safety Council: Accident facts, Chicago, 1986, The Council.

FIG. 7-5. Universal signal used to indicate choking.

this signal. The rescuer, therefore, should take into consideration other factors such as the surroundings before deciding to use the Heimlich maneuver. Studies have shown that over 98% of persons dying suddenly in an eating establishment have choked on food.

Heimlich maneuver. To be safe and effective, the Heimlich maneuver should be performed in one of the following prescribed ways:

1. When the rescuer is standing and the victim is standing or sitting, the rescuer should do the following:
   a. Stand behind the victim and wrap your arms around the victim's waist (Fig. 7-6).
   b. Make a fist and place it thumb side against the victim's abdomen slightly above the navel and below the rib cage (Fig. 7-7).
   c. Grasp the fist with the other hand and press into the victim's abdomen with a quick upward thrust.

FIG. 7-6. Heimlich maneuver with child upright.

FIG. 7-7. Rescuer standing when using the Heimlich maneuver.

   d. This process may need to be repeated several times.
2. When the victim is sitting, the rescuer stands behind the victim's chair and performs the maneuver in the same manner as for a standing victim.
3. When the rescuer is kneeling and the victim is lying face up, the rescuer takes the following steps:
   a. With the victim lying on his/her back, face the victim, and kneel alongside the hips.
   b. With one hand on the top of the other, they are placed on the victim's abdomen slightly above the navel and below the rib cage.
   c. Press into the victim's abdomen with a quick upward thrust (Fig. 7-8).
   d. Repeat several times if necessary.

The standing and sitting positions are used most often; however, it is extremely important that rescuers learn the supine position (victim lying down, face upward). Only in that position, can a small person—one who cannot reach around the victim's waist or who is not strong enough to press a fist upward around the diaphragm with sufficient force—save a heavy victim. In the supine position, the rescuer uses weight, not strength, to press upward on the diaphragm.

The choking victim has 4 minutes to live from the onset of choking; however, when a victim is on the floor unconscious, he/she does not have a full 4 minutes but may only have a matter of seconds. It is necessary therefore to apply the Heimlich maneuver without delay. It is important to remember that the Heimlich maneuver is to be used only in emergency situations. It should not be practiced on people since damage to internal organs could occur.

Serious bleeding

Severe bleeding must be stopped immediately. In addition to danger resulting from the loss of blood, it is likely to bring about serious shock. Furthermore, children are usually frightened by the sight of their own blood if the bleed-

FIG. 7-8. Rescuer kneeling when using the Heimlich maneuver.

ing is serious. Fright may add to the seriousness of shock. If a large blood vessel is severed, a quart of blood can be lost from the body within 1 minute. Consequently, in an emergency of this kind the teacher must act instantly. Direct pressure with elevation is the method recommended to stop bleeding. In most cases hand pressure with a sterile dressing or clean napkin, towel, or cloth is the accepted procedure. A compress directly on the wound with a tight bandage will control the blood flow in a majority of cases. Blood flow from the head and face can usually be controlled in this way. If bleeding cannot be controlled using direct pressure and slight elevation, the rescuer should apply pressure on a main artery that supplies the wound area with blood. Pressure is applied on the artery against an underlying bone.

If a large artery of the arm or leg is cut, it may be necessary under rare circumstances to apply a tourniquet. Because a tourniquet is an extremely dangerous piece of equipment in the hands of the average first-aider, its use is highly restricted and should be viewed in the light that a limb may be sacrificed to save a life. Some results of improper use of a tourniquet are the following:

1. The artery may be permanently damaged through crushing by too much pressure.

2. Keeping the supply of blood from a part of the body too long may cause loss of the limb.

3. Additional bleeding resulting from removing the tourniquet too soon may prove serious.

4. Removing the tourniquet after an extended period of application may increase shock.

A tourniquet is seldom needed for bleeding below the knee or elbow since wounds in these areas can usually be controlled by direct pressure in conjunction with use of a pressure point. If a tourniquet is needed anywhere on an extremity, it should be applied; as close to the wound as possible, on the nearest uninjured tissue, and only tight enough to stop or slow bleeding so that direct pressure on the wound will be effective. Any material fairly thick and soft that can be tied around the arm or leg and twisted tight enough to stop the bleeding can be used as a tourniquet. *It must not cut or bruise the flesh.* Such materials as wire or rope should never be used as a tourniquet.

It is important to remember that a tourniquet should be used *only in case of serious bleeding that threatens life* and cannot be stopped by other recommended means. A tourniquet is seldom necessary and if a tourniquet is applied, it should not be released other than by a physician or properly trained medical personnel. When a tourniquet is applied, the time of application should be attached to or, if possible, written on the forehead of the victim.

Shock

In a state of shock the body processes are usually greatly reduced. Broken bones, poisoning, severe burns, hemorrhage, perforation or inflammation of internal organs, reactions to drugs or proteins, or strong emotions may cause shock. Intense pain, loss of blood, tissue destruction, and sometimes strong emotions may interfere with the nervous system's control of the circulatory system. Blood pressure may fall to a level so low that circulation is inadequate. The brain fails to get enough blood to supply sufficient oxygen and nutrition, and, as a result, consciousness may be lost.

Shock may not be clearly noticeable following most minor injuries. However, some degree of shock may follow any injury, particularly if it is accompanied by strong emotional reactions.

Some people are much more subject to shock than others. An injury that causes only slight or moderate shock in one person may cause serious shock in another. Severe shock usually follows serious injury. Consequently, the teacher should always be alert and expect shock in giving first aid to pupils who are accident victims. Shock may appear soon after an injury, or it may appear many hours later.

It may not be possible to prevent shock, but the proper first-aid care may greatly reduce its seriousness. There are a number of ways by which shock can be detected. Some of the signs are the following:

1. The lips and fingernails are blue or grayish
2. The skin is cool to the touch, yet it is covered with moisture, making it feel clammy
3. The injured child may be nauseated
4. The injured child may vomit
5. The victim may be partially conscious and complain of feeling cold
6. The face becomes pale, almost gray

First aid for shock consists of keeping the person lying in a supine position with the head lower than the feet. Precaution should be taken, however, in placing the head lower than the feet. *In head or chest injuries, or if breathing becomes more difficult* with the head low, the *child's head and shoulders should be raised a few inches* higher than the feet. This can be done by placing a pillow or coat under the victim's head and shoulders. If the child develops difficulty in breathing with the head and shoulders elevated, lower them. The pupil should be kept comfortably warm with blankets or coats *but not overheated.* Pain contributes to shock. Unnecessary movement of an injured person makes unnecessary pain. Fear may increase shock. The child should be reassured and should not be bothered with unnecessary questions. The first-aider should never give a person in shock any kind of liquids or stimulants.

Poisoning

Once poison is swallowed and reaches the stomach, it is only a matter of time until it is absorbed. In most cases of poisoning it is important that the poison be diluted and as much of it as possible emptied from the stomach by vomiting. Poisoning from foods occurs often. Food poisoning may be caused by spoiled or partially spoiled foods. Certain types of mushrooms, wild berries, roots, and some types of leaves are poisonous. The poisonous type of mushrooms are often called toadstools. Small children are often poisoned by aspirin and petroleum products, such as kerosene and gasoline.

The symptoms of poisoning may vary greatly, depending on the substance swallowed and the time elapsed after ingestion. Some of the general symptoms are nausea, stomach cramps, pain, and sometimes vomiting. Sometimes posions are absorbed before symptoms become evident. The corrosive poisons, such as acids and alkalis, may burn the lips and mouth and cause very marked shock. Poisoning caused by foods may cause vomiting, diarrhea, and collapse. There is usually some degree of prostration present.

When first aid for poisoning is given, the first step is to call the hospital emergency room or the nearest poison control center. When first aid is administered for poisoning from other than strong acids, petroleum products, and alkalis, an attempt should be made to dilute the poison and induce vomiting. Fluids suitable for use in diluting the poison and filling the stomach are plain water and milk. A few teaspoons of baking soda if available should be added to each glass of water because it tends to induce vomiting. Although water is always the most readily available fluid, milk is good to use because it gives some protection to the lining of the digestive tract. Four or five glasses of fluid should be given. Vomiting should not be induced if acids or alkalis were swallowed because the poison coming up may do further damage to the lining of the food passages.

With the rapid increase in the number of over-the-counter and prescription drugs available to children in the home, opportunities for poisoning or dangerous overdose are much greater today than in past years. Sometimes children will ingest medicines or drugs in the home, yet effects may not be noticed until later in the day at school.

Diabetic reactions

Diabetic reactions occur as the result of too much (insulin shock) or too little (diabetic coma) insulin. In insulin shock the first sign noted in the child is general irritability. The student may be despondent, cry readily, or be exuberant or belligerent. In addition, the student may be hungry, perspire excessively, tremble or be unable to concentrate, and complain of dizziness. The symptoms vary in duration and will often disappear in 10 to 15 minutes by providing the child with any of the following: sugar cube, soda pop, candy, raisins, fruit juice with sugar, or any other carbohydrate. If the symptoms do not subside after this action, the pupil's parents should be notified. A diabetic coma, a rather rare condition, is caused by the failure to take insulin, an illness, or neglect of a proper diet. It is slow in onset and may be observed by these symptoms: thirst, frequent urination, flushed face, labored breathing, nausea, and vomiting. The teacher should keep the child in a resting state and maintain body temperature. In addition, the school nurse, the principal, and the parents should be immediately notified.

Epileptic convulsions

Most elementary school classroom teachers at one time or another are confronted with the problem of dealing with epileptic convulsions in children. The minor form of epilepsy is not a particular problem for the teacher. The seizures in major or grand mal epilepsy require emergency care on the part of the teacher. The seizures are usually marked by loss of consciousness, convulsions, and thrashing about. The convulsive state is then followed by prolonged stupor.

In giving a child first aid for a seizure, the teacher should not resist his/her thrashing about. Keep calm and let the convulsion run its course, which it will do in 2 to 5 minutes. The child should be kept in the open where he/she will not be injured by striking any hard or sharp objects. *Do not force anything between the child's teeth*. The child's collar should be loosened to prevent breathing from being obstructed. Turn the victim's face to one side so that liquid emitted does not fall back into the throat. Place something soft, such as a rolled-up coat, beneath the person's head. After the convulsion the child should be taken to the emergency room to lie down and sleep. However, the parents should be notified because they may wish to call for the student at once. Ordinarily, if it is known that the child is epileptic, arrangements should be made with the parents and physician concerning the routine to follow.

Fainting

Just before fainting, a child is likely to feel weak and dizzy. Vision becomes blurred, the face becomes pale, and the victim may be covered with a cold sweat. When a child faints, he/she should be placed in a supine position. The color of the face indicates to some extent the amount of blood being supplied to the brain. If the face is pale, slightly lower the head until the color of the face improves. If, on the other hand, the face is extremely red, it may be desirable to keep the head slightly raised. After the fainting victim has recovered consciousness, the victim should lie quietly for a few minutes. The child should then sit up for a few minutes before taking a standing position. The fainted person should have plenty of fresh, cool air. After regaining consciousness, a cool, wet cloth may be applied to the face or chest as a stimulant to recuperative action.

Nosebleed

A nosebleed frequently results from a blow on the nose, although there may be other causes. Some of the small blood vessels in the mucous membrane of the nose can be ruptured easily. It is often unneccesary to give first aid for a nosebleed, as many, if not most of them in children, will stop without emergency care. For minor cases pressure can be applied by pinching the nostrils closed with the fingers and tilting the head back. In giving first aid for a more persistent nosebleed, it is preferable to place the child flat in a prone position. This keeps the blood from flowing back into the throat. Cold packs may be applied to the nose, or it may be temporarily packed with sterile gauze. If a nosebleed cannot be readily stopped, a physician is required.

Wounds

Any injury to the skin or tissue is classed as a wound. The person giving first aid is primarily concerned with wounds in which the skin or mucous membrane is broken. Any tiny break in the skin is considered a wound if germs are allowed to enter.

Wounds may be classified according to the way the injury occurs, the type of wound made, and the kind of first aid required. The general types of wounds with which the first-aider is likely to be concerned are incisions or clean-cut wounds torn or lacerated wounds, abrasions or scraping, or rubbing types of wounds made by the body sliding on the floor or on a rough surface. Puncture or stab wounds are made by such objects as pins, needles, and nails.

Clean-cut wounds usually bleed freely and are not likely to become infected. Wounds made by machines or other rough objects, however, are more likely to become infected. They may not bleed freely, and often there are dirt and grease in the wound. Puncture wounds are ordinarily more serious than other types of minor wounds. They usually do not bleed freely and are hard to cleanse properly. Furthermore, there is danger of tetanus, or lockjaw, from puncture wounds.

Infection is a danger from a majority of wounds. Although thousands of organisms may enter even a tiny wound, not all wounds become infected. The body may resist and overcome the organisms, depending on a number of factors, or the organisms may not have the strength to grow and multiply.

In giving first aid for wounds in which serious bleeding is not a factor, a main purpose is to prevent infection if possible and to keep germs from entering the wound. If a physician will be available soon, all the first-aider will need to do as far as the wound is concerned is cover it with a sterile dressing. Never try to clean a wound or apply an antiseptic if the services of a physician are needed and readily available. If it is necessary to cleanse a wound, use plain soap and running tap water adjusted to room temperature. The first-aid care of ordinary small wounds requires only that the first-aider apply a sterile compress and bandage to keep dirt from entering the wound.

Punctures and stabs are particularly dangerous types of wounds for the following reasons:

1. Tetanus, or lockjaw germs, may grow readily when there is a lack of air, such as in a puncture wound.

2. Punctures do not bleed freely; consequently, dirt and germs are not washed out, as in an open wound.

3. It is extremely difficult to clean the wound, and germs may have been deposited in the bottom of it by the instrument making the wound.

A physician is needed to treat a puncture wound as protective measures may be needed against tetanus. If a physician cannot be secured for some time, the first aider should encourage bleeding without bruising the tissue.

Eye injuries

Since the eyes are delicate organs, they should be treated with the greatest of care. Children should not be allowed to use most sharp-pointed instruments because of the danger of injuring the eye or falling on the instrument. The following points should be remembered in caring for eye injuries:

1. If any type of chemical gets into the eyes, it should be washed out immediately with plenty of water.

2. The first-aider should *never* attempt to remove an embedded object from the eye.

3. If a foreign object gets into the eye, the eye should not be rubbed. Rubbing the eye with a foreign object in it, especially if it is a sharp particle, such as a cinder, may drive it into the eyeball tissue.

4. If a child gets a small, foreign object in the eye, the teacher should attempt to remove it

with a sterile cloth. If the object cannot be removed readily, a physician is needed.

5. The use of any kind of sharp object should be avoided in removing foreign particles from the eye.

Burns

There are three general types of burns— *chemical, thermal,* and *solar*. Burns and scalds are from heat of such a degree as to cause injury to the skin and tissue of the body. Burns from hot liquids or steam are classified as scalds. Burns are sometimes classified as follows: first-degree burns are those in which the skin is reddened; second-degree burns are those in which the skin is blistered; third-degree burns are those in which there is destruction of deeper tissue and are serious, since growth cells that form new skin are destroyed.

Giving first aid for a burn depends somewhat on the extent of the burn. If it is extensive or if tissue has been destroyed, a physician is needed as soon as possible. The main duty of the first-aider in this case is to try to prevent and care for shock until a physician is in charge of the individual. Nothing should be put on the burned area. However, relief of pain and control of tissue damage can often be achieved in first- and second-degree burns by immersion in cold water. Chemical cold sprays should not be used because of the danger of frostbite and possible tissue damage. Be careful not to use ice since this has been known to aggravate shock in the victim.

Fractures

Although there are many classifications of fractures, for the purpose of first aid they can be classed as (1) simple or closed fractures, in which a bone is broken but the skin is not broken, and (2) compound or open fractures, in which a bone is broken and a wound extends from the break through the tissue and skin.

The symptoms of fracture include swelling, pain, and bruising. If a portion of a limb swings

FIG. 7-10. Splint and sling for fracture of upper arm.

FIG. 7-9. Pneumatic splint for fractured arm.

in any direction that it could not do unless the bone were broken, that is sure proof that there has been a fracture. If a bone that ordinarily appears straight suddenly assumes an angular position, the irregularity of the line indicates a fracture. Not all symptoms will necessarily be present in every fracture.

If fracture is suspected, a physician is needed. The usual policy of the school should be followed in this case. Shock may follow a broken bone. The first-aider should give first aid for shock. If medical aid is readily available, the child should not be moved. If it is necessary to move the patient, a splint should be applied if the arms

or legs are involved. If possible, pneumatic splints (plastic inflated sleeves) are best for the extremities since they are easy to use (Figs. 7-9 and 7-10).

If the neck or back is involved, extreme care should be used in handling the person. An injured person should be moved only if more danger is imminent. However, if it is necessary to move the injured person with a neck or back injury before medical aid is available, it should be remembered that the body should never be allowed to sag, especially the head or neck. The child should be prevented from moving in any way if at all possible. Rigid material should be used to move the person. A wide flat board or door will keep the body straight and prevent it from sagging. Be sure the person is securely strapped to the back board. Plenty of help should be available for carrying the injured person.

Skull fracture may result from any type of hard blow on the head or by the head striking a hard surface. Some of the symptoms of skull fracture are bleeding from the nose, mouth, or ears; unconsciousness; pupils of the eyes unequal in size; face flushed or pale, depending on the seriousness of the injury; and evidence of a blow on the head, such as a cut or a bump. All of the symptoms may not be present in every case.

First aid for skull fractures involves keeping

the person in a lying position with the head and shoulders *slightly elevated if the face is flushed*. If the face is pale or ashen, the head and shoulders should not be elevated. The child's body temperature should be maintained, but no heated object should be applied. A physician should be secured as soon as possible. If a person must be moved before medical aid is available, the victim should be kept in a lying position.

Dislocations

A dislocation is a bone out of place at a joint. The ligaments are injured and torn or stretched. The blood vessels and nerves may be injured, and the ends of the bones may be chipped. A physician is needed to reduce a dislocation safely (this should never be done by a teacher). The parts of the body that may be dislocated are the fingers, shoulders, jaw, elbows, knees, and hips. The first-aid care for a dislocation consists of placing an ice bag or cold compresses over the joint and securing a physician. There should be no movement of the joint, since there is danger of chipping the bone.

Frostbite

In some areas of the country, school children may occasionally suffer from frostbite. It results from loss of circulation because of constriction of arteries at low temperatures. Consequently, the tissues are deprived of oxygen. Injury from frostbite varies with circumstances and the kind of emergency care given.

The fingers, toes, nose, ears, and cheeks are the parts of the body most likely to be frostbitten. The signs of frostbite are a sensation of intense coldness followed by numbness, then finally almost complete loss of sensation in the frozen part. The frostbitten part may be flushed at first and then become very white or grayish white. Because of numbness and loss of sensation, people may not realize that their nose, cheeks, or ears are frostbitten until someone calls attention to it.

In giving first aid for frostbite, the teacher should be careful not to damage the tissue. Rubbing or careless handling of a frozen part may bruise the tissue and cause further damage. If a person is outdoors, the frozen part should be covered with the hand or with cloth, preferably woolen. The child should be brought indoors and placed in a warm room, the frostbitten part should be covered with a warm cloth and immersed in water that has been heated to 102° to 105°F. However, hot objects of any kind should be kept away from the frostbitten part.

Sprains

In sprains, ligaments and other tissues may be damaged. Wrists and ankles are most often sprained. In giving first aid for a sprain, the teacher should apply cold compresses or an ice bag for 20 to 30 minutes after the injury. The injured part should be kept elevated and the child not allowed to put any weight on the sprained part. A sprained ankle may be helped by a crisscrossing bandage, elastic bandage, or adhesive around it to keep it immovable. The usual school procedure in contacting the parents concerning a physician should be followed.

First-aid supplies

Every elementary school should have adequate first-aid supplies, depending on the enrollment as well as the location of the school and the availability of medical assistance. In most elementary schools the first-aid supplies are likely to be under the care of the principal. They should be kept in a central place, such as the health service room, the emergency room, or the principal's office. Periodic stock taking should be done to assure that first-aid kits are complete and up to date. The following list shows the usual first-aid supplies needed by the school:

Absorbent cotton
Adhesive tape
Compresses of various sizes
Sterile gauze of various sizes

Roller bandages of various sizes
Triangular bandages
Cotton swabs sterilized in packages
Scissors
Eye dropper
Aromatic spirits of ammonia
Tourniquet
Tincture of green soap
Meat tenderizer (for bee stings)
Wooden applicators
Hand brushes
Elastic bandages, 2 and 3 inches wide
Blankets
Splints (pneumatic type preferably)
Pillows
Paper cups
Safety pins
Tweezers
Hot-water bottle
Ice bag
"Instant cold" chemical bags

It is important to remember that *no medicines of any kind* are part of a first-aid supply cabinet!

SUMMARY

The concept of school safety has received a great deal of attention over the past few years. Whenever a child is injured at school, the question, "Who is going to pay for this injury?" arises. There is an increasing trend for people to recover costs from accidents, and the attitude has begun to emerge that parents expect teachers to pay for accidents resulting in injuries to students.

The teacher has a duty to care for those who are injured and ill but must realize that the possibility of litigation exists. In general, teachers should carry personal liability insurance even though school boards may increasingly be sued for damages in injury cases.

Although it is best if all teachers are trained and certified in first aid and that these personnel be on duty whenever children are present at school, techniques for handling select emergency situations have been presented in this chapter. It is hoped that these suggestions will motivate the individual to seek additional first-aid training and that any certification acquired will be kept up to date.

QUESTIONS FOR DISCUSSION

1. Whose responsibility is the promotion of safety in the elementary school?
2. What are the basic components of a school's emergency care procedures?
3. Why should the school emergency plan be a written document?
4. How would you characterize the role of the teacher in emergency care?
5. What is meant by the phrase, "a reasonable and prudent individual?"
6. What is probably the best way to avoid becoming involved in liability litigation?
7. Under what circumstances is the teacher liable in the event of pupil injury?
8. What are the major legal defenses a teacher can use in a possible negligence lawsuit?
9. Briefly discuss the basic principles that should be followed in administering first aid to the injured.
10. What legal duties would a teacher be expected to perform in terms of a school safety program?
11. Do you feel that the school board should be exempt from legal liability in cases of pupil injury? Why or why not?
12. Some individuals maintain that school boards should be required to purchase personal liability insurance for all employees. What is your viewpoint on this issue?
13. Why is it desirable that a person certified in first aid be present at all times that students are in the school facility?
14. Why should all pupil accidents be reported on accident report forms?
15. What is meant by "The ABC of Life Support?"
16. Why are school personnel admonished not to give a pupil any type of medication unless that medication has been specifically prescribed by a physician?

SELECTED REFERENCES

Airhihenbuwa, C.O.: First aid and emergency care: procedure and practice, Dubuque, Iowa, 1986, Kendall/Hunt.

American Alliance for Health, Physical Education, Recreation, and Dance: Safety education review, Washington, D.C., published annually, The Alliance.

American National Red Cross: Advanced first aid and personal safety, ed. 2, Garden City, N.Y., 1979, Doubleday and Co., Inc.

Amercian National Red Cross: Standard first aid and personal safety, ed. 2, Garden City, N.Y., 1979, Doubleday and Co., Inc.

Hafen, B.Q.: First aid for health emergencies, ed. 3, St. Paul, 1985, West Publishing Co.

Heimlich, H.J., and Uhley, M.H.: The Heimlich maneuver, Clinical Symposium, CIBA **31**(3):1979.

National Safety Council: Accident facts, Chicago, published annually, The Council.

National Safety Council: School safety magazine, Chicago, published quarterly, The Council.

Parcel, G.S.: Basic emergency care of the sick and injured, ed. 3, St. Louis, 1986, Times Mirror/Mosby College Publishing.

Rinke, C.M., editor: Standards and guidelines for cardio-pulmonary resuscitation (CPR) and emergency cardiac care (ECC), Journal of the American Medical Association **255**(21):2905-2894, 1986.

Trubitt, H.: Legal responsibilities of school teachers in emergency situations, The Journal of School Health **36**:Jan., 1966.

PART

IV

HEALTH EDUCATION

CHAPTER
8

HEALTH EDUCATION TODAY

Effective health education early in life can help to prevent the major diseases of adulthood . . . as children grow older, we must teach them how to become responsible informed consumers of health care . . .

JOSEPH A. CALIFANO, JR.
Former Secretary of the U.S. Department of Health, Education, and Welfare

KEY CONCEPT: Comprehensive school health education programs contribute to the well-being of students.

Health education in America's schools has been slowly approaching a threshold of awareness, growth, and emphasis that should have a profound future influence on the children and youth of the United States. Acceptance of the need for preventive health care with a focus on adopting lifestyle behaviors that promote good health is now widely advocated by all leaders in the health and medical community. The concept has received general approval by parents and the public at large.

Elementary school health education is supported by governmental, professional, and health and educational organizations, voluntary health agencies, commercial companies, and parents. In 1975 the Comprehensive School

Health Education Act was under consideration by the U.S. Congress to provide financial support for the development of programs in elementary and secondary schools. Although the act was never passed, recognition of need and public awareness were greatly increased.

Approximately 30% of the 50 states have mandated school health education, but its definition varies widely. Other states have required specific curriculum areas such as alcohol, tobacco and other drugs, safety, and sexually transmitted disease. Still others have additional permissive legislative provisions. The introduction of health education into schools has been advocated by the American Academy of Pediatrics, the American Association of School Administrators, the

American Dental Association, the American Medical Association, the American Public Health Association, the American School Health Association, the Association for the Advancement of Health Education, the Council of Chief State School Officers, the National Association of State Boards of Education, the American Cancer Society, the American Heart Association, and the American Lung Association. The National Dairy Council, the United Way, the Kellogg Foundation, the Henry J. Kaiser Family Foundation, the Robert Wood Johnson Foundation, Metropolitan Life, and Blue Cross and Blue Shield, among others, have supported financially the development of programs in various U.S. communities.

A significant position paper adopted by the Governing Council of the American Public Health Association in 1974 states that:

The school is a community in which most individuals spend at least twelve years of their lives . . . the health of our school-age youth will determine to a great extent the quality of life each will have during the growing and developing years and on throughout the life cycle.*

In 1981 the Education Commission of the States† proposed that state education agencies should do the following:
1. Encourage local school boards and administrators to include health education in the curriculum in elementary and secondary schools
2. Promote health education as a responsibility shared by the family, school, and community
3. Promote the development of comprehensive school health education programs

In 1985 the Metropolitan Life Foundation made $400,000 available to local school districts for the recognition and promotion of comprehensive health education programs (see Chapter 10).

Despite the legislative provisions and the efforts of the various organizations and agencies previously identified, health education programs are neither common nor universally found in schools in the United States. The paucity of curricula is caused primarily by the lack of understanding of the need for and the significance of such programs of learning. It is estimated that only several hundred formal health instruction programs may be in operation in the 1,500 school districts and 58,000 schools in the United States. However, the number of programs has been increasing in recent years. Most health education programs were probably introduced within the past 20 years. Where programs have started, many are fragmented or piecemeal in scope. Some may be broad based (include a variety of topics) but few are what might be considered comprehensive. Some lose their priority status and become obsolete a few years after their initiation. Little has been done to assess the effectiveness of such programs on children's behavior. The situation is best described by the U.S. Department of Health and Human Services in its publication *Better Health for Our Children:*

Many school health education programs at present are neither sufficiently comprehensive nor sufficiently attuned to the influence of peer culture and other important determinants of youthful behavior to be truly effective in promoting good health habits.*

Teachers, nurses, administrators, and others who may desire to or have a duty to develop curricula for their classrooms and schools or those who wish to assume leadership to promote the introduction of health education programs in their districts will find practical material in this text. Programs may be prepared from the information found in the chapters that follow or from the illustrations and sources identified in this chapter.

---

*Governing Council of the American Public Health Association: Education for health in the school community setting; a position paper, New Orleans, Oct. 23, 1974. (See Appendix C.)
†Education Commission of the States: Recommendations for school health education: a handbook for state policymakers, Denver, 1981, The Commission.

---

*U.S. Department of Health and Human Services, Public Health Service: Better health for our children: a national strategy, vol. 1, major findings and recommendations, Washington, D.C., 1981, Superintendent of Documents.

WHY IS HEALTH EDUCATION NEEDED?

Education regarding health should be an essential component of the school curriculum at all grade levels.*

Julius B. Richmond, M.D., former Surgeon General of the United States, advocated that efforts of the Public Health Service (PHS), of the U.S. Department of Health and Human Services, could best serve Americans through a preventive approach to health. As a result, the PHS has supported health programs in schools for a number of years by providing funds for curriculum development and demonstration projects and through evaluative studies.

The need for education about health and health care has been growing in recent years and has reached a high level of acceptance. There is increasing awareness among the public in general of the need for increased information and actions that will help persons, families, and communities. Federal and state laws have been passed that mandate instruction in various aspects of health in curricula. Parents and many community organizations have supported and actively campaigned for the inclusion of health education in school programs. The numerous student health problems and conditions identified in Chapter 1, many of which can be reduced by preventive action, clearly demonstrate the need for health education. There are a variety of specific reasons that justify the inclusion of school health instruction.

High cost of illness and medical care

In 1983 the expenditure for health care in the United States was approximately $335.4 billion,† and it has been rising each year. This sum represents 10.8% of the gross national product. The per capita outlay of funds for health care was in excess of $1,459. The cost of room and board for a day in a hospital can exceed $327, and the average cost per hospital stay is $2,501. The so-called working poor and the elderly are the people chiefly affected when a continuing or catastrophic illness causes a severe financial burden.

However, middle-income families also pay a heavy price for health services because long and expensive illnesses may reduce them to poverty. It should be obvious that information provided at an early age that aids in preventive action could help reduce the costs of illness and medical care.

Gullible public

It is estimated that at least $10 billion annually is spent on worthless health products and services, many of which may even be harmful. Millions of dollars each year are wasted on valueless cancer and arthritis remedies. Approximately $150 million is spent on useless and fake remedies ordered through the mails. Over $1 billion is spent on questionable foods, fraudulent weight-reduction schemes, and fad diets, and another $2 billion goes for vitamins and minerals. In 1983 over $13 billion went for over-the-counter drugs and drug products, many of which were unnecessary. Quacks and quackery are rampant throughout the United States. Children and young people need to learn to make intelligent decisions regarding the purchase and use of health products and health services and know how to identify charlatans.

Health misconceptions

Children as well as adults lack accurate scientific health information. Although almost two decades old, one of the largest and most respected efforts to study health practices* and

---

*U.S. Department of Health and Human Services, Public Health Service: Better health for our children: a national strategy, vol. 1, major findings and recommendations, Washington, D.C., 1981, Superintendent of Documents.
†National data book and guide to sources, statistical abstract of the United States 1985, ed. 105, Washington, D.C., U.S. Department of Commerce, Bureau of Census.

---

*Food and Drug Administration: A study of practices and opinions, Springfield, Va., 1972, National Technical Information Services, U.S. Department of Commerce.

opinions still merits attention. The study, conducted by the U.S. Food and Drug Administration, identified many commonly held misconceptions, among which were the following:

1. Extra vitamins give more pep and energy
2. The major reason for bad health is that people do not eat the right foods
3. Substantial weight loss can occur through perspiring
4. A daily bowel movement is necessary for good health
5. Most things that advertisements say about health and medicines are true
6. Most things people buy in drugstores to treat themselves are practically worthless

The 1985 National Health Interview Survey* conducted by the Center for Health Statistics of the U.S. Department of Health and Human Services reported gaps in Americans' practice and knowledge of health habits concerning such things as stress, exercise, tooth decay and tooth loss in children, and alcohol and its relation to throat cancer.

These inaccuracies expressed by adults are unquestionably related to the lack of information they received as children.

Health information confusing

Health information that people read or receive from friends, neighbors, and family members may be inaccurate or never clearly defined for a variety of reasons. Testimony from individuals may be based on opinions rather than scientific data. Often factual information becomes distorted in transmission. The causes, prevention, and treatment of many illnesses including arthritis, cancer, and heart disease have not been completely identified. The media often dramatize the significance of preliminary data from limited scientific studies and mislead the public to believe the information is conclusive. The tremendous expansion of newspapers, magazines, books, and radio and TV stations has produced an overwhelming amount of health information that is difficult for people to understand and interpret. This information often contains unproved claims. The dissemination of false and inaccurate information by authors and writers is protected by the constitutional provision of "freedom of speech." One study conducted by the American Council on Science and Health* rated 19 popular magazines on the accuracy of nutrition information provided and revealed that 5 were reliable, 8 were inconsistent in reliability, and 6 were unreliable. These factors make it virtually impossible for consumers to determine the reliability and validity of what they read and hear. The question may be asked, "How does one determine fact from fiction?" Young people must learn to locate and use reliable sources of information to be able to identify truths from falsehoods.

Media influence on behavior

What people read or hear through the media influences their decisions to purchase and use health products and services. Advertising, however, is often unclear, misleading, and deceptive—often deliberately so. The intent is to capitalize on the ignorance of the consumer by describing a product in terms of a mystical ingredient physicians are said to recommend rather than in terms of specific contents and value. Advertising claims have multiple meanings, one or more of which may be false or unsubstantiated from a technical standpoint.

Children need help in learning how to analyze advertising to be able to determine the accuracy of information provided by the media.

Lifestyle and disease

American lifestyles contribute to the high incidence of certain diseases such as cancer, heart

---

*Gaps found in Americans' knowledge of health habits as reported in the Nation's Health (American Public Health Association):1,17 July, 1986.

*Hudnall, M.: ACSH survey: how popular magazines rate on nutrition, American Council on Science and Health News and Views **2**:1-2 Jan./Feb., 1982.

disease, diabetes, and dental decay. Data reveal that people who exercise regularly, eat nutritious foods, obtain proper sleep and rest, control their weight and the use of alcoholic beverages and drugs, eliminate cigarette smoking, and reduce stress increase their potential to live longer. People who expose themselves to the identified risk factors increase their chances for ill health. One study that assessed the relative contributions of a variety of factors to the 10 leading causes of death suggested that about one half of the deaths were caused by unhealthy behavior and lifestyles.* Schools can help children to eliminate or reduce the risk factors involved through a health education program.

Peer and adult pressures

Young people are under pressures by their peers to conform to group behavior patterns in such activities as smoking, alcohol and drug use, and sexual activity. In addition, young people wish to become adults and emulate adult behaviors. Students need to be prepared to know how to deal properly with these pressures as well as those they will encounter as adults. A comprehensive school health instruction program will help pupils acquire the skills needed to cope with the health problems and pressures confronted by both teenagers and adults.

Self-care

The focus on preventive aspects of health places emphasis on wellness rather than illness. Since good health has a high correlation with lifestyles and behaviors, the concept of self-care needs development and implementation in the health instruction program. Children must learn to assume responsibility for their own bodies. They must be taught at an early age to make intelligent decisions on ways to reduce or eliminate risk factors that lead to ill health.

---

*Healthy people: the Surgeon General's report on health and disease prevention. Washington, D.C., 1979, U.S. Department of Health and Human Services.

WHAT IS THE CURRENT STATUS OF HEALTH EDUCATION?

Despite the greatly increased awareness of the need for health education, the implementation of programs into local schools and school districts continues to leave much to be desired. Comprehensive curricula are being advocated, but their numbers are not rapidly increasing. Most programs continue to be piecemeal and fragmentary. They consist of one or several health subject areas at selected grades. However, the outlook for improvement in the future is optimistic. Events at national, state, and local levels support the positive outlook for school health education.

National

A chronology of recent significant legislation, activities, and offices established in support of health education includes:

1973: President Richard Nixon's Committee on Health Education reported that school health education in elementary schools was not, or was poorly, provided.

1974: The Bureau of Health Education (now the Center for Health Promotion and Education) was established in the Center for Disease Control, U.S. Public Health Service.

1975: The National Center for Health Education, a nongovernmental agency, was established to promote health education.

1975: A variety of federal agencies including the Public Health Service of the U.S. Department of Health, Education, and Welfare established as priorities for national health planning and resources development the prevention of disease and the development of effective methods for health education of the public.

1975-1976: The U.S. Congress gave consideration to the passage of the Comprehensive School Health Education Act. The bill did not pass but it gave health education greater visibility, which was reflected in the amendments to the Elementary and Secondary Education Act in 1978.

1976: The Office of Health Information and Health Promotion was created in the U.S. Department of Health, Education, and Welfare (now the Department of Health and Human Services).

1978: Amendments to the Elementary and Secondary Education Act of 1965, Title III, authorized funds for states and local districts to develop and implement comprehensive school health education programs. Local school districts now have legal authority to expend funds awarded to states by the federal government under the so-called block grants provision for health education programs.

1979: The Office of Comprehensive School Health was established in the U.S. Department of Education to coordinate the variety of efforts in school health services, instruction, and environmental programs. The office is not currently operative.

1975-1980: The National Parent-Teacher Association Comprehensive School/Community Health Education Project was contracted for by the Bureau of Health Education (now the Center for Health Promotion and Education) to increase community awareness and understanding of health education needs and to develop support for more effective health education.

1980-1981: The U.S. Surgeon General's Office* expressed support for school health education programs.

1982: The Centers for Disease Control reorganized and now includes a School Health Section illustrating a continued federal commitment.

1982: National School Health Education Coalition (NASHEC) was formed as an effort of voluntary health agencies and others to cooperate on a national level for the improvement of school health.

1983: The federal government held an interagency meeting and identified 140 different federal agencies responsible for some

respect in the health of the school-age child.

1984: The American School Health Association (ASHA) completed and made available a national marketing kit for school health programs.

1984: The Office of Disease Prevention and Health Promotion (ODPHP) entered into a cooperative agreement with the American Association of School Administrators to disseminate the Oregon model health conference known as the Seaside Health Conference.

1985: ODPHP entered into a cooperative agreement with ASHA to develop model strategies to relate the 1990 health objectives for the nation to the school population.

1985: ODPHP entered into a cooperative agreement with ASHA, Association for the Advancement of Health Education (AAHE), and the Society for Public Health Education (SOPHE) for an ongoing national survey of knowledge, attitudes, and practices in school health.

1985: National School Health Education Evaluation study completed and published.

1986: ODPHP approved a study to follow up the 1985 National Youth Fitness Study by evaluating the health status of 6- to 9-year-olds.

1986: National Center for Health Education cooperates with ASHA and AAHE to publish an evaluation manual for school health programs.

State

In most states, laws require health instruction as part of the curriculum. This requirement is usually general in nature and not adequately defined in terms of scope, sequence of topic, grade, and time allotment. However, most state departments of education have prepared recommendations, guidelines, and frameworks for health instruction.

A summary of state requirements is found in Chapter 1. Every state requires certain health topics to be taught. This has led to fragmented rather than comprehensive programs. Alcohol,

*U.S. Department of Health and Human Services, Public Health Service: Better health for our children: a national strategy, vol. 1, major findings and recommendations, Washington, D.C., 1981, Superintendent of Documents.

tobacco, and drug education is required in 38 states but the quality of instruction is not known.

Local

It is estimated that 300 to 400 health instructional programs may be found in the 1,500 elementary school districts (over 58,000 schools) in the United States. These vary in nature from individual topical programs to broad-based, comprehensive ones. Their impact on children has not been adequately evaluated. They have been financed by federal, state, and local district funds as well as by voluntary health agencies, private foundations, and a few industrial corporations.

The National Center for Health Education* prepared a report that contained limited information about 102 instructional programs, of which 78 were for elementary schools. Eleven of the 78 were developed by voluntary and government agencies and organizations and were not identified with specific school districts. A review of elementary programs, in which 30 states and the District of Columbia were represented, revealed the following types of programs:

41 broad-based (several topics covered)
9 comprehensive
28 individual topics: nutrition, 5; drugs, 5; vision, 4; heart, 3; human sexuality, 3; emotional health, 2; alcohol, 2; epilepsy, 1; fire safety, 1; parenting education, 1; dental, 1

Preschool children

The introduction of early education and day-care programs for children 3 to 5 years of age has resulted in new opportunities for health-related education for 3 million pupils. The federal government has advocated instruction and has developed health instruction materials for

*National Center for Health Education: A compendium of health education programs available for use in schools, San Bruno, Calif., 1982, The Center (Revised 1984).

use in such programs as Head Start. Stress has been placed on the development of habit patterns relating to such areas as nutrition, safety, disease control, and dental health. In this text, the content material for teachers in Chapter 11 and the teaching/learning activities in Chapter 12 are useful in the development of health instruction programs for preschool children.

Special services for handicapped children

The passage of Public Law 94-142, the Education for All Handicapped Children Act of 1975, has placed greater emphasis on providing equal educational opportunities for handicapped young people. The act enables handicapped children to be integrated (mainstreamed) into regular academic classes. A number of school districts are now giving consideration to providing health instruction for these students. Suggestion for content may be found in Chapter 11. Many of the activities in Chapter 12, with modification, are useful.

WHAT ARE THE ADMINISTRATIVE PROBLEMS?

The major administrative problem is the low priority given to health education as a subject field by superintendents and school boards despite the increased recognition of need and the progress made in program development. The problem is compounded by these concerns now facing all U.S. public schools: (1) the questioning by the community of the quality of education, (2) the desire of parents for a return to an emphasis on basic subjects (reading, writing, arithmetic) in the curriculum, and (3) the curtailment of federal and state financial support.

These difficulties are formidable but are not insurmountable. Health instruction can be introduced into school curricula despite existing problems. School boards make the decisions regarding the adoption of health instruction as well as any other curriculum. As community representatives school board members are expected to serve the people they represent. Coordinated pressures by parents and health professionals can affect such decisions.

The presence of a health instruction program in a school is no assurance that it will have a positive effect on children. A quality program is dependent on the thorough consideration of a variety of administrative problems that follow.

How should health instruction be included in the curriculum?

The question of whether to have a pattern of instruction that includes *direct* teaching or *integrative* teaching or both must be answered.

Direct teaching. The direct teaching approach is one in which health is identified as a separate subject in the curriculum with a specified amount of teaching time allocated in the school day similar to that given to other subjects. Direct teaching provides status to health instruction as a necessary curriculum area. Its inclusion more likely provides the opportunity for a sequential program of learning throughout the grades. Direct teaching in health education allows for the attainment of attitudes and practices of healthful living by students that will enable them to develop lifestyles conducive to good health.

The direct method of teaching must receive priority as the best approach to use in health instruction.

Integrative teaching. The integrative teaching approach is one in which health is taught throughout the many subject fields in the curriculum. For example, social studies may include information about health organizations and personnel—health departments, physicians, and nurses. When covering addition, subtraction, and multiplication in arithmetic, the teacher can relate these procedures to the numbers of oranges and apples in boxes or to determining the cost of 1 day's food supply; the structure and function of muscles and body organs may be included in science; language arts may include reading and writing about "Who am I?"

or a show-and-tell visit to the dentist; and the physical education program may cover safety on apparatus or on the playground. Actually, health-related matters can be integrated with any school subject.

The integrative approach presents two important problems for health instruction: (1) the major emphasis in the learning may be on a special subject area rather than on health, and (2) the learning objectives stressed may be on the acquisition of information, factual data, or the skills of writing, reading, or computation rather than on healthful living. By way of illustration, a lesson in reading from a nutrition text may focus on teaching students how to read rather than on eating the proper foods. If the health program's objective is to get pupils to eat nutritious foods, reading may be used to help students analyze the nutritional content of breakfasts, lunches, and dinners.

The integrative method can provide positive health learning especially when used for reinforcement and repetition. It should not be the basic, nor the only, approach to the teaching of health.

Integrative health teaching is the only health program found in many schools that claim to have a health education program. The quality of such programs in terms of their impact on student health lifestyles can often be questioned.

Informal teaching. Informal health teaching has always existed in schools when, for example, students go to visit the nurse or ask a teacher about a specific health problem. This generally occurs incidentally, on an unplanned basis. Although the word *informal* connotes actions that take place spontaneously, there is need for a limited amount of planning. In recent years, except perhaps in drug education, little informal health instruction has occurred. Drug counselors or people knowledgeable about drugs have been available to meet with students individually or in small groups on a voluntary basis for information or guidance. In a few schools, voluntary student group meetings, in which opportunities are provided for pupils to ask questions or merely listen to discussions on specific health problems, have been held after school hours. Informal gatherings of this nature need to be included in health instruction programs, although planning will need to be limited in an informal learning setting. These gatherings should be correlated with the direct teaching program. Presently there are no guidelines for conducting this kind of instruction.

What about grade placement?

The determination of grade placement for any or all of the health instruction areas in the curriculum is a complex task. It has not been clearly defined by professional health educators or by curriculum specialists. The reason is probably the variety of pupil and community health problems that must be locally identified and introduced. In addition, grade placement is an imperfect but expeditious manner of organizing schools. There is no single grade arrangement that will function best for all school districts. The pattern to be used must be selected on an individual basis. The suggestions that follow are based on our many years of curriculum experience.

Grade placement in health education is determined through the use of several curriculum principles and a number of additional factors. Three principles in need of attention are that (1) student needs and interests are fundamental, (2) instructional areas should be sequentially organized through the grades, and (3) repetition of subject areas is necessary for the reinforcement of learning.

Students may not always be able to identify health needs and interests for use in curriculum development. Therefore in addition to pupil involvement through surveys and other means, information must be derived from state laws (some mandate specific content areas by grades or grade level groups), review of the growth and developmental characteristics of children; examination of local community health problems; identification of ethnic, religious, and racial factors; observations of pupils by parents; and data from physicians, dentists, and other health professionals.

The sequence of subject areas in health instruction through the grades must follow a pattern that is related to children's growth, development (for example, dental health at the first grade level because of the appearance of the 6-year molar; menstruation for girls at the fourth, fifth, or sixth grade level), and to their felt and unfelt needs and interests. The curriculum information presented to pupils must flow from simple facts to more complex concepts as students move upward in grade level.

The content and objectives provided in the sequence of learning must give consideration to reinforcement of learning without repetition throughout the grades. It may be advisable to space or cycle some health areas. For example, nutrition can be introduced in kindergarten or earlier and repeated in grades 1, 3, 5, and 7. Not every health area needs to be taught at every grade. There may not be enough time in the total school curriculum for such consideration.

Adequate amounts of time are needed in the formal instruction program for direct teaching to have a positive effect on student lifestyles. Such provision will enable the spacing procedure to be introduced into the health curriculum and help reduce the problem of excessive repetition of information, yet allow for the necessary reinforcement of learning to take place.

The chart found in Table 11-1 provides an illustration of grade placement for health instruction. The content areas were determined through a survey of pupil needs and interests, with consideration given to growth and development characteristics, and through the use of a variety of other information and procedures. The areas have been cycled and are not taught at every grade; however, the individual teacher in any given grade can use judgment to repeat health areas in immediate higher grades depending on student needs. This curriculum provides for direct teaching in the formal instructional program.

How much time should be allotted?

The amount of time needed to teach health instruction adequately at any given grade level or throughout the grades has not been adequately researched. Therefore most of the information available today is based solely on professional opinions.

There is, however, one recent study that provides excellent insights about many important questions concerning implementation of effective health education programs including how much time should be allotted to the teaching of health for effective results. In 1985 results of the School Health Education Evaluation (SHEE) were reported.* This study involved more than 30,000 children (grades 4 to 7) in 1,071 classrooms from 20 states.

Fig. 8-1 represents a summary of the SHEE data that shows the relationship between classroom hours of health education and the extent of the resultant effects on student health knowledge, practices, and attitudes. The information in this figure highlights several items of interest in relation to the question of "How much time should be spent in health instruction?":

1. More classroom hours are required to produce significant attitude change than are needed to produce either knowledge or practice change.
2. "Large" effects (greater than 0.8 standard deviation) are achievable for general health knowledge gain, but only after more than 50 classroom hours. Conversely "large" gains in specific subsets of health knowledge are achievable in far fewer hours.
3. "Medium" effects are achievable for general health practices when more than 30 hours of classroom instruction is provided.
4. "Small" effects are achievable for general health attitudes, but these emerge only after 40 hours of classroom instruction is provided.
5. Effects for all three domains reach generally stable levels at about 50 classroom hours.*

*Connell, D.B., Turner, R.R., and Mason, E.F.: School health education evaluation, final report, vols. I-VI, Washington, D.C., 1985, Centers for Disease Control and Office of Disease Prevention and Health Promotion, Public Health Service, U.S. Department of Health and Human Services.

Thus the data from this study suggest that there is a definite association between student effects and classroom hours across all three domains. Furthermore, the evidence seems to indicate that a minimum of 50 hours of instruction time is required to reach the maximum total effect. This is not unreasonable since there are usually 36 weeks in a school year.

Traditionally most health education experts have recommended instructional time configurations ranging from 40 hours per year in the primary school grades, to 75 to 80 hours in the middle school grades. Although local schools and school districts must individually determine the amount of time to allot for health instruction, data from the SHEE and expert opinion do provide excellent guidance.

Who is responsible for the program?

The development, maintenance, and continuance of a health instruction program will take place most effectively if one person in the school or school district has supervisory or administrative responsibility. This individual should be professionally qualified in the field of health education. A person designated as the health coordinator, supervisor, or consultant could be a health educator, a physician, a nurse, or a teacher. Someone is needed who has access to the school superintendent and the school board. This person must be given the responsibility and authority to (1) develop the curriculum, (2) seek funds for support of the program, (3) conduct inservice teacher preparation programs, (4) communicate with parents and community organizations and agencies, (5) order and help select teaching aids and equipment, and (6) supervise and administer the program. Unfortunately, except perhaps in some large districts, there are not many such people employed in local school districts.

Many school nurses have become qualified in the field of health education and have assumed health education responsibilities in schools. These are some of the ways nurses may provide assistance:

FIG. 8–1. Relationship of effect size and instruction hours for health knowledge, attitudes, and practices. (*From Connell, D.B., Turner, R.R., and Mason, E.F.: Summary of finding of the school health education evaluation: health promotion effectiveness, implementation, and cost, Journal of School Health,* **55:**320-321 *Oct., 1985, Copyright, Kent, Ohio, 1985, American School Health Association.*)

1. Help with the selection and location of teaching aids
2. Locate resources for community materials and speakers
3. Assist in lesson planning
4. Teach classes on occasion
5. Serve as school health committee members
6. Consult with teachers regarding instructional possibilities of health services programs
7. Aid in evaluation of the programs
8. Assist in curriculum development

Despite the lack of administrative or nurse assistance in schools that have no program, competent individual teachers who wish to introduce health instruction into their classrooms will find sufficient information in this text to develop a program. These teachers should also understand that the variety of state and local government offices, health departments, and voluntary and professional health agencies and organizations in the local community have many services to provide on request.

Who should teach health education?

At the elementary level the primary responsibility for the teaching of health should rest with the classroom teacher. This person is familiar with teaching methods and is in the best position to maintain, coordinate, and integrate the program into the curriculum. Where nurse services are available, teachers should not hesitate to use them as a resource in many ways, including bringing them into the classroom to discuss specific health topics.

Although some nurses are qualified to teach health education, for them to serve on a full-time basis and in all classes would be logistically impossible. Many districts may provide only limited nurse services. Besides, if nurses are expected to be involved in the health services program and possibly the environmental health aspect of the program, their multiplicity of responsibilities would not permit them to participate extensively in health education.

In-service training programs should be pro-vided for teachers who are expected to teach health but are not qualified. Those teachers who wish to become prepared in health education or desire to upgrade their competencies can do so by taking college and university courses and workshops, reading current health literature, attending conferences and seminars, and seeking help from the many available community health resources.

What about financing?

School districts must provide funds in their budgets for the development, supervision, personnel, and teaching aids needed for health instruction programs. No program can exist without adequate financial support.

The present economic situation may necessitate that schools seek community help for the development and maintenance of health instruction programs. Two sources of funds that have been used with varying degrees of success by some districts are (1) voluntary health agencies, local health departments, and other governmental offices, and (2) solicitations from industrial corporations. In recent years more businesses, including banks and insurance companies, have been providing funds for school health instruction programs.

Should parent education be included?

The need for both formal and informal education of parents is justified on the basis that many health behaviors occur outside the classroom, in the home and the community. Without parental support and cooperation, the effectiveness of school health instruction will be greatly reduced. Parents should have the opportunity to review and comment on the objectives of the program. They need to understand the nature of the school program.

Parent education, although difficult to make operational, can be achieved through planning and concerted effort. Formal education can take place through lectures, films, group discussions, newsletters, and other procedures. Information regarding the inclusion of controversial areas must be communicated to parents.

Informal education may occur through parent-teacher, nurse-parent, or nurse-parent-teacher conferences; special bulletins; telephone calls; notes home; newspaper articles; radio and TV presentations; and in many other ways. Counseling and guidance can be effective in handling individual student problems.

The extent of parent health education is believed to be sporadic in U.S. schools, and its effectiveness is not known.

What controversial areas should be included in the curriculum?

Sex education and education about sexually transmitted diseases, drug education (including alcohol and tobacco), and values education are curriculum areas parents generally have the greatest concern about including in the health instruction program. The primary arguments raised in the controversy are as follows:

1. Students will be encouraged to experiment with sex and drugs.

2. The home and/or church should be responsible for this education.

3. Schools are not capable of dealing with moral and ethical issues, that is, with values education.

4. Schools may teach values that are in conflict with the home or church.

5. Parents generally prefer teaching abstinence in the use of drugs and sexual involvement rather than moderation or intelligent decision making.

6. Teachers are not competent to teach these subjects.

Many student problems are connected with these controversial areas. Unfortunately, numerous parents are unable, unwilling, or lack the information to provide the counseling and guidance their children need. Schools have a responsibility to attempt to help students and parents cope with these problems through pro-

grams of instruction and in other ways. Should schools decide to introduce any or all of the controversial areas into the curriculum, these factors must receive consideration:

1. Parents, with community support from health departments, physicians, voluntary health agencies, churches, and others, should give input to the inclusion of those curriculum areas identified. Involvement of these individuals and organizations in the preparation of the curriculum will provide understanding and enhance the chances of approval by the school board.

2. Curricula must be approved by the school board. School board members are representatives of the people and will supply the funds to implement and support the program.

3. Teachers must be qualified to teach the subject areas. In-service programs may be necessary to develop curricula and teacher competencies. Teachers must be interested in, feel comfortable with and be capable of teaching the subject to which they are assigned.

4. Teachers should be well-adjusted, emotionally stable, mature persons with a wholesome and positive outlook on life. Parents should be provided the opportunity to meet the teachers who will conduct the instructional programs. Parents need to feel comfortable and assured that these teachers will give proper professional treatment to the instructional program.

5. Parents should be provided the opportunity to view teaching materials. This is mandatory for sex education in some states.

6. The curriculum objectives, content, and materials should be periodically reviewed by parents and appropriate community groups. School districts cannot expect that a program approved in any given year will have support in later years. The needs and problems of students and the nature of families and community representatives are constantly changing.

Controversial areas have been approved for inclusion in the curriculum and have generally been successful in school districts where these factors have received adequate consideration.

What should be the role of the community?

The school as a part of the community must involve parents and health and safety organization representatives in the development, maintenance, implementation, and assessment of health instruction programs. The extent and nature of their specific participation must be determined by each school or school district.

Parents can provide valuable assistance in a variety of ways that include (1) identification of student health problems, (2) help in conducting pupil need and interest surveys, (3) service on health instruction committees, (4) organization of community support for instructional programs, (5) persuasion of school boards to develop and conduct health education, and (6) assistance with evaluation procedures. Health departments, voluntary health agencies, medical and dental organizations, and individual physicians and dentists can participate in parent activities and in addition can help to (1) determine the nature and accuracy of the curriculum content, (2) determine the feasibility of the program objectives, and (3) provide, recommend, and assess teaching aids.

Is evaluation necessary?

The health instruction program periodically should be quantitatively and qualitatively evaluated to determine the extent to which objectives have been achieved. Quantitatively it is important to know whether the curriculum is adequate. Some of the questions that should be answered include:

Are the subject areas provided sufficient to meet student needs?
Is the curriculum guide useful?
Are the teaching aids effective?

It is more important, however, to discover the quality of the program in terms of its impact on the student behavior. It is necessary to learn lifestyle changes in terms of student practices, attitudes, and knowledge.

The evaluation process in health education has not been greatly used or adequately developed. Qualitative assessment of the health program has rarely occurred except to determine the extent of knowledge students have acquired. Chapter 14 provides information that will help with the evaluation process.

SUMMARY

The awareness of the need for health instruction programs, although fairly well-established, continues to require development. Many parent and community health organizations and agencies support the inclusion of health education in school curricula. Despite the establishment of several national and governmental health education agencies and organizations, as well as the existence of numerous state requirements, few comprehensive health instruction programs may be found in schools. Fragmented curricula consisting of one or more content areas are evident in many school districts. Health instruction programs may be justified because of the spiraling costs of medical care, health misconceptions, a gullible public, confusion about health information, the media influence on behavior, the relation of lifestyle to disease, and the need for self-care. The implementation of effective programs in schools can be achieved through the resolution of a variety of administrative problems.

QUESTIONS FOR DISCUSSION

1. What evidence exists that indicates there is increased support for health instruction programs in U.S. schools?
2. What factors identify the need for the health education of elementary school children?
3. What is the current status of health education in the United States today at the national, state, and local levels?
4. What are the administrative problems in need of school attention to ensure effective health instruction programs?
5. Identify and describe the patterns of health instruction that may be used in schools. What are the advantages and disadvantages of their use? Illustrate their application to health instruction.
6. What principles are used in the determination of the grade placement of health education in schools? Illustrate their application to the health instruction program.

7. How much time should be provided in the elementary school curriculum for health education? What factors are used in determining the amount of time for health education?

8. Who should teach in the elementary school health instruction program? Why?

9. Why should parents be included in the elementary school health education program? How can this be achieved?

10. Why are some topics considered to be controversial in health education? What factors need school consideration for decisions to include these topics in the instruction program?

SELECTED REFERENCES

American Academy of Pediatrics: School health: a guide for health professionals, Evanston, Ill., 1981, The Academy.

American Public Health Association, School Health Section: Education for health in the school community setting, Washington, D.C., 1975, The Association.

Connell, D.B., Turner, R.R., and Mason, E.F.: School health education evaluation, final report, vols. I-VI, Washington, D.C., 1985, Centers for Disease Control and Office of Disease Prevention and Health Promotion, Public Health Service, U.S. Department of Health and Human Services.

Connell, D.B., Turner, R.R., and Mason, E.F.: Summary of findings of the school health education evaluation: health promotion effectiveness, implementation and cost, Journal of School Health **55**(8):Oct., 1985.

Cornacchia, H.J., and Barrett, S.: Consumer health, a guide to intelligent decisions, ed. 3, St. Louis, 1985, Times Mirror/Mosby College Publishing.

Cornacchia, H.J., and Barrett, S.: Shopping for health care: the essential guide to products and services, New York, 1982, Mosby Medical Library.

Creswell, W., Newman, I., and Anderson, C.,: School health practice, ed. 8, St. Louis, 1985, Times Mirror/Mosby College Publishing.

Culliton, B.J.: Preventive medicine, legislation calls for health education, Science, Sept. 26, 1975.

Education Commission of the States: Recommendations for school health education: a handbook for state policy-makers, Denver, 1981, The Commission.

Food and Drug Administration: A study of practices and opinions, Springfield, Va., 1972, National Technical Information Service, U.S. Department of Commerce.

Hudnall, M.: ACSH survey: how popular magazines rate on nutrition, American Council on Science and Health News and Views 3:1-2 Jan./Feb., 1982.

Joint Committee on Health Problems in Education: Why health education in your school? Washington, D.C. and Chicago, 1974, National Education Association and the American Medical Association.

Kolbe, L.J., et al.: School health in America: an assessment of state policies to protect and improve the health of students, ed. 4, Kent, Ohio, 1987, American School Health Association.

Levin, H.M., editor: Community control of schools, New York, 1976, Simon and Schuster.

McGavran, E.G.: The role of primary prevention in public health, Health Education, July/Aug., 1977.

National data book and guide to sources; statistical abstract of the United States 1985, ed. 105, Washington, D.C., U.S. Department of Commerce, Bureau of Census.

Noak, M.: State policy support for school health education: a review and analysis, education commission of the states, Report No. 182-1, Washington, D.C., 1982.

Russell, R.D.: Health education, Washington, D.C., 1975, Joint Committee on Health Problems in Education of the National Education Association and the American Medical Association (available from the American Alliance for Health, Physical Education, and Recreation and Dance, Washington, D.C.).

Sliepcevich, E.M.: School health education study: a summary report, Washington, D.C., 1964, School Health Education Study.

U.S. Department of Health, Education and Welfare: Health services and mental health administration: the report of the President's Committee on Health Education, Washington, D.C., 1973, Superintendent of Documents.

U.S. Department of Health and Human Services: Healthy people: the Surgeon General's report on health and disease prevention, Washington, D.C., 1979, Superintendent of Documents.

U.S. Department of Health and Human Services, Public Health Service: Better health for our children: a national strategy, vol. 1 major findings and recommendations, Washington, D.C., 1981, Superintendent of Documents.

CHAPTER

9

THE LEARNING PROCESS AND HEALTH EDUCATION

Health education programs must be theoretically consistent. . . . they should be designed so that their goals, objectives, interventions [methods and techniques], and evaluative measures are consistent with the basic theories of learning.

M. A. VOJTECKY*

KEY CONCEPT: Utilization of fundamental learning principles will have a favorable impact on student health behavior.

Although favorable progress is taking place, health education continues to be criticized for its failure to help individuals develop practices and habits that prevent illness and maintain and promote good health. Health education often is accused of providing only information or knowledge of a physiological nature. Human health behavior, however, is a complex process resistant to change and influenced by a variety of factors previously identified in the concept of

health (see also Chapter 1). These factors include physiological, psychological, social/cultural, and spiritual components (holistic health*). Home atmosphere; racial, ethnic, or cultural background; peer influences; self-image; adequacy of housing and food intake; affection received; achievements; self-respect; and bias and prejudice all have a specific impact on children and youth. Pupil needs, motivations, beliefs, values, experiences, and environmental influences all affect their health habit patterns. These influences affect the ability of people to make re-

---

*Vojtecky, M.A.: An adaptation of Bigge's classification of learning to health education and an analysis of theory underlying recent health education programs, Health Education Quarterly **103**:247-261 Fall/Winter, 1984.

---

*Holistic health refers to the health of the total person and not merely the physiological aspects.

sponsible health decisions and to cope with or adjust to problems they face in the society in which they live. These factors are in need of recognition and use if educational programs are to achieve high levels of wellness in individuals.

Modification of health behavior in terms of health knowledge, attitudes, and practices is necessary to enable individuals to live in a healthful manner. However, the problem of whether to try to modify the health behavior of people and more important how to modify it has not been adequately resolved. Health behavior involves an internal process that is influenced by personal needs and environmental exposures. It is not something done to pupils but rather includes educational procedures or methods used to help individuals adapt, adjust, solve problems, or cope with situations in regard to their health. Health education should attempt to aid students in making intelligent and responsible decisions.

The question of the extent to which educators should try to modify health behavior is moot. Should the use of alcohol or tobacco, including smokeless tobacco, be condemned or condoned? Should all individuals exercise at regular intervals and in the same manner? Should the use of contraceptives be promoted? Should pupils reduce their consumption of foods containing high levels of sugar and cholesterol? Should the flossing and brushing of teeth be universally advocated? Hochbaum* states that in controversial aspects of health behavior, no attempt should be made to make modifications in line with rigid criteria (not to drink, not to smoke). He believes that students should be informed adequately and accurately and helped to develop skills and motivation that will enable them to arrive at rational and intelligent decisions.

It is the purpose of this chapter to help the reader gain insight into the behavior modification problem by providing information that will (1) help teachers become better informed in regard to the learning process, and (2) introduce

---

*Hochbaum, G.M.: Behavior modification, School Health Review **2**:Sept., 1971.

and apply the essential principles of learning needed in the selection of methods and materials (see also Chapters 12 and 13) for effective health instruction programs.

WHAT IS LEARNING?

Learning is a complex process that depends on factors taking place both inside and outside the individual. It refers to the physical, intellectual, and emotional changes that occur in human organisms as a result of their interaction with the environment. It is the growth and development process that goes on within individuals as a result of their participation in a variety of experiences, feelings, attitudes, and interests. The health-educated pupil, having been exposed to a variety of health opportunities and activities, is better able to promote and maintain good health.

The process of learning happens within the individual but is influenced by the experiences to which pupils are exposed through the teaching methods, techniques, and material aids (see also Chapters 12 and 13) selected by the teacher. Knowledge of the nature and conditions of learning is basic to an understanding of the teaching process in the health instruction program.

HOW DO CHILDREN LEARN?

The exact nature of learning is not known. However, the process does involve a series of rewards and punishments. Positive reinforcers may include money, candy, privileges, grades, peer approval, praise, attention, and self-interest. Negative reinforcers that result in the elimination of behavior may include loud sounds, disapproval, punishment, poor grades, and use of unpleasant substances. It is believed that learning takes place most efficiently and effectively when someone *wants* to learn something (positive learning). This person is then said to be motivated to action—to be goal directed. A diagram best illustrates the learning process as it probably occurs (Fig. 9-1).

The process of learning may be illustrated by

FIG. 9–1. Schematic diagram illustrating the learning process.

the example of the teacher who desires to have a student learn procedures that will help prevent and control communicable disease. The goal is established whereby students will know and realize the importance of, and will behave in a manner to control and prevent disease. The teacher selects a variety of activities to aid in the achievement of this objective. These experiences may include reading about germs, demonstrating how bacteria grow and may be transmitted, stressing the importance of washing hands before lunch and at other times, and having students look at bacteria under a microscope. The activities may create emotional tension or conflict in the students. The amount of tension or conflict will depend on a number of factors such as the intensity of the motivation, the difficulty encountered in reaching a solution (numerous errors), the amount of work required, and the desire for a good grade. In the process the teacher guides the pupils individually or collectively to try to reduce the errors. If the activities and guidance are appropriate, the goal

will be reached and pupils will return to the equilibrium desired. Should the goal not be reached, pupils may react through a variety of adjustment mechanisms by making excuses as: "There was too much work to do." "The teacher didn't help me enough." "I didn't understand what to do."

Learning occurs when a learner encounters new experiences in the environment. Pupils can learn without teachers, however, teacher guidance serves to motivate this learning and reduce the errors a pupil may make in the learning process by controlling, manipulating, and selecting the appropriate kinds of activities.

LEARNING AND THE CONCEPT APPROACH TO HEALTH EDUCATION

One effective approach to teaching health is through the emphasis on concepts. It is important to help students develop big ideas or reach conclusions about health that will enable them to take positive action and make wise decisions regarding their own, their families', and their community's health. Teachers must be aware of these generalizations and help students to achieve them. Such concepts—smoking may be harmful to the human body, drugs are mood modifiers, certain foods are needed for proper growth and development, there are ways to protect ourselves from disease—help teachers determine more relevant and effective health education goals (see also Appendix B, Partial Health Units). These "big ideas" are more likely to be remembered and hopefully will provide greater potential for pupil action.

LEARNING AND THE GOALS OF HEALTH EDUCATION

Knowledge of the objectives of health education is important to the learning and teaching processes. Goals give direction to the learning and enable pupils to acquire the concepts needed for healthful living. It is necessary therefore that teachers clearly understand the purposes of health education for the most effective teaching. Precisely defined health objectives have particular meaning since learning should be centered on behavior outcomes as well as on factual achievements. Learning should lead students to the acquisition of health education concepts.

The present aim of health education is to develop practices and attitudes of safe and healthful living through the understanding of scientific health information. Individuals should be able to make intelligent decisions about the physical, mental, and social aspects of health. Health behaviors are therefore related to and dependent on the cognitive learning acquired by pupils. It is important that children develop a correct understanding about health. Attitudes also affect health habits.

The precise interrelationships of knowledge and attitudes to practices are not known today. Phi Delta Kappa's Center on Evaluation, Development, and Research recently stated there had been no significant research to indicate the consistent nature of these relationships.* Present evidence, however, indicates interdependency and reveals that the possession of understanding by itself does not necessarily result in good health habits. Knowing how to brush the teeth does not mean that this practice will be followed. Knowing that some snack-time foods are more nutritious than others is no assurance that they will be eaten. Knowing that immunizations protect against diseases does not always result in these preventive measures being obtained. Knowing the physiological effects of drugs does not necessarily reduce their usage. *Although knowing may not always lead to doing, there will be no doing without knowing.*

Lawrence and McLeroy† advocate the importance of attitudes in health teaching as a means of bridging the gap between "knowing" and "doing." They claim that self-efficacy (one's belief in the ability to do a specific behavior) is the principal connection because it usually precedes behavior. Appreciations and feelings about actions may or may not lead to favorable health behaviors. A person who is interested in preventing dental decay is more likely to brush one's teeth or visit a dentist on occasions. Someone who believes or values these practices will probably behave appropriately. A hierarchy of attitudes, ranging from those of lesser to greater intensity, is presented in Table 9-1. This hierarchy should receive consideration in the health instruction program. Those strong attitudes that have been internalized, such as beliefs and values, and are of great significance probably will have the most impact on health actions. Teachers must be aware of the importance of the emotions in learning about health.

Research has shown that health habit patterns frequently may be developed without attitudinal involvement and with little or no knowledge. This evidence is particularly applicable to young children, especially those in the lower grades.

---

*Practical application of research, Newsletter of Phi Delta Kappa's Center on Evaluation, Development and Research **5:**4 June, 1983.

†Lawrence, L., and McLeroy, K.R.: Self-efficacy and health education, Journal of School Health **56:**317-322 Oct., 1986.

TABLE 9-1. Hierarchy of attitudes

	Attitude	Definitions	Behavioral manifestations
Overt action	1. Interest	Emotional responses to stimuli; feelings	1. Attention, awareness, appreciation by listening, talking, reading, writing, and other ways
	2. Opinion	—	2. Verbal or written expression
Internalization	3. Belief	Emotional acceptance of a concept, proposition, or doctrine; a preference; a decision about something; a conviction to or about something	3. Willingness to be identified with a proposition, or concept; self-expression with verbal, written or performance action
	4. Value	A high, deep, and long-lasting degree of emotional acceptance and commitment to a concept, proposition, or doctrine; to cherish or prize; a faith; a potential goal	4. Pursues, seeks, and wants; takes action in satisfying ways through participation—convincing others, spending time, effort, and funds

Modified from Rosser, J.M.: Journal of School Health 41:386-390, 1971; and Cornacchia, H.J., Smith, D.E., and Bentel, D.J.: Drugs in the classroom: a conceptual model for school programs, ed. 2, St. Louis, 1978, The C.V. Mosby Co.

In the home, the nutritional, dental, sleep and other behaviors are usually established by parents. In school, habit patterns may occur through rules and regulations issued by the teacher or principal as they relate to safety (bicycle, playground), nutrition (school lunch, snack machine contents), and control of disease (washing hands before lunch and after toilet use, sneezing, coughing).

Consideration must be given to the fact that behavioral and attitudinal changes in health do not necessarily take place immediately after teaching. Cultural, social, and other values and beliefs that pupils bring from home and community relating to health habits are extremely difficult to change within short periods of time. However, some behavior changes may be observable in the classroom and are subject to measurement; those occurring in the home and elsewhere outside of school may not be seen and may be extremely difficult to assess. It should be recognized that the impact of health learning often takes time to have its effect on children. Despite these difficulties, health education must provide correct information if appropriate health behaviors are to be acquired by pupils.

Good health behavior is significant only in terms of its effect on the lives of pupils. Good health therefore should be a means to an end and not an end in itself. Being healthy should enable children to obtain a better education, be happier, have fun, be able to play for longer periods of time without undue fatigue, be more productive in the world, and be better citizens in the community. When good health is an end in itself, pupils are likely to become overly concerned about their health and become health neurotics.

Teachers should be aware of the fact that all students may not be able to acquire the same health levels because of hereditary and environmental factors. Children who are blind or deaf may never have these senses restored. Pupils who are paralyzed from poliomyelitis may never be able to walk as others do. Boys and girls with uncorrectable heart defects may never have the stamina to play in strenuous games. Students without food may be hungry and malnourished. Despite these handicaps, students need to maintain the best health status possible for themselves within their own limitations. Numerous illustrations of handicapped people leading well-adjusted, happy, and productive lives are found in society. The goals in health education therefore may need to be modified to fit the individual differences of children.

Inspection of the specific outcomes of health education that teachers seek to achieve reveals them to be categorized into the following:

1. Practices, habits, skills—action domain
2. Attitudes, feelings, ideals, interests, appreciations—affective domain
3. Knowledge, understanding, information—cognitive domain

The *decision-making process* (see "Ability to solve problems," p. 184) must receive attention by teachers in the health instruction program. Pupils are growing and developing organisms who are exposed constantly to environmental influences affecting health and about which decisions must be made. Young people must have the opportunity to make their own decisions and not be expected to follow the dictates of the teacher. However, such decisions must be based on complete awareness of the consequences. To make wise decisions, it is important that students be exposed to the possible alternatives for action without teacher bias or prejudice. Such teacher consideration is vital to health teaching because it aids in the establishment of credibility, it allows for the free choice of action, and it prepares students to think and act for themselves. It is teaching for the future. By way of illustration, young people find cigarettes available in their communities and are constantly being persuaded to use them. If these individuals are to be able to determine intelligently whether to smoke or not to smoke, they must learn the positive as well as the negative effects of smoking on the human organism. Merely condemning cigarettes may create distrust among students who talk to peers and adults and obtain conflicting evidence regarding the beneficial or detrimental aspects. This is not to imply the use of tobacco is not hazardous but rather to emphasize that wise decisions will more likely come about when the total spectrum of tobacco's effects is provided.

HOW CAN TEACHERS RELATE KNOWLEDGE TO BEHAVIOR IN THE INSTRUCTION PROGRAM?

The importance of health practices and habits points out the need for the use of teaching procedures that will help bridge the gap between the knowledge and behaviors to preserve and maintain health. Unfortunately, the precise methods are not known today. However, there is significant evidence that indicates that attitudes play an important role in student health behaviors. It is believed that the acquisition of feelings, interests, and appreciation will lessen the time needed to convert the basic understanding that pupils receive into desirable practices.

An attitude refers to a mind set to action; it is an internal readiness to perform or behave. Therefore what pupils believe, feel, or value affects what they do. Children who feel they are not susceptible to diseases may not think it necessary to be immunized against these diseases. Pupils who do not believe that excessive sugar consumption might lead to dental decay may not attempt to eat nutritious snack-time foods. Boys and girls who do not realize the dangers of jaywalking may not cross streets at the proper places. Young people may need to be helped to develop an interest in the concept of self. Effective learning in health education therefore must give consideration to including teaching methods that will attempt to develop appropriate student health attitudes as well as proper understanding.

A health education program that tries to stress the development of health attitudes is difficult to achieve, particularly since children are coming to school with ideas, interests, values, and feelings developed and influenced by their home and community experiences. For example, in arithmetic or spelling the child may come to school lacking any information. Yet in matters relating to health and safety the child may not only lack scientifically sound information but also, and more important, may have strong beliefs affirmed by family and community that are false and perhaps even dangerous. Getting pupils to take responsibility for their own lives, whereby they seek to protect and maintain good health, takes much teaching skill and thoughtful planning. It involves initiative, ingenuity, creativity, and fortitude on the part of teachers who aspire to reach this goal.

Learning about health and safety does not always start with the provision of information or knowledge. There will be occasions when students will be expected to behave in certain ways and develop habit patterns of conformity that precede understandings from which positive or negative attitudes will emerge. These will be situations in which adults take authoritative or arbitrary action that is considered to be in the best interests of students. For example, when a fire breaks out in the school, the candy and soft drink machines are removed from the halls, a school lunch program is provided for all children, or an accident occurs to the school bus that is taking pupils home.

Many theories have been advanced by psychologists about learning. Numerous health educators and other health specialists have conducted research on segments of the learning process. They have generalized about its application to health behavior. Despite these efforts, however, a consistent approach to learning applied to health instruction has not been forthcoming.

The principles of learning contained in this chapter attempt to provide a consistency of approach for use in health education. They represent the result of a thorough and careful review of pertinent literature and the extensive school health experiences of the authors. They have been found to be successful in the development and implementation of health education curricula. They will enable teachers to improve learning and thereby help students to acquire favorable health practices and attitudes.

WHY ARE PRINCIPLES OF LEARNING IMPORTANT IN HEALTH?

Knowledge of the principles of learning is important to teachers in health instruction programs because:
1. Learning is a complex process
2. Behavior-centered emphasis in learning compounds the complexity of the learning process; attitudes are difficult to assess, and many practices are nonobservable in the classroom

3. Understanding about motivation and behavior is necessary for effective teaching
4. Teaching methods and learning are interrelated

WHAT ARE THE PRINCIPLES OF LEARNING?
Motivation is essential to learning

Health behavior is determined by individuals' motives and beliefs or values about various courses of action open to them. Since all behavior is motivated, the extent to which health behavior of individuals can be understood, predicted, or controlled depends on the ability of teachers to identify these motives and beliefs and to use them in their health teaching.

Positively, motives refer to those drives, needs, urges, or inner compulsions that stimulate individuals to want certain things. They are classified as the following:
1. Physiological needs, such as food, water, sleep, rest, air, sunshine, and exercise
2. Psychological needs, such as security, love, achievement, independence, responsibility, and authority

Motives may also be considered in a negative sense, as barriers that individuals must overcome.

Values are the strong beliefs or attitudinal concerns that have influence on positive or negative motives. The use of alcohol and tobacco, the significance of immunization, periodic visits to physicians, daily exercise, playing safely, and support for health departments depend on individual beliefs of the importance of these actions on their lives. People have to feel that their practices will enable them to play longer, have more fun, and be more productive citizens.

Values are acquired from a variety of sources including the family, social groups, TV and other mass media, adults admired by children, and peer cultures in school. When they are consistent with the goals of health education, they will reinforce learning, but when they are in conflict, learning may be limited or restricted. They are not completely resistant to change despite the cultural and social factors that may have influenced their formation. The earlier in the lives of children that attempts are made to acquire proper health behaviors, the greater are the possibilities that these practices will be highly valued by pupils. The school therefore has both a responsibility and an opportunity to modify beliefs and attitudes as well as develop new ones that will promote and maintain good health.

Principles of motivation. Several principles of motivation based on current research provide some important information about health behavior:

Preventive health action is determined by the degree to which a person sees a health problem as threatening in terms of the following:

1. Its probability of susceptibility or occurrence. Will smoking cause lung cancer?

2. Its seriousness, severity, or urgency of the consequences. Is dental caries sufficiently important to warrant attention? Will an infection be painful?

3. Its benefits or courses of action open that will reduce or remove the threat to the individual's health. What health practices should individuals follow, and will these practices be beneficial? Are vision screening and hearing tests important, and will they reveal important findings? How much will they cost?

Individual motives and beliefs about various courses of action are often in conflict with each other, and behavior emerges as the conflicts are resolved. The kinds of conflicts referred to include the following:

1. When two motives compete with each other for dominance, the one of greater importance or the more highly valued one will become dominant. A family may spend what little money it has for food, shelter, and necessities rather than on medical or dental visitations. A child who must wear glasses because of poor eyesight may not wear them because the peer group at school ridicules this practice. A pupil will smoke cigarettes to gain social acceptance.

2. If a pupil is motivated to act in a healthful manner (sees a course of action open), but the action is unpleasant, painful, time-consuming,

or inconvenient, the pupil may not complete the action.

3. A pupil may not accept a teacher's beliefs or opinions that there are ways to prevent or help a specific health condition and therefore does not see an effective way (course of action) to resolve the problem. For example, a girl with a boil on her leg may have been advised to visit a doctor but fails to do so because she may not believe the condition is serious or because she does not see how this action can help her. She may try self-medication, but as the infection grows worse she may find that her concerns and fears increase because she is not sure what action she should take.

Health-related motives may sometimes lead to behavior unrelated to health, and conversely some behavior that has the appearance of being health related may in fact be determined by motives unrelated to health. A hungry child may not reveal hunger to a teacher and may be untruthful when asked whether he or she has eaten any food. An illustration of the converse part of this principle is one in which a child may drink milk in class because other students are drinking it.

It should be evident that teachers play an important role in health instruction programs by motivating children to seek appropriate health goals as well as by helping boys and girls to acquire beliefs and values related to these motives. Teachers must provide pupils with experiences and activities that will improve their values of good health so that they will be better prepared to resolve conflicts in motives when they occur.

Fear can lead to rational as well as irrational behavior. It serves to protect, and it can be destructive to individuals. The fear of cancer may help students to refrain from smoking. The fear of becoming overweight may lead pupils to reduce food intake, However, a teenager with a genital sore or infection may be afraid to learn that a sexually transmitted disease has been contracted and may not have the condition checked by a physician.

Risk-taking is normal and necessary and de-

mands selectivity on the part of individuals after determination of benefit and harm. Everything people do involves risks of varying degrees. The decision to take them depends on whether the rewards outweigh the penalties. Crossing the street or eating food in a restaurant or lunchroom involves risk. However, they are minimal in comparison to the advantages. Surgery is hazardous, but if the chances of survival are increased, the benefits predominate in the decision. The dangers of using cocaine or driving an automobile when under the influence of alcohol may be greater than the pleasures derived. Young people need to be taught to compare the advantages and disadvantages of risk-taking behavior in order to make responsible decisions.

Subprinciples of motivation. The subprinciples of motivation that follow will point out additional aspects valuable in both the learning and teaching processes.

Cultural and social factors may be barriers to learning. The traditions and practices in the home, at play, in social groups, with adults, in the peer culture at school, and in the total environment in which children live affect and influence the values, prejudices, and perceptions that pupils bring to class. Families that rank highest economically generally spend more of their income on health services and products. Some families may not have funds to purchase glasses, toothbrushes, or food or to provide health examinations for children. Some parents may be concerned with immunizations or dental care. The nutritional and dress habits of certain ethnic and racial groups may differ somewhat from those advocated in school. Working parents may not be able to adequately supervise the eating habits and behaviors of their children. Certain religious groups may not believe in health examinations and appraisals, treatment, services, or fluoridation of the water supply. If both parents smoke cigarettes, the smoking rate among their children is higher than among those whose parents do not smoke. Social pressures of peers, parents, or the media have an influence on children's use of alcoholic beverages.

Teachers should be cognizant of these cultural and social factors and realize that they may have an effect on the health education program. They may support the health instruction program, or they may adversely affect it.

Size of objects, use of color, and movement in instructional materials may aid in attracting attention and developing interest in learning. The principle concerning size, color, and movement emphasizes the importance of using a variety of teaching aids in the health instruction program. These materials aid in gaining attention, increasing interest, and helping make teaching more effective, therefore making learning more concrete and specific.

The use of a variety of films, filmstrips, tape recorders, TV and radio programs, phonograph records, exhibits, flannelboards, magnetic boards, objects, specimens, graphs, and charts will stimulate interest in the learning experiences provided by the teacher.

The use of such models as the human torso, heart, eyes, ears, and teeth serve as valuable teaching tools. Exhibits of the contents of first-aid kits or the hazardous objects found in the home help to create interest in the area of safety. Use of food models and flannelboards will increase attention when nutrition is being taught.

Chapter 13 provides detailed information about teaching aids usable in the health instruction program.

Extrinsic motivation is less effective than intrinsic motivation. Should children perform good health habits because of some material reward they will receive or because of the inherent values of the practices performed? Should teachers award gold stars to children who come to school with clean handkerchiefs, when they have brushed their teeth, and for other such reasons? Is it advisable to present a special scroll to classrooms that report 100% attendance of their pupils? Should pupils receive candy or toys as rewards for visits to dentists or doctors? The external stimuli described may obtain the health action desired, but the results are usually temporary. Also, learning may be prevented because the reward becomes the motivation. The procedures described are questionable practices because:

1. Some parents do not give their children clean handkerchiefs to bring to school.

2. Some parents do not buy toothbrushes for their children, nor do they take them to physicians.

3. Pupils not able to have clean handkerchiefs or brush their teeth may be embarrassed when special note of these practices occurs in class. The mental health implications may be of greater importance than the rewards themselves.

4. Children who are ill may infect others in school.

Many educators believe that the best motivation is self-motivation. Teachers should motivate children to good health practices through the use of meaningful experiences and other approaches that develop intrinsic values for good health rather than through the use of artificial stimuli. This kind of health teaching will more likely provide the lasting behaviors desired. Further illustrations of this point will be found in other principles of learning.

Moderate tension facilitates learning, but severe tension may inhibit learning. Individuals generally perform better under some tension. However, the degree of pressure that pupils can handle is an individual matter. Teachers often question the degree to which they should pressure children into desirable health behaviors and practices. The illustrations that follow provide examples that give some guidance.

The cause of a child's dislike for or never having tried celery and carrot sticks may be related to some unpleasant home experience involving pressure or punishment. This same pupil, however, is more likely to try these foods in the classroom during a tasting party where the pressures of group approval are not quite as severe and there is an accompanying pleasant experience.

The teacher who is consistently sarcastic, rude, and unfair, who expects absolute quiet at all times, or who seldom has a sense of humor or permits pupil planning or decisions in the classroom undoubtedly provides a mental health environment that is less conducive to learning. However, the teacher who is generally courteous and fair and who frequently uses democratic procedures in class presents a more permissive atmosphere that probably provides a better balance of tension that will facilitate learning.

The fear approach in health education, in which the teacher exhorts and admonishes children by saying, "If you don't do this, here's what will happen," may create tensions that will inhibit the acquisition of the desired health behaviors. The teacher who strongly urges poliomyelitis shots because failure to do so will bring on the dreaded disease may create such great tensions that fewer pupils participate in the program. Although children may be afraid of having a needle injected into the skin, they are more likely to obtain these immunizations if some understanding of their nature and values is provided in a positive manner and if their classmates are obtaining them.

Learning is generally greater when praise is used more often than blame or reproof, when success occurs more often than failure. Success and praise reinforce learning, but constant frustration and failure adversely affect learning. The importance of the application of this statement to the mental health of children is extremely significant for classroom teachers. It emphasizes the need for teachers to recognize improvement based on individual standards rather than on general levels of achievement. Pupils with poor vision, defective hearing, or other physical ailments may need special praise or opportunities for success experiences in the classroom or on the playground. The balance between success and failure differs with individuals.

Achievement standards should be individual. From a mental health viewpoint, the expectation level of children toward the health goals established should be constant with their powers of accomplishment. A few specific illustrations of the application of this principle to a behavior-centered health education program are the following:

1. Children's needs for sleep may vary in amount.

2. The brushing of teeth after meals may not be possible in those homes that do not provide toothbrushes or dentifrices.

3. Some children may be allergic or diabetic and should not be expected to drink milk or eat all the foods prepared by the cafeteria at lunch.

Knowledge of results is a strong incentive to learning. The principle of knowledge as a strong incentive to learning refers to evaluation of the instructional program in terms of the achievement of the health education goals discussed earlier. Teachers as well as pupils want to know whether they are progressing toward the attainment of these purposes. They will want to know whether the practices, attitudes, and knowledge of healthful living have been acquired. This assessment of learning serves as a stimulus as well as an aid in redirecting the learning when necessary. Through the use of paper and pencil tests, demonstrations, observations, surveys, and other such techniques, some of the following questions may be answered:

1. Are children receiving the appropriate immunizations?

2. Do children know what to do when injured or ill at school?

3. Can children identify hazardous play areas?

4. Do children know how to administer simple first aid?

5. Are children getting adequate sleep, rest, and exercise?

A more complete discussion of evaluation can be found in Chapter 14.

It should be noted that motivation is related to all of the principles that follow.

Maturation and readiness of the child affect learning

Heredity, or the constitution of the pupil, sets the limits of learning of that individual by determining the individual's native intelligence and other capacities as well as physical and mental disabilities. However, maturation, or the physiological growth and development of the pupil, is a determining factor whether the pupil is mentally, physically, socially, or emotionally ready to learn. It provides a state of readiness important in health education as well as in all learning.

In dental health 6- and 7-year-old children may have difficulty learning the proper toothbrushing technique. This coordination involves use of the small muscles of the fingers and hands, and pupils may not be ready to learn this difficult procedure as completely or as accurately as desired. Although the brush is a fairly large implement, expertness of performance will take time and may be delayed until the child physically matures. Nevertheless, the brushing habit needs to be started early, and teachers should introduce this motor skill in school.

In the area of safety, children may not be ready to learn to manipulate sharp-pointed implements, use apparatus safely, operate bicycles safely, or perform other motor skills. Teachers need to be aware of these pupil limitations in their educational programs.

The taking of heights and weights in school is a time when pupils are ready to learn about their individual physical and emotional growth patterns. Pupils will be able to better understand their hereditary limitations in weight, height, size, and shape at this time.

The menstrual process generally begins in girls in the fifth and sixth grades, and an educational program is appropriate when this growth change appears.

Adolescence is a time when students are interested in the growth changes taking place in their bodies.

In the early grades especially, pupils are not completely ready to learn to be social individuals. However, it becomes necessary for children to learn to get along with others, respect authority, and cooperate in school if they are to grow into emotionally healthy individuals (see also Appendix L).

Experiences and the environment affect learning

Despite the variety of health behaviors that children bring to school, provisions must be made for learning experiences and environmental conditions that are conducive to good health. Teachers and other personnel have responsibilities to control the daily activities and conditions under which pupils learn. Some of the health experiences and conditions that should be included are the following:

1. The curriculum should include opportunities for children to learn how to live healthfully and safely.

2. Nutritious snack-time foods should be sold at lunchtime or used at parties and social gatherings, rather than candy, cakes, and soft drinks that may not be conducive to good dental health.

3. Provision of a hot lunch at noon may help develop good nutrition habits.

4. Playgrounds, classrooms, halls, and other places should be free of hazardous conditions and should be safe areas for learning.

5. Classrooms, halls, and playgrounds should be maintained in a neat, clean, and sanitary fashion.

6. Lavatories should provide soap and water for use when necessary.

7. Teachers should be free of communicable diseases and in good physical and mental health.

8. Adequate lighting, heating, and ventilation should be provided.

9. A democratic atmosphere in the classroom and the school will result in greater learning than an autocratic atmosphere where discipline is severe or nonexistent.

Guidance is necessary for the most effective learning

Health instruction must be a part of the school curriculum if the greatest health learning is to occur. A comprehensive health education program is necessary if children are to learn to play fairly and get along with others, understand fears, know how to prevent and control diseases, know what to do when injured, realize the importance of adequate sleep and rest, and follow numerous other health practices and attitudes. Inclusion of this program means that schools must make teachers available to teach the subject area and must also provide materials that will enable them to carry out this teaching responsibility. These items should include teachers' guides or units that have been developed around pupils' health problems as well as a variety of teaching aids and materials.

The teacher aids children in the health instruction program by motivating them to learn, selecting the goals to be achieved, determining the content to teach, and choosing and arranging the experience or activities to be used. Teachers help children learn to wash their hands properly, brush their teeth properly, assume responsibilities, have success experiences, and ride bicycles safely by using a variety of experiences and techniques including dramatizations, demonstrations, experiments, and discussions.

The teacher facilitates learning by providing motivation, distributing the learning at appropriate intervals, and organizing the learning process. Use of the learning principles found in this chapter will aid in this organization process.

Learning is a self-active process

The behavior-centered emphasis of health education makes the active participation of the learner particularly important and appropriate. Merely telling pupils "you should eat the proper foods," "you should take the safest route home," or "you should play fairly" will not achieve the desired health behaviors. Bridging the gap between knowledge and practices is more likely to come through pupil participation. Children must feel, see, discuss, act out, manipulate, and even taste things if the attitudes that affect good health practices are to be developed. The teacher has the important role of determining the nature of the experiences to be used in the learning process. Whenever possible, children should have two, three, or more of their senses involved in learning. It is believed that the greater the pupil participation, the greater will

Health Claims:
Separating Fact From Fiction

Checklist
For Choosing a Doctor

FLYING WITH A COLD: SAVE YOUR EARS

Hands-On Health Fair

Prescription drugs: How your doctor can cut your medicine bill in half

Sex and Schools

Relief from Canker Sores

Hospital Stays Most Expensive In California

NUTRITION LABELING AND HEALTH CLAIMS

FIG. 9-2. Learning is a self-active process—students prepare bulletin board of current newspaper/magazine articles with topical headings: "What's In The Health News."

be the possibility of developing the appropriate behaviors (Fig. 9-2).

To illustrate the application of this principle, the following specific activities are listed:

1. Have children learn about good snack-time foods by conducting a tasting party in which they eat appropriate nutritious foods.

2. Have children learn the proper way to brush their teeth by actually performing the exact procedure in class. Merely demonstrating this technique will not be satisfactory.

3. Have children make a survey of the unsafe conditions in the school and help develop solutions for their elimination.

4. Take the class on a field trip and actually follow the safest way to the home of one class member.

5. Teach fair play, honesty, getting along with others, or waiting turns by including these values in a softball game, a tag game, or as part of apparatus play.

6. Have pupils collect and analyze a variety of advertisements relating to health products.

Most effective learning occurs when there are good personal relationships between the pupil and the teacher

The dominant factor in any learning situation is the combination of personal and social relationships that exist between the pupils and the teacher in the classroom. Learning should take place in a democratic setting with the opportunity for free expression and participation by all children. Consideration must be given to the fair, just, and humane treatment of all pupils, regardless of race or ethnic background. The school and classroom should provide a warm, comfortable, and friendly environment. The teacher should be understanding and permissive but must also provide guidance and security. The emotional climate that pervades a school is extremely important to the effectiveness of the learning process.

Teachers should realize that their personal values, beliefs, prejudices, enthusiasms, and perceptions of health are brought to the classroom. They may affect the human relationship's atmosphere if they conflict with those of their pupils, peer groups, or families. They may influence the health behavior of children in a way that is contrary to best practice. Illustrations of these differences include the following:

1. Cleanliness and appropriate clothing
2. Amount of sugar consumed and significance to dental health
3. Appropriate foods for parties and snack times
4. Food faddism—use of vitamins and other food supplements
5. Food aversions—spinach, milk, liver
6. Fluoridation of the water supply
7. Use of alcohol and tobacco
8. Exercise and play
9. Choice of medical practitioner or health adviser

Teachers who make conscious efforts to avoid permitting their prejudices to influence pupils' health and who are willing to objectively permit children to look at scientific evidence do not necessarily have to compromise their own beliefs and values. This approach should enable teachers to maintain the good relations previously established.

Much learning is soon forgotten, and only a fraction of what was once learned is ultimately remembered

Studies reveal the greatest forgetting by pupils occurs when emphasis in learning is placed on the recall of factual material; evidence shows that meaningful information related to attitudes and practices is more easily learned and is remembered more completely and for longer periods of time. Understanding and knowledge should be provided in a context other than that of unrelated, isolated, factual information. Mere memorization or regurgitation of the names of the teeth, the digestion of foods, or the body systems will not be remembered unless the facts are more closely associated with the attitudes and habits of healthful living. They should lead to the acquisition of big ideas or generalizations, to concepts of health.

This principle emphasizes the need to stress the psychological approach over the logical or structure-and-function approach to teaching. It indicates the importance of the greater use of problem solving in the health instruction program. It demonstrates the importance of learning centered around health needs and problems of pupils. Here are several illustrations to demonstrate this principle:

1. Pupils' appreciations of the possible hazards of using tobacco and other drugs must be more meaningfully related to the ingredients of tobacco and various drugs. Pupils must feel that these substances may affect their performances in athletics, in recreation, and in school as well as their growth and health.

2. Pupils' interests in immunizations against diseases and the prevention of infections' spread will be greater if the diseases considered are those they or their parents may acquire or have acquired.

3. Pupils' appreciation for eating the proper foods will be increased if the lack of vitamins, minerals, and other substances is related to their own or their families' food needs or deficiency diseases.

Well-organized, meaningful material is more easily learned and is remembered longer than meaningless or nonsense material

The content of the health education program should be based on the needs and interests of pupils if it is to be meaningful. Various studies indicate the following areas to be representative of these needs and interests: cleanliness and grooming; community health; consumer health; dental health; control and prevention of disease; care of the eyes, ears, and feet; exercise and fitness; family health; growth and development; mental health; nutrition; rest, sleep, and fatigue; safety; and alcohol, tobacco, and drugs. Learning organized around these areas will result in the most effective health behaviors.

Schools should have teacher guides to health education containing units of instruction focused around the health areas identified in the previous paragraph. These manuals should define the learning that should take place at the various grade levels. They should provide a sequence of learning that avoids excessive overlapping and duplication of content.

Teachers should capitalize on incidents that occur at school or in the home and use these "teachable moments" (see Chapter 12) in their instruction programs, thus making health education practical as well as functional. Such incidents as the following are usable:

1. The class is going to use the playground apparatus
2. The nurse is coming to do the vision screening
3. Fire Prevention Week is emphasized in the community
4. A child reports a visit to the dentist
5. Children wash their hands before lunch and after going to the lavatory

The ability to solve problems, to reason, to make intelligent decisions, and to do reflective thinking involves training and must be learned

Reasoning ability does not appear suddenly, but rather it develops gradually with age and experience. Differences in the reasoning ability of children and adults are differences in degree and not in kind. Children should be taught how to think rather than what to think. In the primary grades this process can be done more simply using questions that challenge pupils' thoughts.

Duryea* identifies these steps in decision making (problem solving): (1) appraise the challenge (review of problem), (2) survey alternatives, (3) weigh alternatives (advantages/disadvantages), and (4) determine commitment (select alternative). The decision then needs to be implemented and evaluated.

The many quacks, charlatans, and pseudo-medical people who live in our communities to-

---

*Duryea, E.J.: Decision making and health education, Journal of School Health **53:**29-30 Jan., 1983.

gether with the millions of dollars spent yearly on unnecessary drugs, vitamins, and patent medicines make it necessary that children begin to be able to do reflective thinking in health as they do in other phases of learning. Children and adults need to know whether health information they are hearing is valid and to know reliable sources of health facts.

Illustrations of problems that teachers may use for children to solve may include the following:

1. What should you do when you are injured?
2. What should you do when you are ill?
3. Who can help you when you are ill or injured?
4. How can you make friends?
5. What kinds of clothing should you wear to protect your body?
6. How does the health department protect the health of the people?
7. Should we believe what we read and hear about health products?
8. What hazards in the home may cause accidents?
9. Where can you get help if you have a sexually transmitted disease?

The learning process must specifically include teaching for transfer of training or learning if this transfer is to occur

Health knowledge that carries over into or transfers to pupil activities outside of school is the most significant kind of learning. Transfer does not happen by chance but rather by design. Teachers must include teaching for carryover in their planning if school health activities are to occur in the home and community.

The most effective transfer of learning happens when the learning in school is as near real-life situations as possible. Learning, therefore, must be lifelike to obtain the greatest transfer.

When teaching pupils about safety at street corners, it may be necessary either to go to the corner itself and perform the safe behavior or to simulate a street corner on the school grounds using traffic lights, small cars, and other props with the children participating in a role-playing activity.

To obtain the greatest safety in the home, it may be necessary for children to survey the hazards therein and suggest ways to reduce or remove these hazards.

To expect children to eat balanced meals at home, it may be advisable to provide such meals in schools at noontime.

To expect children to reduce their consumption of sugars and sweets, it will be necessary to curtail, or remove, their availability at lunchtime, at snacktime, during parties, and during other social occasions in school. However, some health educators believe that foods containing sugars should be available but controlled as an educational means of teaching children their proper use.

Parental involvement in the identification of two ways to leave the house when a fire occurs should be part of home fire safety.

The use of repetition and reinforcement is necessary in learning

Health learnings must be repeated and reinforced if they are to have the greatest effect on the health behavior of individuals and if they are to be useful in the children's daily lives. A brief exposure in a classroom, or elsewhere, to a discussion, demonstration, or report of the safest way home from school, the safe way to act on the bus, the use of hand signals when riding a bicycle, the importance of eating the proper foods, the hazards of smoking, what to do when someone is injured, or the proper way to brush teeth does not assure that these actions will be followed consistently for any length of time. Activities used to achieve health and safety objectives must be used on several occasions either during the unit, during the semester, or during the entire school year. Where skills such as proper toothbrushing, and first-aid and safety procedures are involved, repetitive practice becomes necessary for reinforcement. These skills

TABLE 9-2. Principles of learning and their reference to text information

Principles	Text references by chapter
Motivation	
Principles	
Preventive action threatening	1 - Prevention
	8 - Gullible public, health misconceptions, health information conflict, media influence, peer pressure
Conflict in beliefs	1 - What is health? Factors influencing pupil health
	2 - Controversial areas
	8 - Controversial areas, lifestyle
	11 - Values
Health-related motives, unrelated behavior, etc.	1 - Social and lifestyle-related problems
Fear: rational/irrational behavior	8 - Prevent action, peer pressure
Risk taking	1 - Social and lifestyle-related problems
	8 - Controversial areas, peer/adult pressure
Subprinciples	
Cultural/social factors	1 - What is health? Factors influencing pupil health, social and lifestyle-related problems
	2 - Controversial areas
	8 - Lifestyle and disease, peer/adult pressure, media influence, self-care, Why health education?
	11 - Values
	12 - Incidents as methods
Size of objects, etc.	13 - Instructional aids (see also Appendixes D, E, F, and I)
Extrinsic/intrinsic	8 - Why health education?
	12 - Methods and techniques
Moderate tension	11 - Taxonomy of objectives, units (objectives)
	12 - Methods and techniques
Praise/blame	12 - Methods and techniques
	14 - Evaluation (see also Good personal relations)
Individual achievement	2 - Individual differences
	6 - Guidance, adjustment of program
	12 - Methods and techniques
	13 - Instructional aids
Knowledge of results	14 - Evaluation
Maturation/readiness	1 - Health problems of children
	5 - Appraisals—growth and development characteristics
	11 - Interest/needs of students, values
	12 - Incidents as methods
Experiences/environment	3 - Environment—physical aspects
	4 - Emotional climate
	5 - Emergency care
	8 - Role of community
	11 - Values, Why health education?
Guidance	2 - Individual differences
	6 - Guidance/counseling
	8 - Patterns of instruction, grade placement, time, concepts
	10 - Health education approaches
	11 - Taxonomy of objectives, unit teaching, lesson planning, scope and sequence
Self-active process	12 - Methods and techniques
	13 - Instructional aids (see also Appendixes E, F, G)
Good personal relations	2 - Health of personnel
	3 - Environment—physical aspects
	4 - Emotional climate (see also Guidance)
Much learning soon forgotten	11 - Taxonomy of objectives
	12 - Methods and techniques
	13 - Instructional aids

TABLE 9-2. Principles of learning and their reference to text information—cont'd

Principles	Text references by chapter
Well organized/meaningfulness	1 - What is school health? What is health?
	10 - Health education approaches
	11 - Scope and sequence, unit teaching, lesson plans
	12 - Incidents as methods (see also all other principles)
Problem solving (decision making)	11 - Needs/interests of pupils
	12 - Methods and techniques
	13 - Instructional aids
	9 - Units, lesson plans (see also all other principles)
Transfer of training	11 - Needs/interests of pupils (see also all other principles)
Repetition/reinforcement	11 - Scope and sequence, units, lesson planning
	12 - Methods and techniques
	14 - Evaluation (see also Guidance, and Well organized/meaningfulness)

must be transferred to the home and community for effective health education. There is evidence to show that prevention programs that increase social skills (for example, "learning to say no") have promise of curbing tobacco smoking.

In psychological terms, this type of learning is often referred to as spaced learning—a repetition of what has been taught after intervals of time have elapsed. These time intervals may occur during or at the end of a lesson, in the middle or end of a unit, or during the semester, or there might be longer spacing. To illustrate, when teaching the proper technique for brushing the teeth during a unit on dental health, a demonstration of the correct procedure might have to be made again during the lesson and followed by the pupils actually performing the correct technique. The entire sequence, or some modification, may have to be repeated one time or more during the unit and possibly reviewed during the semester. Had this learning occurred in the first or second grade, it may be advisable and necessary to repeat or reinforce it in the third or fourth grades and possibly again in the fifth, sixth, or seventh grades. In a comprehensive health education curriculum this procedure is referred to as cycling—sequential placement of specific health areas at a variety of grades throughout the school years.

The extent and degree of repetition will vary and depends on any or all of the following:

1. The individual differences in pupil abilities
2. The health values pupils bring to school
3. The nature of the health environment in the home and in the community
4. Parental cooperation and assistance

SUMMARY

Learning is a complex process that occurs when it is internalized and when it is influenced by external experiences in individuals. How children learn is not clear, but it is clear that pupils learn when teachers motivate students, select the appropriate goals, and choose activities and experiences that will enable pupils to live in a healthful manner. This learning must involve more than the provision of health knowledge. Bridging the gap between health practices and health knowledge probably occurs through the development of favorable attitudes. However, some practices may be learned without attitudinal involvement. The variety of principles of learning described in the text will be helpful to teachers when planning and teaching health education. Application of the learning principles to the information found in this book is presented in Table 9-2.

QUESTIONS FOR DISCUSSION

1. What are the factors involved that help students prevent illness and maintain and promote health?
2. What is learning and how is it believed that children learn?
3. What are the basic goals of health education? What are their relationships to learning? Illustrate.

4. What is the hierarchy of attitudes and its relationship to learning about health?
5. What is meant by the term *teaching for decision-making*? Illustrate its application to health education.
6. How can teachers relate knowledge to behavior in health education?
7. What is meant by "bridging the gap" between health knowledge and health behavior?
8. Why are the principles of learning important in health teaching?
9. What are the principles of learning that will help the teacher in the health instruction program? Provide illustrations of the application of each principle to health education.
10. What are the principles of motivation that have an effect on learning in health education?
11. Why are good teacher/student relationships important and necessary for effective health teaching?
12. What are several illustrations of ways the teacher can make health learning a self-active process?
13. What is the significance of fear and risk taking in behavior modification in health education?
14. What is the meaning of "spaced learning?" Illustrate its application to health education.

REFERENCES

Bernard, H.W.: Psychology of learning and teaching, ed. 3, 1972, Oregon State System of Higher Education.
Clarke, K.S.: Values and risk-taking behavior; the concept of calculated risk, Health Education 6: Nov./Dec., 1975.
Duryea, E.J. Decision making and health education, Journal of School Health 53:29-30 Jan., 1983.
Flay, B.R., DiTecco D., and Schlegel, R.P.: Mass media in health promotion: an analysis using an extended information-processing model, Health Education Quarterly 7:127-147, 1980.
Fodor, J.T., and Dalis, G.T.: Health instruction: theory and application, ed. 3, Philadelphia, 1981, Lea & Febiger.
Gagne, R.M.: Some new views on learning and instruction, Phi Delta Kappan 7:May, 1970.
Galdston, I., editor: The epidemiology of health, New York, 1953, Health Education Council, New York Academy of Medicine.
Gilchrist, L.D., et al.: The relationship of cognitive and behavioral skills to adolescent tobacco smoking, Journal of School Health, 55:132-134 April, 1985.
Goodstadt, M.S.: School-based drug education in north america: What is wrong? What can be done? Journal of School Health 56:278-281 Sept., 1986.
Hochbaum, G.: Research in behavioral sciences, presented at the Regional Institute on the Science of Health Education at the University of California at Los Angeles, June 12-14, 1961.

Hochbaum, G.: Learning and behavior: alcohol education for what? Alcohol Education Conference Proceedings, March 1966, U.S. Department of Health, Education, and Welfare.
Hochbaum, G.: Effecting health behavior, presented at the annual meeting of the New York State Public Health Association, Buffalo, May 23, 1967.
Hochbaum, G.: How we can teach adolescents about smoking, drinking, and drug abuse? Journal of Health, Physical Education, and Recreation 39: Oct., 1968.
Hochbaum, G.: Changing health behavior in youth, School Health Review, Sept., 1969.
Hochbaum, G.: Health behavior, Belmont, Calif., 1970, Wadsworth Publishing Co., Inc.
Hochbaum, G.: Human behavior and nutrition education, Nutrition News 40:Feb., 1977.
Hochbaum, G.: Should health behavior change be the objective of health education? Journal of School Health 51:379-380 May, 1981.
Katz, J.: Responsible decision making, Health Education 6: March/April, 1975.
Lawrence, L., and McLeroy, K.R.: Self-efficacy and health education, Journal of School Health 56:317-322 Oct., 1986.
Lewis, C.E., M.D., and Lewis, M.A.: Peer pressure and risk-taking behaviors in children, American Journal of Public Health 74:580-584 June, 1984.
Motivations, practical applications of research, Newsletter of Phi Delta Kappa's Center on Evaluation, Development and Research, 5:1-3 Sept., 1982.
Nolte, A., Smith, B.J., and O'Rourke, T.: The relative importance of parental attitudes and behavior upon youth smoking behavior, Journal of School Health 53:264-271 April, 1983.
Ripple, R.E., editor: Learning and human abilities, education psychology, New York, 1964, Harper & Row, Publishers, Inc.
Rosenstock, I.M.: Motivation bases for health education practices, presented at the fifty-first annual meeting of the Wisconsin Anti-Tuberculosis Association in Milwaukee, April 24, 1959.
Rosenstock, I.M.: Psychological forces, motivation, and nutrition education, American Journal of Public Health 59: Nov., 1969.
School Health Education Study: Health education: a conceptual approach to curriculum design, St. Paul, 1967, 3M Education Press.
Schunk, D.H., and Carbonari, J.P.: Self-efficacy models. In Matarazzo, J.D., et al. editors: Behavioral health: a handbook of health enhancement and disease prevention, New York, 1984, John Wiley and Sons.
Sunseri, A.J., et al.: Reading, demographic, social and psychological factors related to pre-adolescent smoking and non-smoking behaviors and attitudes, Journal of School Health 53:257-262 April, 1983.

HEALTH EDUCATION APPROACHES

Health education works; it works better when there's more of it; and it works best when it is implemented with broad-scale administrative and pedagogic support for teacher training, integrated materials, and continuity across grades.

THOUGHTS FROM THE
SCHOOL HEALTH EDUCATION ADVISORY
PANEL TO THE NATIONAL SCHOOL
HEALTH EDUCATION EVALUATION STUDY

KEY CONCEPT: Comprehensive health education curricula, despite varied approaches, need a consistent and sound educational philosophy.

SELECTED CURRICULA IN ELEMENTARY SCHOOL HEALTH EDUCATION

Many elementary school health education programs in the United States have been developed by health education and curriculum specialists among others (including voluntary health agencies and commercial companies) without the use of a consistent procedure or educationally sound philosophy. Few individuals, including health educators, understand completely the process of curriculum development;

know how to prepare functional programs using pupils, teachers, and community resources; have been engaged in successful experiences in terms of completion and implementation; or have been able to assess the effectiveness of their programs. Often programs and curricula have been prepared based on what others have done without adequate consideration of their quality or the nature of their impact on children. A basic set of principles and procedures that are universally acceptable or that can be generally implemented by professionals has not emerged. The development of health education curricula cannot take place without such guidelines. The first major organized effort in this regard that used talented health education experts occurred in the 1960s in the School Health Education Study (SHES) project directed by Dr. Elena Sliepcevich. Since that time several curricula have been prepared at national, state, and local levels. These curricula have been found useful, have gained popularity, and show promise of fulfilling the basic principles for development found in Chapter 11.

The purpose of this chapter is to provide illustrations of selected programs that should receive study by schools. It is hoped the resources provided will encourage the examination of additional curricula before the adoption of one in particular.

Numerous approaches to curriculum development have been used, and many programs are available. However, each program must be reviewed in terms of its particular strengths and weaknesses. Therefore schools wishing to introduce a health education curriculum should peruse other successful programs to be certain they are sufficiently flexible to meet local student and community needs and interests as well as the legal mandates of the state. It is important therefore to become familiar with the National Diffusion Network, a federal dissemination system designed to assist schools in locating exemplary programs in all areas of curriculum, including health instruction programs.

NATIONAL DIFFUSION NETWORK

The National Diffusion Network (NDN) is a federally funded system that makes exemplary and proven educational programs available for adoption by schools, colleges, and other institutions. It was formed in 1973 under the Elementary and Secondary Education Act (ESEA) of 1965, and it has become the nation's primary means of sharing proven educational programs.

Whereas many locally developed programs have proven to be extremely successful in helping children learn, few of these projects have been used away from the sites where they were first developed. Because of this, a need exists for a nationwide means of disseminating information about the programs. The NDN was formed in response to the desire of Congress to formulate such a dissemination system.

The basic purpose of the NDN is to offer local schools the chance to adopt high-quality, cost-effective education projects that have been developed by classroom teachers.

The goals of the NDN are as follows:
1. To stimulate positive educational change in local schools
2. To help parents, teachers, and administrators find programs for children that match local needs
3. To move programs quickly and cost-effectively to classrooms nationwide
4. To help public and private schools secure information about new programs and support for their implementation in the district
5. To ensure that nationwide communication about these programs continues among local school districts, intermediate service agencies, and state departments of education

By achieving these goals, the NDN supports the flow of new ideas and increases the impact of educational investments that have already been made.*

The NDN can provide limited funds to help create an awareness of exemplary school programs, aid schools with adoption decisions, provide in-service training and follow-up assistance, and in selected instances, purchase teaching aids for classroom use. At present, over 380 exemplary programs are available through the NDN.

What is an exemplary program?

To be considered "exemplary" by the NDN, a program must have proved itself educationally effective for children and be cost-effective with reasonable per pupil cost. If a program devel-

*The information contained in this section comes in part from a filmstrip and cassette on the National Diffusion Network prepared in 1979 by the U.S. Office of Education. It is available from the U.S. Department of Education.

oper feels that the program meets these criteria, the developer can submit the program to the NDN for consideration.

The Joint Dissemination Review Panel

Before being accepted for inclusion among the more than 380 NDN-approved programs, the program is reviewed by the Joint Dissemination Review Panel (JDRP). The JDRP was first appointed in 1972 and was created specifically to review evidence (generally research) presented by program developers who state that what they developed was effective in attaining the goals set forth for that particular program.

Consisting of approximately 50 education and evaluation experts from the U.S. Department of Education and other areas of educational research practice, the JDRP convenes periodically to review programs that have been nominated as exemplary. The method used for program nomination depends on the source of funding for initially developing the project. If federal funding was used for project development, the state officer responsible for administering the federal funds can nominate it. A second means is for those who develop a program using state funds to contact the state program officer and request nomination. If other than federal or state funding sources were used for project development (such as foundation or other agency support), or if the original funding program no longer exists, the person responsible for developing the program can send it directly to the U.S. Department of Education Recognition Division, which administers the NDN.

Once a program nomination has been received, it is reviewed by a program-significance panel to be sure that the program materials are grade level–appropriate. If everything is in order, the project is scheduled for review. This review can be conducted either by mail or by a special panel convened in Washington, D.C. A minimum of seven experts, appointed by the Secretary of Education, review the evidence submitted and vote to determine if the nomi-

nated project does, in fact, do what it purports to do. This decision is made immediately following the review discussion.

If a project is approved, it becomes eligible for diffusion funds either from the NDN or through other federal funding programs. If the program is not approved, the reasons for rejection are explained. In the case of rejection, the project can be revised or new evidence of effectiveness can be prepared and the project resubmitted for consideration at a later date.

An approved program receives several direct benefits including (1) recognition of the program by both professionals and the public through awareness workshops, (2) increased chances for obtaining competitive federal funds, and (3) entry into a federal diffusion system.

NDN state facilitators

Each state has at least one individual specifically designated as State Facilitator for the NDN. This person is in a key position to aid local school district planners who want to examine a variety of approaches to a given curricular area before the development of a local curriculum. The state facilitator is often in close communication with the ESEA Title IV director for the state and will be able to convene an awareness workshop of proven programs for districts that ask to see exemplary projects available through the NDN. These "showcases" are conducted several times each year in each state at no cost to the local district. They generally prove quite useful since they provide information about a wide range of programs in any given curricular area.

The state facilitator may also help a local school district match its needs with appropriate NDN projects, help develop and plan local workshops, help search for alternate sources of funding, and help local program developers prepare the information needed to nominate a program for review. Furthermore, the state facilitator has limited funds to support school personnel who wish to visit sites of demonstration projects.

SELECTED ELEMENTARY SCHOOL HEALTH INSTRUCTION PROGRAMS

Presented here are some examples of the more widely known elementary health education programs available in the United States. This listing is in no way meant to be exhaustive. It should also be pointed out that inclusion of a given program does not suggest our endorsement of the program nor does omission of a program suggest our rejection. These programs are presented as examples of nationally validated programs (included in the NDN), state-based programs, locally based programs, programs available through various health-related agencies, and commercially prepared programs. A listing of sources of selected programs may be found in Appendix D.

Programs included in the NDN

In May, 1979, the School Health Curriculum Project became the first health instruction program to be nationally validated for inclusion in the NDN. One year later, the Primary Grades Health Curriculum Project, a companion to the School Health Curriculum Project, was also approved for inclusion in the NDN. These two programs subsequently merged to form Growing Healthy. This program is the only comprehensive health instruction program approved for inclusion in the NDN. However, some programs have been approved that emphasize individual subject areas and include content dealing with nutrition, cardiovascular health, fitness, smoking, and alcohol and drug abuse.

Growing Healthy. Originally called the Berkeley Project and the Seattle Project, and subsequently the School Health Curriculum Project and the Primary Grades Health Curriculum Project, these two companion projects have merged to form Growing Healthy, a K through 7 program that is student focused and broad based in scope.

The goals of Growing Healthy are to:
1. Increase students' knowledge and decision-making abilities about a wide range of behaviors and in a number of health education areas
2. Help students learn how their bodies function and how their personal choices affect their health
3. Integrate classroom learning with other life situations
4. Offer students and teachers an experience-based understanding of the physical, mental, and emotional dimensions of their own health

Designed primarily as a direct method of teaching health, the units of instruction also lend themselves to integration with other elementary school curricular topics. Growing Healthy is a broad-based program that includes an intensive 30 to 60-hour teacher-training component; a wide variety of teaching methods; strategies for involving both parents and the community; and a variety of useful teaching aids. It has been called a student-centered, hands-on, multimedia approach to health instruction.

The program content at the various grade levels has been developed around central themes with these titles:

Kindergarten: Happiness is Being Healthy
Grade 1: Super Me
Grade 2: Sights and Sounds
Grade 3: The Body: Its Framework and Movement
Grade 4: About Our Digestion and Our Nutrition
Grade 5: About Our Lungs and Respiration
Grade 6: About Our Hearts and Circulation
Grade 7: Living Well With Our Nervous System

The pattern for health teaching at each grade level follows this organizational sequence: introduction (motivational activities), awareness (body interactions), appreciation (proper function of body parts contribute to well-being), structure and function (in a healthy state), diseases and disorders, prevention, and culmination (overview of learned concepts presented by students at a special parents' night).

Growing Healthy has developed an ongoing program of research to determine its effectiveness. The K through 3 segment of the program has been evaluated in selected demonstration centers across the United States. Reports of this evaluation are available from the American Lung Association. More recently, the 4 through 7 component was included in the national school health education evaluation conducted by Abt Associates, Inc., of Cambridge, Massachusetts, under a contract with the Centers for Disease Control of the U.S. Department of Health and Human Services.

The K through 3 segment of Growing Healthy has been adopted in over 300 school districts in more than 30 states, and the 4 through 7 segment has been adopted in over 400 school districts in more than 40 states. The program (in a somewhat modified form) is also being used in the Sheffield, England schools, as well as in the Arabian American Oil Company schools in Saudi Arabia.

Have a Healthy Heart. Have a Healthy Heart has been included in the NDN since December, 1980. This limited-focus program designed for grades 4 through 8 deals with cardiovascular health. It was developed by Model Classrooms, a corporation that develops educational programs in cooperation with business and industry as well as with public and private schools. Presented as a supplement to existing programs, this project utilizes an aerobic fitness component designed to be taught 1 to 2 hours per week during a 2- to 3-month period. The basic goal of the program is to help students learn and practice health habits that will help decrease their risk of incurring heart disease.

A 1-day workshop for teachers was developed to acquaint them with the philosophy and materials used in the curriculum. The American Heart Association and the American National Red Cross often participate in the workshops and help provide follow-up services for workshop participants.

The classroom implementation phase begins with the administration of a walk-run test and the studying of a fitness booklet developed specifically for the program. Students participate in aerobic exercise 3 times each week for 15 to 20 minutes. At the end of each month, the walk-run test is readministered so students can see the progress they have made relative to cardiovascular fitness. On completion of the fitness booklet, students begin working on a lifestyle booklet that is designed to acquaint them with cardiovascular risk factors and the methods they can use to reduce those risk factors in their personal lives.

The results of various evaluations of Have a Healthy Heart suggest that student knowledge about cardiovascular risk factors and performance on general fitness tests increase significantly as a result of exposure to the program.

State-based programs

A number of states require some sort of health instruction to be included in the curricula of their schools. In 1976 when the first edition of *School Health in America* was published by the American School Health Association, it was reported that 16 states had mandated comprehensive school health education. However, selection of subject matter to be included was an individual school district decision. It should also be noted that there was no universally accepted definition of "comprehensive school health education" at the time the report was published. In 1985 when the survey used in *School Health in America* was repeated, health education was required to be taught at some time during grades K through 12 for a specific number of hours in 27 states, but there was no mention of whether these programs were considered "comprehensive."*

School health education is currently included in state education codes or other legislation in 45 states, but there is a great deal of latitude in how it is viewed by school districts. Commonly the teaching of drug, alcohol, and tobacco use and misuse is mandated, although for varied

---

*This information and the information that follows is from: Kolbe, L.J., et al.: School health in America: an assessment of state policies to protect and improve the health of students, ed. 4, Kent, Ohio, 1987, American School Health Association.

amounts of time. Going beyond merely stating that health education should be taught, 39 states have developed guidelines for local school districts to use when developing health education programs. Some states have passed legislation allowing the State Superintendent of Public Instruction to set minimum guidelines for the development of health instruction programs. Still others, such as California and Pennsylvania, have developed rather detailed frameworks for health instruction. In many states there is a validation process for recognizing exemplary programs within the state.

California Framework. The Framework for Health Instruction in California Public Schools* was originally published in 1972 by the California State Department of Education. The Framework incorporates a conceptual approach with an emphasis on the achievement of selected behavioral objectives and the development of health knowledge and attitudes. The document is an attempt to provide a comprehensive set of guidelines for school districts so that with minimal effort, through the addition of teaching/learning activities, teaching aids, and evaluation procedures, a health instruction curriculum can be developed.

The Framework evolved from an assessment of the health needs of school-age children in California and was developed by a team of health instruction experts. The needs assessment included literature reviews and numerous discussions with various health authorities from around the state. Ten content areas emerged: consumer health; mental-emotional health; drug use and misuse; family health; oral health, vision, and hearing; nutrition; exercise, rest, and posture; disease and disorders; environmental health hazards; and community health resources. The Framework is organized to include an overview, major concepts, specific grade level concepts, and suggested behavioral objectives and content for each content area.

The publication is updated periodically to in-

*California State Department of Education: Framework for health instruction in California, Sacramento, 1972, The Department.

clude new developments in the health field as they arise. The document has been distributed widely in California as well as elsewhere across the United States. It forms the basis for many of the health instruction programs that have been developed by local school districts in California as well as in other states. This document is presently in the process of revision.

Pennsylvania Progression Chart. Beginning in the mid-1970s and designed to end in 1981, the Pennsylvania Department of Education initiated Project 81, which had as a goal, determining what health abilities and skills a student graduating from high school should possess. Previously 12 goals of quality education had been identified in such areas as communication, mathematics, self-esteem, analytical thinking, understanding others, citizenship, arts and humanities, science and technology, work, family living, health, and environment.

After identifying 10 major content areas (community health, consumer health, disease prevention and control, family health, safety and first aid, fitness, growth and development, nutrition, personal health, and tobacco, alcohol, and other drugs), specific student skill objectives were developed for each of the content areas using the quality education goals as a basic framework. The specific health goals that emerged represented an adaptation of the goals developed for the School Health Education Study (SHES) and the Health Education Curriculum Progression Chart (originally developed for Growing Healthy). Across the state, leaders in both health and education were questioned concerning essential health skills for graduating seniors. Numerous curriculum materials from other states were also reviewed.

After many months of work, the Pennsylvania Health Curriculum Progression Chart emerged as a guide for local school districts to use when developing their own scope and sequence outline in health education. Divided into four segments (K through 3, 4 through 6, 7 through 9, and 10 through 12) the progression chart focuses on objectives that will facilitate desirable lifestyles and behaviors deemed important for functioning as a healthy adult. It is also responsive to the immediate health needs of the students.

Locally based programs

A number of local school districts have developed programs that are said to be comprehensive in scope. For example, Project Prevention in The Dalles, Oregon; It's Up to You, in Brattleboro, Vermont; 3 R's and HBP in Atlanta, Georgia; the Hazelwood School District in Florissant, Missouri; Project CHEK in Lansing, Michigan; and "Here's Looking at You, 2000," in Seattle, Washington.

Project Prevention. Primary prevention of health problems through a comprehensive framework of health instruction is emphasized in Project Prevention. This health instruction program was initially developed in The Dalles, Oregon, using funds from ESEA Title IV C. This was one of the development and demonstration grants provided through the NDN process.

The program was designed for students in grades K through 12. An advisory committee consisting of parents, grade level teachers, medical specialists, school administrators, social workers, counselors, clergy, and students from grades 6 through 12 developed the guiding philosophy for the program. Program goals, scope and sequence, and lesson plans were then developed. The program can be entirely or partially adopted and integrated into the existing instructional program. It is designed primarily as a program of direct instruction, although many of the activities integrate well with other topics in the curriculum.

Emphasis is placed on each student developing a positive self-concept, applying decision-making skills in a variety of situations, developing effective communication skills for effective, healthful living, and evaluating various health resources and services available in the community. Teachers who use the program must participate in an intensive 2-day training program designed to acquaint them with the various methods and materials to be used. The teacher's guide includes lesson plans, a guide to free or inexpensive health materials, a guide for adopting the program, individual test booklets designed for each lesson plan, 35-mm slides, audiotapes, and overhead transparencies. Approximately 150 teachers in approximately 30 schools in eastern Oregon and southeastern Washington are using the program.

It's Up to You! It's Up to You is a state-validated broad-based 1 through 6 grade health education program that was developed in Brattleboro, Vermont. Initially developed under a Title IV C grant, the program has attained a regionalized status. The program focuses on the concept that individual responsibility and awareness of one's values is paramount to the development of a health-promoting lifestyle. The program is "hands on" oriented with both content and concepts developed from grade to grade in a sequential fashion. The program incorporates a "cookbook" core approach that teachers have found excites students. Included in each grade level teacher's guide are activities and materials that can extend the basic core activities so that health can be integrated into other areas of the curriculum. The program has stated goals in the areas of physical, social, and mental health areas.

3 R's and HBP. Developed through local funding from the Georgia Affiliate of the American Heart Association, 3 R's and HBP is a limited focus program specifically designed for grades 5 and 6. The program is aimed at helping students understand high blood pressure and incorporates a parental outreach component whereby students have the opportunity to borrow medical equipment from their school so that they can talk with their parents and other family members about high blood pressure while actually measuring the blood pressure of the family members. A 6-hour teacher in-service program is designed to show the teachers how to implement the curriculum most effectively and teach the process of measuring blood pressure. Knowledge inventories, skills tests, and community involvement, including hospital tours for classes involved in the curriculum, are incorporated into the program.

Hazelwood School District Comprehensive School Health Education Program. The Hazelwood School District Comprehensive School Health Education Program was developed using local school district funding in Florissant, Missouri. This K through 6 broad-based health education program includes eight major content areas (substance abuse, safety and first aid, mental and emotional health, personal health, drunken driving, nutrition, environmental health, and community health). As with other health education programs, individual responsibility is stressed at each grade level. Unique to this program is a segment designed to foster an appreciation in the students of the progress that has been made in health research and the health professions.

A detailed scope and sequence outline identifying the major areas of content for each grade level is central to the program. Specific grade level objectives, learning experiences and evaluative activities have been developed for each unit within each grade level. The program uses community resources as well as 16-mm films, slides, filmstrips, overhead transparencies, posters, and games.

Project CHEK. Project CHEK is a broad-based, state-validated K through 8 health education program developed under a Title IV C grant in the Lansing, Michigan public schools. The program is based on Michigan's Essential Performance Objectives.* The central purpose of the project is to develop and reinforce student health awareness, knowledge, and practices so that the student can make informed choices about health matters. For the K through 3 segment, five modules are repeated in a sequential format each year. The five modules are as follows:

Module 1: About Me
Module 2: The Way I Grow
Module 3: The Food I Eat
Module 4: The Choices I Make
Module 5: How I Stay Healthy

---

*Michigan State Board of Education: Essential performance objectives for health education, Lansing, Michigan, 1974, Revised, 1982, The Board.

The K through 5 component is designed to cover 10 major topic areas over the course of the year of instruction. The 6 through 8 grade sequence builds on what has occurred in grades K through 5 and a 4-week health education experience is integrated into the program at the grade 6 level for inclusion in a Life Science unit. This extends the course beyond direct health instruction. At grade 7, the course covers one full semester (20 weeks) and includes eight major units of instruction. The grade 8 segment contains five units that focus on the health needs and concerns of the adolescent.

A teacher training component is central to the total project. The component includes a grade level curriculum guide that contains grade level objectives, learning activities, and worksheet masters for pretests and posttests for each unit. Two health service manuals and two management training manuals for the teacher are also included. A complete listing of materials and suggested sources for these materials accompany the package. The program draws on such resource persons as the school nurse, dental hygienist, food service director, counselor, and physical education instructor. The program is recognized as a model program through the Michigan School Health Association's Recognition Standards for Identification of Comprehensive School Health Education Models.

Here's Looking At You, 2000. Here's Looking At You, 2000, is a nationally recognized K through 12 alcohol and drug education program. It is based on recent research studies that identify characteristics of potential drug users. These "risk factors" include early drug use, association with friends who use drugs, lack of positive social skills, chemical dependency in the family, and failure in school, among others. Each lesson focuses on one or more of these risk factors.

Here's Looking At You, 2000 was created with input from subject area experts. It has been extensively pilot tested by master teachers and is being used throughout the nation. Teachers are guided through at least 15 lessons at each grade level. The program includes strong "no use" messages, opportunity for parental involvement, focus on "gateway" drugs (tobacco, alcohol, and marijuana), social skill training, and opportunities for cross-age teaching.

A kit containing all the materials necessary to teach each lesson is available for each grade level. The program can be taught as a 3-week unit in a regular health instruction program or can be integrated throughout the school year. A 3-day teacher-training workshop for classroom teachers, school counselors, nurses, and school administrators is designed to acquaint these persons with the methods, materials, activities, and content of the program.

Programs available through various health-related agencies and associations

The American Heart Association, the American Cancer Society, the National Dairy Council, the National Fire Protection Association, the American Health Foundation and the United Way are some of the many health agencies that have developed programs that can be integrated into an existing health instruction program.

Putting Your Heart into the Curriculum. Putting Your Heart into the Curriculum, developed by the American Heart Association, is specifically designed as a series of teaching modules and strategies to be used in grades K through 12 by teachers as an addition to their regular health instruction program. It is designed to affect those attitudes and value judgments of young people that may have an effect on their behaviors.

The following areas are included:
1. Choosing not to smoke
2. Making informed and healthy food choices
3. The importance of having a blood pressure within normal limits
4. Recognizing the various risk factors of cardiovascular disease and how to lessen their impact on the individual
5. Developing and keeping a regular program of weight control and physical exercise

In-service training for teachers is available from the Association or through selected universities that participate in the program. Teaching aids and materials are available free of charge from local chapters of the American Heart Association.

An Early Start to Good Health. An Early Start to Good Health instruction program for grades K through 3 developed by the American Cancer Society consists of four separate units and includes teacher guides, filmstrips, posters, phonograph records, and activity sheets. It is designed to develop health awareness and to supplement existing programs.

The four units of instruction include the following:

Unit 1: My Body—introduction to basic body organs

Unit 2: My Self—the difference between the inner and outer self

Unit 3: My health—activities needed to maintain health

Unit 4: My choice—personal choices and the effects of those choices

Health Network. Health Network was also developed by the American Cancer Society and is designed as a companion to the Early Start to Good Health program. Health Network consists of three units of instruction designed specifically for use in grades 4, 5, and 6. Each unit contains a filmstrip and either a phonograph record or tape cassette that provides the story for the unit. Also included are a teacher's guide with an introductory lesson and several group activities, reproduction masters to make handouts for the students, and either a game or poster that exemplifies the basic content of the unit.

The three units of instruction each have objectives for students that aid the teacher in planning to use the program. The three units of instruction are as follows:

Unit 4: Special People—cigarettes don't improve one's self-image and one need not be a "star" to be a valuable person

Unit 5: Health News—a simulated television news broadcast that reports on how the respiratory system uses oxygen in the process of breathing

Unit 6: Starga's World—a girl from outer space visits Earth and learns how to make decisions about herself and her health

Food: Your Choice. The National Dairy Council designed Food: Your Choice, a nutrition education program, for students in grades K through 6. The program is sequential and activity oriented. Its purpose is to: (1) foster an understanding of key concepts of nutrition, (2) convey the importance of nutrition in preventing health problems, and (3) encourage maintaining a healthy body.

The program consists of three levels:

Level 1: Specifically designed for use in grades K through 2, nutrition concepts are learned through hands-on experiments and meal preparation.

Level 2: Designed for use in grades 3 and 4, this level is designed to further expand the concepts learned in Level 1. Students have the opportunity to examine more closely the role of food in society. They classify foods and learn the consequences of poor food selection and eating habits.

Level 3: Designed for grades 5 and 6, this level focuses on a study of nutrients in food as well as analysis of those factors that influence eating patterns, food selection, and food advertising. Special materials have been developed to integrate nutrition teaching into social studies, science, and home economics.

Most state dairy council office staff members will conduct teacher-training workshops designed to acquaint school personnel with the program.

Learn Not to Burn. The Learn Not to Burn program was developed between 1975 and 1978 by the National Fire Protection Association (NFPA) to provide a comprehensive fire prevention program for grades K through 8. A survey revealed that little coordination between fire departments and school districts in terms of fire prevention curricula existed in the United States. The program is unique in that it involves parents as well as fire department personnel.

The basic goals of the program are as follows:
1. Protection of persons from fires
2. Prevention of fires
3. Motivation of persons to practice fire prevention and safety

The program consists of three major segments that are reflected in the program goals. It includes 25 key fire prevention and protection behaviors in the three major segments of protection, prevention, and persuasion. Each of the 25 behaviors has at its core an action domain determined to be the most direct means of saving life and property together with knowledges and attitudes necessary to achieve the action.

The NFPA* reports it has documented evidence that 73 lives have been saved with over 1 million pupils in 43,000 classrooms having been exposed to the curriculum.

Know Your Body. Know Your Body is a broad-based, nationally available curriculum developed by the American Health Foundation through funding provided by the National Cancer Institute, the National Heart, Lung and Blood Institute, and the W.K. Kellogg Foundation. Developed for grades 1 through 9, this program is designed to:
1. Increase student health knowledge about selected health factors
2. Develop values and attitudes that promote a healthy lifestyle
3. Promote behavior that will enhance personal health
4. Increase student ability to alter personal health practices

The overriding objective of Know Your Body is to provide health education that helps students realize that health is a personal, relevant, and enduring concept. Based in social learning theory, such things as role modeling, goal orientation, and positive health behavior reinforcement are central to the program. Each student participates in a personalized health screening program to learn about basic concepts of wellness and health behaviors. Through this process they are encouraged to alter their behavior through personal decision making so that their total well-being is enhanced. The concepts of self-responsibility and self-care are stressed as they relate to decision making in the areas of nutrition, physical fitness, and avoidance of use

---

*Powell, P., Manager, Public Education, National Fire Protection Association: Personal communication, Oct. 29, 1986.

of tobacco, alcohol and drugs. Instruction in how to prevent some of the major health problems of today (accidents, cancer, and heart disease) is also stressed.

A sequentially arranged spiraled scope and sequence has been developed to better articulate grades 1 through 3, 4 through 6, and 7 through 9. As students progress through the curriculum, new concepts are introduced and prior learnings are reinforced. Printed teacher's guides and student worksheets for each grade level are available for teachers who participate in the training workshops conducted by Know Your Body staff.

Health Education Curriculum Guide. Developed in 1974 by a committee of teachers, health educators, health agency personnel, and parents, the Health Education Curriculum Guide is a special project of the United Way of Central Stark County, Ohio. The main content areas of this K through 6 broad-based curriculum include family living; growth and development; alcohol, drugs, and tobacco; safety; environmental, community, and mental health; and nutrition. A teacher's guide containing content, learning activities, and suggested evaluation activities and resources for each of the six content areas is available for each grade level. Nearly 400 learning activities across the seven grade levels are presented in the program.

Commercially prepared programs

Many school health instruction programs rely on commercial companies for the teaching aids and other materials they use in their programs. Therefore some of these business firms have prepared curricula that incorporate the variety of teaching aids they manufacture for sale. Two such programs are Beltman, developed by Film Loops, Inc., and the Health Activities Project, distributed by the Hubbard Scientific Company.

Beltman. Beltman is a multimedia program specifically designed for students in grades K through 2. Designed for 9 to 10 lessons, the purpose of the program is to teach young children pedestrian safety and to increase their seatbelt use. The program objectives include:

1. Teaching children how to use seatbelts and motivating them to use the belts
2. Teaching children proper pedestrian behavior including the safe way to cross streets
3. Developing within children an appreciation of safety as a lifestyle

A teacher's guide, five cassette tapes, three filmstrips and other teaching aids are included in the kit. Such things as iron-on decals are included as motivational devices. Independent evaluation of the Beltman program indicated that when it was combined with parental involvement, the program could develop safety consciousness and more consistent use of seatbelts in children.

Health Skills for Life. Although developmental funding for Health Skills for Life, a skill-based, comprehensive K through 12 health education program came from the Oregon State Department of Education and from a Title IV C grant, it is now available through a private, commercial company that carries the same name as the project. The project itself consists of 118 separate teaching packages. For grades K through 8 there are 7 to 12 units per grade level and there are 35 high school units included. Each of the grade level units is packaged separately so a school system can select those units that are responsive to the specific needs of the district.

The purpose of the program is to provide students with opportunities to practice health behaviors in the areas of physical, mental, social, and emotional health. Each of the 118 skills were written as competencies that were to be demonstrated by the student exposed to the units of instruction. This facilitates the evaluation of the unit of instruction. Combined with the skills are performance indicators, health content, and a set sequence of activities that help direct the student toward the skill. Suggestions for integrating the specific skills and content with other curriculum areas such as mathematics, reading, and writing are included.

A detailed scope and sequence chart is available, as are administrator's guides and optional resource materials that could be included in the program. A 3½ hour teacher training program and a 2-hour administrator training program are offered by the project developers.

Health Skills for Life has been validated by the Oregon State Department of Education and was selected in 1985 as 1 of the 20 programs honored by Metropolitan Life Foundation as an exemplary health education program in the United States.

Health Activities Project. The Health Activities Project gets students involved with personal health and safety using hands-on, discovery-type activities. It is assumed that students can realize how to improve their health and safety by learning how their bodies function.

The program uses a variety of teaching aids for the 58 different activities. The teacher's guide contains a description of each activity, the health background for it, the space requirements necessary to conduct the activity, and the materials that are needed. The activities are specifically designed to supplement and enrich existing school health, physical education, and science curricula.

SUMMARY

The programs described in this chapter represent but a few of the different types of health instruction programs available in the United States. The critical elements in each program that must be identified are its flexibility in terms of meeting student and community needs and how local teachers can use the program in terms of direct and integrated health instruction. For those persons faced with having to develop a health instruction program, these illustrations provide suggestions for use in newly developed curricula.

We recognize that anyone who is not familiar with health education curriculum development and desires to develop a program should obtain expert assistance before undertaking such a project. This aid might be obtained from the state department of education, professional health educators in colleges or universities, or neighboring school districts. Programs should be developed that are responsive to student and community needs and that are based on sound principles of curriculum development such as those presented in Chapter 11.

It should also be noted that the Metropolitan Life Foundation, in 1985 initiated their Healthy Me awards program to recognize exemplary public school health education programs and community coalitions devoted to promotion of comprehensive health education in local school districts. In the initial phase of the program, 20 innovative programs and 20 coalitions were judged by a panel to meet the criteria established for the awards. These 20 health education programs and 20 community coalitions were given special recognition awards by Metropolitan Life Foundation in November, 1985.*

QUESTIONS FOR DISCUSSION

1. Why do you think that no clear-cut procedures for developing and implementing health instruction curricula in U.S. schools have been developed?
2. What do you perceive is the value of the National Diffusion Network?
3. Why might state National Diffusion Network facilitators be considered the most important links in the network?
4. What are the different ways a program might be considered for inclusion in the National Diffusion Network, and what is the basic process for including a program in the network?
5. Briefly critique the process and procedures used by the Joint Dissemination Review Panel in reviewing "exemplary" programs.
6. How would *you* define an "exemplary" health instruction program? How does your definition differ from that used by the Joint Dissemination Review Panel?
7. What benefits might accrue to a program that is included in the National Diffusion Network?
8. You have been asked to make a recommendation to a school district about how to initiate a comprehensive school health instruction program. How would you go about formulating your recommendation and what basic advice would you give to the school district about curriculum development?
9. What factors appear to have been key elements in the

---

*For additional information about the Metropolitan Life Foundation Healthy Me Awards, contact Metropolitan Life Foundation, One Madison Avenue, New York, NY 10010. A videocassette, "Healthy Me," about many of the programs is available free of charge from Modern Talking Picture Services, Inc., 5000 Park Street North, St. Petersburg, FL 33709.

success of the specific programs illustrated in this chapter?

10. What factors do you feel have kept many state legislatures from enacting comprehensive school health instruction legislation?
11. What factors exist in common between the six locally based health instruction programs presented in the text?
12. What factors exist in common between the seven programs available through health-related agencies that are discussed in the text?
13. In your opinion, why have commercial companies produced health education programs?

SELECTED REFERENCES

American Heart Association Subcommittee on Health Education of the Young: We've put our heart into the curriculum, Health Education 13:20-23 Jan./Feb., 1982.

American School Health Association: Teaching about drugs: a curriculum guide, K-12, Kent, Ohio, 1984, The Association.

Bailey, W.J.: Ten smoking education programs for schools, Journal of School Health 55:33-34 Jan., 1985.

Birch, D.A., and Nybo, V.: Promoting school health education in Maine: the Maine school health education program, Health Education 15:67-68 Aug./Sept., 1984.

Brooks, C.H., and Howard, D.J.: The response of special education students to an activity-centered health curriculum, Journal of School Health 53:527-530 Nov., 1983.

Byrd-Bredbenner, C., et al.: A nutrition curriculum for health education: its effect on students' knowledge, attitude and behavior, Journal of School Health 54:385-388 Nov., 1984.

California State Department of Education: Framework for health instruction in California, Sacramento, Cal., 1972, The Department.

Connell, D., et al.: School health education evaluation, International Journal of Educational Research 10:245-345, 1986.

DuShaw, M.L.: A comparative study of three model comprehensive elementary school health education programs, Journal of School Health 54:397-400 Nov., 1984.

Folio, S.B., et al.: A survey of elementary school health education in West Virginia, Journal of School Health 54:401-402 Nov., 1984.

Frager, A.M.: Toward improved instruction in hearing health at the elementary school level, Journal of School Health 56:166-170 May, 1986.

Gielen, A.C., and Radius, S.: Project KISS (Kids in safety seats): educational approaches and evaluation measures, Health Education 15:43-47 Aug./Sept., 1984.

Hammes, M.: Guidelines to assist classroom teachers in designing and implementing student involvement techniques, Health Education 17:48-50 Aug./Sept., 1986.

Health education curriculums in action, Health Education 10:Nov./Dec., 1979.

Journal of School Health: Recipients of the 1985 Metropolitan Life Foundation "Healthy Me" awards, Journal of School Health 56:117-119 March, 1986.

Kitttleson, M.J., and Ragon, B.M.: Project panther[2], Health Education 15:16-18 Dec., 1984/Jan., 1985.

Kolbe, L., et al.: School health in America: an assessment of state policies to protect and improve the health of students, ed. 4, Kent, Ohio, 1987, American School Health Association.

Kupsinel, N.: A look at state health curriculum guides, Health Education 11:25-27 May/June, 1980.

Livingood, W.C.: Backwards and not very humanistic: The Pennsylvania health curriculum progression chart, Health Education 15:49-52 Oct./Nov., 1984.

Marty, P.J., Banks, R.L., and McDermott, R.L.: Arnie the aardvark: an innovative cancer education program for the primary grades, Health Education 15:41-44 Mar./Apr., 1984.

McNab, W.L.: Staying alive: A mini-unit on child molestation prevention for elementary school children, Journal of School Health 55:226-229 June, 1985.

Michigan State Board of Education: Essential performance objectives for health education, Lansing, Michigan, 1974, Revised 1982, The Michigan State Board of Education.

Miller, D., and Davis, L.: An evaluation of the Beltman traffic safety program for children, Health Education 15:51-53 Aug./Sept., 1984.

National Parent-Teacher Association: Comprehensive school/community health education project, Chicago, 1981, The Association.

Olsen, L., Redican, K., and Krus, P.: The school health curriculum project: a review of research studies, Health Education 11:16-21 Jan./Feb., 1981.

Parcel, G.S., and Coreil, J.: Parental evaluations of a sex education course for young adolescents, Journal of School Health 55:9-12 Jan., 1985.

Pennsylvania Department of Education: Pennsylvania health curriculum progression chart, Harrisburg, 1981, The Department

Pigg, R.M., et al.: Evaluation of American Cancer Society elementary school public education programs, Journal of School Health 55:156-160 April, 1985.

Price, J.: Learn not to burn: a K-8 curriculum, Journal of School Health 51:543-547, 1981.

Renick, N.L., and Botvin, G.J.: Enhancing junior high school students' life skills as a smoking prevention strategy, Health Education 16:45-51, June/July, 1985.

St. Pierre, R.W., Shute, R.E., and Jaycox, S.: Youth helping youth: a behavioral approach to the self-control of smoking, Health Education 14:28-34 Jan./Feb., 1983.

Taylor, M.E.: Qualitative and quantitative strategies for exploring the progress of sex education for the handicapped, Health Education 16:16-19 June/July, 1985.

Terhune, J.A., and Shaughnessy, J.: Health skills for life, Health Education 14:27-32 Sept./Oct., 1983.

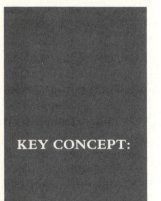

CHAPTER
11

ORGANIZING FOR
HEALTH TEACHING

Instruction for healthful living is essential for every student.

AMERICAN MEDICAL ASSOCIATION MEDICINE/EDUCATION COMMITTEE
ON SCHOOL AND COLLEGE HEALTH

KEY CONCEPT: The development and teaching of comprehensive health education programs are shared responsibilities of teachers, administrators, and community members utilizing basic principles of curriculum development and instruction.

There is general agreement among authorities on the importance of planning and organizing for health education. This is critical if objectives are to be attained in the cognitive (knowledge), affective (attitudes), and action (behavior) areas of child development in schools. Clear definitions should be provided in curricula in terms of what pupil goals teachers should be seeking, what content should be included, what methods and materials are to be used, and whether the purposes established have been achieved. Ideally, experiences for pupils should be both scientifically fact oriented and student centered. The purpose of this chapter is to provide information and direction to this end.

Health education must be organized in both formal and informal ways if the differing needs

and interests of students are to receive proper consideration. Pupils with drug problems (including alcohol and tobacco), sex concerns, and emotional and psychological difficulties often cannot be helped except on a one-to-one or small group basis. To date, insufficient attention has been given to the informal approach in schools. Chapter 6 provides a variety of ways to guide and counsel young people. This chapter and succeeding chapters focus on organizing for formal health teaching.

Curriculum development and implementation is basic to organizing for formal health teaching. A variety of tasks needs attention, including determination of what shall be taught and the preparation or selection of units for teacher reference and use. In addition, teachers need help in developing their own plans for teaching and guidance through illustrative units.

Before presenting material in this text in regard to curriculum development and teacher planning, it is important the reader understand some basic principles involved, be familiar with the conceptual approach, be aware of the usefulness of values clarification as a strategy in health education, and have knowledge about personal responsibility for the preparation of the curriculum.

WHAT ARE THE BASIC PRINCIPLES FOR CURRICULUM DEVELOPMENT IN HEALTH EDUCATION?

For any educational function to proceed on a sound basis, it must be predicated on certain valid principles or assumptions. If we begin with a firm foundation of fact and philosophy, we cannot stray far from the path of excellence. To choose learning experiences on the basis of established principles is to assure worthwhile education for pupils; to make the selection on the basis of popularity, newspaper headlines, tradition, personal bias, or yesterday's problems is to run the risk of failure in preparing children to live and function in a complex, changing society.

Fundamentally, a sound curriculum must be based on the needs, problems, and opportunities of society and the individual. Beyond this broad approach are certain principles and assumptions that may be used as guidelines for curriculum planning and development in health education:

1. Provision for a sequential, comprehensive program of instruction that includes the ascending spiral effect allowing for an increasing depth of information from kindergarten through grade 12
2. Provision for repetition of content areas without excessive duplication through the cycling of content areas, or in other appropriate ways
3. Adaptability and flexibility to allow for changes and modifications; introduction of new content, new information, and new materials as they develop and emerge in society
4. Use of the concept approach in curriculum development with particular emphasis on health concepts and objectives
5. Emphasis on the preventive aspects of health in the instructional program with a focus on self-care responsibilities
6. Health emphasis that includes physiological, sociological, psychological, and spiritual aspects
7. Emphasis on the needs and interests of students in forming the basis for the curriculum so it will be appropriate to the local community or communities and the social climates in which pupils reside; special consideration must be given to the problems of minorities and those with ethnic and cultural differences
8. Provision for writing goals in behavioral terms, including cognitive, affective, and action domains*
9. Provision for goals observable in the classroom, nonobservable, and delayed in their attainment in the action domain where it is appropriate and possible
10. Provision for goals, with the following differential emphasis at the grade level groups indicated whenever possible:
    a. Primary grades—focus on physiological aspects of health with limited psychological and social aspects
    b. Intermediate grades—focus on physiological aspects of health with greater in-

---

*The student drug problem resulted in new educational terminology (such as affective and confluent education), and emphasis being introduced in schools. The need for students to develop positive self-concepts, express feelings and aspirations, reach social maturity, and participate in values clarification has led authorities to support affective education. It is believed such emphasis will enable persons to more effectively cope with life's problems. Confluent education refers to the integration of affective and cognitive elements in learning. These are worthwhile directions for inclusion in health education. The clearly written objectives found in the units in Appendix B include these new ideas.

clusion of psychological and social aspects and limited spiritual emphasis

    c. Upper grades—focus primarily on psychological and social aspects with decreasing emphasis on the physiological aspects but with concern for the spiritual phases

11. Provision for inclusion of all the possible alternatives to action so that students can make intelligent decisions regarding behavior

12. Allowance for students to make their own decisions regarding behavior

13. Current content, accurate and nonbiased, derived from scientific sources; both positive and negative aspects to be included whenever possible

14. Use of the principles of learning (see Chapter 9) in the selection of the methods or techniques of teaching for behavioral changes that stress student involvement, decision making, critical thinking, discussions, problem solving, self-direction, clarification of values, and responsibility

15. Use of a variety of resource materials that are interesting, current, accurate, carefully screened, and appropriate for the grade level intended

16. Involvement of students, parents, and community representatives in the development and evaluation of the curriculum

17. Provision for periodic assessment of various aspects of the curriculum

These principles and assumptions may seem to be self-evident, yet often elementary school programs of health education omit one or more of these guidelines. The material that follows is based on these principles and their application.

THE CONCEPTUAL APPROACH

For many years researchers in psychology and education have attempted to increase their knowledge of how children learn so they can help pupils learn more effectively. The concept approach is one of the more promising methods to evolve from their efforts.

Concept formation

Learning involves **thinking**. The thinking process may include **one or more** of these six types of thinking: *perceptive, associative, inductive-deductive, creative, critical,* and *problem-solving*. The formation of concepts involves the use of the perceptive **process**.

Percepts are simplified conclusions that students obtain from seeing, hearing, touching, tasting, and smelling. They are the raw materials of thinking that result from environmental stimuli. In the classroom these stimuli are generally provided and controlled by the teacher and may include the teacher's oral presentation, other pupils' comments, content of health textbooks, films, bulletin board information, and many others. Perception is essential to concept formation.

Inhelder and Piaget* indicate that children's ability to understand broad concepts or generalizations, and abstractions depends on their ability to have direct sensory experiences. These experiences help them construct and reconstruct percepts. Modern research shows that sensory-motor experiences (for example, manipulation and construction) are most effective in developing percepts. Then, through use and application of these raw materials of health instruction, children can understand and deal with more abstract concepts. For example, "use of substances that modify mood and behavior arises from a variety of motivations," is a concept. It is a rather obtuse statement that necessitates specific sensory experiences for understanding and comprehension. Pupils may need to have discussions, hear comments by recovering drug abusers, and review literature about why people use drugs to grasp the meaning of the concepts.

Thus children are exposed to, screen, and select stimuli. The stimuli produce percepts that lead to the formation of concepts, which are conclusions or generalizations.

*Inhelder, B., and Piaget, J.: The growth of logical thinking from childhood to adolescence, New York, 1958, Basic Books, Inc., Publishers.

Concepts applied to health education

The concept approach to health education was introduced in the mid-1960s and emerged from the School Health Education Study (SHES) conducted under the leadership of Dr. Elena Sliepcevich.* It continues to be a valid and useful procedure for use in curriculum development. An innovative project, the study was prepared using up-to-date educational philosophy. It was also the first attempt to scientifically develop a health education curriculum that followed the basic principles used for all other educational curricula. Many health curriculum efforts since publication of the SHES have direct roots in this landmark work. It is fundamental to the eclectic plan identified in this text, which gives consideration to a variety of other significant prevalent ideas, including holistic health (physiological, psychological, social, and spiritual), student needs and interests, prevention, and ecology.

Health concepts are conclusions or generalizations that result from learning experiences to which students have been exposed. They cannot be taught directly. They emerge from exposure to the variety of activities introduced by teachers from which students derive perceptions. They serve as the organizing framework to use in determining the content and in preparation of the objectives of the curriculum. Thus after students have completed their learnings, they should be able to conclude that, "use of substances that modify mood and behavior arises from a variety of motivations."

Examples of realistic and effective applications of the conceptual approach are the health education curriculum illustrative partial units, which are represented in Appendix B.

VALUES IN THE CURRICULUM

Family lifestyle changes, the influence of the mass communications media, technological innovations, world events, materialism, conflict of conformity and self-reliance, ethics, and affluence are among the factors creating difficulties in the establishment of values by young people. As a result, youth are searching for meaning in life. They are asking themselves questions such as, "Who am I? Why am I here? What really matters?" They desire to cope with daily problems, develop life-coping skills, understand themselves, and be able to make wise decisions. Because of the failure to answer these questions a variety of patterns of behavioral problems have been appearing in school-aged children. Such problems include apathy, inconsistent behaviors, drifting, dropping out, overconforming, and overdissenting. Schools have a major role in helping children and youth at early ages begin to clarify their values.

Leaders in the field of psychology have indicated the need for individuals to have a sense of purpose in their lives. People actively search for meaningfulness and identity in life, although some may never be able to clearly define or achieve such a goal. The achievement or failure of achievement of a sense of purpose may affect an individual's mental health either positively or negatively.

There is no single, clear definition of values. They have been said to be deep, long lasting commitments to a concept or doctrine that is highly prized and about which action will be taken in satisfying ways. They are characteristics or attitudes about human experiences that are strongly desirable to an individual or group of individuals. Values give direction to life and may be considered determinants of behavior. They aid in the making of decisions and judgments. They have been identified in the concept of health described in Chapter 1 as part of the *spiritual* aspect of health (Fig. 1-2). They have been included in the units in Appendix B in the affective domain objectives.

Values may be learned through a variety of meaningful experiences and through interaction with the environment. Thus the sources of values are adults, peer cultures, the family, religious leaders, the communications media, friends, social groups, and the school.

---

*Lieberman, E.J., editor: Mental health: the public health challenge, Washington, D.C., 1975, American Public Health Association.

Raths, Harmin, and Simon* believe the focus—probably starting in the intermediate grades—should be on *value* clarification and not on the teaching of values per se. They believe values will emerge through this process. Didactic value clarification involves a series of strategies or methods for helping students learn to identify values. They state that a value must meet these seven criteria:

Choosing

1. Choosing freely—individual should not be coerced and should have freedom of selection
2. Choosing from alternatives—a variety of alternatives must be provided
3. Choosing thoughtfully—consideration should be given to the consequences of each alternative
4. Affirming—when something is cherished, it is publicly and verbally supported: doing something

Prizing

5. Prizing and cherishing—choice has a positive tone and is held in high esteem

Action

6. Acting on choices—life is affected through reading, spending money, and budgeting time
7. Repeating—persistency and endurance become a pattern of life

Value clarification has a place in health education as part of both content and methodology. It has particular application to the areas of mental health, drugs, human sexuality, alcohol, smoking, health care, and environment; but it is also useful in other health areas. The outlines of content found in the illustrative units in Appendix B contain suggestions. Some of the strategies that are useful for value clarification are found in Chapter 12.

The inclusion of value clarification in health teaching may be considered controversial by some parents. Things to be considered when deciding on whether to include them in the cur-

riculum are found in Chapter 8, p. 167.

Beane* claims that the value clarification process may only superficially treat values. It cannot be assumed that students will evaluate or decide on their own values. The conceptualization and organization of values may require cognitive elements for analysis, synthesis, and evaluation. The method does generate interest and stimulate student discussion, but Beane raises serious questions about the contribution of the method of values education.

WHO IS RESPONSIBLE FOR DEVELOPING THE CURRICULUM IN HEALTH?

Curriculum development and improvement have become major functions of modern education. Not too long ago the curriculum was shaped largely by experts in the various disciplines. However, in recent years these experts have been joined by teachers, pupils, and lay citizens in planning curricula. This does not mean that the opinions of experts are minimized or disregarded. It means that a curriculum can be developed to fit a certain school and community best if opportunity is provided for teachers, pupils, and lay groups to adapt the curriculum to local interests and needs.

For example, an elementary school in Florida might want to give time in the curriculum to hookworm infestation and "creeping eruption" (a skin infestation caused by dog and cat hookworms), instead of spending time on frostbite and winter sport safety. An impoverished area school in the inner city might decide to stress the problems of unwanted pregnancy and sexually transmitted disease at an earlier grade level than a suburban school. A rural school might emphasize the importance of water purity and sanitation, whereas an urban school might take more time for air pollution. A school whose pupils come from families where ethnic and racial

*Raths, L.E., Harmin, M., and Simon, S.: Values and teaching; working with values in the classroom, Columbus, Ohio, 1966, Charles E. Merrill Books, Inc.

*Beane, J.A.: The continuing controversy over affective education, Educational Leadership, Dec., 1985/Jan., 1986.

backgrounds shape their daily meals would surely want to stress the place of Italian, Mexican, Asian, Indian, and "soul" foods as they apply in choosing a balanced diet.

Thus we find real need for adapting the curriculum to best meet local problems in many areas of health. Yet fundamentally the subject matter is the same for all schools and all children. It is the fringe areas and the manner of illustrating basic concepts that offer the best opportunity for adaptation.

Curriculum development is a shared responsibility. Even though the approach may differ from one community to another, the curriculum in health and safety should reflect the interests, concerns, and efforts of teachers, pupils, parents, physicians, dentists, public health specialists, law enforcement officials, civil defense authorities, school board members, fire department officials, representatives of voluntary health agencies, school nurses, principals, curriculum specialists, and school health coordinators. These people, working together at the local level, can fashion the most fundamental and functional curriculum for their local school situation while retaining the common learnings in health and safety. Often the local group will need to make only a few minor changes in a course of study that has been prepared by the state department of education, county school office, or some other school district.

Again, the matter of cooperative planning and action can be helpful. The school health council at the district level, under the direction and guidance of the health coordinator or consultant, can give considerable support to the curriculum development program. The health council usually represents the thinking of most, if not all, concerned persons and organizations. Moreover, it provides a ready-made mechanism for resolving many variances in philosophy and for implementing group decisions.

Experience in the national SHES showed that few school districts throughout the country have the personnel resources to develop a sound, up-to-date health education curriculum on their own. If a health coordinator is not available, schools should seek guidance from state or local colleges and universities or private consultants.

Critical analysis of the curriculum in health education must be a continual process if the instructional program is to be truly functional in the lives of children. The rapid advances in the health sciences no longer permit the schools to "stand pat" for very long on content. Sequence also is affected by the increasingly frequent medical and health science developments and problems. These are in the main accurately and promptly reported in newspapers, magazines, telecasts, and other media. Often such health science reporting provides the teacher with a "teachable moment"—a time when pupils are more likely to be motivated—for a topic that had not been planned. Examples are many: new vaccines for the prevention of communicable diseases, the sexually transmitted diseases, zero population growth statistics, elimination of smallpox vaccination from the standard schedule, toxic shock syndrome and tampon use, the energy crisis, radiation hazards, new drugs being used and abused, quackery and fraud in the health marketplace, and a host of others.

The wise teacher will be flexible enough to depart from the lesson plan and take full advantage of the heightened interest of pupils when these stories "break." The unimaginative teacher will cling steadfastly to the planned sequence and, ignoring publicized fresh facts of importance, plow ahead with the predetermined unit on a less relevant topic.

HOW IS THE CURRICULUM DETERMINED?

Many factors must be considered in determining a district's health education curriculum. The most significant factors are those directly related to the students. Therefore to determine what should be taught in health education, it is necessary to identify the health interests and needs of pupils. Once they have been identified, a scope and sequence chart is prepared. This chart is used to determine which units need to be constructed at each grade level.

Samples of scope and sequence charts from state and district levels are found in Tables 11-1 and 11-3. It is important to note that developing a scope and sequence chart provides the logical basis for further program refinements for the general student population, but consideration must also be given to the special problems and unique needs of minority, non–English speaking, economically deprived, handicapped, and other special groups.

Interests and needs

The following is a variety of information sources useful in determining the scope and sequence of the curriculum.

Pupil interests. Pupils learn better when they have interest in the subject matter. In essence, interest is an attitude favorable to learning. Beyond this, interest hinges on the values, desires, wants, and purposes of the pupil. As children perceive the relationship of a topic to their personal advantage and well-being, they become interested. The *active interests* are those that relate here and now to the child's daily life and world. *Latent interests* are those that the child may have had at an earlier age, but that were stifled because parents and other adults would not or could not encourage and develop them.

Finally, since interests depend heavily on past experiences, there are many areas in which pupils have practically no interest. It is one of the central purposes of education to amplify and diversify the interests of children. Thus pupil interests, although vital to motivation, cannot be considered in themselves as complete indicators of the relative importance of topics in health and safety.

Yet teachers should identify pupil interests and emphasize those already developed. This is simply good motivation. Latent health interests (for example, "What makes me grow?" "Where do I go when I sleep?" "Where do babies come from?") will have to be further developed and

new interests will need to be created if health teaching is to be effective.

A 1984 report* by the Washington State Department of Education provides remarkable insight into the health interests, concerns, and problems of elementary school pupils. This study involved more than 5,000 students from kindergarten through the twelfth grade. It showed, among other things, that basic health interests were common to all pupils whether they lived in a city, rural, suburban, or high socioeconomic environment. The questions and comments of elementary school-age children were grouped according to grade level.

Responses were obtained by structured and unstructured methods. Written questionnaires were the source of the structured data. The sources of unstructured data were:

1. Classroom observations by teachers and Washington State Medical Association Auxiliary volunteers
2. Audio tapes and open classroom discussions stimulated by questions
3. Voluntary responses by individual students
4. Voluntary oral comments made after students finished the written questionnaires

Sample summaries of structured and unstructured responses follow to illustrate, on a grade level basis, some of the findings of this study.

KINDERGARTEN PARTIAL SUMMARY OF INTERESTS
Human body/growth and development— a high interest

Unstructured:

In kindergarten, a big interest was the human body. Questions related to parts of the body, systems of the body, physical handicaps, the kindergartners' own growth, and prenatal growth and development.

Structured:

The number one interest, as shown on the written questionnaire, was about the body and its parts. Tied for third in interest was how the kindergartners' ears and eyes are made and work, and how they grow as human beings.

---

*Trucano, L.: Students speak, Seattle, 1984, Comprehensive Health Education Foundation.

Safe living/first aid—a high interest

Unstructured:

The most frequently recited responses centered around accident prevention, what to do in case of a fire, and first aid; there was also interest in poisoning.

Structured:

Of the six written questionnaire items on safe living/first aid, all are in the top fifteen interests: What to do if there were a fire (tied for first in interest); what to do when one is hurt at school or home (tied for second); how to prevent younger brothers and sisters or neighbor children from eating and drinking things that could poison them (tied for second); what to do if one is lost, how to prevent accidents at school, and how to prevent getting hurt going to and from school (all tied for fourth).

Physical well-being—a high interest

Unstructured:

When asked about topics relating to their physical well-being, kindergartners seemed to be interested in everything—especially dental care, sleep, and exercise.

Structured:

Tied for first in interest to kindergartners on the written questionnaire was how to stay healthy. Tied for fourth was how to take care of one's teeth and what foods one should eat to play, learn, and grow.

FIRST GRADE PARTIAL SUMMARY OF INTERESTS
Human body/growth and development— a high interest

Unstructured:

This health area was of highest interest to first graders. They wanted to know all about such things as how the body looks, works, breaks down, heals, and grows inside and out.

Structured:

The written question receiving the highest percentage of interest by first graders was the one dealing with the body and its parts. In fourth place was how ears and eyes are made and work.

Safe living/first aid—a high interest

Unstructured:

First aid and accident prevention was an area of high interest to first graders. They imagine all kinds of circumstances in which they might find themselves and wonder what they should do. They were even concerned about preventing accidents from rockets.

Structured:

Four of the six written questions on safe living/first aid were in the top fifteen interests of first graders. These four were: preventing younger brothers and sisters from ingesting poisonous substances (tied for first place); what to do in case of a fire (second most interesting item); what to do if lost (in third place); and how to prevent harm to themselves as they go to and from school (tied for sixth place).

Mental health—a high interest

Unstructured:

First graders were interested in understanding why people behave as they do, causes of feelings, and dealing with feelings. Friendship and decision making also held concern for them.

Structured:

The six written questions on mental health show 82% to 86% interest by the students.

SECOND GRADE PARTIAL SUMMARY OF INTERESTS
Human body/growth and development— a high interest

Unstructured:

The health area, human body, held an interest at all elementary grade levels, but second graders' responses seemed to indicate that this was *their* main interest. Second graders wanted to know all about body parts, how they work, how they grow, and how babies grow inside mothers. They wanted details; including limits of vision, why wrinkles occur, how one learns to talk, how organs relate to each other, and how a cell starts. Types of handicaps and the reasons for them also brought forth a lot of questions. They were interested in their own beginnings and endings. Typical questions were, "How does God invent people?" "How long can you stay alive?" and "Why do people die early?"

Structured:

Three of the four written questions for this health area were in the top fifteen interests. The questions were how the ears and eyes work (95%); about the body and its parts (93%); and how one grows (92%).

Mental health—a high interest

Unstructured:

Four topics brought forth the most questions: friendship, death, feelings and behavior. On the topic of behavior, second graders wanted to know why they act as they do and how to control behavior that is negative.

Structured:

The mental health question in the top fifteen interests concerned why people act the way they do. Not in the top fifteen, questions second graders wanted answered, but with an 85% interest, concerned how what one does or says affects other people, and what makes one feel good and bad; 89% of the second graders were interested in ways to get along with others; 87% in how handicapped people feel; and 86% in getting over sad, angry, or fearful feelings.

Physical well-being—a high interest

Unstructured:

Second graders were most interested in how to stay healthy, exercise, and keep teeth healthy.

Structured:

The number one interest of second graders was in learning how to stay healthy, with 97% of the students indicating they were interested. Other items in the top fifteen were: what foods one should eat so one can play, learn, and grow (93%); how food affects teeth (92%); and why one needs to rest and exercise (90%).

THIRD GRADE PARTIAL SUMMARY OF INTERESTS
Human body/growth and development— a high interest

Unstructured:

Third graders wanted to know much about the body and its parts, especially the brain and heart, and about their own growth and development. They were interested in fetal development. They wanted to know what happens to make things go wrong and cause handicaps such as deafness, dumbness, and paralysis. There was some interest in aging, senility, and how and why people die.

Structured:

Written questionnaire items appearing in the top fifteen interests were: learning about your body and its parts (95%); how the ears and eyes are made and work (90%); and how one grows (88%).

Safe living/first aid—a high interest

Unstructured:

Although there were a lot of questions and comments by students on accident prevention—from snake bites, to lead poisoning—no one topic dominated this health area.

Structured:

Five of the six written questions in this health area were in the top fifteen interests. What to do if lost had 95% interest; preventing younger brothers and sisters from ingesting poisonous substances had 95% interest; knowing what to do if hurt at home or school had 94% interest; what to do in case of a fire had 93% interest; and preventing accidents at school had 87% interest.

Disease control/preventing health problems— a high interest

Unstructured:

Disease was another area where there was a considerable number of questions but no pattern except for a commonly expressed interest in how people become sick or why some people get one disease and not another. There were many questions about specific diseases—especially about arthritis, cancer, and heart attacks. Several questions also were voiced on immunization

Structured:

Three written questions concerning this health area appear on the list of the top fifteen interests. One question concerned home medicines—how they may help or hurt a person (90%); a second indicated an interest in certain illnesses, like colds (87%), and the third concerned immunizations (87%).

FOURTH GRADE PARTIAL SUMMARY OF INTERESTS
Mental health—a high interest

Unstructured:

Fourth graders showed much concern about their own feelings and the feelings of others. They wanted to help others feel good about themselves. They wanted to like themselves, make friends, and avoid excessive worry and fear. Several commented on the deaths of friends, family members, and pets. They were concerned about how to make the right decisions.

Structured:

In the written questions, how a good friend should act was one of two mental health items in the top fifteen. The reasons why people might misuse drugs was the other item.

Family relationships—a high interest

Unstructured:

Fourth graders had a lot of interest in family. There was deep concern for the happiness of their families—how they could help make the family happy and keep the family together. Many questions were asked about divorce and the effect of divorce on them. They were interested in how babies come about, develop, and are born.

Structured:

Two written questions on family relationships were considered of top interest to fourth graders. They were concerned about how to help their families be happy; and closely tied to this was the concern of how problems may affect their families.

Drugs—a high interest

Unstructured:

Fourth graders were interested in the effects of drugs on the human body and mind and on relationships; they wondered why people use them; they were concerned about the dangers and whether or not experimentation is dangerous and leads to habituation or addiction.

Structured:

All four written questions on drugs appeared in the top fifteen interests of fourth graders: they wanted to know about drugs and what they do to the body; why people misuse drugs; how drugs affect the way people act; and how the wrong use of drugs may affect the family and community.

FIFTH GRADE PARTIAL SUMMARY OF INTEREST
Mental health—a high interest

Unstructured:

Students asked about reasons for and how to deal with feelings. They were concerned about friendships, self-concept and decision making. Of lesser interest were how people are alike and different, and how to deal with death and grief.

Structured:

Written questionnaire items on mental health from the top fifteen interests were: reasons people misuse alcohol and medicine, how drugs affect how people act, how a good friend should act, and how the wrong use of drugs may affect the family and community.

Human body/growth and development—a high interest

Unstructured:

Fifth graders wanted to know how the body works and why it does—from why there is swelling after an injury to how the body heals. Prenatal growth patterns and their own growth patterns brought forth many questions.

Causes of handicapping conditions and problems relating to the handicapped were mentioned often. Many questions on heredity also were asked.

Structured:

The top fifteen interests that fifth graders expressed on the questionnaire included the causes of handicaps, changes occurring at puberty, the development of the unborn, and the mechanics of the human body.

Family relationships—a high interest

Unstructured:

One of the most frequently recited responses concerned family happiness. Students wanted to know how to keep a family happy, how to prevent divorce, and how to get over the hurt of divorce. There was some interest in how babies come to be. There was a beginning recognition of boy-girl relationships. There was also concern about child abuse.

Structured:

How to help the family be happy and how problems affect the family were in the top fifteen interests from the written questionnaire.

Drugs—a high interest

Unstructured:

Fifth graders' individual responses were numerous about legal and illegal drugs. Mostly they were interested in the effects of drugs on the mind and body, and in why people take drugs. They were interested in the reasons drugs exist, which drugs were illegal and which ones were harmful, and in how to help people stop taking drugs.

Structured:

All written questions on drugs related to other health areas and appeared here as well as in the other areas. Questions relating to drugs from the top fifteen interests were: about drugs, and what they do the body; why people misuse alcohol and medicine; how drugs affect how people act; and how the wrong use of drugs may affect the family and the community.

SIXTH GRADE PARTIAL SUMMARY OF INTERESTS
Mental health—a high interest

Unstructured:

The major interests of sixth graders in the area of mental health concerned personal relationships (liking and being liked), fears and worries (about family, dark, crime), suicide (causes, prevention, helping friends), and feelings (helping others, controlling emotions, effects on health, releasing emotions without hurting others, and understanding behavior of others).

Structured:

The item, "Ways to say no if your friends are pressuring you to use drugs," was the second highest item of interest on the written questionnaire.

Family relationships—a high interest

Unstructured:

Teenage pregnancy concerned sixth graders; they wanted to know why it happens and the effect on all concerned. A high interest topic was family; family harmony, parenting (caring for children), and child abuse. There was some interest in boy-girl relationships.

Structured:

Appearing in the top fifteen interests from the written questionnaire were the effects of pregnancy on the unwed teenage girl, the responsible boy, and others.

Drugs—a high interest

Unstructured:

The interest in drugs, including alcohol and tobacco, was high. The topics of concern centered on the effects of drugs and why they are being used. Sixth graders expressed concern about why drugs are sold and how to avoid them, or how to help others avoid them.

Structured:

The top two interests of sixth graders on the written questionnaire concerned how drugs, including aspirin, alcohol, and speed affect people's minds and bodies, and ways to say no if friends are pressuring one to use drugs.

Physical well-being—a high interest

Unstructured:

The major topics that emerged were exercise (its effect, types, how much), grooming (skin care, evaluating products, relationships to health and stress), and being healthy in general (how one becomes healthy and how one knows if one is healthy).

Structured:

How to be physically fit was the third most popular item on the written questionnaire.

Human body/growth and development—a high interest

Unstructured:

Sixth graders wanted to know about prenatal growth and development (how food, drugs, and disease affect healthy development), and about how they themselves mature (the differences, reasons for changes, and the effect these changes will have on their future). They asked about the structure and function of the body (how it grows, looks, works, and changes—especially the reproductive system). There was high interest in the handicapped person (what help is available, including changing environmental barriers; how handicaps affect people's lives and their families, and how they all cope emotionally and physically). There was expressed interest in genetics (inherited diseases, feelings about incurable hereditary diseases, birth defects, and what one can inherit).

Structured:

In the top fifteen interests of sixth graders from the written questionnaire was the item, "What causes changes in the body when a girl becomes a woman and a boy becomes a man?"

SEVENTH GRADE PARTIAL SUMMARY OF INTERESTS
Mental health—a high interest

Unstructured:

Seventh graders seemed to have a preoccupation with suicide. They wanted to know why people do it, how to prevent it, and how to talk people out of it. They stated high interest in stress—its causes, effects, and prevention—and in coping mechanisms. Many comments appeared on worries and fears: how to get rid of them, facing them, and whether or not to share them. How to be a good friend was high on the students' interest list. They wanted to know how to select a good friend. Other topics that received comments were: self-concept, feelings, coping with problems, peer pressure, and relating to others.

Structured:

Two items appeared in the top fifteen interests from the written questionnaire: the causes and preventions of suicide, and ways to say no if one's friends are pressuring the use of drugs.

Family relationships—a high interest

Unstructured:

The biggest topic of concern for seventh graders was the unmarried pregnant teenager. They were concerned about why such pregnancies occur, how to help a friend who is pregnant, the effect on all involved, and having healthy babies. Family relationships were of high interest. They wanted to understand problems families have, how they could help and not hurt family members, and how they themselves affect their families. Areas of medium interest were child abuse, babies, and child care.

Structured:

Two written questionnaire items relating to family were on the list of the top fifteen interests of seventh graders. One item was the effects of pregnancy on unmarried teenagers and all concerned. The other item was what love is and how one might know if he/she is really in love.

Drugs—a high interest

Unstructured:

Seventh graders were interested in the effects of drugs, including alcohol and tobacco. They were interested in why people use drugs and abuse drugs. They wanted to know about types of drugs and about the legal controls on drugs.

Structured:

Three questionnaire items were in the top fifteen interests of seventh graders. The number one interest was how drugs, including aspirin, caffeine, alcohol, and speed affect people's minds and bodies. The other two items concerned ways to say no if friends are pressuring one to use drugs; and how drugs, including alcohol, tobacco, tranquilizers and marijuana, might cause injury to self or others.

EIGHTH GRADE PARTIAL SUMMARY OF INTERESTS
Drugs—a high interest

Unstructured:

Eighth graders wanted to know everything about legal and illegal drugs, especially how they affect the mind and body. The impression given by the students' comments was that they wanted information, not advice. They were not too eager to try drugs, but they wanted to know what drugs really do, why people take them, how to help people in trouble with drugs.

Structured:

Three written questionnaire items were on the list of top interests of eighth graders. They were how drugs, including aspirin, caffeine, alcohol, and speed affect people's minds and bodies; ways to say no when friends are pressuring one to use drugs; and how drugs might cause one to injure oneself or others.

Nutrition—a high interest

Unstructured:

Eighth graders wanted to know the effect foods have on the body, which foods are best, the amount needed, how food and disease are related, and the effect of nutrition on a developing baby. There was special interest in weight control, such as why people have trouble controlling weight, how to diet for physical fitness, how to lose weight in a healthy way, why some labels do not list calories, the effect of dieting, what are healthy snacks, how to diet when eating out, and the effects of candy on appetite. Another topic of some interest was world hunger.

Structured:

Questionnaire items of most importance to eighth graders included: how to determine if one is eating so one will grow and stay healthy; how exercise, work, and stress affect food eaten; world hunger and its effects; the importance of breakfast; and fast foods, food processing, and food additives.

Family relationships—a high interest

Unstructured:

Eighth graders were extremely interested in family, the effect on one's lifespan, how families influence children, how to promote closeness, exploration of "rules for fighting" to prevent hurting family members, how to be honest among family members, how to raise children properly, effective discipline, divorce and its effects on family members, child abuse (why it occurs, options, where to go for help), and adoption.

Another big topic of interest was human sexuality. The topic of most concern dealt with problems surrounding pregnancies of unmarried teenagers. Students wanted to know how it affects the child, the parents of the teenagers, and the teenagers themselves—including the boy. There was some interest in birth control; that is legality, types, vasectomy. They recognized the need to know the consequences of early sexual behavior, they wanted some understanding of how changes in feelings occur and how to handle them. They also wanted to discuss responsible boy-girl relationships, and especially how to say "no" to sexual activity.

Structured:

Two written questionnaire items appeared on the list of the top fifteen interests: the effects of pregnancy of unmarried teenagers on all concerned, and what love is.

Mental health—a high interest

Unstructured:

Students were interested in suicide, stress, relating to others, coping skills, and understanding feelings. They wanted to know causes and preventions of suicide, indications that someone might try suicide, and how to cope after a friend has committed suicide. In regard to stress, they wanted to know both the physical and mental effects, how to overcome it, and how peer pressure creates it. Relating to others seemed to revolve around brother-sister relationships, coping with bullies, what love is, making and keeping friends, and expressing oneself comfortably. Coping skills related to peer pressure, shyness, understanding oneself (what is normal, how to be happy), and how to reduce fears and worries were important. Understanding feelings included how to express them responsibly, how to control one's temper, depression, and causes of fears and worries.

Structured:

Eighth graders placed the causes and prevention of suicide in their top fifteen items of interest. Also of concern were ways to say "no," if one's friends are pressuring one to use drugs.

Student needs. Student needs may be considered as falling into two groups: those that are *felt* by children and those that are prevalent health and safety problems but are *unfelt* by children. *Felt needs* are the wants and desires of students that can be expressed in *interest surveys* such as the one completed in Washington state. *Unfelt needs* are health problems and concerns from other sources and those expressed by people other than pupils. Such information comes from mortality and morbidity statistics; accident statistics, growth and development characteristics of children; state laws regarding health instruction areas; local, state, and national health departments; voluntary, commercial, and professional health agencies and organizations; pupils' health and absenteeism records; and other sources. Some of the people who can provide information about health problems of children include parents, teachers, nurses, physicians, dentists, and health officials in health departments and health agencies.

Using the wide variety of sources and people identified may be logistically difficult if not impossible to handle in determining the nature of the health instruction curriculum, even with computers. Local schools and school districts may find it more convenient to select a sampling of procedures to provide the best representative information on the needs of their pupils. However, large districts and statewide curriculum projects may find it advantageous to conduct extensive surveys of student interests and needs.

The illustrative units found in Appendix B include a broad approach to pupils' interests and needs.

SCOPE AND SEQUENCE

To determine the scope and sequence of health teaching in the elementary school program, it is necessary to consider the needs and interests of children at all age levels from kindergarten throughout the elementary school. Many state departments of education produce a sample scope and sequence chart to provide guidance to local school districts. These state level documents are usually based on research, literature reviews, and advice from teachers, parents, and other experts. They provide an excellent point of reference for people charged with the responsibility of developing health education programs in local districts. Table 11-1 contains an illustrative scope and sequence chart published by the Wisconsin Department of Public Education.*

Organized health instruction should be provided at all grade levels throughout the elementary school. There are a number of impor-

---

*Wisconsin Department of Public Instruction: A guide to curriculum planning in health education, Madison, Wis. 1985., The Department.

tant reasons why it should be offered at all levels. First, the body of knowledge concerning health and healthful living in the modern world is so extensive that it is necessary to offer it over a period of years to adequately impart the knowledge needed. Second, there is a need for a certain amount of health knowledge at all grade levels, including kindergarten. The degree of maturity of children in the elementary grades is such that they cannot be given the extensive knowledge needed for adult life. Yet it is highly important that instruction be given and that the various phases of health and healthful living be introduced to the children as rapidly as their maturity and level of intelligence will permit.

From the viewpoint of psychology it is much easier to establish proper habits of health and healthful living early in the child's life. Also, the child needs to practice good health and safety habits just as much at an early age as later. Therefore it seems psychologically sound to teach as much as possible about health as early

TABLE 11-1. Wisconsin state level scope and sequence and recommended time allotment for specific grade levels

School health education Major content areas for classroom instruction	Recommended number of periods per year* 1 year = 34 weeks				Recommended number of periods per semester	
	K	1-2	3-4	5-6	7-8-9	10-11-12
	45 min. per wk. 1 period = 15 min.	75 min. per wk. 1 period = 25 min.	100 min. per wk. 1 period = 25 min.	125 min. per wk. 1 period = 50 min.	1 course, meeting 90 periods in a semester. 1 period = 50 min.	1 course, meeting 90 periods in a semester. 1 period = 50 min.
	Grade levels					
	15-min. periods	25-min. periods			50-min. periods	
	K	1	2	3	4	5	6	7-8-9	10-11-12

School health education Major content areas for classroom instruction	K	1	2	3	4	5	6	7-8-9	10-11-12
I. Accident prevention and safety	15	12	12	15	15	6	5	5	14
II. Community health	0	0	0	6	6	5	5	5	5
III. Consumer health	0	0	0	6	6	5	5	10	8
IV. Environmental health	0	0	0	6	6	5	5	10	10
V. Family life education	6	9	9	12	12	10	10	15	12
VI. Mental and emotional health	18	18	18	18	18	13	15	12	8
VII. Nutrition	18	18	18	18	18	10	10	5	5
VIII. Personal health	18	18	18	18	18	13	12	10	9
IX. Prevention and control of disease	6	6	6	6	6	3	3	3	4
X. Substance use and abuse	6	9	9	15	15	15	15	10	10
Total periods	87	90	90	120	120	85	85	85	85

Reprinted with permission from the Wisconsin Department of Public Instruction.
*The recommended periods for a year or semester *do not* necessarily mean that all instruction should be completed in that specific content area in consecutive lessons.

as possible, considering the stages of maturity of the children. An example of this is in the area of nutrition, which is a phase of the health education program at practically all grade levels. The subject of nutrition should be introduced and developed as far as the ability of the children at any particular age level permits, for nutrition is a functional part of the life of the primary-age child just as it is of an older child. If by educating children in nutrition to their capacity at the primary level we can better assure their optimum nutrition, then it is obvious that the subject should be introduced in school just as early as possible. Even though primary-age children are not mature enough to be given all the safety information they need for life, it is highly important that they know as much about safety as possible to safeguard their lives while growing up. As an example, the failure to teach elementary school children certain facts about traffic safety could result in a child's death or permanent disability.

What then can we consider to be properly included in the course of study for health and safety in our elementary schools? As we know, the needs of communities, states, and regions may differ somewhat in that some problems are specific for certain localities.

In general, research, experience, and surveys have shown that the elementary health curriculum should include units on nutrition; consumer health; growth; exercise; sleep; rest and relaxation; dental health; eyes and ears; family life and health; mental health; safety; first aid; alcohol, tobacco, and other drugs; body mechanics; structure, function, and care of the body; control of diseases; medical and dental care; community health problems; and chronic diseases. Many of these areas are covered in the illustrative material found in Appendix B.

Special education

Although often mainstreamed into regular classrooms, students in special education need to be provided learning experiences in health education. They have problems and interests similar to those of the so-called normal students. For those who are mentally retarded, much of what is used in the regular program in sex education can be adapted to a simpler presentation. Also the use of more visual aids and repetition is necessary. For those who have cerebral palsy, special toothbrushes and prophylactic implements can be prepared for oral health. For blind students, braille materials should be provided. Teachers will need to develop their own items, make adaptations, or explore community resources for assistance.

A suggested health education program usable in a classroom where there are different types of handicapped children is found in Table 11-2.

Health education curriculum for preschool programs

Children regardless of their ages should be exposed to educational programs about health. Many habit patterns are established early in life, and numerous health problems are preventable in the formative years. The preschool setting offers opportunities to influence the development of behaviors and reduce problems. Preschool programs should include curricula in health education. The information in this chapter including the unit materials that are categorically listed in Appendix B as well as the activities in Chapter 12 at the primary grade levels are useful. Teachers will need to extrapolate the applicable sections and adapt and organize them into suitable units and lessons. However, the U.S. Office of Child Development Project Head Start prepared a curriculum guide useful to teachers. The following represents a suggested content outline adapted from that reference.*

All about me
My body (inside, outside, functions of body systems)
Who am I? (sex, race, ethnic group)
Real me (How do I feel inside? happy, sad, angry, afraid, lonely, and so forth)

---

*Adapted from the U.S. Office of Child Development Project Head Start: Healthy that's me: a health education curriculum guide for Head Start, Washington, D.C., 1971, U.S. Department of Health, Education, and Welfare.

TABLE 11-2. Health education for special children

Areas	Levels*				
	I	**II**	**III**	**IV**	**V**
Safety	*Emergencies* Awareness and simple first aid Communication Report	*Traveling* Pedestrian Passenger Bicycle	*School* Classroom Building Playground	*Home* General Fire and electricity Appliances and equipment	*Recreation* Environment Use of equipment and games Bicycle and camping
Mental health	*Self-acceptance* Physical abilities and limitations Mental abilities and limitations Cultural and social differences	*Acceptance of others* Physical abilities Mental abilities and limitations Cultural and social differences	*Values* Personal Home and school Community and national	*Adjustment to stress* School Home Community	
Family living	*Roles in family* Recognizing roles Learning roles Accepting changing roles	*Home management and maintenance* Supervised responsibilities Simple independent responsibilities Self-directed responsibilities	*Family and child care* Supervised responsibility Simple independent responsibilities Self-directed responsibilities	*Sex education* Sex organs Reproduction	
Nutrition	*Foods* Sources Types Components	*Diet* Selection of basic food Planning of daily menus Effects of components	*Preparation and preservation of foods* Cleaning and storing Preparation of food for meals Preservation of foods	*Health problems* Weight Vitality Allergies	
Body care and personal hygiene	*Cleanliness* Routine Grooming Body changes	*Respect and protection of body parts* Dental care	*Rest and exercise* Awareness of need Understanding of need Ways and means	*Proper clothing and shelter* Awareness of need Understanding of need Ways and means	
Disease and illness	*Communicable disease* Symptoms Causes Treatment	*Sanitation* Personal Home and school Community	*Personal care* Awareness Communication Treatment	*Health services* Knowledge of community Knowledge and location of services When and how to use	

Prepared by a group of special education teachers in Ellensburg, Washington.
*Refers to stages of learning progression. Children move from level to level upward when ready regardless of grade.

Accident prevention and first aid
Home
Fire
Playground
To and from school
Dangerous strangers

Disease control
Germs
Infections
Colds
Coughs
Immunizations and other control

Dental health
Decay
Brushing and flossing
Sugar foods

Nutrition
Selection of nutritious items

Rest, sleep and exercise
Need for and adequate amounts

Who helps to take care of health
Family (parents, physician, teacher, school nurse; vision and hearing testing, and others)

THE UNIT IN HEALTH TEACHING

Few concepts in education are less understood by teachers than is the unit or the unit method. Unit teaching is basically a good way of organizing for teaching.

It is common for both prospective and certified teachers to become confused about the definition, concept, nature, and purpose of the unit approach. This is entirely understandable when one reviews the educational literature. It seems that each writer places his or her own interpretation on the unit and its use in improving instruction in the classroom. But through the fabric of a multitude of definitions is woven the common thread of organization. Both topics and learning experiences are organized in such a manner that they are related to a central theme or problem. Thus units in health are built around fundamental concepts in health and the major

problems of children and society in safe and healthful living.

Most statements of unit organization and content include certain essential elements: objectives, content, teaching aids, activities, and evaluation procedures.

Certainly the unit is far superior to teaching in a hit-or-miss fashion. Yet the most carefully planned and thoroughly detailed health unit falls short of its purpose and potential if it deals with trivia. Occasionally teachers may be led to believe that the process is more important than the learning products. When this happens, teachers may become so infatuated with the procedures and techniques of the unit approach that they fail to pay enough attention to the significance of the knowledges, attitudes, and practices they seek to develop among pupils.

The unit approach is one of the best means available for organizing more meaningful learning experiences. Beyond this, the unit helps assure a sound, logical presentation of subject matter. It represents an effective blending of psychological and logical organization of topics and concepts.

In the preparation of the objectives for the units found in this chapter, the taxonomy (classification) of educational goals that was developed by Bloom and associates* and widely utilized in curriculum development in the United States was used. Today it continues to be one of the most effective ways to prepare objectives.

TAXONOMY OF OBJECTIVES

Cognitive domain (knowledges/understandings)
  Know—define, name, relate, list, recall, explain, state, recite, tell
  Comprehend—predict, draw conclusions, diagram, illustrate, discuss, classify, recognize, identify, report, review, describe

---

*Adapted from Bloom, B., editor: Taxonomy of educational objectives. Handbook I: Cognitive domain, New York, 1956, David McKay Co., Inc. and Krathwohl, D.R., Bloom, B.S., and Masia, B.B.: Taxonomy of educational objectives. Handbook II: Affective domain, New York, 1964, David McKay Co., Inc.

Apply—solve, translate, demonstrate, dramatize, illustrate

Analyze—identify, distinguish, establish criteria, conclude, interpret, translate, classify, criticize, debate, question, examine

Synthesize—plan, integrate, summarize, develop, compare, design, create, prepare, construct, formulate, compose

Evaluate—compare, contrast, differentiate, judge, rate, appraise, select, assess, measure, estimate

Affective domain (attitudes: feelings, appreciations, values)

Attend (be receptive)—talk about, be supportive, listen, display interest, be attentive

Respond (be impressed)—ask questions, react, give opinions, bring things to class

Value (rate highly)—accept, support

Action domain (practices)

Act, eat, wash, brush, buy, avoid, refrain from, demonstrate, choose, place, obey

Illustrative partial units for primary, intermediate, and upper grades

The illustrative partial units in Appendix B cover many of the important health content areas teachers may use in planning for health instruction. Included in the appendix are such areas as consumer health; dental health; disease control; exercise, rest, and body control; drugs; family health; mental health; nutrition; safety and first aid; and vision and hearing. Note that they follow the basic principles previously identified and give consideration to the new definition of health, the concept approach, and values.

Appendix B is designed to ease the burden on those new to teaching elementary health. It saves many hours of work by providing an outline of general content in each area plus hundreds of sample concepts and objectives. In essence it provides the raw material for each teacher to begin planning for his/her basic health lessons. This material has the additional advantage of covering the entire K through 8 grade sequence. Thus a teacher who faces a grade level assignment change can turn to the material in Appendix B to ease the burden of creating health units appropriate for his/her new assignment.

HOW DOES THE TEACHER PLAN?

There are a variety of ways teachers can plan for health instruction programs in schools. They involve procedures that organize learning experiences into a number of useful patterns. The materials presented in this chapter together with those provided in Chapter 9 and 12 through 14 and Appendixes B, D, E, F, and G will be helpful. These guidelines should be followed in the sequence listed for the *direct* teaching of health in classrooms where there are no health curricula:

1. Identify the needs and interests of students and use this information to establish a scope and sequence of content
2. Identify student learning objectives
3. Identify school and community resources for health instruction curriculum guides, teaching aids, and health education specialists
4. Prepare a series of units from the scope and content previously identified
5. Prepare lesson plans or modules from the units

In those school districts where curriculum guides are available, teachers may wish to start with procedure 2 or 3 in this list.

Classroom scope and sequence

A health instruction program should be related to the specific needs and interests of children in a particular school or school district. Using the material or one of the procedures described in this chapter will enable a teacher to identify these needs and interests. A meeting with the school nurse may help to obtain this information quickly. These data can then be grouped into topical areas as illustrated in Table 11-1 and Table 11-3 (under *Area*). The sequence in terms of a monthly schedule as seen in Table 11-3 is merely illustrative and may need modi-

TABLE 11-3. Second grade scope, sequence, and teacher plans for health education, Ellensburg, Washington, public schools

Month	Area	Concepts	Learning activities	Teaching aids	Integration
September	Mental health	New experiences may give satisfaction Home, school, church, and community can be warm, safe places	Have children act as "big brother" or "big sister" to new students Encourage drawings about things they love, how it feels when hurt or scared, how to be helpful Encourage art work to relieve tensions Discuss leaders and followers, forgiveness, and other topics Dramatize putting self in others' shoes Films	Films: We play and share together Courtesy at school Health text: second and third grade	Language arts: write short experiences Music: listen to quiet music if tense Physical education: suggest activities to relax Social studies: discover community helpers
October	Dental health	Daily care promotes dental health Dentists help maintain healthy teeth Community resources provide for dental care	Demonstrate (using model) brushing teeth Make toothpowder in class Show films and filmstrips and discuss them Survey for number of dental visits Have vocabulary bingo game Write creative story about detergent foods	Films: The beaver tale Learning to brush Salt and baking soda Toothbrush dental kit Pictures: detergent foods and other foods	Mathematics: count teeth; subtract missing teeth Social studies: characterize dentist as community helper Art: make detergent-food mobile
November	Family health	Families help each other in the community	Make pictures of the family Tell experiences List ways neighbors can be helpful Arrange bulletin board about good neighborhood	Health text Record: Community helpers, Bowman Family fun with familiar music	Language arts: employ creative dramatics Music: play records and songs Art: draw pictures
January	Consumer and community health	Doctors and dentists who help us are our friends Hazards of the environment can cause discomfort and problems Many people keep water and air safe Individuals can improve their surroundings	Keep home duty chart Use atomizers to show how odors disperse Show films and filmstrips Make notebook on community helpers' relation to environment Dramatize how children help at home Locate on map local family and health agencies	Film: Magic touch Filmstrip: Dentist School nurse Record: Community helpers Personal pictures Map of community	Social studies: relate to community helpers unit Language arts: encourage reports or notebooks Art: make mural of community helpers

Month	Unit	Concept	Activities	Audiovisual materials	Correlation
February	Nutrition	There are many kinds of foods / Some foods may be better than others for you	Decorate flannelboard with creative story with characters / Leave food out, covered and uncovered, to relate to improper storage / Try new foods at tasting party / Experiment with white rat / Make vegetable soup / Make grocery store; use food models and shop for nutritious foods / Make clay or paper maché fruit / Select basic 4 foods, using magazine pictures	Film: Eat for health / Filmstrip: The food we eat / Transparencies: See unit / Food models of cardboard cutouts / Health text	Art: draw basic 4 food groups; prepare mural / Mathematics: sell items in grocery store and add costs / Science: Experiment with white rat / Social studies: take trip to store
March	Anatomy-physiology	Good posture helps prevent fatigue, enables the body to work better, and makes you more attractive	Use horizontal ladder for proper alignment / Use plumbline to check posture / Decorate bulletin board with stick figures or pipe cleaners / Show film and discuss	Film: Beginning good posture / Filmstrip: Let's stand tall	Physical education: relate to apparatus activities / Art: make silhouettes and individual pictures / Language arts: show and tell
April	Disease control	Good health habits help to keep us well / When ill, certain practices help us get well / We depend on others for good health	Use poster to illustrate ways to protect others / Stage choral reading and speaking / Use chart to show ways germs are transmitted / Write reports / Grow germs on cloth in warm and cool places / Dramatize going to doctor for help / Experiment with potato and agar in petri dish	Films: Common cold; Soapy the germ fighter / Milne: We are six (Wheezie and Sneezie)	Language arts: relate to experiences when sick, effects of care, creative stories / Science: experiment with potatoes and agar
May	Family health	An egg grows into a baby	Discuss charts of mammal reproduction / Prepare chart on life cycle of animal reproduction / Hatch egg in incubator / Chart and discuss fish egg development / Make mural of animals caring for own babies / Show films and filmstrips	Eye Gate charts of mammal reproduction series and fish egg development / Films: Baby animals; Animals growing up / Filmstrip: The zoo trip	Science: hatch egg: relate to insect unit / Art: prepare mural

fication during the school year. The mental health unit permeates the entire school curriculum, and portions may be covered whenever it is deemed appropriate. Teachers should feel free to modify this arrangement if a teachable moment arises that will permit introduction of an area when it will have greater student interest and motivation.

Unit construction

By definition, unit construction refers to a procedure that organizes the learning experiences that are related to a particular topic or unifying purpose—for example, nutrition or dental health. The content of a unit generally includes these elements: topic, grade level, number of lessons or time, concepts, goals or objectives, content, teaching/learning activities, teaching aids, evaluation, and integration relationships. The partial illustrative units in Appendix B contain the content, concepts, and objectives. The teaching techniques, the teaching aids, and the evaluation suggestions can be selected by the individual teacher from the material found in Chapters 12 through 14.

Table 11-3 is a partial illustrative unit or a series of units that is also a yearly scope-and-sequence arrangement prepared by an individual teacher. This unit outline can help teachers plan a health instruction program for a semester or for an entire year. It will be necessary to develop lesson plans or modules from this material that will also include the objectives to be achieved and other relevant information.

It might be advisable to provide information about ways to integrate this unit into language arts, social studies, science, and other curriculum areas. Table 11-3 provides an illustration of how this material might be included.

In planning the development of the unit, the teacher should check local school and community resources for material that will help in unit construction or lesson planning. These are some of the items that need to be identified: resource personnel, curriculum guides, films, filmstrips, models, charts, books, pamphlets, and other teaching aids. School nurses can often be of considerable help in this regard.

Lesson plans/modules

Lesson plans or modules are step-by-step procedures to be followed by the teacher in one session or for a given period of time. A lesson or module therefore may not be completed in one day. Lesson plans/modules are segments of instruction that are related to a particular subject matter area. They are prepared from the units previously discussed in this chapter, and their content may include concepts, objectives, content, and other information. They should also provide for a presentation or learning sequence that enables teachers to know exactly what to do at any time, how to introduce content, how to use the teaching aids, and how to involve students. A module may differ somewhat from a lesson plan in that it contains all of the teaching aids such as charts, illustrations, tests, and other materials ready for use by any teacher. A teacher may have to prepare a lesson plan without all of the items found in a module and therefore must develop them before using the lesson plan. In some instances a single unit around an instructional area may not be prepared, but rather several modules centering on a given subject area are developed. This arrangement could be considered to be equivalent to a unit in organization.

The following pages contain illustrations of lesson plans containing varying degrees of detail, beginning with a minimum of information and progressing toward a greater amount of detail.

ILLUSTRATION OF A LESSON PLAN

Unit: Prevention and control of disease
Level: Grade 6
Specific topical key: Major killers
Approximate time: 50 minutes
Objective: The students will name the four major killers of Americans today.
Activities: Following a lecture on the four major killers of Americans—heart disease, cancer, stroke, and accidents—the students will create an advertising campaign with the theme "May the 'Fours' Not Be with You."

   The students can work in pairs to construct posters advertising the healthy behaviors that can help prevent the four major killers. Encourage the students to use the *Star Wars* theme to add drama and flair to their advertisements.
Source: Jon Hisgen, School District of Pewaukee
Resources needed: Magazines, *Star Wars* memorabilia
Evaluation focus:

   ☒ Knowledge   ☒ Attitude   ☒ Problem Solving
Teacher's notes (Things to change):

Reprinted with permission of Wisconsin Department of Public Instruction.

ILLUSTRATION OF A LESSON PLAN

Unit: Mental and emotional health
Level: Grade 1
Specific topical key: Self-concept
Approximate time: 50 minutes
Objective: The students will recognize positive qualities in themselves and others.
Activities: Read the story *The Little Rabbit Who Wanted Red Wings* by Carolyn Sherwin Bailey to your class or, if you prefer, show them the filmstrip that is available.

  Afterward, discuss the book and ask children to fill out the answer sheets.
Script: Do you remember the story of *The Little Rabbit Who Wanted Red Wings?* He always wanted to be anything but what he was. He found out that the best thing to be was himself—a rabbit! There was only one rabbit like him and he decided to be the best he could be. Your job is to be the best that you can be. Just think, there is only one person like you in the whole world. Isn't that great? Now, the little rabbit would like to know more about that special you. Please fill out your answer sheet for him.

Answer sheet:
  1. My first name is _____
  2. My last name is _____
  3. I am _____ years old
  4. I am in _____ grade
  5. (Really think about this before you write your answer down.) I am special because

  _____

  _____

  6. Draw a picture of "that special me"

Teacher note: This can lead to a discussion about positive qualities others display.
Resources needed: The book and/or filmstrip entitled *The Little Rabbit Who Wanted Red Wings*.
Evaluation focus:
  ☐ Knowledge   ☒ Attitude   ☐ Problem Solving
Teacher's notes (things to change):

Reprinted with permission of Wisconsin Department of Public Instruction.

ILLUSTRATION OF A LESSON PLAN

Unit: To smoke or not to smoke
Level: Grade 7 or 8
Time needed: About 45 minutes
Previous lesson: Strategies used in advertising
Concept: Advertising may influence the use of tobacco
Objectives: The student:
1. Identifies the appeals and slogans used to influence the use of cigarettes
2. Realizes the importance of slogans and advertisements in influencing the use of cigarettes

Content: Advertising appeals: attractive people; glamour and elegance; sex or love; macho image; better taste; beautiful scenery; better filter; low tar and nicotine; sign of adulthood
Slogans: "You've come a long way, baby"
"The coolest taste around"
"Where a man belongs"
Some reasons for use: sell more cigarettes by trying to appeal to people's psychological needs through social influences—adulthood, peer acceptance, love, beauty, less hazardous to health, strong/powerful/controlled person
What are advertisers trying to sell? Hope; to be like others

Learning activities/procedures:
1. On chalkboard teacher introduces some slogans and appeals obtained from cigarette advertisements brought to class by students.
2. Organize class into small discussion groups with one student as chairperson in charge of each and provide each group with three advertisements. Ask each group to take 20 minutes to analyze the advertisements in terms of: (1) identification of the advertising appeals and slogans and (2) the reasons why these slogans and appeals are used.
3. Reassemble the class, have chairpersons report their information, and tally the findings on the backboard.
4. Teacher summarizes the essential points and students put information in notebooks.

Evaluation: Teacher observations of student interest in lesson together with the extent of pupil participation
Materials and resources needed: Numerous magazine and newspaper cigarette advertisements; chalkboard
Assignment: Students bring empty cigarette containers to class and are prepared to orally comment on the meaning of the "warning against smoking" found on the package. Also identify the amount of tar and nicotine in the brand of cigarettes. Read appropriate chapter in the assigned text.
Next lesson: Alternatives to use of cigarettes: develop own personality; better self-care; self-image; success in school, job, and recreational skills.
Vocabulary: glamour, elegance, beautiful, nicotine, advertisements, adulthood, attractive

Adapted from Middleton, K.: Back to some basics in health lesson planning, Health Education **12:**4-8 Jan./Feb., 1981.

A DRUG THAT'S NOT A MEDICINE
Grade 3

READY
The student will demonstrate the ability to

1. Describe the physical and behavioral effects of nicotine.

2. List reasons why people use and don't use drugs.

SET
Resources
From the kit
Message poster, "Be smart—don't start"
Definition card, "Nicotine"
Nicotine puzzle and outline
From the guide
Fact sheet, "Nicotine"
Read the **fact sheet**

New vocabulary
stimulant a drug that speeds up the functioning of the body
tobacco a plant made into products that are often smoked or chewed
nicotine a stimulant drug found in tobacco

GO
Review

1. Remind the class that yesterday they learned about some of the medicines that are used a lot in your community.

Introduction

2. Explain that today you have a special puzzle that will help them learn some important facts about a drug found in tobacco that isn't used as a medicine.

3. Ask students if they have ever put something in their mouth that tasted terrible. Ask:

   • What was it?
   • Would you put it in your mouth again?

   Explain that tobacco is like the substances they named because it tastes terrible, but people keep using it because it's hard to stop using it once you start.

Objective

4. Explain that today students will learn about a drug found in tobacco; the drug is called *nicotine*. Explain that they are also going to learn why people use nicotine.

Activity

5. Explain that tobacco has been around for a long, long time. Ask students what products have tobacco in them (*cigarettes, pipes, cigars, chew, snuff, etc.*).

6. Explain to students that nicotine is a *stimulant* drug, which means that taking it speeds up the body.

7. Distribute pieces of the **puzzle** to students in the class so that each student has at least one piece.

8. Place the large **puzzle outline** sheet on the floor (or large table) so that students can gather around the sheet and have easy access to it. Have students come around the puzzle and look over the outline to try and locate where their piece should be placed.

9. Have students start at the head and place their pieces on the outline until the head and messages around the head are complete. Have the students whose pieces made up this area of the puzzle read the statements they created out loud and in unison to the rest of the class. Continue this process for the other parts of the anatomy.

Closure

10. Ask students to share a new fact they learned about tobacco (nicotine). Encourage them to make positive, healthy choices like not smoking. Show the **message poster**, "Be smart—don't start." Display the **definition card**.

Extension

11. Have students talk with any adult in his/her home who has used nicotine, asking when and how the adult got started. Have students write down the reasons. If there is no one at home who has used nicotine, the student can ask an adult to share any stories about people he/she knows who have used it. Make a list of the reasons and talk about them with the students. Discuss ways of avoiding starting to use nicotine.

From: Here's Looking at You, 2000. (Courtesy of The Comprehensive Health Education Foundation.)

SUMMARY

Effective health teaching in the classroom revolves around a well-organized curriculum conceived from a scope and sequence based on known growth and developmental patterns and student needs and interests. The curriculum itself must be founded on sound principles applicable to all subject area disciplines. It must also include those factors that are unique to the teaching of health such as physiological, sociological, psychological, and spiritual aspects of health.

The conceptual approach, first applied to health teaching by a team of health educators under the leadership of Dr. Elena Sliepcevich, has produced a number of landmark papers and documents that still serve as the basis for much of today's curriculum work in health. The conceptual approach is fundamental to the eclectic plan identified in this text. It legitimizes the inclusion of value clarification, holistic health, and decision making into the curriculum.

A relatively new approach to health curriculum development teams content area authorities with teachers, nurses, and parents in collaborative efforts to develop subject matter. This allows for the development of curriculum tailored to specific local needs. However, the fundamental subject matter in health is primarily the same for most schools.

The needs and interests of students are basic sources of information for determining the health curriculum, including the scope and sequence. Local surveys can be undertaken or reference can be made to existing data such as those contained in Students Speak. Another benefit of using these data is that misinformation and misconceptions are often revealed. Attention should be given to all grade levels and to the needs of all students, including children enrolled in preschools.

The unit is a method of organizing lessons within a specific health program. Hundreds of sample concepts and objectives are included in

Appendix B for the teacher. Content is outlined in general, but each teacher must seek out additional content for his/her own lessons. This is as it should be, since content in health topics changes rapidly and teachers need to consistently upgrade their knowledge.

Illustrations of lesson plans containing varying degrees of detail are provided to assist the teacher in deciding which might work best. The samples share one common philosophy—they are all student centered. Information contained in this and succeeding chapters has been developed to provide guidance and aid for the teacher in making every lesson important, relevant, and student centered.

QUESTIONS FOR DISCUSSION

1. Who should be responsible for curriculum development in the school?
2. What are the basic principles on which the health curriculum should be based?
3. Why is both formal and informal health education necessary in schools?
4. What is the meaning and significance of the inclusion of values in the curriculum?
5. What is the meaning of the concept approach, and how can it be applied to health education?
6. Who should be responsible for the development of the health and safety education curriculum?
7. How is the curriculum in health education determined?
8. To what extent would you use the health interests of children as shown by the Washington study?
9. What are some of the sources of helpful information in determining health content for elementary pupils?
10. What are the procedures to be followed in determining the health education curriculum for elementary schools?
11. What is the fundamental purpose of the unit in health teaching?
12. What is the meaning of the phrase *scope and sequence?*
13. What are the common, essential elements of a good *teaching* unit?
14. What should be the nature of the health education curriculum for students in special education and preschool programs?
15. What must the teacher do to plan for health instruction?
16. How can the broad concept of health (holistic) identified in Chapter 1 be utilized in the development of the health education curriculum?
17. What does the phrase *taxonomy of objectives* mean as identified by Bloom and others, and how can it be used in health education?

SELECTED REFERENCES

Anderson, C.L., and Creswell, W.H.: School health practice, ed. 8, St. Louis, 1985, Times Mirror/Mosby College Publishing.

Beane, J.A.: The continuing controversy over affective education, Educational Leadership 43(4): Dec., 1985/Jan., 1986.

Bloom B., editor: Taxonomy of educational objectives. Handbook I: Cognitive domain, New York, 1956, David McKay Co., Inc.

Bradley, C., editor: A guide to curriculum planning in health education, Madison, Wis., 1985, Wisconsin Department of Public Instruction.

Byler, R.V., Lewis, G.M., and Tottman, R.J.: Teach us what we want to know, New York, 1969, Mental Health Materials Center, Inc.

Cornacchia, H.J., and Barrett, S.: Consumer health: a guide to intelligent decisions, ed. 3, St. Louis, 1985, Times Mirror/Mosby College Publishing.

Cornacchia, H.J., and Barrett, S.: Shopping for health: an essential guide for products and services, St. Louis, 1982, Mosby Medical Library.

Costa, A.L., editor: Developing minds, Alexandria, Virginia, 1985, Association for Supervision and Curriculum Development.

Felt, M.C.: Improving our schools, Newton, Mass., 1985, Education Development Center, Inc.

Havighurst, R.J.: The values of youth. In Issues in American education, New York, 1970, Oxford University Press.

Hoyman, H.S.: Health ethics and relevant issues, Journal of School Health 42:Nov., 1972.

Krathwohl, D.R., Bloom, B.S., and Masia, B.B.: Taxonomy of educational objectives. Handbook II: Affective domain, New York, 1964, David McKay Co., Inc.

Lieberman, A.: Collaborative work, Educational Leadership 43(5):Feb., 1986.

Lieberman, E.J., editor: Mental Health: the public health challenge, Washington, D.C., 1975, American Public Health Association.

Loggins, D.: Values clarification revisited: clarifying what and how well, Health Education 7:March/April, 1976.

Middleton, K.: Back to some basics in health lesson planning, Health Education 12:4-8 Jan./Feb., 1981.

Perry, C.L.: A conceptual approach to school-based health promotion, Cooperative Edition, Health Education, 15(4), and The Journal of School Health 54(6):1984.

Raths, L.E., Harmin, M., and Simon, S.: Values and teaching: working with values in the classroom, Columbus, Ohio, 1966, Charles E. Merrill Publishing Co.

Roberts, H.C., et al.: Here's looking at you, 2000, Seattle, 1986, The Comprehensive Health Education Foundation.

School Health Education Study, Inc.: Health education: a conceptual approach, St. Paul, 1967, 3M Educational Press.

Sliepcevich, E.M.: Curriculum development: a macroscopic or microscopic view? The National Elementary Principal **48:**Nov., 1968.

Stenner, A.J., and Katzenmeyer, W.G.: Self-concept development in young people, Phi Delta Kappan **58:**Dec., 1976.

Trucano, L.: Students speak, Seattle, 1984, The Comprehensive Health Education Foundation.

Tyler, R.: Basic principles of curriculum and instruction, Chicago, 1969, University of Chicago Press.

Wang, M.C., Rubenstein, J.L., and Reynolds, M.C.: Clearing the road to success for students with special needs, Educational Leadership **43**(1):Sept., 1985.

PART V

METHODS AND MATERIALS IN HEALTH EDUCATION

CHAPTER 12

METHODS AND TECHNIQUES IN HEALTH TEACHING

Health cannot be given to people, it demands their participation.

RENE SAUD

KEY CONCEPT: Achievement of positive student health attitudes and practices is increased through the use of pupil-centered methods and techniques in health instruction.

Having discussed the learner and health education in Chapter 9 and having covered ways to organize for health teaching in Chapter 11, it is now necessary to look at the role of the teacher in changing behavior with specific reference to the learning process.

The teacher is the most important factor in the health education program. The responsibility for organizing, guiding, and directing the learning toward health objectives rests with the teacher. This is accomplished through a familiarity with a wide assortment of teaching activities and experiences. The selection of those methods and techniques that will most efficiently and effectively aid learning and lead to health-educated pupils is necessary. The variety of procedures used by teachers to achieve the practices, attitudes, and knowledge goals of healthful living are called methods or methods of teaching.

WHAT IS METHOD?

Method is a broad term in teaching referring to the organized and systematic ways used by teachers to achieve purposes or objectives. Method is often said to be the "how to" of teaching. *Technique* is a concrete word describing more specific ways to attain goals. Techniques may be called activities, experiences, or teaching/learning activities. In health education, these procedures help to interpret and translate scientific information to pupils.

The mere selection of appropriate activities or

experiences by the teacher does not ensure effective learning. These related factors must also receive consideration:

1. The maintenance of good pupil relationships provides an atmosphere conducive to learning. Understanding children's physical, emotional, social, and intellectual characteristics, treating pupils fairly and firmly, and using democratic procedures contribute to an appropriate social climate in the classroom.

2. Teachers must recognize and provide for differences in abilities, aptitudes, and achievements in pupils. For example, some students may need more help in learning how to floss and brush their teeth, whereas others may require special guidance to complete survey and research projects.

3. Methods may be teacher or pupil centered. Teacher-centered methods are those dominated by the teacher and are usually more formal in approach. They may include recitations, question-and-answer sessions, and lectures. Pupil-centered methods refer to the nondirective processes that allow for greater student participation. They may include demonstrations, excursions, constructive activities, and peer group involvement. Greater emphasis must be given to those activities involving pupils if health attitudes and behavior changes are to occur.

WHAT ARE THE TYPES OF METHODS?

Methods are difficult to categorize because the variations and combinations used by teachers are so numerous. In addition, their close relationship to instructional materials adds to the complexity of grouping. Nevertheless, the types listed here are classifications that have been found effective and useful in health instruction programs in elementary schools.

1. Problem solving
2. Construction activities
3. Creative activities
4. Demonstrations
5. Discussions
6. Dramatizations
7. Excursions and field trips
8. Experiments
9. Individual and group reports
10. Illustrated presentations
11. Resource people—guest speakers
12. Show and tell time
13. Surveys

Problem solving

Problem solving is a very important and practical method available for teacher use in the development of pupil health behaviors—in helping students make decisions. It is a general process whereby children learn to solve personal and community health problems through the use of the scientific approach. Pupils learn how to investigate, reason, and think reflectively so that they can differentiate facts from fiction and truth from superstition.

Several illustrations of health problems that may be solved are: How can we protect ourselves from disease? Who are some of the people who help us stay healthy? What foods do we need for growth? How can we prevent accidents? How can we deal with the pressure to use drugs and alcohol? (See Fig. 12-2.) What can be done to stop people from using tobacco products?

The sequential steps that teachers can use to guide pupils in solving health problems are as follows:

1. Recognition of the problem
2. Definition of the problem
3. Selection of methods of procedure
4. Collection of pertinent data
5. Selection, interpretation, and organization of data
6. Preparation of conclusions or alternatives
7. Application of conclusions or alternatives to the solution, problem, or plan of action
8. Evaluation of solution or solutions

Brainstorming, a type of problem solving. Brainstorming is a group attempt to solve a well-defined problem by offering any solution that comes to mind, no matter how extreme. It attempts to generate ideas quickly and in large quantity by the free association of ideas.

These procedures should be followed:

1. Encourage a free flow of ideas no matter how far out; permit free thinking
2. Do not permit critical judgments, negative comments, or evaluations
3. Restate the problem and start sorting out and refining ideas
4. Evaluate the ideas objectively and narrow them to one or more solutions
5. Summarize and assign responsibilities

These problems are illustrations of ones suitable for brainstorming. How can we encourage pupils to refrain from smoking cigarettes? How can we improve safety at school? How can we convince pupils to refrain from the use of drugs?

This procedure has value because it allows for freedom of expression, an exchange of ideas, and creative thinking. It has limitations in that the teacher may find it difficult to maintain class control, and it may not be productive if the class is too large. It also demands clarification of ideas, well-planned organization, and follow-up for effective results.

Values clarification, a type of problem solving. Values clarification involves a series of strategies or methods for helping students learn about values. It does not attempt to teach values per se.

Values clarification will help students review their own as well as society's values. It will help pupils identify the concept of self and search for meaning in life.

Construction activities

Construction activities involve pupil and teacher planning as well as pupil participation in the preparation of a variety of items (using paper, wood, cardboard, glue, crayons, and other materials). Illustrations of specific items that may be made include a fire alarm box; a traffic light standard with stop and go signals; papier-mâché models of fruits and vegetables;

plaster-of-paris models of teeth, the heart, and other organs of the body; and construction of paper models. These items have use in dramatic play, exhibits, bulletin board displays (see Fig. 12-5), and other techniques of teaching.

Creative activities

The free expression of children's thoughts, ideas, and feelings through such media as stories, poems and verses, dramatic plays, murals, and other creative activities may be useful and productive in the health instruction program. (See Teaching Techniques, pp. 251 to 329 for illustrations.)

Construction and creative activities offer the additional advantage of providing meaningful learning opportunities for those students who tend to learn more efficiently by manipulation of objects and creative thought processes. This important fact has gained considerable attention through recent research on how people learn, and it holds great promise in the teaching of thinking skills. Good teachers have long known that creative and constructive activities work and have applied this knowledge to health activities, as well as other subjects.

Demonstrations

Demonstrations are methods that help make abstract verbal descriptions and symbols more concrete and meaningful in health education. They may include involvement of the visual, tactile, and auditory senses (Fig. 12-1). They are helpful ways to improve the teaching process and may be performed by teachers or pupils.

Five important reasons for the use of demonstrations in teaching are the following:

1. They stimulate interest and thereby motivate learning
2. They help clarify learnings
3. They help improve and speed up the learning process
4. They may be used to initiate a unit

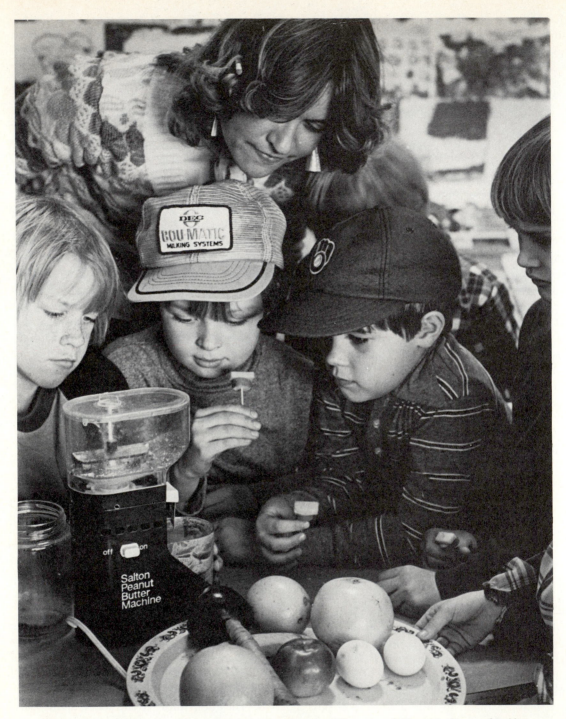

FIG. 12-1. Tasting Party—making peanut butter. *(Courtesy of Wisconsin Dept. of Public Instruction, Madison, Wis.)*

5. They provide a visual image helpful in the retention of things learned

Some demonstrations usable in health education are (1) the importance of oxygen in fires; (2) the proper way to brush teeth; (3) the safest way to ride a bicycle on sidewalks, streets, and highways; and (4) the proper use of fire extinguishers.

Discussions

The discussion as a method of teaching is probably the most familiar and commonly used procedure in health instruction. All activities and methods include or should include some type of discussion. These methods generally permit children to ask questions, make recitations, perform surveys, and participate in numerous other ways in the learning process. They provide opportunities for the exchange of information between pupils and teachers. Group discussion is especially valuable since it is conducive to helping children gain understanding and respect for each other's feelings and viewpoints.

Discussions need teacher guidance, and the following points should aid in directing the conversation along constructive channels:

1. Encourage and stimulate pupil questions since they provide information about needs, interests, and concerns. Pupils should be helped to think through their own experiences and relate them to the discussion.

2. Try to get all children in the class to participate or be involved.

3. Do not hurry the discussion.

4. Listen carefully to all contributions and relate them to the topic. Compliment and encourage children who make remarks. It may be necessary to have students amplify their statements.

5. When groups are reluctant to engage in discussions, mention of a personal experience or anecdote may help get children to participate.

Discussions may take place in a variety of ways, and the suggestions that follow merely serve to illustrate the numerous variations and formats that may be used in the health instruction program.

Questions and answers. Questions may serve not only to introduce a health area, they may also be part of the teaching process used during the presentation of a unit or lesson, and they may serve as a review or summary of a class discussion.

The best results are obtained when careful thought, planning, and organization are given to building sets of questions. As a general rule, question-and-answer periods and sessions should be planned in detail and in advance as carefully as other teaching procedures.

QUESTION BOX. Occasionally, children are reluctant to ask questions in class because they fear embarrassment or for other reasons. This situation can be solved by having a receptacle of some kind available where pupils may anonymously place questions of interest or concern. This procedure may be especially appropriate when the topic of sex education or social hygiene is being considered in class.

QUIZZES. Quizzes can be oral, written, or performance based. They have value when used for drill, review, or grading purposes. They serve to motivate learning and are important in the instruction program. They have evaluation limitations since they tend to measure only the cognitive learning (understandings) acquired by pupils.

SELF-TESTS. Self-tests are a series of teacher-prepared, easily answered questions that help stimulate discussion about a particular health topic. The number and difficulty of questions can vary depending on the purpose of the test and the grade level in which it is used.

These tests are not given for grading purposes. They have value because they can be duplicated and distributed at the start of the class and immediately get all pupils participating and thinking about the lesson. They may also be used to initiate a unit as well as to help determine additional class activities.

The following is an illustration of a partial self-test:

What do you know about tobacco?

Please circle the correct answer to the statements that are listed below. If you do not know the answer, circle the letter "D."

1. The drug in tobacco is caffeine   T   F   D
2. Smoking has been linked to lung cancer   T   F   D
3. The use of tobacco increases the heart rate   T   F   D
4. Smokeless tobacco has no bad health effects   T   F   D
5. Smoking cigarettes irritates linings in the body   T   F   D
6. Smoking has no link to heart disease   T   F   D
7. Nicotine is a drug that slows the body down   T   F   D
8. Blood pressure goes down when a person smokes   T   F   D

Experience charts and records. Experience charts and records are lists of phrases or brief stories that are dictated by children to the teacher who records their suggestions, ideas, or thoughts on the blackboard or on large sheets of paper. This procedure has been used in the primary grades to introduce reading, but it also serves as a good technique when teaching health education. It is usable at other grade levels as a way to list or record questions that need to be answered about a particular health topic. It may be considered part of the problem-solving technique in teaching.

Buzz groups. The buzz group method is one in which the class is divided into groups of from five to eight pupils to discuss a specific problem or series of problems for a limited time, usually 3 to 5 minutes. Each subgroup selects a chairperson to keep the discussion on the topic and give everyone an opportunity to speak. A recorder is chosen who not only will jot down key points but will also be prepared to present these orally to the entire class on request. The teacher's role during the buzzing is to move from group to group to be certain that the topic is being discussed, see that students know what is expected of them, and clarify questions relating to the problem under discussion. At the conclu-

sion of the buzzing the teacher permits the spokespersons to report their answers, and a pupil summarizes the main points on the blackboard. Further discussion is encouraged by the class members during the summary period.

This technique has a number of important advantages for use in the health instruction program:

1. It provides a way to have several committees in class study different aspects of a given topic
2. It allows greater pupil participation in the discussion
3. It provides an atmosphere conducive to discussion
4. It may serve as a diagnostic procedure to find out what pupils know about a particular topic
5. It may lead to further pupil activities or experiences

Buzz groups may be used to (1) discuss a particular problem or question, (2) determine what action to take regarding a particular problem or question, and (3) determine questions to ask a resource person who may be coming to class the following day.

This procedure has limitations, especially if pupils have no background information about the discussion topic; it may result in a rehash of ignorance. Also, a buzz group takes careful planning for the optimal results, for the prevention of a few students dominating the conversation, and for confining of the comments to the topic being discussed. Selection of a subject about which students have controversial and varying opinions increases the chances of success for this method.

Problem solving—answers to questions. Problem solving is a teaching technique whereby children are presented with specific health questions or situations and they attempt to provide solutions through class discussions. For example, a teacher may present the following situations for pupil reactions:

1. What would you do if you were injured at school?
2. What would you do if you were injured a long way from home?

3. What would you do if a friend tried to persuade you to smoke a cigarette?

A modification of this procedure would be to present a problem in written form, such as the following:

You were playing in the school yard at lunchtime and cut your leg on a sharp object. The wound was bleeding quite a bit, and you were in pain. Place a check in the box beside the statement below that would best describe what you would do. Be prepared to tell why you would take this action.
1. Take out my handkerchief and wrap it around the cut ☐
2. Wash the cut with water ☐
3. Press my hand on the cut to try to stop the bleeding ☐
4. Report to the nurse or to my teacher ☐
5. Wait until I arrived at home before doing anything ☐
6. Not do anything ☐
7. Go home ☐

Critical review of quotations found in the literature and analysis of newspaper articles, lyrics from popular songs, scenes from movies, and value strategies are additional problem-solving possibilities.

Dramatizations

Dramatizations are ways for children to express their feelings and urges through make-believe, imitation, and imagination. It is believed that children are more likely to remember facts when they are portraying them. These procedures are interesting to children and apparently contribute to the development of health attitudes and values since pupils tend to identify themselves with characters in the situations.

Dramatic play. Dramatic play is an informal, spontaneous, natural way for children to act out what they have been reading, discussing, or seeing in health.

Children who have visited a fire station or read about one may construct an imaginary station in the classroom and play fire fighter. A visit to a grocery store may result in such a store being established in school. The presence of the school doctor may encourage children to establish a corner in the room as a physician's office.

Role playing. Role playing is a more formalized procedure than dramatic play. The teacher determines the focus and assigns the roles. It is spontaneous and unrehearsed and focuses on a health problem of interest or concern. It provides a considerable amount of emotionalism and realism that apparently communicates to individuals.

The steps to follow in conducting role playing generally include the following:
1. Selection of a problem of interest and importance to children
2. Explanation of the technique in simple terms
3. Provision of enough of the story to set the scene
4. Selection of children to participate
5. Definition of the problem and role of each pupil
6. Definition of the audience role
7. Provision of cues to begin or opening remarks needed by first actors to get started
8. Cessation of role playing at the point where action drops or when discussion should be started (may be after a 2- or 3-minute presentation)
9. Conduction of discussion afterward, asking such questions as: "What was being presented?" "What was good about the way the situation was handled?" "What might have been changed in the situation?"

Illustrations or dramatizations suitable in health education include (1) walking across the street, (2) riding a bicycle on the street, (3) helping a person who is lost, (4) showing how a person behaves when teased by someone, and (5) describing how to say "no" without losing friends (Fig. 12-2).

Plays. Plays are more formal because they have a prepared script and involve memorization of dialogue. They may or may not be pupil written. They can serve as culminating activities with presentations made to parent groups or school assemblies.

FIG. 12-2. Problem solving—learning to say "no" to drugs. *(Courtesy of Jay Schupack, Seattle, Wash.)*

Puppet shows. When children are involved in making the puppets and planning the stories for puppet shows, the result on health behaviors can be beneficial. These experiences are enjoyed by young children both as spectators and as participants. They have great attitudinal effects on pupils. Puppets may also be used in dramatic play or with spontaneous dialogue.

Many areas including mental health, nutrition, and safety provide suitable materials for these shows.

Stories and storytelling. Children enjoy stories and storytelling* to the extent that various health topics can serve as themes. They can be used to initiate a unit in health, or they may be part of the ongoing activities. They help stimulate questions and answers.

Some illustrations of how this procedure may be used are (1) read stories about fear, courage, honesty, truthfulness, and other phases of mental health; (2) read stories about fire and traffic safety; (3) prepare a puppet or a construction

_____
*See Appendix E for specific story references.

paper character having some such name as Bozo the dog, Chippy the chipmunk, or Ronny the raccoon and create a story in which this animal discusses mental health or nutrition; (4) prepare a flip chart with a series of humorous or otherwise interesting drawings that relate to how to take care of the eyes, ears, or feet; and (5) show pictures of toothbrushes, wash cloths, combs, and other such items and encourage pupil discussions relative to the importance of these items to health.

Excursions and field trips

Excursions are designed to enrich classroom teaching procedures by making health more meaningful. Field trips may be limited to the school plant and the school neighborhood, or they may be distant journeys requiring bus transportation.

Some places to visit that may be part of the health instruction program are the school lunchroom, the school grounds, a grocery store, the corner crosswalk, the first-aid station, a dairy, a

FIG. 12–3. Teacher helps students study cancer-risk reduction. *(Courtesy of Jay Schupack, Seattle, Wash.)*

hospital, a dentist's office, and the health department.

Experiments

Experiments are procedures that use the scientific method to test suggested truths or to illustrate known truths (Fig. 12-3). They are ways to solve problems and may also be classified as demonstrations. They differ from demonstrations because the techniques employed are more exacting and precise, and controls are used to ensure valid results. The specific sequential steps may include the following:

1. Define the problem to be solved or the hypothesis to be tested
2. Select the methods of procedure to be used
3. Identify and assemble the necessary materials
4. Conduct the experiment
5. Collect and record data
6. Select, organize, and interpret the data
7. Prepare conclusions

Experiments stimulate interest and attention in learning. They provide realism to abstract concepts and make learning more meaningful.

Following are illustrations of experiments that have been helpful in the health instruction program:

1. The effect of good and poor diets on growth development may be shown by the white rat feeding experiment, details of which are available from the National Dairy Council.* This demonstration may be done with kindergarten or first-grade children to encourage the drinking of milk and discourage the consumption of excessive sweets.

2. The importance of washing hands with soap may be demonstrated through the use of a series of sterile agar plates (petri dishes from science department). Children touch one dish

---

*National Dairy Council, 111 N. Canal St., Chicago, Ill. 60606.

with fingers before washing with soap and water and a second dish after washing. The dishes are then incubated or kept in a warm place for 24 hours or longer, and the extent of germ growth can be compared in the two dishes.

Individual and group reports

Individual and group reports are methods whereby oral or written reports, or both, are made about assigned or special interest health topics by individual pupils or groups of pupils. They involve critical reading and analyses, research, independent study, interviews, investigations, and excursions or field trips. Questions and answers become necessary since they may precede, be part of, or follow the reports. They may include panel and forum presentations and independent study.

Illustrated presentations

Illustrated presentations are activities whereby teachers present phases of health using audiovisual materials such as charts, models, pictures, and specimens. Children should be encouraged to participate in discussions and ask questions.

An example of this procedure would be the use of food models on a flannelboard to illustrate the basic four food groups or appropriate breakfasts, lunches, and dinners.

Chalk could be used effectively to make cartoons, sketches, and schematic drawings of germs, body parts, foods, maps, illustrated slogans (such as "Germs hate soap"), charts, and a variety of other valuable and useful visuals presentations.

Resource people—guest speakers

The use of community resource people who are experts in their chosen fields often enriches the health instruction program. Such individuals may include physicians, dentists, health officers, police officers, fire fighters, and nurses.

The following points should be discussed with resource people or guest speakers who are invited to schools:

1. The choice of a topic appropriate to that being covered in class
2. The grade level of the class
3. The material covered in class before and what will happen after the speaker departs
4. The nature of the vocabulary to use
5. The use of audiovisual aids whenever possible
6. The use of demonstrations, experiments, and illustrations whenever possible
7. Permission for children to ask questions; pupils should prepare their questions in advance

Peer group and cross-age teaching. This is a method whereby students prepare materials for use or are able to discuss one or more health topics with their peers in formal and informal educational settings. By way of illustration, these procedures may include preparing audiovisual materials for presentation, conducting rap sessions, participating in and leading a variety of discussions, and writing and producing newspaper articles and special bulletin materials for distribution.

Some lessons are readily adaptable to cross-age teaching. The teacher may find it a rewarding change of pace, as well as an opportunity to get a different perspective, by bringing in an older student to help teach some health lessons (Fig. 12-4). Older students who have successfully recovered from operations, who are drug free, or who have other health-related experiences can share their experiences with great influence. A senior high or junior high class can stage a health-related play for younger children. Refusal skills, making friends, and staying out of trouble are topics that lend themselves well to cross-age teaching. This idea is worthy of consideration in the upper grades and possibly also in the intermediate grades.

Show and tell time

Show and tell is an appropriate time to discuss health matters as well as other topics. This ac-

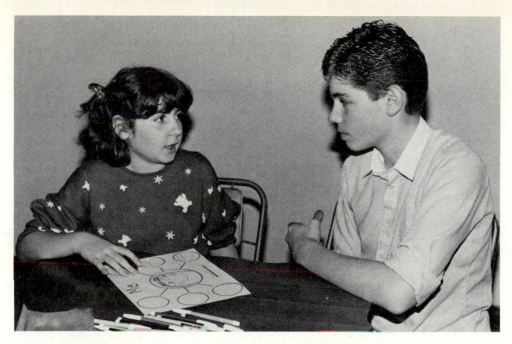

FIG. 12–4. Cross-age teaching. *(Courtesy of Jay Schupack, Seattle, Wash.)*

tivity is especially useful in the primary grades for children to tell about visits to dentists or physicians, accidents at home, or fires that happened in the community. Some children with parents who are physicians, dentists, fire fighters, police officers, or health officers may have special health items, such as stethoscopes, teeth, models, charts, books, and pamphlets, that they will bring to school and share with their classmates.

Surveys

Surveys are procedures in which students use checklists, interviews, questionnaires, and opinionnaires to collect information about the nature and extent of pupil or community health problems or practices. They may be considered part of the problem-solving process.

The survey provides excellent opportunities to integrate health with language, art, and mathematics. The survey forms will need to be prepared by pupils, and oral and written reports and research may also be necessary. In addition, mathematic tabulations and computations must be completed.

Some areas in health that lend themselves to surveys are (1) the types and amounts of snack-time foods consumed by pupils; (2) the amount of candy and soda consumed daily, or weekly, by children; (3) the kinds of foods eaten for breakfast, lunch, and dinner by children; (4) the extent to which students smoke cigarettes or use drugs; and (5) the safety hazards in the school or home.

Others

There are many variations of the methods of teaching described in this chapter that can be used in health education. Teacher ingenuity and creativity are necessary to develop the variety of other possible techniques. Communication media including television, radio, tape recordings, films, filmstrips, videotapes, and slides, as well as models, charts, exhibits, displays, bul-

FIG. 12-5. Bulletin board display of attractive posters purchased or pupil prepared.

letin boards (Fig. 12-5), posters, flannelboards, and other audiovisual aids may be combined with the procedures just presented to provide numerous additional activities and experiences. Chapter 13 contains details on the use of these teaching aids in the school health program.

WHAT METHODS SHOULD TEACHERS USE?

There is no one best method or combination of methods to use in the health instruction program. If any procedure is to be singled out as a basis from which to start selecting, perhaps the problem-solving approach must be given first consideration. This is a meaningful and scientific way to teach health education, it involves other activities, and it is behavior centered, as well as pupil centered.

The process of developing health-educated individuals is complex and difficult. The techniques teachers employ should help pupils understand the concepts needed to acquire the practices, attitudes, and knowledge for healthful living. It is important therefore that teachers be familiar with the nature, values, and limitations of many methods so that they may choose those that will aid pupils to achieve their objectives.

Teachers should review the following questions and use them as criteria when selecting procedures for the health instruction program:
1. Will the objectives be achieved?
2. Will they have educational value?
3. Will pupils participate actively?
4. Will their interest be attracted and maintained?
5. Will information be communicated to pupils?
6. Will the teacher feel comfortable using the procedures?
7. Will the methods be appropriate for the abilities and aptitudes of pupils?
8. Will the methods be suitable for the grade level?
9. Will the methods be adaptable to the supplies, equipment, and facilities that are readily available?

Kindergarten and primary grades

The health education program in kindergarten and the primary grades should be centered around daily activities in school, the home, and the community, such as safety, disease control, nutrition, rest and sleep, the doctor, the police officer, the fire fighter, and the nurse.

Health can be integrated easily into other areas of the curriculum, such as language arts (Fig. 12-6), social studies, and science; however, there will always be the need for direct teaching.

The methods selected for these grades should be those that include doing, experiencing, and observing. The techniques that will achieve the best results will probably include reading, stories, games, problem solving, excursions, discussions, show and tell periods, creative activities, construction activities, questions and answers, experience charts and records, and dramatizations.

Intermediate grades

Children in intermediate grades have acquired a new level of curiosity and enthusiasm. They begin asking more questions and want to know the "why's" of health. They are seeking more exact answers to their questions.

The growth changes occurring in pupils provide the need for learning about the structure and functions of the human organism. Girls particularly need information about menstrual hygiene.

The beginning of group activities and the wider use of community resources and problem-solving procedures become possible and should be considered for use by teachers in their health instruction programs.

Health continues to be integrated to some extent with other subjects, but more direct teaching is necessary.

The methods that teachers may use in their programs include discussions, problem solving, educational games, surveys, excursions, illustrated lectures, role playing, experiments, demonstrations, resource people, and individual and group reports.

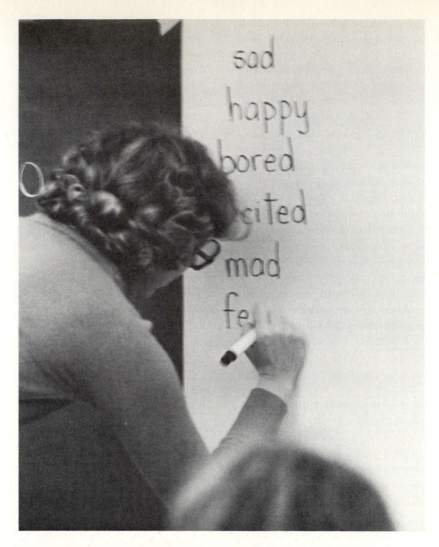

FIG. 12–6. Integration of mental health into language arts. *(Courtesy Mary Wilbert Smith, Educational Service District #121, Seattle, Wash.)*

Upper grades

Children in the upper grades are adventuresome, want to experiment, and desire more activity than ever before in their lives. Therefore the health experiences must go far beyond the confines of the textbook. Pupils can be involved in cooperative planning and sharing of experiences (Fig. 12-7).

The early adolescent period indicates the need for additional content areas to be included in the health instruction program. Tobacco, alcohol, and the use of drugs begin to have added meaning for these children, although these areas should receive consideration in the lower grades. In addition, exercise takes on importance, with dental and nutritional problems and sexually transmitted disease having special significance.

FIG. 12-7. Dissecting—examining an animal heart.

Some of the methods that may be included in the health instruction program are surveys, panels, debates, excursions, peer group action, exhibits, tape recordings, independent and group work, demonstrations, experiments, buzz groups, and problem solving.

ARE INCIDENTS METHODS?

Incidents by themselves are not methods. However, they are teachable moments that stimulate learning by setting the stage for meaningful health education. They can serve to initiate units or lessons. They may be considered as health problems that lend themselves to solutions through the use of the problem-solving process and other procedures. They lend themselves to both formal and informal educational approaches. Therefore they may be considered a part of method.

Teachers must be constantly alert for the numerous occasions that happen in schools, homes, and communities and that are usable in health instruction programs. The newspapers, magazines, and TV are sources of these incidents, as are student and adult reports. Teachers who consistently capitalize on these motivating events will undoubtedly be more successful in getting children to acquire the appropriate health behaviors.

The teacher must recognize that there are values as well as limitations in the use of incidents in health teaching. When they are improperly used, they may result in serious emotional disturbances among children. A teacher who discusses the cleanliness habits or the decayed teeth of a particular pupil in class not only may embarrass the child but also may make the child unnecessarily conspicuous before the other students. From a psychological viewpoint, therefore, this action may be harmful to the child. The teacher must use discretion in choosing incidents, as well as the appropriate occasion for capitalizing on such situations. Incidents in health teaching may be used in several ways:

1. To discuss individual health problems with pupils in private or with parents.

2. To discuss health and safety problems that have been observed in school or elsewhere without reference to any special pupil or groups of pupils.

3. To discuss special events or occasions involving health and safety that will take place in the school or community.

4. To discuss a particular pupil health problem when the child is not in the room. This is probably the rare occasion but may be necessary for the protection of the child. For example, if a child has had an epileptic seizure in class, it will be necessary for the teacher to seek the support of the child's classmates to help the pupil when necessary. This attack could occur on the playground or on the way home when the teacher or other adult is not nearby. Therefore a brief explanation of the nature of seizures and first-aid procedures is important. This action may help to prevent the pupil from being injured and being rejected by the other classmates.

The following incidents that occur in the school setting illustrate opportunities available for health instruction:

1. Students using tobacco products in school
2. Many children absent because of the flu
3. Pupils come to school with colds
4. Children prepare refreshments for a party at school
5. A student tells how a friend's hand was burned while playing with matches
6. The school conducts a fire drill
7. A child reports a visit to the dentist
8. Pupils make fun of children wearing eyeglasses or hearing aids
9. The food served for lunch at school
10. Children have their vision and/or hearing screened at school
11. A student asks about dental health or nutrition claims in TV commercials
12. A child is bitten by a dog on the playground
13. A student has an epileptic seizure in class
14. An accident occurs to a student on the way to or at school
15. Students eating candy and sweets in excess

A third-grade teacher who took advantage of a report in the newspaper of a bicycle accident that occurred to a school child and resulted in a broken arm will serve to illustrate how to use an incident in the instruction program. The morning after the accident the teacher asked the class how it happened. Discussion brought out such matters as careless riders, unsafe conditions, and unsafe equipment. The conversation led the pupils to list the actions that often lead to accidents: bicycle riding, car driving, walking, behavior in school, and behavior at home. The teacher then asked the question: "If these may lead to accidents, how can we act safely?" The pupils began to mention safety rules but finally decided they needed more information to be able to answer this question satisfactorily. At this point the teacher suggested that continued planning go on the next day.

When the discussion resumed the following day, the children decided to participate in a variety of experiences to learn more about safety. These are some of the activities that they selected:

1. Read stories in safety books and pamphlets
2. Create bulletin board displays of safety posters
3. Create a checklist of "Ways to make my home safe"
4. Invite a police officer to visit the class to discuss safety
5. Conduct a culminating activity that dramatizes a typical day of children who do not practice safety and a typical day of children who do

Special community and school events are also important occasions to motivate for health education in schools. The Monthly Health Specials Calendar approach that follows offers useful suggestions.

MONTHLY HEALTH SPECIALS

September
National Rehabilitation Month
National Sickle Cell Month
National Sight-Saving Month
Grandparents Day
Cystic Fibrosis Week
National Farm Safety Week
National Rehabilitation Week
Citizenship Day

October
National Family Sexuality Month
National Spinal Health Month
National Sudden Infant Death Syndrome Awareness Month
Spina Bifida Month
Child Health Day
National Community Health Center Week
Fire Prevention Week
National Running and Fitness Day
National Handicap Awareness Week
World Food Day
National Lupus Awareness Week

November
National Alzheimer's Disease Month
National Diabetes Month
National Epilepsy Month
Great American Smokeout

December
National Home Care Week
National Autism Week

January
March of Dimes Birth Defects Prevention Month
National Volunteer Blood Donor Month

February
American Heart Month
National Children's Dental Health Month
National Child Passenger Safety Awareness Week
National Cardiopulmonary Week

March
National Nutrition Month
Hemophilia Month
Mental Retardation Month
National Kidney Month
Red Cross Month
Save Your Vision Week
National Poison Prevention Week
Children and Hospitals Week

April
Cancer Control Month
Health Fair Month
National Child Abuse Prevention Month
World Health Day
Bike Safety Week
Save the Children Week

May
Better Hearing and Speech Month
Correct Posture Month
Foot Health Month
National Arthritis Month
National Mental Health Month
Older Americans Month
National High Blood Pressure Month
National Physical Fitness and Sports Month
National Nurses Day
National Digestive Disease Awareness Week
Mother's Day
Memorial Day

June
National Safe Boating Week
National Physical Therapy Week
Father's Day

Other seasonal events offer opportunities for health education: (1) when children return to school in September may be the appropriate time to discuss safety to and from school, bicycle safety, and playground safety; (2) fall and winter may be significant times to discuss respiratory diseases and other communicable diseases; and (3) spring may be the time when camping, picnic, and water safety become important.

IS THE USE OF THE HEALTH TEXTBOOK A METHOD?

The health textbook is an important teaching aid that should serve as a reference or resource to provide information necessary to solve health problems. It should be used in conjunction with pupil activities and experiences and therefore may be considered a part of or related to method. It may be used in the preparation for discussions, panels, individual and group work, and so on. It can help provide continuity and direction to learning experiences.

A textbook, however, should not be used as a passive reading lesson. Children will not acquire the necessary health behaviors if their experiences are limited to a 10- or 15-minute daily reading assignment in a health text. This procedure is contrary to the principles of learning discussed in Chapter 9. Teachers must be more imaginative and creative and use a variety of the methods and activities described in this chapter if the goals of health education are to be achieved. Additional information on textbooks is found in Chapter 13 and Appendix E.

WHAT ARE THE RELATIONSHIPS BETWEEN METHOD AND MATERIAL AIDS?

Material or teaching aids, such as models of the teeth, health films and filmstrips, flannelboards, exhibits, or displays of the contents of first-aid kits, are valuable supplementary items that enrich learning experiences. They are aids to learning that make abstract health concepts specific, concrete, and meaningful in the lives of students; they serve to attract and maintain attention; they help to stimulate interest in the teaching process; and they assist in encouraging greater student participation in the learning process. Teachers should be familiar with the variety of such items that are available and use many of them in their teaching. Chapter 13 provides comprehensive coverage of the nature of these aids.

Instructional aids should not be considered teaching methods in themselves. However, they are important supplementary and complementary aspects of the procedures used in learning. They are part of the "how to" methods of teaching.

At times it is difficult to distinguish between methods and teaching aids. An example or two best illustrates this point. A film by itself is a teaching aid. When children are expected to look for specific information as they view the film and, after its showing, discuss what they saw, then it becomes part of the teaching process. Therefore discussion may be the method

used in the learning, with the film being a part of this procedure. A flannelboard and food models are teaching aids. When these items are used in a discussion to demonstrate the food items needed for an adequate breakfast, they become a method.

Using a variety of teaching aids can greatly contribute to the emphasis on pupil-centered teaching. They will assist in providing more pupil participation in the learning process.

WHAT TEACHING TECHNIQUES ARE USABLE IN HEALTH INSTRUCTION?

The wide variety of specific teaching techniques* that are presented next will aid the teacher in the achievement of the objectives in health education. They include more than 1,200 ideas for use in the instructional program. They are organized alphabetically into 15 subject areas, and the appropriate grade level group for each activity is identified.

When the procedures for health teaching are selected, it will be helpful to keep in mind these essentials:

1. The purposes of health education go beyond an emphasis on information alone; they also consider the development of health attitudes and practices.

2. The principles of learning described in Chapter 9 are important.

3. The specific technique or combination of techniques to be used should help achieve a desired goal or goals.

4. Activities should be continually evaluated to determine the extent of learning taking place.

Despite the many types of activities presented, the procedures that follow do not provide a comprehensive coverage of all health teaching experiences, nor do they include the use of films and filmstrips. Rather they serve a fourfold purpose:

---

*An excellent culminating activity that involves much student, parent, and community participation is a *health fair*. The references at the end of this chapter related to health fairs are worthy of review.

1. To provide specific, tested techniques that will give spark and vitality to the health instruction program (the numerous experiences listed have been used by many teachers in their classrooms)
2. To provide a broad selection of activities
3. To provide suggestions of teaching techniques that will stimulate the creative and imaginative teacher to modify, change, or devise completely new procedures
4. To provide methods that may be used to initiate new units or as culminating activities

It should be noted that the following teaching procedures have been organized in a functional and practical manner for easy reference by the teacher. The letters or numbers found on the right of the page in the activities or experiences that follow refer to the *suggested* grades or grade level in which they may be used: P, primary; I, intermediate; U, upper.

ALCOHOL

			Grades
Bulletin board	1	Illustrated display of accidents and other losses attributed to alcohol.	U
	2	Illustrated display of the alcohol content of the various kinds of beverages.	U
Buzz group	3	Conduct a buzz session on the questions "What should be the punishment for driving while intoxicated?" "Why do people drink alcoholic beverages?"	U
Chart	4	Prepare a chart or poster that shows the effects of alcohol on the body and the level of alcohol in the blood after beverages with alcohol are consumed.	U
Demonstration	5	Place a small (3-inch) goldfish in a solution of ½ ounce of alcohol in ¾ pint of water (the amount in a 12-ounce bottle of beer). In almost 20 minutes the fish will be "under the influence" (floating to the surface). When the effect of the alcohol can be seen, remove the fish and place it in fresh water to be revived.	I, U
Discussion	6	The physiological, psychological, and sociological effects of alcohol on the human body.	U
	7	The nutritional elements of a glass of milk, an ounce of whiskey, and a bottle of beer.	U
	8	The nature of the alcohol content in beer, wine, and whiskey.	U
	9	Collect ads from newspapers and magazines on alcoholic beverages and analyze them in class.	U
	10	Safe and unsafe use of alcohol.	U
	11	Predisposing factors to alcoholism.	U
	12	Effects on families of individuals with alcohol problems.	U
Dramatization	13	High school drama class depicts scenes of pressures put on sixth-, seventh-, and eighth-grade students to drink alcoholic beverages. Follow with discussion of junior high school pupils' suggestions for handling such situations.	U
Exhibit	14	Display whiskey, wine, and beer glasses and discuss the amount of alcohol contained in each beverage and in each glass.	U
	15	Display a variety of magazines, pamphlets, and other materials for students to read, do research, and prepare oral and written reports on alcohol.	U

ALCOHOL—cont'd

		Grades
Exhibit— cont'd	16 Pupils display labels taken from medicine bottles and other containers and prepare a list of the amount of alcohol found in these substances.	U
Graph	17 Compare the amount of money spent nationally on alcohol and the amount spent on education, cancer, tuberculosis, and other health projects.	U
Guest speaker	18 Invite a member of Alcoholics Anonymous to discuss the services rendered by this organization to help alcoholics.	U
	19 Invite a physician to discuss the physiological effects of alcohol on the human body.	U
Individual and group reports	20 Pupil committees write letters to organizations having materials on alcohol and request copies for use in class.	I, U
	21 Pupils prepare oral and written reports on recent magazine articles about alcohol.	I, U
	22 Pupils prepare oral and written reports on the effects of alcohol on a person participating in sports, driving an automobile, flying an airplane, typing, and using industrial skills.	U
	23 Pupils prepare individual and group reports on such topics as the preserving quality of alcohol, alcohol as a fuel, alcohol in medicine, and alcohol as a disinfectant.	U
Interview	24 Interview a member of the sheriff's office or police department to find out the effect of alcohol on the crime rate and the accident rate in the community.	U
	25 A pupil committee interviews a physician and the health officer on the benefits and adverse features of the use of alcohol.	U
Panel	26 Have a panel discussion on the topic: "Why people drink alcoholic beverages."	U
Problem solving	27 Pupils do research and prepare oral and written reports about a series of problems such as: "Why do people drink? Why do some people pressure others to drink? What effect does alcohol have on the body? What effect does alcohol have on the mind? Is alcohol a food? What are the uses of alcohol?" These may also serve as introductory questions to stimulate student discussion to determine ways to find solutions.	U
Reports	28 Pupils prepare reports on Alateen and Alanon programs; relationships of alcoholism and nutritional problems; state laws; community resources to treat alcoholism; and alcohol and its use in religious ceremonies.	U
Resource persons	29 Have police officer talk about alcohol intoxication tests.	U
Role playing	30 Saying no when offered an alcoholic beverage.	U
	31 Pressures of peer groups to consume alcoholic beverages.	U
Scrapbook	32 Pupils make scrapbooks to include pictures, magazine and newspaper articles, stories, and other items about the use and effect of alcohol.	U
Self-test	33 Pupils complete a self-test and conduct a discussion afterward.	U
Survey	34 Conduct a survey among pupils to find out their views on alcohol use.	U
Tape recording	35 Have students interview a recovering alcoholic about attitudes toward use of alcoholic beverages.	U

COMMUNITY HEALTH

			Grades
Bulletin board	1	Display illustrated drawing or pictures of the functions of various community health agencies.	I, U
	2	Show the life cycle of the mosquito or the fly.	I, U
Chart	3	Make illustrated charts and posters about community health helpers.	P
	4	List ways the children can help promote good health in the community.	P, I
	5	Make a chart listing the professional, official, and voluntary health agencies in the community.	I, U
Checklist	6	Prepare a checklist for use in rating the school health environment and the community health environment.	U
Construction	7	Make a bear's head out of papier-mâché and a large ice cream carton; have the mouth open for paper deposits—"Litter Bear."	P, I
Demonstration	8	The correct way to use the drinking fountain.	P, I
	9	How water may be purified by filtration as illustrated in Fig. 12-8.	I, U
	10	Have pupils examine some swamp water under a microscope and a second sample of this same water after it has been treated with chlorine.	U
	11	Show how a small amount of oil on water forms a thin layer that causes mosquito larvae to die because they cannot penetrate the film to breathe. Obtain swamp or other stagnant water containing mosquito larvae for this demonstration.	U
Diorama	12	Prepare a diorama showing the locations of the agencies and the helpers involved in community health.	P
Discussion	13	Discuss and illustrate with pictures and stick-figure drawings the various kinds of community helpers who take care of our health, such as the fire fighter, the police officer, the doctor, the nurse, and the dentist.	P
	14	Collect pictures of ponds, lakes, rivers, and reservoirs and ask the class whether they think it is safe to drink water out of or swim in these places.	P, I

FIG. 12-8

COMMUNITY HEALTH—cont'd

			Grades
Discussion— cont'd	15	The proper use and maintenance of drinking fountains and lavatories.	P, I
	16	The maintenance of a healthful school environment including cleanliness, lighting, heating, and ventilation.	P, I
	17	The danger of petting strange animals and the procedures to follow if bitten by one.	P, I
	18	The importance of sanitation including the disposal of lunch papers and refuse in the school and classroom.	P, I, U
	19	The community rules and regulations concerning garbage and rubbish disposal.	I, U
	20	The relationship of water supply to the sewage disposal systems in schools, homes, and rural areas.	I, U
	21	The importance of restaurant sanitation.	I, U
	22	The responsibilities of individuals to keep public places clean, such as picnic grounds, parks, campgrounds, and lavatories.	I, U
	23	The effects of water pollution and how local health laws protect against pollution.	I, U
	24	The need for periodic health examinations.	I, U
	25	The use of chemical sprays and dusts in agriculture and the possible dangers involved.	I, U
	26	Ways used by the city to remove and dispose of garbage and trash.	I, U
	27	The sanitary procedures necessary for swimming pools.	I, U
Dramatization	28	Prepare and present a play to a parent group on the work of the health department.	I, U
	29	Prepare and present a play to a school assembly that will dramatize community health problems with possible solutions.	I, U
Drawing	30	Make drawings showing the sanitary procedures used in the school cafeteria.	I
Excursion	31	Take an excursion to the lavatories in the school and discuss use and maintenance.	P
	32	Visit a grocery store or food market to observe how perishable foods are stored and how cleanliness is practiced.	P
	33	Take a trip to a dairy to observe the sanitary procedures used in the handling of milk.	I, U
	34	Visit a water purification plant, a sewage disposal plant, or a health department.	I, U
	35	Visit food markets, restaurants, and other establishments to observe sanitary ways of handling and dispensing food.	I, U
	36	Visit a local hospital.	I, U
Exhibit	37	Display larvae, eggs, pupae, and adult mosquitoes and flies to observe development.	I, U
	38	Display pamphlets, books, and other reading material relating to community health.	I, U
Experiment	39	To demonstrate the need for refrigeration in preserving foods, obtain two glasses of milk and cover them. Put one in the refrigerator and leave the other outside at room temperature. Compare the milk in each glass for several days, noting the differences in appearance, texture, and odor.	I, U
Guest speaker	40	Invite the custodian to discuss ways used to protect the health of pupils in school.	I, U

COMMUNITY HEALTH—cont'd

		Grades
	41 Invite a member of the mosquito abatement office to discuss the control of mosquitoes and flies in the community.	I, U
	42 Invite members of the health department staff such as sanitarians, laboratory technologists, statisticians, and health officers to discuss community health.	I, U
	43 Invite a sanitarian from the local health department to discuss health laws regarding public eating places, public lavatories, and the sale of food in the community.	I, U
	44 Have a guest speaker from the community health council or committee describe the organization and its functions.	U
	45 Have a panel of speakers discuss possible health careers, such as nurses, physicians, dentists, and dietitians.	U
Individual and group reports	46 Write an individual or group letter to the city water department requesting literature on how water is filtered and purified.	I, U
	47 Write a group letter to the health department asking about its role in the health of the community.	I, U
	48 Write a group letter to the local health officer requesting materials that tell how he/she helps to protect the health of the community.	I, U
	49 Pupils prepare a list and conduct a study of the common insects and animals that carry disease and create sanitation problems.	I, U
	50 A pupil committee writes to the mosquito abatement office for information concerning the control of mosquitoes and flies.	I, U
	51 Report on the procedures used to make water safe for drinking in the community.	I, U
	52 Investigate the nature of air pollution and the role of the health department in this problem.	I, U
	53 Pupils write to the World Health Organization, the U.S. Public Health Service, and their state department of public health for information about their services and activities.	U
	54 Consult the local health officer and report on the morbidity and mortality statistics of the community.	U
	55 Pupils report on the health heroes in history and their contributions to community health.	U
	56 Investigate ways that the community is protected against disease from people who come from foreign countries by ship and plane.	U
	57 Report on the services rendered to the community by such agencies as the heart and cancer organizations.	U
	58 Pupils write reports on the methods of sewage disposal in the community and the problems related to these procedures.	U
	59 Write reports on ways to purify water and compare them with the procedures used in the community.	U
Interview	60 Pupils interview parents on the major community health problems.	I, U
	61 Interview health officials and obtain information about food poisoning.	I, U
	62 A committee of pupils visits the cafeteria manager to discuss ways used to sanitize dishes, dispose of garbage, and store food.	I, U
	63 A committee of pupils interviews someone from the county or city health department for information about housing laws.	U

COMMUNITY HEALTH—cont'd

		Grades
Mural	64 Draw a mural showing the location and functions of the various community health helpers.	P, I
Panel	65 Have a panel discussion of the major community health problems and present viewpoints of the nurse, physician, health officer, and others.	U
Posters	66 Make illustrated posters and charts about keeping clean public places, such as parks, lavatories, and campgrounds. Include slogans: "Did you use the garbage can?" "Did you leave the campground clean?"	I, U
	67 Pupils prepare drawings and posters after a trip to the dairy to observe the procedures used in the sanitary handling of milk.	I, U
Scrapbooks	68 Prepare scrapbooks containing pictures of and newspaper and magazine articles on community health helpers.	I, U
	69 Make illustrated booklets of the work of the health department or a local hospital or both.	I
Show and tell	70 Have a child tell of a recent visit to a hospital.	P
Role play	71 Children dramatize an unclean classroom or improper sanitation in the cafeteria or a restaurant.	I
Story	72 Write a cooperative story about "Jeremiah Germ" who delights in bad health habits that help him get around the community.	P
Survey	73 A pupil committee surveys the school environmental conditions, such as light, heat, and flies, that influence health.	I, U
	74 Have a committee survey the community to determine its "clean-up" needs and plan a campaign.	U

CONSUMER HEALTH★

		Grades
Attitude opinionnaire	1 Prepare a series of statements as illustrated below:	U

Check the appropriate box for each statement below (SA = strongly agree; A = agree; N = neutral; D = disagree; SD = strongly disagree).

	SA	A	N	D	SD
1. A physician is the best person to see when ill.	☐	☐	☐	☐	☐
2. Nurses provide reliable health information.	☐	☐	☐	☐	☐
3. People should treat themselves when ill.	☐	☐	☐	☐	☐
4. Acupuncture helps people with certain illnesses.	☐	☐	☐	☐	☐
5. Special foods and diets help people with arthritis.	☐	☐	☐	☐	☐
6. Books and pamphlets are good places to find out about health.	☐	☐	☐	☐	☐

		Grades
Bulletin board	2 Display health products advertised in newspapers and magazines for student review and analysis.	I, U
	3 Display magazine and newspaper articles related to consumer health that students bring to class.	I, U
	4 List local consumer health agencies and organizations and the services they render. Include addresses and telephone numbers.	I, U

★Teacher information is available in Cornacchia, H.J., and Barrett, S.: Consumer health: a guide to intelligent decisions, ed. 3, St. Louis, 1985, Times Mirror/Mosby College Publishing.

	CONSUMER HEALTH—cont'd	
		Grades
Discussion	5 Pupils bring a variety of labels from health products to class for discussion.	I, U
	6 Pupils bring advertisements of health products to class for critical analysis.	I, U
	7 TV and radio advertisements of health products.	I, U
	8 The Pure Food, Drug, and Cosmetic Act.	U
	9 Health food fads and fallacies.	U
	10 Superstitions and quacks in health.	U
	11 Role of the physician, nurse, dentist, and other health practitioners.	P, I, U
	12 Use of products in the medicine cabinet at home.	P, I
	13 Alternative healing philosophies—acupuncture, faith healing, chiropractic, and others.	U
	14 Self-diagnosis and self-medication.	I, U
	15 The intelligent health consumer.	P, I, U
	16 Reliable sources of health information.	P, I, U
	17 Community agencies and organizations to protect the health consumer.	U
	18 Food fads—vitamins, wheat germ, yogurt, and others.	I, U
	19 Use of aspirin and aspirinlike compounds.	P, I, U
Excursion	20 Visit a Food and Drug Administration laboratory.	I, U
Exhibit	21 Display a variety of items that are available in the various health food stores and discuss.	I, U
	22 Display labels of a variety of over-the-counter drugs available in drugstores.	I, U
	23 Have a place in the classroom where pamphlets and publications relating to consumer health are available for pupil use.	I, U
	24 Have the Food and Drug Administration, the Arthritis Foundation, or other organizations display gadgets and items sold by quacks in the community.	U
Guest speaker	25 Invite the school nurse or a physician to discuss answers to such questions as "How can I choose a competent physician?" "Should I choose my own medication at the drugstore?" "What are the various kinds of specialists who can help me when I am sick and what do they do?"	I, U
	26 Invite a speaker from the Food and Drug Administration to relate how that organization protects the health of the consumer.	I, U
	27 Invite speakers from such organizations as the Federal Food and Drug Administration, the Better Business Bureau, the state Food and Drug Administration, the U.S. Postal Service, the Federal Trades Commission, or the American Medical Association to discuss how they protect the health of the consumer.	I, U
Individual and group reports	28 Children prepare lists of the health products, or the products that affect health, advertised on radio and TV as well as in newspapers and magazines.	I, U
	29 Pupils collect lists of superstitions, sayings, or customs related to health and health practices.	I, U
	30 Pupils prepare reports on the meaning of the terms *quack* and *nostrum*.	I, U
	31 Write to the Food and Drug Administration, the Better Business Bureau, the American Medical Association, and other organizations for information and materials about consumer health.	U

			Grades

CONSUMER HEALTH—cont'd

			Grades
Individual and group reports —cont'd	32	Pupils write reports on the different kinds of health specialists found in the community.	U
	33	Pupils prepare individual and group reports on consumer health found in current magazine articles.	U
	34	Compile a list of community sources from which reliable and accurate health information can be obtained.	U
	35	Students prepare a list of services rendered by community health agencies and organizations protecting the consumer.	I, U
	36	Students prepare reports analyzing health publications available for sale.	U
Interview	37	A committee of pupils interviews a member of the Food and Drug Administration, the Better Business Bureau, the U.S. Postal Service, and other agencies that play a role in consumer health.	U
	38	A pupil committee interviews a representative from the advertising department of a local newspaper to learn whether newspapers have criteria for accepting advertising for health products and services.	U
Panel	39	Have a panel discussion of the question "What are the dangers of self-medication?" Present viewpoints of parent, nurse, and physician.	I, U
	40	Have a panel discussion on the question "How should I choose a physician?" Present viewpoints of parent, nurse, and physician.	I, U
Self-test	41	Prepare a self-test on superstitions, quackery, or health fads.	U

Nutrition facts or fiction?

Place a check mark in the box under the appropriate answer.

	FACT	FICTION	DON'T KNOW
1. Dry cereals are necessary for body energy.	☐	☐	☐
2. Raw eggs are more nutritious than cooked.	☐	☐	☐
3. Eating an egg a day is harmful.	☐	☐	☐
4. Fish and celery are brain foods.	☐	☐	☐
5. Frozen orange juice has less nutritive value than fresh.	☐	☐	☐
6. Vegetable juices have magic health-giving qualities.	☐	☐	☐
7. All fruits and vegetables should be eaten raw.	☐	☐	☐
8. It is dangerous to leave food in a can that has been opened.	☐	☐	☐
9. Water is fattening.	☐	☐	☐
10. Drinking ice water causes heart trouble.	☐	☐	☐
11. Wine makes blood.	☐	☐	☐
12. If one vitamin pill a day is good, two or three are better.	☐	☐	☐
13. Meat is fattening.	☐	☐	☐
14. Toast has fewer calories than bread.	☐	☐	☐

			Grades
Survey	42	Students ask parents and friends about the kinds and extent of use of over-the-counter drug products purchased in drugstores.	U
	43	Students ask parents and friends about the kinds and extent of use of foods purchased in health food stores.	U

DENTAL HEALTH

		Grades
Bulletin board	1 Display a collection of magazine pictures about dental health.	P, I
	2 Display illustrated captions on dental health such as the following:	P, I

> Here is little Billy
> Doesn't he look silly?
> He was pulled out by Carol
> When he fell in a barrel.
>
> I would have been just fine
> If I had kept my place in line
> To the faucet I did run
> Broke this tooth and that's no fun.
>
> Here's a tooth so very loose
> As you can see it's not much use.
> 'Cause Tommy refused to look ahead
> And ran into someone else's head.

		Grades
	3 Prepare posters or displays on dental health as illustrated in Figs. 12-9 to 12-13.	P, I, U
	4 Students help the teacher in the preparation of a health chart of practices that contribute to dental health as follows:	P, I

PRACTICES	PRODUCTS NEEDED	SERVICES NEEDED
Brush teeth	Brush	See dentist twice yearly
	Toothpaste	or when problem de-
Floss teeth	Dental floss	velops

FIG. 12-9   FIG. 12-10

DENTAL HEALTH—cont'd

FIG. 12-11

FIG. 12-12

FIG. 12-13

DENTAL HEALTH—cont'd

			Grades

Brush-in **5** Provide toothbrushes and toothpaste to be used in practicing tooth-brushing procedures. Use disclosing tablets to determine effectiveness. **P, I**

Checklist **6** Children prepare a daily brushing chart to be taken home and hung in the bathroom to record when their teeth have been brushed. **P, I**

7 Have students complete and discuss "How do I rate?" **I, U**

How do I rate?

	YES	NO
1. I have had a thorough examination of my teeth in the last 6 months.	☐	☐
2. All dental treatment recommended by my dentist has been completed.	☐	☐
3. I brush my teeth or rinse my mouth with water soon after eating.	☐	☐
4. I understand the importance of having missing teeth replaced.	☐	☐
5. I do not eat sweets between meals.	☐	☐
6. I have my teeth cleaned by a dentist or dental hygienist regularly.	☐	☐
7. I know that sugar in candy and soft drinks can lead to tooth decay.	☐	☐
8. My teeth have been treated with a fluoride solution at the recommended ages.	☐	☐

Construction **8** Children make large construction paper toothbrushes. Each day the child reports the removal of plaque from brushing, the child may hang the brush on the wall-long toothbrush holder. **P**

Debate **9** Have a debate or panel discussion on fluoridation of the water supply. **U**

Demonstration **10** Teacher demonstrates the proper way to brush teeth, and students practice the technique using the flexed fingers of one hand on the cheeks and lips. Distribute toothbrushes and small tubes of toothpaste for all children to take home and use. **P, I**

11 Make tooth powder in class. Students mix the following ingredients in the proportions indicated: 1 teaspoon salt, 2 to 3 teaspoons baking soda, and 1 or 2 drops of oil of peppermint, wintergreen, or cinnamon. Pupils take home some of the mixture to use when brushing teeth. **P, I**

12 Demonstrate proper way to use dental floss and have students practice this skill in class.

13 Demonstrate the proper way to brush teeth using a large toothbrush and a large set of teeth. Children participate in a toothbrush drill using tongue depressors instead of toothbrushes. Pupils also practice rinsing their mouths and swallowing—"swishing and swallowing." Pupils may also be given disclosing tablets to take home and use.*

14 Show spoonful amounts of sugar found in candy, soft drinks, and other foods by placing equivalent quantities in test tubes or other containers. Each container should be labeled and placed on exhibit. **I, U**

Discussion **15** The value of certain foods, such as apples, celery, carrots, and oranges, as tooth cleaners. **P**

---

*Your dentist or local dental society can provide information about securing a supply of these tablets.

DENTAL HEALTH—cont'd

			Grades
Discussion— cont'd	16	Display and discuss magazine pictures brought by children showing good and bad foods for teeth using "the happy and sad tooth" chart.	P
	17	The loss of primary teeth (deciduous) as a normal process unless there is tooth decay or an accident.	P
	18	The importance of teeth in speaking after having children pronounce such words as thirsty, thank you, thistle, and sister Susie sitting on a thistle.	P
	19	Show and discuss pictures of people smiling. Illustrate how some of these people would look with missing teeth by blackening a few teeth.	P
	20	The reasons why the dentist is a friend.	P
	21	Have the class discuss how teeth grow by examining a model of the teeth and jaw.	I, U
	22	The types and functions of teeth, using models: incisor—cuts; cuspid—tears; bicuspid—crushes; molar—grinds.	P, I
	23	The qualities and care of a good toothbrush. Draw on blackboard or bring models of toothbrushes to school.	P, I, U
	24	During discussion of teeth have pupils label mimeographed diagrams.	I, U
	25	The value of the use of toothpastes or tooth powders.	I, U
	26	Fluoridation.	U
	27	Discuss the decay process using the illustration in Fig. 12-14.	P, I, U
Dramatization	28	Children set up a dentist's chair and dramatize cleaning teeth and visiting a dentist. A discussion should precede this activity on how to clean teeth and why visits to the dentist are necessary.	P

FIG. 12-14

DENTAL HEALTH—cont'd

Grades

29 To show that acid will weaken substances containing calcium (such as tooth enamel), place a whole egg in a bowl of vinegar (acetic acid) for about 24 hours. The eggshell should become soft as the vinegar decalcifies the shell. — P, I, U

30 Have class write a play on dental health and present it to a parent group or at a school assembly. — P, I, U

Drawing

31 Children draw, color, and possibly animate different teeth as well as different parts of teeth. — P, I

Excursion

32 Visit the community water plant and observe how water is fluoridated. — U

Exhibit

33 Display pencils, unshelled nuts, buttons, and other hard objects and discuss the dangers to teeth when these items are bitten or chewed. — P, I

34 Display an explorer and mouth mirror and other implements used by the dentist to examine the teeth and discuss them. — P, I

35 Build a toothbrush holder and supply each child with a new toothbrush for noon brushing. Be certain that each brush is properly labeled with each child's name on it. — P, I

36 Display several types of toothbrushes. — I, U

37 Display booklets, pamphlets, teeth, models, and other items relating to dental health. — I

38 Display x-ray films and discuss their use in dental care. — I, U

39 Obtain extracted teeth from a dentist and display to illustrate decayed teeth. — I, U

40 Display models of orthodontia showing before and after results. — U

41 Exhibit mouth protectors used in sports such as football and boxing. — U

42 Show the relative amounts of sugar in different foods, such as candy bars and soft drinks. — U

Experience chart

43 Prepare an experience chart or record listing significant points about dental health, such as: — P

> Teeth are our helpers.
> Teeth must be cleaned.
> Teeth help us to chew.

44 Prepare a chart listing the foods that are good for teeth. — P

Experiment

45 Observe the progress of decay in two apples by breaking the skin of one and leaving the other intact. Place both apples in a place where they can be seen for a few days and relate to what happens in the dental decay process. — P, I

46 Have each child eat a cracker and with the tongue feel the coating of food on the teeth. Then have each student eat a piece of carrot, celery, or apple and note how much cleaner the teeth feel. — P, I

47 To show the presence of bacteria in the mouth, sterilize some gelatin (sweetened with sugar) in a pressure cooker for 15 minutes (or heat in oven at 100° to 120° F for 1 hour). Prepare two shallow dishes of the gelatin. Carefully scrape between the teeth and near the gum line to remove food debris (may use a toothpick). Place these scrapings in one dish. Cover both dishes, label, and place in a warm place. After several days fungus growth should appear in the dish exposed to the mouth bacteria, but little or none will be seen in the uncontaminated dish. — I, U

	DENTAL HEALTH—cont'd	Grades
Flannelboard	48 Compose a story of how a rabbit or other animal took care of its teeth and illustrate the procedures using a flannelboard.	P
	49 Prepare models to compare the parts of a tooth with a hard-cooked egg or an apple. *Enamel*—skin of apple or egg shell *Dentin*—white of apple or egg white *Pulp*—core of apple or egg yolk	P, I
	50 Discuss appropriate foods for dental health by preparing models for use on the flannelboard and include poor food (candy and soft drinks) models, but do not put sandpaper on the backs of these items. When an attempt is made to place them on the board, they will fall off, indicating their poor quality.	P, I, U
	51 Show the parts of the tooth and how decay proceeds by using colored flannel cutouts with black for decay, gray for a filling, pink for the pulp, yellow for the dentin, white for enamel, and red for infection and abscess. Use name tags (enamel, dentin, crown, and others) made of paper with sandpaper backing to identify the flannel parts.	P, I, U
	52 Illustrate the decay process (Fig. 12-14).	P, I, U
	53 Illustrate the progressive stages of dental caries.	P, I, U
Field trip	54 Students visit a dentist's office.	P, I
Flip chart	55 Make a flip chart that shows the importance of retaining all of one's teeth. Show pictures of appetizing foods, such as steak, apples, oranges, and celery. Also illustrate types of baby food that would have to be eaten if children did not have teeth.	I, U
Guest speaker	56 Invite a dentist or dental hygienist to class to discuss dental care.	P, I, U
Individual and group reports	57 Children write brief summary paragraph in answer to the question "What must we do to take care of our teeth?"	P, I, U
	58 Children prepare lists of good dental snack-time foods.	P, I, U
	59 A pupil committee sends a composite letter to the American Dental Association requesting materials on dental health.	I, U
	60 Pupils write reports on the values of x-ray films in dental health.	I, U
	61 Pupils investigate the use of fluoride in preventing tooth decay.	U
	62 Pupils write a group letter to the water commission requesting information about the natural supply of fluoride in the water supply.	U
	63 Students identify foods consumed in 1 day and determine the amount of sugar in each item and total the daily intake. Provide plans for reduction of amount eaten.	I, U
Kit	64 Prepare a plaque control kit containing a toothbrush, flossing material, and disclosing tablets for use at school or at home.	P, I, U
Mural	65 Make a mural in which each child draws a self-portrait and writes a slogan under the picture describing good dental health practices.	I

	DENTAL HEALTH—cont'd	

		Grades

Poems

66 Create original poems.   P

> We brush the teeth as they grow
> Down from the top and
> Up from below.
> Your teeth look swell
> When you brush them well.
> But your teeth decay
> When you keep the brush away.

Puppets

67 Children participate in puppet shows emphasizing a visit to the dentist, brushing the teeth properly, or eating the proper foods for dental health.   P

Scrapbooks

68 Children prepare scrapbooks of picture cutouts showing good and bad teeth, as well as proper and improper foods for dental health; also drawings of toothbrushes, dental floss, and toothpaste.   P, I

Show and tell

69 Children share a visit to the dentist or the experience of losing a tooth.   P

Songs

70 Create simple toothbrushing or dental health songs.   P

> TUNE: *A Hunting We Will Go*
> A brushing we will go,
> A brushing we will go,
> We'll brush our teeth so white and clean,
> A brushing we will go.

> TUNE: *Mulberry Bush*
> This is the way we brush our teeth,
> Brush our teeth, brush our teeth,
> This is the way we brush our teeth
> Right after eating food.

Stories

71 Have children make up a short story about the care of teeth.   P

Survey

72 Survey the class to determine how many pupils have visited the dentist within the past year.   I, U

73 Have children keep records of the amount of candy, soft drinks, and other such items consumed and estimate the total amounts of sugar being eaten.   I, U

Tasting party

74 Have a bunny rabbit party in which celery, green peppers, and carrot sticks are served and discuss their importance in helping to clean teeth.   P, I, U

75 Plan a dental health program for parents and serve nutritious snacktime foods.   P, I, U

DISEASE CONTROL AND PREVENTION

		Grades

Bulletin board

1 Display a list of good health rules and practices that will protect children from disease. — P

2 Display illustrations of animals and insects that carry disease. — P, I

3 Display pictures or drawings showing how to cover the face when coughing or sneezing. — P, I

4 Prepare posters to illustrate ways to protect others from communicable diseases, such as: — P, I

> Catch that sneeze (use of handkerchief or tissue)
> Cut the apple to share it (rather than taking a bite)
> Use your own comb or towel or washcloth

5 Display the signs, symptoms, control, and treatment of a particular disease. Different diseases can be featured. Community health organizations often have materials to help with the bulletin board. — U

6 Prepare pictures of such items as soap, washcloth, toothbrush, comb, and towel. Place caption below reading "We need these to keep clean." — P

7 Display the hands of all the children in class by tracing them on paper and making cutouts. Place the caption below to read "We wash our hands." — P

Chart

8 Prepare a chart that lists the ways germs are transmitted from one person to another: talking, sneezing, coughing, dirty hands and objects, carelessness in handling foods, utensils, and dishes. — P, I

9 Make a "Good health habits" chart to include statements with illustrations of the following: — P

> My hair is combed.
> My face is clean.
> I wash my hands and nails often.
> My clothes are neat and clean.
> My shoes are clean.

Choral speaking

10 Children participate in choral speaking. — P

My hanky

> See my hanky white as snow,
> I use it when my nose I blow,
> It's not to play with,
> Oh, my, no!!

Construction

11 Prepare a disease prevention railroad train for bulletin board display using construction paper. The various freight cars should be hauling a comb, toothbrush, handkerchief, washcloth, soap, and other items needed. Each car can be labeled "Comb car," "Toothbrush car," and other appropriate names. The total train might be called "The disease prevention train" or the "Getting ready for school train." — P, I

12 Construct a TV box and prepare a series of panels on various aspects of cleanliness. Children or teacher could make the panels, which might include soap, comb, washcloth, children washing, and others. Have a TV show when everything is ready. — P

DISEASE CONTROL AND PREVENTION—cont'd

		Grades
Demonstration	13 The proper way to blow the nose.	P, I
	14 The way to cover coughs and sneezes.	P, I
	15 The proper way to wash hands.	P, I
	16 The proper use of handkerchief or tissue.	P, I
	17 How to use a paper bag as a sanitary way to discard disposable tissues and other contaminated objects.	P, I, U
	18 Darken the classroom and flash the light from a movie projector on the wall so that the dust particles in the air may be seen. This will show how germs may be spread by the dust to which they attach.	I, U
	19 Have a member of the health department demonstrate different types of disease testing.	I, U
	20 The use of the clinical thermometer in class and its importance in illness.	I, U
	21 Demonstrate how germs may be transformed by putting fluorescent dye on some coins or other appropriate objects with several pupils handling the items. Have one or two of these pupils wash their hands with soap and water. Using "black light" (ultraviolet) in a darkened room, observe the hands of the children who handled the objects as well as those who washed their hands. If the dye remains on the hands, it will be clearly visible by glowing in the "black light" and thus showing how germs may be spread. The washed hands may or may not fluoresce, depending on the thoroughness of the washing. Ultraviolet light may be damaging if shone directly into the eyes. The nurse may have a Wood's light for use in this demonstration.	I, U
	22 Show pictures of a boy washing hands, a girl washing hands, and hands being washed with soap. Discuss how and when to wash hands. Demonstrate the proper way and follow by having all children practice the proper way to wash hands (Fig. 12-15).	P

FIG. 12-15

DISEASE CONTROL AND PREVENTION—cont'd

			Grades
Demonstration —cont'd	23	Demonstrate the proper way to wash the hands and face.	P
	24	Make soap in the classroom.	P, I
	25	Show the proper way to clean and file fingernails.	P, I
	26	Have children use a magnifying glass to examine the creases and folds of the skin and the dirt on one hand. After washing the hand have pupils again examine the skin.	I
	27	Examine samples of different kinds of clothing material with magnifying glass. Discuss seasonal appropriateness of each.	I
	28	Demonstrate "hidden dirt" on the skin of a child who appears to be clean but has perspired by washing an area of the skin with rubbing alcohol using a piece of cotton. Show the cotton to the class after the demonstration.	I, U
	29	Display two beakers containing warm water in one and cold water in the other with each having a tablespoon of oil and a tablespoon of liquid soap. Stir both beakers and compare the results. Warm water disperses the oil globules more effectively and hence is better for washing.	I, U
	30	Using charts and models, study the structure of the skin and relate this to cleanliness and disease control.	I, U
Discussion	31	Disease control in terms of sleep and rest requirements.	P
	32	Briefly discuss some of the common childhood diseases, their symptoms, prevention, and control.	P
	33	The need for immunizations.	P
	34	Why children should stay at home when not feeling well.	P, I
	35	How to protect ourselves and others from contracting contagious diseases.	P, I
	36	The importance of washing hands before lunch and after using the toilet. Have children practice these habits at the appropriate times.	P, I
	37	Cleanliness in handling and consuming food; washing of fruits and vegetables before eating and refusing to share bites of food or to eat food that has been dropped on the floor.	P, I
	38	The causes of disease.	P, I
	39	Colds and other contagious diseases in terms of prevention.	P, I
	40	Beneficial and harmful germs. Beneficial germs give cheese its flavor, make bread rise, and turn apple juice to cider. Harmful germs cause disease and illness.	P, I
	41	The importance and significance of poliomyelitis immunization.	P, I, U
	42	The use of disinfectant in the control of disease.	I, U
	43	The methods that help to destroy bacteria; soap and water, pasteurization, sterilization, light, and air.	I, U
	44	Tuberculin test and its meaning.	I, U
	45	Food poisoning and how it may be prevented.	I, U
	46	The heart and heart disease using a model of the heart and a chart of the circulatory system.	U
	47	Weather and seasonal changes that require different kinds of clothing.	P, I
	48	Pictures of appropriate shoes and clothing for work and play, as well as for different kinds of weather.	P, I

DISEASE CONTROL AND PREVENTION—cont'd

			Grades
	49	The correct disposal of tissues.	P, I
	50	Such questions as "Why should I keep clean?" "What should I do before I eat?"	P, I
	51	Need, frequency, and methods of bathing.	P, I
Dramatization	52	Dramatize a visit to the doctor to be immunized or to obtain treatment for a contagious disease.	P
	53	Getting ready for school using towels, soap, nail file, mirror, nail brush, comb and brush, cloth to wipe shoes, toothbrush, and clean handkerchief.	P
Excursion	54	Visit the school health office and meet the school nurse.	P
Exhibit	55	Display pamphlets and materials on communicable diseases for student use.	I, U
	56	Display samples of clothing for use in different kinds of weather. Have children discuss and select appropriate apparel for the weather indicated by the teacher or by pupils.	P
Experience chart	57	Prepare an experience chart about good health rules and practices in preventing and controlling communicable diseases.	P
Experiments	58	To show the existence of germs on the hands, wash with soap and water and place salt on them. Try to rub off the salt until none is visible. By touching the tongue to the hands it can be shown that salt still remains. Wash hands again with soap and water and touch tongue to hands to show that the salt has been removed.	P, I
	59	To discover the conditions that may affect the growth of germs, have pupils wet two pieces of cloth and place one in a dark, warm place and the other in sunlight and air for 1 week. The results will show that warmth, moisture, and darkness help molds and bacteria to grow whereas sunshine prevents this process.	P, I
	60	To discover that hands are germ carriers, have pupils with dirty hands touch a piece of bread and place it in a labeled jar. Have children with freshly scrubbed and dried hands touch another piece of bread and place it in a second labeled jar. After a week or more, the piece of bread that was touched with the dirty hands will have much more mold than that touched with clean hands.	P, I
	61	To discover how germs are spread, push a needle into the moldy part of an orange. Pierce a second orange with the contaminated needle. Clean and sterilize the needle by boiling and pierce a third orange. Label all oranges and observe the changes that occur daily for a week or more. Mold will grow on the contaminated orange.	I, U
	62	To discover the presence of germs, wash, dry, and sterilize (heat directly on an electric plate at medium temperatures for 1 hour on each side) two petri dishes (may use metal lids and glass squares). Prepare a sterile solution by dissolving ½ ounce of plain gelatin in 1¾ cups of water and boil for 1 hour. Pour this substance into the petri dishes. Cough into one petri dish and cover. Merely cover the second dish. Place these dishes in a warm dark place and observe them daily for 1 week. Colonies of bacteria will develop in the contaminated dish.	I, U

DISEASE CONTROL AND PREVENTION—cont'd

		Grades
Experiments —cont'd	63 To discover that sunlight kills bacteria, inoculate two petri dishes (prepared as previously described) from a dish where bacteria are growing. Place one dish in the open sunlight and the other in a warm dark place. After one dish has been in the sunlight for several hours, place it in the dark, warm, place with the other dish. Examine the two dishes each day for several days.	I, U
	64 Using a magnifying glass, study the molds that have grown on stale bread, fruit, or other material. Bring a microscope to class for each child to view this mold.	I, U
	65 To show the growth of germs, boil some small, peeled potatoes, keeping them firm, and place one in each of four sterile pint jars with lids. Maintain one jar as a control, but contaminate the potatoes in the other three jars by (a) rubbing with dirty hands, (b) rubbing with hands after washing with soap and water, and (c) rubbing with tissue after blowing nose. Put lids on all jars, label, and place in a warm but visible location. Observe daily the growth of bacteria and compare with the control potato.	I, U
	66 Touch different articles in the classroom with swabs and touch these to petri dishes containing agar. Incubate the dishes so that the germs will grow. Ask a laboratory technologist from the health department to identify some of the germs.	I, U
	67 To teach the importance of cleanliness, put some dust on a sterile agar petri dish (may use gelatin if agar not available), cover, and place in a warm, dark place. Use a sterile petri dish as a control, cover, and place with the first dish. Observe results daily for about 1 week and compare the growth of germs.	I, U
	68 To show how flies spread disease, have one crawl across a sterile agar petri dish (may use thin layer of gelatin if agar not available), cover, and place in a warm, dark place. Use a sterile petri dish as a control; cover, and place with the first dish. Observe results daily for about 1 week and compare the growth of germs.	I, U
Finger plays	69 Children participate in finger plays.	P

Here is my little washcloth,   Here is Johnny, ready for bed;
Here is my bar of soap.   Down on the pillow he lays his head.
This is the way I wash my face,   He pulls up the covers over him tight,
Until it's clean, I hope.   This is the way he sleeps all night.
This is the way I brush my teeth,   Morning comes, the sun is bright,
Until they are so white.   Back with a kick the covers fly.
I drink my milk and eat my cereal   He jumps up and gets dressed
So when at school I feel just right.   And goes to school to play with the rest.

		Grades
Flannelboard	70 Use paper dolls on a flannelboard to illustrate the appropriate clothing for school and different kinds of weather.	P, I
Guest speakers	71 Invite the health officer or nurse to discuss communicable diseases.	P, I, U
	72 Invite guest speakers from the heart, cancer, and tuberculosis associations to discuss the nature of chronic diseases.	U
	73 Invite a nurse, dermatologist, or other physician to discuss skin problems or care of the skin.	U

DISEASE CONTROL AND PREVENTION—cont'd

		Grades
Individual and group reports	74 Children write a brief summary paragraph or two in answer to the question "Why is it necessary to wash our hands and when should this be done?"	P, I
	75 Children write a brief report on "Why I should stay home when I am ill."	I, U
	76 Pupils read about such health heroes as Antonie van Leeuwenhoek, Robert Koch, and Louis Pasteur and write about their contributions to the control of disease.	I, U
	77 Pupils read and write reports about communicable diseases transmitted by insects or animals to man including methods of control.	I, U
	78 Pupils write to the health department, requesting materials about the control of diseases.	I, U
	79 Pupils prepare written reports for publication in the school newspaper on tuberculosis, poliomyelitis, colds, and other communicable diseases.	I, U
	80 Form pupil committees to report on diseases such as tetanus and smallpox.	I, U
	81 Pupils read and write about harmful bacteria in drinking water, milk, or food.	I, U
	82 Pupils write reports on TV or radio programs they have seen or heard on the control of disease.	I, U
Interview	83 A pupil committee interviews health department officials about the prevention and control of disease in the community.	I, U
Mobile	84 Make a mobile showing a toothbrush, comb, washcloth, nail file, and other items needed for cleanliness and disease control.	P
Pantomime	85 Discuss the various procedures a child should follow when getting ready for school. Have children pantomime these procedures and let the class guess the activities being dramatized.	P
Poem	86 Children or teacher or all create poems.	P, I, U

Dirt

Dirt is fine:
    For gardens and roads,
    For worms and toads,
    For puppy to dig—
    And maybe for pig—
    For cats
    For rats
    For night-flying bats,
    For lambs
    and clams
    and even for dams,
    For slugs and snails,
    but
       Under my nails,
    Not mine!

DORIS HAMMER

DISEASE CONTROL AND PREVENTION—cont'd

Poem—cont'd

If you cough,
Or if you sneeze,
Cover your mouth
With a tissue, please.

Cover your mouth when you sneeze,
'Cause if you don't
Someone might get the disease.

The man with the flying sneeze

Germs fly through the air with the greatest of ease,
Whenever you cough or whenever you sneeze.
So don't be a goose,
A clean handkerchief use,
Anytime with a flying sneeze.
   Ah - - Choooooooo - - - - - -

Good food we should eat,
And get plenty of sleep.
When water is deep,
Away from it keep.
Be on the alert
And don't be a jerk
Anytime with a flying sneeze.

		Grades
Posters	87 Children make posters about the control and prevention of communicable diseases.	P, I, U
Problem solving	88 Jimmy and his parents are going on a camping trip for a week where there are no modern facilities such as tap water, electricity, or other conveniences. Help Jimmy answer the following questions: How can we keep clean? How can we obtain safe drinking water? What should we do if we get a cut knee? What other things must be done to protect ourselves from disease?	I, U
Puppets	89 Make two puppets and call them "Healthy Harry" and "Sick Sam." Dramatize children coming to school who feel sick.	P
Quiz	90 Show students a series of pictures and have them tell or write the answers to these questions.	P, I

PICTURES	QUESTIONS
Washing hands	1. When do we do this?
Brushing teeth	2. When do we do this?
Going to bed	3. How much sleep do we need?
Coughing or sneezing	4. What must we do?
Wearing raincoat	5. Why do we need this?

		Grades
Research	91 Children read and write reports on how disease germs are spread and controlled.	I
	92 Committees prepare oral and written reports on the following diseases: heart, cancer, diabetes, asthma, allergies, and arthritis.	U
Riddle	93 Make up riddles such as "I'm thinking of something we should do after we play and before we eat. What is it?"	P, I
Scrapbooks	94 Prepare scrapbooks of magazine and newspaper articles and pictures relating to communicable diseases.	I

DISEASE CONTROL AND PREVENTION—cont'd

		Grades
	95 Pupils collect magazine articles, pictures, and other information on chronic diseases and prepare scrapbooks.	U
Self-test	96 Prepare a self-test on the prevention and control of disease.	I, U
Show and tell	97 Children report experiences about illnesses at home.	P
Role play	98 The school health examination.	P, I
	99 The immunization procedure.	P, I
	100 The procedures for the proper handling of foods.	P, I
	101 The role of the nurse and the physician in the prevention of disease.	P, I
Stories and songs	102 Prepare creative stories and songs about the physician, nurse, and health habits.	P
Survey	103 Survey the nature of illness and the extent of immunizations of the children in class.	I, U

DRUGS*

		Grades
Advertise-ments	1 Students bring drug advertisements to class for analysis.	U
Brainstorming	2 Have students identify ways they can contribute to the control of drugs in the school and the community.	U
Bulletin board	3 Display magazine and newspaper articles brought to class by pupils.	U
	4 Display illustrations of popular drugs used and abused.	I, U
	5 Display pamphlets and other reading materials and permit students to select items they wish to read or report on.	U
	6 Display of ways to say no (see Fig. 12-3).	I, U
Buzz groups	7 Discussion questions: Why should students not use drugs? Why should marijuana not be legalized? Does "everybody's using drugs" mean everyone should do so?	U
Comparative analysis	8 Have students seriously think about something they like to do above all else—art, music, reading, football—and ask them to jot down in several brief, concise phrases their feelings of what this activity does to and for themselves. Teachers list all the phrases on the chalkboard without reference to the activity. Give students a copy of a list of phrases extracted from drug abusers about their feelings of what drugs do for them. Compare this list with the chalkboard list, which might include:	U

It makes you aware.	It gives you a sense of awe of nature.
My mind is broadened.	It's an intense total experience.
It does something to my perception.	You appreciate your senses better.
I notice differences more.	It puts me in a world by myself.
It increases my potential.	I don't understand why people find boredom in living.
The world is more interesting.	I am totally involved in the environment.

*For additional techniques, see Cornacchia, H.J., Smith, D.E., and Bentel, D.J.: Drugs in the classroom: a conceptual model for school programs, ed. 2, St. Louis, 1978, The C.V. Mosby Co., or "Here's Looking at You, 2000," 1986, The Comprehensive Health Education Foundation, 20832 Pacific Highway So., Seattle, Wa. 98198.

DRUGS—cont'd

		Grades
Comparative analysis— cont'd	Ask students to identify the similarities and differences in the two lists and give the reasons why. This procedure should encourage a discussion of alternatives to drugs rather easily and profitably.	
Discussion	9 The kinds of medicines that are used by members of the family such as cough medicine (codeine), sleeping pills, aspirin, and others. Also talk about the effects of these drugs on the body: sleep induction, sedation, and relief of pain.	I, U
	10 Read current newspaper articles about drugs and have pupils prepare questions that they wish to have answered. List these questions on the blackboard and have pupils determine how to find answers.	U
	11 The importance of taking prescription drugs under parents' and doctors' supervision.	P, I
	12 The effect of coffee, tea, and cocoa on the body.	P, I
	13 Why people use drugs.	U
	14 The physiological effects of drugs such as marijuana, heroin, morphine, barbiturates, amphetamines, volatile chemicals, hallucinogens, and others on the body.	I, U
	15 Sociological factors, including laws of drug use and abuse.	U
	16 Drug usage by students in schools.	U
	17 Poisonous substances in the home.	P, I
	18 Emergency procedures when poisonous substances are ingested.	P, I, U
	19 How young people are introduced to drugs.	I, U
	20 The federal and state regulations concerning the sale and use of drugs.	U
Dramatization	21 A student is urged by friends to ingest an unknown substance.	I, U
Exhibit	22 Display a variety of containers that contain drugs obtainable at drug stores.	U
	23 Display a variety of pamphlets, magazine articles, and other materials for pupil use in writing and preparing reports.	U
Field trip	24 Students attend a court session involving illegal drugs.	U
	25 Students visit and talk with recovering drug abusers.	U
	26 Entire class visits a rehabilitative resource center for teenagers.	U
Guest speaker	27 Invite a member of the sheriff's office, the local police department, or the state narcotics office to discuss narcotic drugs.	U
	28 Invite a physician or pharmacist to come to class to discuss the effects of drugs on the human body.	U
Individual and group reports	29 Vocabulary lists and definitions of such drugs as narcotics, heroin, morphine, marijuana, barbiturates, amphetamines, hallucinogens, volatile substances.	U
	30 Use of drugs by individuals and their effects on the body.	I, U
	31 Oral and written reports on the uses of drugs in medicine.	U
	32 Origins of drugs.	U
	33 Federal, state, and local laws about the sale and use of drugs.	U
Music	34 Have students relate rock music, or music in general, to the drug scene.	U
Newspaper articles	35 Students collect articles about drugs for discussion in class.	I, U
Interview	36 A committee of pupils interviews a physician to obtain information about the values, dangers, and abuses of the use of drugs.	U

DRUGS—cont'd

			Grades
Panel	37	Have a panel discussion describing the effects of such drugs as aspirin, sleeping pills, and tranquilizers on the human organism.	U
Peer group	38	Upper-grade students prepare presentation for sixth-grade pupils or seventh and eighth graders.	U
Posters	39	Students plan a drug education program for schools using a variety of posters (see Fig. 12-5).	U
Pretest	40	Give a pretest to determine the extent of pupils' knowledge about drugs.	U
Problem solving	41	Place the following terms on the blackboard (or assign pupils to locate their meaning): *bennies* (benzedrine pills), *coke* (cocaine), *cook a pill* (heat opium for smoking), *fix* (injection), *get high* (smoke marijuana), *hemp* (marijuana), *horse* (heroin), *junk* (narcotics), *mainliner* (addict), *pusher* (peddler), and *weed* (marijuana cigarette). Ask pupils to identify these words. Continue the discussion by defining the terms and providing additional information about drugs. Pupils may raise further questions that need exploration.	U
	42	Procedures to be followed to ensure the proper use of medicines.	P, I
	43	If you discovered your brother, sister, or friend using drugs, what would you do? What should you do?	U
	44	What might be the consequences if you are attending a party or are in a car where drugs are being used?	U
Puppets	45	Prepare stick or other types of puppets and dramatize use of medicine in the home.	P
Questions and answers	46	Pupils prepare anonymous questions that they would like answered about drugs.	U
	47	Provide opportunities for students to meet voluntarily in small groups or on a one-to-one basis with a school person who communicates easily with students and is knowledgeable about the drug scene.	U
Reports	48	Have students prepare reports on: my philosophy of life; what I value; peer pressure and drug use; drug laws and minors.	U
Records	49	Play records of rock bands related to drugs. Prepare verses to songs and discuss contents.	U
Role playing	50	Students dramatize a parent giving medicine to a sick child.	P
	51	Students dramatize someone refusing an offer to smoke a marijuana cigarette.	I, U
Scrapbook	52	Pupils make scrapbooks containing drawings, newspaper and magazine articles, and written reports on drugs.	U
Sociodrama	53	Conduct a sociodrama of a peddler who approaches a group of pupils and tries to sell them marijuana cigarettes.	U
Student information center	54	Establish a location in school manned by students where pupils seeking information may go for help.	U
Survey	55	Students attempt to discover the extent of the use of drugs in school.	U
Television	56	Students view a current program about drugs and prepare a report for class.	U

CARE OF THE EARS

		Grades
Bulletin board	1 Display drawings or pictures that show how the ears help us to hear.	P, I
	2 Prepare a bulletin board showing the head of a clown and place a large pupil-drawn ear on the clown. Put a caption at the top of the display "We use our ears to:" and then put various other statements around the clown, such as "use the telephone," "hear bells," "hear danger signals," and "enjoy music."	P, I
Cartoons	3 Draw cartoons illustrating rules about the care of and hazards to the ears.	P, I
Demonstration	4 The proper way to wash the ears.	P
	5 The proper way to blow the nose. Have children practice the procedure following the demonstration.	P
	6 Show a drum and relate it to the functions of the eardrum and sound vibrations.	P, I
	7 Demonstrate lip reading to show how handicapped a deaf person might be. Discuss the importance of protecting one's hearing.	P, I
	8 How a drum head may be punctured from a severe blow and relate the possibility of this occurring to the eardrum from a loud noise or blow.	P, I, U
	9 Sound vibrations using a tuning fork. Drop a rock in water to show how vibrations travel in all directions.	I, U
	10 Test hearing using the whisper and watch test.	I, U
Discussion	11 How infections, accidents, and foreign objects may affect hearing.	P, I
	12 How the ear helps us to hear.	P, I
	13 The need for reporting pains or other symptoms of ear problems.	P, I
	14 The dangers of putting objects in the ear.	P, I
	15 How we hear. Use rhythm instruments to produce sounds and relate these to hearing.	P, I
	16 How to protect ears from loud noises such as yelling in someone's ear, and the TV or radio turned on too loud.	I, U
	17 The structure and function of the ear using charts and models to illustrate.	I, U
	18 The prevention of ear injuries when swimming, blowing the nose, cleaning the ears, playing, and receiving blows to the ears.	I, U
	19 How colds and other diseases may result in deafness.	I, U
	20 How to help the person with poor hearing: hearing aids, talking into the good ear, making distinct words for the lip reader, and removing wax from the ears.	I, U
	21 Motion sickness.	I, U
Dramatization	22 Dramatize hearing testing or a doctor's examination of the ears.	P
	23 Have children dramatize the following procedures: proper way to blow nose, wash ears, whispered conversation, loud voice, and normal conversation.	P, I
	24 Dramatize a situation in which a person is wearing a hearing aid and is overly conscious of it. Bring out the relationships of hearing problems to emotional stability and the importance of understanding on the part of friends.	U
Exhibit	25 Display an otoscope (instrument to look into ears) and discuss how the doctor uses this instrument.	P, I

CARE OF THE EARS—cont'd

			Grades
	26	Permit children to examine an ear model.	P, I
	27	Display several types of hearing aids.	I, U
Experience chart	28	Prepare an experience chart on the care of the ears.	P
Game	29	Play "listening" game. Have each child blindfolded or with closed eyes and ask individual players to identify different sounds: bell, bottle half full of water being shaken, horn, clock, crumpling of paper, and others.	P
	30	Have pupils prepare a list of common terms relating to the ear and use these words to construct a crossword puzzle.	I, U
Guest speaker	31	Invite an audiometrist to demonstrate hearing testing and discuss care of the ears.	P, I, U
	32	Invite a teacher for the hard-of-hearing to discuss hearing.	I, U
Individual and group reports	33	Pupils prepare written reports on care of the ears.	I, U
	34	Pupils prepare oral and written reports about people who have succeeded in life despite hearing difficulties.	U
Posters	35	Prepare a series of posters showing how the ear may be injured.	I, U
	36	Prepare drawing of the ear and label the major parts.	I, U
Pretest	37	Give a pretest to determine the extent of pupil understanding of the structure, function, and care of the ears.	I, U
Story	38	Children and teacher cooperatively write stories about the care of the ears.	P

EXERCISE AND BODY MECHANICS

			Grades
Bulletin board	1	Display drawings or pictures of proper sitting, standing, and walking posture.	P, I, U
	2	Display charts of the muscles and bones (skeleton) with captions or illustrations showing their relation to exercise, movement, and body mechanics.	P, I, U
	3	Display a series of pictures or drawings of beneficial activities and exercises.	I, U
Debate or panel	4	Have a debate or panel discussion on the "Soft American." Bring in viewpoints of physicians, parents, and others.	U
Demonstration	5	Children observe own posture in a full-length mirror.	P, I, U
	6	The correct way to pick up objects.	P, I, U
	7	Correct sitting, standing, and walking posture. Conduct drills in which pupils practice these procedures.	P, I, U
	8	Correct body alignment using a plumb line.	I, U
	9	Have pupils walk attempting to carry a book on their heads after they have assumed the correct posture.	I, U
	10	To show the effect of exercise on pulse rate, have pupils take own pulse while sitting or at rest. Permit them to stand in the aisles and jump up and down about 10 times and again take own pulse rates. Ranges of pulse rates before and after exercise can be noted on board with individual differences and relationships to exercise discussed.	I, U

EXERCISE AND BODY MECHANICS—cont'd

		Grades
Demonstration —cont'd	11 Conduct posture parade monthly in which the class votes on the boy or girl demonstrating the best walking posture. Children should determine in advance how they plan to make their selection.	I, U
	12 To show the effect of exercise on breathing and oxygen intake, have children count the number of breaths they normally take per minute using a watch with a sweep second hand. Have pupils stand in the aisles, jump up and down about 10 times, and count the number of breaths needed after exercise.	I, U
	13 Children stand against a wall and try to make their heads, shoulders, hips, and heels touch the wall. Follow this action by having pupils walk away from the wall retaining this position.	P, I, U
Diorama	14 Prepare a diorama of suitable physical education activities and exercises using pipe cleaners for figures.	I, U
Discussion	15 The importance and need for exercise in the maintenance and development of physical fitness.	P, I, U
	16 The relationship of muscles and bones to good body mechanics.	P, I, U
	17 The factors that influence posture, such as food, sleep, exercise, and mental attitudes.	I, U
	18 The relationship of exercise and eating to good posture.	I, U
	19 The types of exercise and sports activities that are beneficial.	I, U
	20 The importance of muscular strength in preventing fatigue and in performing daily activities.	I, U
Guest speaker	21 Invite the physical education teacher or supervisor to discuss and demonstrate good body mechanics.	P, I, U
	22 Invite the physical education teacher or supervisor to visit the classroom to discuss "keeping in condition" and its importance in daily living.	I, U
Individual and group reports	23 Pupils write or give oral reports on such topics as "How I exercise each day," and "The sport I like best."	I, U
	24 Pupils prepare written or oral reports on the values of exercise.	I, U
	25 Children prepare written reports about their favorite sports and list the parts of the body that are exercised most in these activities.	I, U
Model	26 Pupils make a posture model (use heavy cardboard) for use in the discussion of body mechanics.	I, U
Mural	27 Make a mural of the variety of kinds of beneficial pupil activities and exercises.	I, U
Music	28 Walk to music, exhibiting good posture.	P, I
Poems, songs, and plays	29 Children create poems, songs, and plays about exercise and its values.	P
Posters	30 Make posters showing the importance of exercise in daily living.	P, I
Scrapbook	31 Make a series of drawings and collect magazine pictures and stories demonstrating proper body mechanics.	P, I
Shadowgram	32 Children make shadowgrams of each other. Using a piece of craft paper as large as a child, with two students holding the paper, have a third pupil stand between the paper and a source of light. A fourth boy or girl outlines the shadow of the third child using a piece of charcoal or crayon. Discuss these drawings individually in terms of good body mechanics.	I, U

EXERCISE AND BODY MECHANICS—cont'd

			Grades
Stories	33	Children write illustrated stories of how exercise helps us.	P, I
Survey	34	Survey the amount of exercise pupils receive by completing the following:	I, U

How much exercise do I get?

Fill in the amount of time in hours or in fractions of hours.

	S	M	T	W	Th	F	S
Riding bicycle or walking to and from school							
Playing at recesses							
Playing before school, in the morning, and at noon							
Exercising during the physical education class							
Active playing after school and before bedtime							
TOTALS							

			Grades
	35	Survey the kinds of activities in which pupils participate.	U
Television box	36	Make a TV or motion picture box and have children prepare a series of pictures showing the importance of exercise and body mechanics.	P

CARE OF THE EYES

			Grades
Bulletin board	1	Display pictures and drawings about care of the eyes.	P, I
Chart	2	Prepare a chart containing important terms to know about the eye.	I, U
	3	Have pupils complete the names of the parts of the eye on a mimeographed diagram.	I, U
Demonstration	4	The correct way to carry objects such as sticks, knives, and tools.	P, I
	5	The procedure for removing foreign objects from the eye.	P, I, U
	6	The proper lighting for reading and working.	P, I, U
	7	Have a child read or look at a book or picture in direct sunlight or under a bright light. Discuss such questions as "Why is it difficult to read?" "Do your eyes hurt?" "Must you squint or frown to see?"	P, I, U
	8	Blindfold a child and have him/her try to walk to different places in the room. Discuss blindness.	P, I, U
	9	The importance of sight by having children cover their eyes and explain their reactions to a variety of situations.	P, I, U
	10	Teacher or nurse demonstrates the vision screening procedure.	P, I, U

CARE OF THE EYES—cont'd

		Grades
Demonstration —cont'd	11 Demonstrate the blinking response using one student in class. With the corner of a soft paper, touch the lashes near the inner corner of one eye. Have children note the blinking reaction. Discuss the closure of the eyelid when sand lands on the eyeball, which is accompanied by a flow of tears to try to flush away the particle.	P, I, U
	12 Completely darken the room for a few minutes and then lighten it. Discuss what happens to sight when you first enter a darkened movie theater and also when later you first come into the bright sunlight.	P, I, U
	13 Demonstrate or draw a comparison between the function of the eye and a camera.	I, U
	14 Display various types of paper showing those with low and high gloss and discuss their importance in vision.	I, U
	15 Use a light meter to show the amount of light in the classroom.	I, U
	16 Have students hold one of their thumbs at arm's length and look at it. Have them close their right eyes and line up the thumbs with the corner of the room. Without moving the arm, have them close their left eyes and look with the right eyes. Students should see a different view with each eye, demonstrating that binocular vision helps to adjust to space relationships.	I, U
	17 Have students close one eye and hold a pencil from 12 to 14 inches from the other eye. Have students look at the pencil and then at a distant object and report how the pencil appeared in each instance. Pencil looks blurred when the eye is focused on a distant object or the reverse is true. This indicates the need for occasional resting of the eyes because muscles are involved in eye focusing changes.	I, U
	18 Have students look at a neighbor's eye in a darkened room. Lighten the room quickly and have students note contractions of the pupils of the eye. The eye must adjust to various amounts of light; therefore, a well-lighted room involves fewer eye adjustments and is less fatiguing.	I, U
	19 Where the optic nerve enters the eyeball there is a blind spot that can easily be demonstrated. Have students draw a black dot (¼ inch in diameter) on a white sheet of paper, and about 1½ inches to the right draw a black cross (¼ inch). Have the students close their left eyes and stare steadily at the black dot with their right eyes while the paper rests on the table. Have students pick up the sheet of paper and move it slowly toward the eye while staring at the dot. They will find a point where the image of the cross to the right will disappear. The blind spot for the left eye can be found by closing the right one and staring at the cross. When the sheet is brought close to the eye, the black spot will disappear.	I, U
	20 With curtains or blinds drawn, hold a lighted 40-watt electric lamp exactly 2 feet above an open book. This is approximately the amount of illumination needed for comfortable reading. Show that light rapidly diminishes as the lamp is moved further away. At a distance of about 3 feet a 100-watt bulb is needed to provide the same illumination that a 40-watt bulb gives at 2 feet.	P, I, U
Discussion	21 The possible danger to the eyes of throwing things including sand, rocks, and dirt.	P, I

CARE OF THE EYES—cont'd

			Grades
	22	The importance of vision to animals, showing pictures to illustrate.	P, I
	23	An accident on the playground that resulted in an injury to a child's eye.	P, I
	24	The importance of wearing glasses when necessary.	P, I, U
	25	Show pictures of artists, surgeons, pilots, and others and discuss the importance of vision in their work.	P, I, U
	26	Care of the eyes and TV.	P, I, U
	27	Have children roll a sheet of paper to make a cylinder and look through it with one eye. Discuss tunnel vision.	P, I, U
	28	The importance of symptoms of vision difficulties such as inability to see the blackboard, words look fuzzy, or vision is blurred. Emphasize importance of notifying parent or teacher when these signs appear.	P, I, U
	29	The hazards to vision of looking directly at the sun.	P, I, U
	30	The ways eyes are protected in various sports.	P, I, U
	31	The structure and function of the eye, using charts and models.	I, U
	32	The importance of periodic eye examinations.	I, U
Dramatization	33	Dramatize the school nurse doing the vision screening test on a child.	P, I
	34	Dramatize the correct sitting distance and lighting for various TV viewing.	P, I
	35	Dramatize good reading habits and a visit to an eye doctor.	P, I
Exhibit	36	Display a model of the eye and permit children to take it apart and put it together.	P, I
	37	Display samples of Braille material and discuss how a blind person uses it to learn to read.	P, I, U
	38	Display various materials used in the vision screening program and discuss.	P, I, U
	39	Display pamphlets, magazines, and other reading materials on vision and make available for reading and research.	I, U
	40	Display different styles of glasses including sunglasses and goggles used to protect the eye in various activities.	I, U
Experience chart or record	41	Make an experience chart or record about the care of the eyes.	P
Game	42	Play the game "Pin the tail on the donkey" and discuss the importance of vision.	P, I
Guest speaker	43	Invite the school nurse to discuss vision screening.	P, I, U
	44	Invite an eye doctor to discuss care of the eyes.	I, U
Individual and group reports	45	Students prepare oral or written reports about signs and symptoms of vision problems as well as common eye difficulties.	I, U
	46	Students prepare oral or written reports on eye infections: conjunctivitis, styes, and others.	I, U
	47	Students prepare oral or written reports on the various kinds of eye specialists in the community.	I, U
	48	Students write reports on the various ways eyes are protected in sports.	U
Mural	49	Make a mural on care of the eyes or hazards to the eye.	P, I
Panel	50	Have a panel discussion of the various ways eyes are protected in sports. Get opinions on football, basketball, baseball, and others from appropriate sources.	U

CARE OF THE EYES—cont'd

		Grades
Poems, stories, and plays	51 Create poems, stories, and plays about care of the eyes.	P
Posters	52 Make a series of pictures or drawings about proper lighting for reading as well as care of the eyes.	P, I
Role play	53 Role-play parents and children watching a TV program, a visit to an eye physician, having to wear glasses, and others. Discuss the significance to vision.	P, I
Self-test	54 Give self-test on the structure and function of the eye.	I, U

Self-test illustration

eyeball	pupil	retina
iris	lens	optic nerve

Fill in the blanks using the words above.

_____ Small, dark, round hole in center of eye.

_____ Carries pictures from retina to brain.

_____ Moves up, down, and sideways.

_____ Light passes through lens, falls on lining at back of eyeball.

_____ Front part of eyeball, blue, brown or gray (in color) in circle.

_____ Behind the pupil and inside the eye.

		Grades
Show and tell	55 Children relate a visit to an eye physician or tell how wearing glasses helps those who need them.	P
Survey	56 A student committee determines the amount of light in the classroom, halls, and other areas of the school using a light meter.	I, U

FAMILY HEALTH

		Grades
Bulletin board	1 Collect pictures of boys and girls of approximately the ages of students in class for a display illustrating differences in size and body build among children of the same age.	I
	2 Show pictures of ways families spend their time in recreation and during holidays.	I
	3 Collect pictures on family life and magazine and newspaper articles about birth and display them.	I, U
	4 Show pictures of happy families and have students describe what makes the families happy.	P
Charts	5 Construct a chart showing varying ages when boys and girls mature.	I
Discussion	6 What can I do to help my family be happy?	P
	7 Ways in which the community helps the family.	P
	8 Differences in growth rates between boys and girls.	I
	9 Inherited characteristics, such as eye and hair color, and curly or straight hair.	I, U
	10 Meaning of "growing up."	I
	11 Anonymous questions prepared by students.	I, U
	12 Living things come from living things.	P
	13 Family rules and family problems.	I, U
	14 Home responsibilities.	I, U

FAMILY HEALTH—cont'd

		Grades
	15 What family members can do to show love, especially at certain times.	P, I
	16 Family customs, traditions, religions, and patterns.	I, U
	17 Care of pets.	P
	18 Nature and functions of the endocrine glands.	I, U
	19 Secondary sex characteristics of boys and girls as they relate to body shape, size, and growth.	I, U
	20 Moral and ethical values and their relation to sexual activities.	U
	21 Different ways of reproduction, asexual and sexual.	I, U
	22 Human reproduction.	I, U
	23 Good sources of information on sex, reproduction, and family living.	I, U
	24 Attraction between sexes.	U
	25 Ways to resolve family conflicts.	P, I
	26 Animal and plant reproduction.	P
	27 Compare the development of human babies before birth with animal babies.	P
	28 Family changes caused by death, divorce, or separation.	P, I
	29 Responsibilities at home, at school, and elsewhere.	P
	30 Freedom and responsibility.	I
	31 Puberty and maturity.	I, U
	32 Love—marriage, children, family.	U
	33 Sex drive, birth process, masturbation, behavior on dates, marriage.	U
	34 People, organizations, and agencies that help people with family problems.	U
	35 Steady dating.	U
	36 Determination of personal values.	I, U
Demonstrations	37 Have male and female guinea pigs or hamsters in the classroom. Pregnancy of the female will offer an opportunity to discuss the creation of new life.	P
	38 Hatch chicks from eggs.	P
	39 Observe the growth of seeds in relation to new life.	P
	40 Observe the growth of frog eggs.	P
Display	41 Make available pamphlets and magazine and newspaper articles about sex, reproduction, and values for student optional reading.	I, U
Drawings	42 Illustrate ways in which families have good times together.	P
	43 Children draw their own family groups and list various family patterns.	P
	44 Illustrate pupil's own family or animal families.	P
	45 Depict mother's, father's, or own work.	P
Exhibit and health fair	46 Students prepare bulletin board displays, posters, charts, and other visual materials for display and exhibit these materials at school. Pupils should be available to discuss their projects, provide information requested, and distribute pamphlets.	I, U
Field trip	47 Tour the school building and include a visit to boys' and girls' lavatories. This should lead to a discussion of anatomic differences of boys and girls and correct names of body parts.	P
	48 Visit a farm and observe the animals.	P
	49 Visit a local museum, hospital, or clinic to view exhibits of a baby before and after birth.	P, I, U

FAMILY HEALTH—cont'd

			Grades
Films	**50**	Observe films on birth and growth of animals.	P
	51	See the discuss films on human growth, menstruation, and reproduction.	I, U
Guest speakers	**52**	Invite a physician or nurse to discuss reproduction, childbirth, and other matters.	I, U
	53	Invite ministers, priests, and other religious representatives to discuss moral and ethical values.	I, U
Graph	**54**	Prepare a graph that shows the heights and weights of class members; compare with national norms.	I
Mural	**55**	Develop a mural showing animals and human beings caring for babies.	P
Pretest	**56**	Develop a test relating to puberty, mate selection, reproduction, sex drive, and other matters.	U
Problem solving	**57**	Develop relevant situations with alternative solutions concerning dating, behavior on dates, selection of marriage partners, sexual relations. Use these as a basis for class discussion.	U
	58	Have children try to provide answers to these questions: How do you grow? What helps you grow? Why do you grow?	I
Individual and group reports	**59**	Rh factor, sex drive, marriage, dating, and others.	U
	60	Different ethnic, religious, and cultural backgrounds of people.	I, U
	61	What things do I do that make my family happy or unhappy?	P, I
Puppets	**62**	Prepare a skit to show how parents help us.	P
Question box	**63**	Provide a box in an appropriate location for students' anonymous questions.	I, U
Role playing	**64**	Provide skits relating to family roles of mothers and fathers, getting along with brothers and sisters, and helping to care for a new baby.	P
	65	Develop skits depicting manners and etiquette.	P
Scrapbook	**66**	Include illustrated materials "All about me," with all the items in terms of family, friends, and things that cause different emotional responses.	I
Story	**67**	Prepare an open-ended story about the family, its activities, and responsibilities of children. Allow pupils to fill in some of the words.	P
	68	Read appropriate stories about families and family relations.	P, I

CARE OF THE FEET

			Grades
Bulletin board	**1**	Prepare a bulletin board display using magazine pictures and drawings of appropriate types of shoes for play, school, parties, and other occasions.	P, I, U
Chart	**2**	Prepare a chart listing the important rules to consider when purchasing shoes.	P, I, U
	3	Prepare a chart listing the important rules to consider in caring for the feet.	P, I, U
Demonstration	**4**	The proper way to walk with the feet parallel. Have children practice this method.	P, I, U
	5	The proper way to wash and dry the feet.	P, I, U

CARE OF THE FEET—cont'd

		Grades
	6 To demonstrate the proper way to walk, have a pupil make footprints on paper and make cutouts of these prints. Draw a straight line on the floor with chalk and have the pupil tape the footprints to the floor so that the inside of each print is parallel to the line and the toes point straight ahead. Now permit the child to walk the chalk line stepping in the footprints.	I, U
	7 Have pupils trace the outline of their shoes on a piece of paper. Have them remove the shoes and trace the outline of the foot on top of the shoe outline. Compare the two drawings and determine whether the shoe is the proper size.	I, U
	8 The importance of the feet to posture. Illustrate how walking with pronated or inverted feet may cause undue back and leg pressures with the possible result that posture will be affected.	I, U
	9 High and low foot arches by having pupils walk on pieces of paper with wet feet.	I, U
Discussion	10 The importance of changing shoes and socks when wet.	P, I, U
	11 The proper way to cut toenails.	P, I, U
	12 The importance of drying the feet properly.	P, I, U
	13 The proper care of the feet.	P, I, U
	14 The importance of shoes and socks or stockings that fit well and provide the best protection for the feet.	P, I, U
	15 The signs and symptoms of foot problems and who to see when they appear.	P, I, U
	16 How posture is affected by shoes that do not fit properly or are in poor condition.	P, I, U
	17 How to prevent athlete's foot and what to do about it when you have the condition.	I, U
	18 The importance of the bones and arches of the feet to posture and walking using a chart, drawing, or model.	I, U
Dramatization	19 Dramatize buying a new pair of shoes.	P, I, U
Exhibit	20 Display a variety of shoes for different kinds of activities.	P, I
	21 Display various types of materials found in socks, such as wool, nylon, and cotton, and discuss their significance in foot care.	I, U
Experience chart or record	22 Prepare an experience chart or record to show the proper ways to care for the feet.	P
Guest speaker	23 Invite a shoe salesman to discuss the way to select a properly fitting shoe.	I, U
	24 Invite a podiatrist to discuss the care of the feet.	U
Poems and plays	25 Children write poems, jingles, and plays about the proper care of the feet.	P
Posters	26 Make drawings or posters illustrating the importance of properly fitting shoes and socks.	P, I
Scrapbook	27 Prepare a scrapbook of magazine pictures and drawings of different styles of shoes for various activities and also stories about the care of the feet.	P, I
Story	28 Have children create a story about the kinds of shoes to wear for various types of weather.	P

GROWTH AND DEVELOPMENT

		Grades
Bulletin board	1 Teacher prepares a series of large drawings that show the progressive stages of the development of a chick embryo into a full-grown chick. Appropriate colors may be necessary to make these illustrations more attractive.	P, I
	2 Children collect pictures showing differences in growth patterns of adults for a bulletin board display: midgets and giants, as well as tall and short persons. Discuss these differences as they relate to the pupils themselves.	P, I, U
	3 Pupils bring to class pictures of well-known, important people and prepare a bulletin board display of these individuals. Discuss the differences in body build.	I, U
	4 Teacher prepares a display showing the relationship of cells, tissues, organs, and systems to the organism as shown in Fig. 12-16.	I, U
Buzz group	5 Have a buzz group discussion about the meaning of the term *growing up*.	I, U
Demonstration	6 Put several articles in a bag and observe whether children can identify the articles by merely touching them and not seeing them. This introduces the fact that the nerves send messages to the brain.	I
	7 Bring an earthworm to class and point out that it has no bones and its only means of locomotion is muscular movement. Mention that without a skeletal system human beings would probably move around like an earthworm. This leads to the concept that each part of the skeleton is shaped for its particular function and that muscles are necessary for locomotion.	I, U
	8 Demonstrate what happens when a person breathes by measuring the size of the chest before and after taking in a deep breath.	I, U

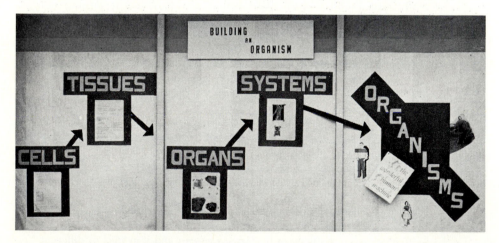

FIG. 12-16. Growth and development bulletin board. *(Courtesy Jefferson Union Elementary School District, Daly City, Cal.)*

GROWTH AND DEVELOPMENT—cont'd

		Grades
Discussion	9 Bring a stethoscope to class to demonstrate how a physician uses this instrument.	I, U
	10 Line up pupils in class and have them note the differences in height. Discuss the fact that children do not have the same growth rate, as a result of many factors: heredity, nutrition, and illness.	I, U
	11 Dissect a hog's or cow's heart and identify its parts (see Fig. 12-7).	I, U
	12 Provide an illustrated discussion of the nervous and digestive systems using suitable charts and models.	I, U
	13 Provide an illustrated discussion of the respiratory system using suitable charts and models.	I, U
	14 Provide an illustrated discussion of the heart and the circulatory system using suitable charts and models.	I, U
	15 Provide an illustrated discussion of the muscles of the body using suitable charts and models. Demonstrate how muscles fasten to bones.	I, U
	16 Discuss the nature and function of the skeletal system using suitable charts and models.	I, U
	17 Discuss the endocrine glands and their role in growth and development.	I, U
	18 Discuss and compare the human body with a machine (automobile). Mention the intake of fuel and the conversion to energy.	I, U
	19 Disassemble a model of the human torso and ask pupils to identify the separated parts. Pupils might also try to reassemble the torso at the conclusion of this discussion.	I, U
	20 Provide pupils with diagrams of the nervous, digestive, respiratory, skeletal, and circulatory systems and have them label the parts.	I, U
	21 Discuss growth as an individual matter and show the differential patterns.	I, U
	22 The story of heredity.	I, U
	23 Ask such questions as: How do you know you have a heart? How big is your heart? What is pulse? Can you feel it? How many times does your heart beat, and how many times do you breathe in 1 minute?	I
Display	24 Bones from a variety of animals including human beings; have students try to identify them.	I, U
Dramatization	25 Dramatize a small boy trying to pick a fight with a large boy. Discuss the implications in terms of growth and development.	I, U
Drawings	26 Children draw, color, and label various systems and organs of the human body.	I, U
Exhibit	27 Display pamphlets and other publications on growth and development in the classroom for review by interested children.	P, I, U
	28 Display animal bones obtained from a meat market. Show some cross sections and longitudinal sections of bones.	I, U
Experiment	29 Demonstrate how baby chicks, ducks, or other animals grow when given the proper food. The white rat experiment (see p. 241) may also be used to illustrate the growth process.	P, I
	30 Provide a flannelboard and a box containing cutouts of the bones of the human body. Permit children to try to build the human skeleton on the flannelboard.	I, U

GROWTH AND DEVELOPMENT—cont'd

			Grades
Films	31	Show and discuss films on human growth and menstruation.	I, U
Game	32	Play the game "Who am I?" A child describes the function of a particular organ of the body and pupils try to identify the organ. Another version of this game is to have children mention bones of the body and then have other pupils name bones to which they attach.	I, U
Graph	33	Construct a giraffe out of heavy paper and place measurements on its neck. Have children periodically measure themselves and record these findings on a graph that they have prepared.	P
	34	Have each child prepare a height and weight graph. Children take their measurements once a month and plot their findings. Separate graphs using height and age or weight and age may also be advisable to make and use.	I, U
Guest speaker	35	Invite the school nurse to meet with the girls to discuss menstruation.	I, U
	36	Invite the school nurse to come to class to discuss the process of human reproduction.	I, U
	37	Invite a physician or other qualified person to class to discuss sexual growth and development.	U
Individual and group reports	38	Pupils compile a list of causes for individual differences in growth.	I, U
	39	Pupils find the meaning of the words *heredity* and *environment*.	I, U
	40	Pupils prepare lists of the characters they have inherited and acquired.	I, U
Model	41	Children make clay models of different organs of the body after they have seen pictures or drawings of these parts.	I, U
	42	Children make a stethoscope using the material shown in Fig. 12-17. Have pupils hold funnel firmly over the heart and listen to heart sounds. Discussion of structure, function, and related diseases could follow.	I
	43	Display plastic models of the heart and other body organs.	I, U
Problem solving	44	Encourage pupils to raise questions about growth and development and list these on the blackboard. Have pupils determine ways to find answers to the listed problems.	I, U
	45	Present these or similar questions to pupils for discussion: What does *growing up* mean? How do individuals grow? Do boys and girls grow at the same rate? Why doesn't everyone grow at the same rate? How does one know when growth is taking place? What factors are involved in growth?	I, U
Question box	46	Provide a question box for pupils' anonymous questions about menstruation, reproduction, and other aspects of growth and development.	I, U
Self-test	47	Prepare a self-test on the various aspects of growth and development, systems of the body, endocrine glands, and heredity.	I, U

FIG. 12-17. Stethoscope model.

MENTAL HEALTH		

		Grades
Bulletin board	1 Collect and display pictures and drawings of happy children and families, as well as of people showing kindness.	P, I
	2 Display work by each child as often as possible to encourage responsibility in doing his or her best work.	P, I
	3 Display a list of class helpers for a week, eventually giving everyone in class a chance to be a leader.	P, I
	4 Prepare a bulletin board of examples found in newspapers and magazines that show good deeds, good sportsmanship, and other qualities.	P, I, U
	5 Display an illustrated list of the hobbies of the children in class.	P, I, U
	6 Prepare a bulletin board with a variety of illustrated mental health phrases such as "Meet friends halfway," "Be cheerful," and "Control your anger."	I, U
	7 Display pictures of a variety of emotions with the caption: "Emotions with which we live."	P, I
	8 Pupils collect for display magazine and newspaper articles that describe mental health problems of concern to pupils.	U

MENTAL HEALTH—cont'd

			Grades
Bulletin board—cont'd	9	Prepare the display illustrated in Fig. 12-18. The teacher can prepare questions in first panel and pupils can bring pictures for second panel and also help to obtain definition and lists for third panel.	I, U
Brainstorming	10	Students prepare lists of problems they consider important and develop plans to resolve them.	I, U
Buzz group	11	Conduct a buzz group discussion on the character traits a pupil likes or dislikes in a person.	U
	12	Have a buzz group discussion of how boys and girls may become better acquainted.	U
	13	Discuss such questions as: What is reality? Does "everybody's doing it" mean everyone should do it?	U
Checklist	14	Pupils complete checklists and teacher either holds individual conferences with pupils or anonymously discusses some of the problems in class. Some sample statements on this list might include: I am often embarrassed when with others. I usually do not know how to act in company. I usually feel inferior to my classmates. I lack self-confidence.	I, U
Consequences	15	Students periodically prepare written statements for discussion of the questions that follow regarding any or all of the actions identified or others deemed appropriate: *Questions*—Do you consider the consequences before taking action? Should you? How frequently? Why? What are the possible consequences of your actions? *Actions*—using tobacco; using marijuana; using heroin; selecting dates; getting angry or emotional with friends or others; refusing the help of parents, teachers, and others when problems arise; sex activities; eating foods that may be harmful to health; racial and ethnic prejudice.	I, U
Demonstration	16	Choose a child to be "big brother" or "big sister" to a new pupil during the first week in school.	P
	17	Demonstrate ways for children to "let off steam" through such activities as play, music, hobbies, creative work, dramatization, and talking about things.	P, I, U
	18	Teacher provides opportunities for all children to have chances in leadership roles.	P, I, U
	19	Teachers provide a warm, friendly atmosphere in the classroom with many centers of interest.	P, I, U
Discussion	20	Children have opportunities to experiment with planning, carry out plans, and evaluate results of a variety of experiences.	P
	21	Talk about how to make friends.	P
	22	Ways to be helpful at home, happy times with the family, and ways to be unselfish about listening to the radio and watching TV.	P
	23	The use of the words *please* and *thank you*.	P
	24	The necessity for proper rules and manners in the cafeteria.	P, I

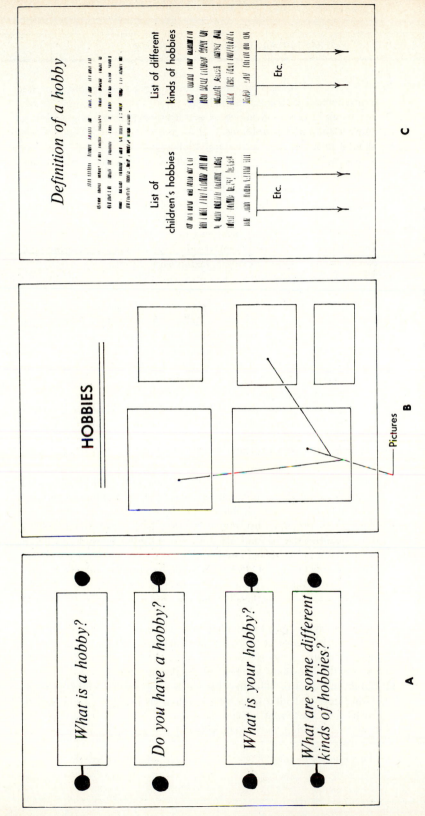

FIG. 12-18. Mental health bulletin board, A, Left panel. **B,** Middle panel. **C,** Right panel.

MENTAL HEALTH—cont'd

			Grades
Discussion —cont'd	25	Children's feelings and the need for control over such actions as crying easily, temper tantrums, and fighting.	P, I
	26	Behaviors in class and in school in terms of getting along with one another and related problems.	P, I
	27	What it means to be a leader and a follower.	P, I
	28	When playing games in physical education, discuss the need to rotate positions to give opportunities for all.	P, I
	29	Discuss what to do when one feels sad, what to do to help others who are unhappy, and ways to behave when something unfortunate happens.	P, I
	30	The need to forgive those who have made mistakes.	P, I
	31	The need for the development of self-responsibility by keeping desk clean, hanging clothes in closet, taking care of pets.	P, I
	32	The quality of friendship.	P, I
	33	How people differ in their abilities to do things.	P, I, U
	34	Ways to cope with and solve problems when they arise. What specific procedures should a pupil follow when faced with a situation for which he/she can find no answer?	I, U
	35	What it means to put oneself in another person's shoes.	I, U
	36	How people can be considerate of the feelings of others and how to handle hurt feelings.	I, U
	37	Honesty and truthfulness.	I, U
	38	Develop standards for acceptable behavior in the classroom, on the playground, to and from school, on the bus, in the library, on study trips, and at home.	I, U
	39	Children who are embarrassed by physical defects and what others can do to help these individuals.	I, U
	40	Inadvisability of keeping emotional tensions, worry, and fear bottled up inside. Discuss the need for friends to talk to, hobbies as outlets, being able to face up to problems, and other solutions.	I, U
	41	Have pupils prepare a list of qualities they like in a person as well as those qualities they do not like and post these on the bulletin board or put them in the school newspaper.	I, U
	42	The following personality traits: kindness, helpfulness, reliability, tactfulness, cheerfulness, good sportsmanship, good manners, intelligence, sense of humor, loyalty, and honesty.	I, U
	43	Evaluate ways boys and girls have of gaining acceptance through such means as conforming to clothing fads, using current slang, forming clubs, and participating in school-sponsored social activities, plays, and other projects.	U
	44	Discuss the question "At what age should one start dating?"	U
	45	Habits and ways of behaving that will give parents confidence in allowing boys and girls increasing freedom to make decisions and to participate in activities outside the home.	U
	46	Reactions to other individuals who do not act, look, or believe as you do.	U
	47	The values of people.	U

MENTAL HEALTH—cont'd

			Grades
Dramatization	48	Dramatize the following: thoughtfulness, courtesy, self-reliance, sharing, playing and working together, helping at school, following directions, respecting each other's property, lost and found, self-control, rudeness, good manners, and criticism.	P, I
	49	Dramatize emotional behavior exhibited such as anger, fear, jealousy, sorrow, hate, love, and temper.	P, I
	50	Dramatize such incidents as the following:	P, I, U

> Things that make me happy.
> Things that make others happy.
> Things that make me sad.
> Problems on playground or in classrooms.
> Things I like to do.
> How to make new friends.
> Other kids can always do things I can't do.
> It's not my fault others won't play with me.

			Grades
	51	Dramatize introductions to and conversations with other people in public places, bus, school, dance, party, theater, and street.	U
	52	Dramatize how it feels to be different from others in terms of race, nationality, beliefs, and customs.	U
Drawings	53	Have children make drawings illustrating: things I love; how I feel when hurt, scared, and angry; when I've wanted something I couldn't get.	P, I
	54	Draw a picture illustrating a way to be helpful to someone.	P, I
	55	Draw pictures of objects or animals that make us afraid.	P
Emotion box	56	Prepare an emotion box and have students periodically complete form in which their names, dates, types of emotion experienced, and the reason for same is identified. Teacher occasionally reviews and uses the material as a basis for class discussion and problem solving without indicating students by name.	I
Exhibit	57	Display pictures brought to class by children of places they would like to visit or where they would like to live. Discuss the reasons these places have been selected.	I, U
Finger paint	58	Provide children opportunities to finger paint to help release tensions and to explore creative abilities.	P
Flannelboard	59	Use the flannelboard to illustrate situations of fair play and good sportsmanship and to create stories about fear, anger, hate, friendship, and others.	P, I
Good-deed box	60	Prepare a good-deed box and have children deposit in writing good things that they have seen classmates do during the day. At the end of the day the teacher reads these to the class without mentioning names.	P, I
Guest speaker	61	Invite a psychologist or psychiatrist to discuss the meaning of the term *personality*.	U
Individual and group reports	62	Children write brief stories or reports on "How to be a better leader or follower."	P, I
	63	Children write a brief summary paragraph or two in answer to the question "Why should we learn to get along with others?"	P, I

MENTAL HEALTH—cont'd

		Grades
Individual and group reports —cont'd	64 Pupils complete an individual written assignment on the topic "When my feelings were hurt."	I, U
	65 Prepare oral or written pupil reports on good manners and courtesy.	I, U
	66 Write a brief paragraph about good citizenship and draw pictures to illustrate.	I, U
	67 Prepare reports on jealousy, prejudice, anger, and others for the school newspaper.	I, U
	68 Boys make up lists of the qualities they like and dislike in other boys and the girls do the same. Discuss the common characteristics found in both lists and their meanings to the pupils.	I, U
	69 Pupils prepare written reports about what they do well and what they would like to improve in themselves.	I, U
	70 Pupils write about and discuss the following: what makes me angry, happy, sad, or afraid; what I wonder about; three persons I love; three wishes; what I would like to change at home or at school; what I like about people; what I like about my friends.	I, U
	71 Pupils write reports about the racial, religious, and other prejudices they have noticed that people have against individuals.	I, U
Murals	72 Make murals, charts, and booklets that emphasize sharing in terms of carrying dishes to the table, going to the store, taking care of pets, making the bed, hanging up clothes, running errands, and putting things away.	P, I
Music	73 Use of various types of music to help calm and relax children to help create a beneficial classroom atmosphere.	P, I
	74 Discuss the meaning of lyrics found in a variety of popular songs.	U
Poems	75 Prepare original poems.	P
	76 Read poems that have positive mental health in messages.	P, I, U
Problem solving	77 Describe a human relations episode to the class, such as lying, stealing, rudeness, or poor sportsmanship, and have children write or orally discuss how they would solve the problem.	I, U
Puppets	78 Make stick, paper bag, or hand puppets and prepare stories or plays around such themes as fear, anger, and jealousy.	P, I
	79 Construct a shadow box or puppet stage with children working together.	P, I
Questionnaire	80 Students complete short answers to the following: Happiness is _____ . Sadness is _____ . I am fearful of _____ . I am angry when _____ .	I, U
Question box	81 Have a question box in class and encourage children to put in questions concerning worries, fears, and other areas of trouble that they would like discussed.	I, U
Role play	82 Students act out such situations as how to make friends; getting along with others; facing dangers; solving problems.	I, U
Scrapbook	83 Children prepare a scrapbook or notebook with illustrated writings on "What to do when I get angry," "How to play fairly."	P, I

MENTAL HEALTH—cont'd

		Grades
	84 Prepare a scrapbook of pictures and magazine and newspaper articles that illustrate good sportsmanship.	I
Self-test	85 Have pupils complete the following:	I, U

Friendliness test	YES	NO
Do you smile easily?	☐	☐
Are you a good listener?	☐	☐
Are you courteous?	☐	☐
Are you a good sport?	☐	☐
Do you refuse to tell tales?	☐	☐
Do you have a hobby?	☐	☐
Can you laugh at a joke on yourself?	☐	☐
Are you usually in a good humor?	☐	☐
Can your friends depend on you?	☐	☐
Do you try to talk about what interests other people?	☐	☐

		Grades
Show and tell	86 Provide time for jokes, funny stories, and riddles.	P
	87 Provide opportunities for all children to show and tell something as often as possible.	P
Sociogram	88 Prepare a sociogram to find out if children in the classroom have friends. Have each child list the three children he/she would like to sit near.	P, I
Stories*	89 Read, make up, and discuss stories showing thoughtfulness of individuals to other individuals, about fears, cooperation, sharing, fair play, courtesy, sportsmanship, honesty, truthfulness, courage, friendliness, and other personality traits.	P
	90 Tell and read stories about helping at home, sharing of toys, caring for baby, and family living.	P
	91 Read and discuss stories of famous people who have overcome handicaps and failures, such as Thomas Edison, Helen Keller, and Louis Pasteur.	I, U
	92 Have students write an ending to an unfinished story. Have several of them read aloud and follow with discussion.	P, I
Survey	93 Conduct a survey regarding the qualities or traits that the pupils like in their friends. Have a committee tabulate the results and prepare a chart for display titled "Our best friends."	I, U
	94 Conduct a survey of interests; tabulate, and prepare a series of discussion questions on the findings. Some sample items that could be included are the following:	I, U

I wish I had better grades.
I wish I didn't get headaches when I read.
I wish I didn't get into trouble at school.
I wish I could change some of my teachers.
I wish my parents got along better.
I wish my parents really loved me.
I wish I could take my friends home.
I wish my father could spend more time with me.
I wish I weren't afraid of things.

*See Appendix E for sample fiction and nonfiction books.

MENTAL HEALTH—cont'd

Grades

Tape recordings 95 Record conversations of a group of children and then have pupils listen   P, I
to the tone of voices. Point out the emotions expressed and consider
ways to modify them.

TV box 96 Make a TV box with a series of drawings illustrating captions such as   P
the following:

> This little girl is too lazy to make her bed.
> Are you a good sport?
> Are you helpful at home and school?
> Do you lose your temper and fight?
> Do you cry easily?
> Are you kind to others?

NUTRITION

Grades

Bulletin board 1 Prepare a display of new foods tried by children. Include the food   P
item, a picture or drawing of the food, and the name of the student
who had eaten the food.

2 From cereal boxes and milk and other cartons construct a food train   P
with an engine and four cars containing the basic four foods. Place food
models made from construction paper, clay, papier-mâché, or cutouts
from magazines in the cars.

3 Prepare a bulletin board display depicting a rocket ship and in the   P, I
pilot's seat insert animated fruits or vegetables. Illustrated caption
might read:

Mr. Carrot: "Fly high with me and grow big and strong."
Mr. Milk: "I fly high and fast because I give lots of pep and energy."

The captions and food items can be changed periodically.

4 Prepare bulletin board displays, showcase exhibits, dioramas, and   P, I, U
others using real foods, food models, attractive pictures, children-made
cutouts, and papier-mâché models showing:

A well-balanced breakfast, lunch, or dinner
Wholesome "snack" foods
Milk products, such as whole milk, skim milk, dried milk, cottage cheese,
   cream, and butter (indicate their importance)
Foods containing vitamins, minerals, proteins, carbohydrates, and fats
Food sanitation including the preparation, serving, cleanup, washing of utensils,
   and storage of food
Meals or foods to be served in the school lunchroom
Recent newspaper and magazine articles
The amount of sugar contained in various kinds of candy, soft drinks and foods
A model of the basic boy and girl with illustrations of the foods they need
   pinned to them
World food problems

NUTRITION—cont'd

FIG. 12-19

Mr. Breakfast

		Grades
		Grades

5 Construct a "Mr. Breakfast" (Fig. 12-19) out of construction or drawing paper as follows: P, I, U
   Hat—bowl of cereal   *Hands*—fruits, eggs, bacon, and bread
   Head—an orange   *Arms*—bananas
   Body—bottle of milk   *Legs*—bacon strips

6 Assign a group of students the responsibility of locating pictures and newspaper and magazine articles related to nutrition. Students should provide statements or comments below each item.   I, U

Chart

7 Prepare a cooperative chart, or charts, on the kinds of foods (carbohydrates, fats, proteins, minerals, and vitamins) with food pictures to illustrate.   P, I

8 Cut pictures of foods from magazines and make a basic four classification chart for the classroom.   P, I

9 Prepare a chart of the food nutrients as follows: U

NUTRITION—cont'd

NUTRIENT	WHAT IT DOES	FOODS IN WHICH FOUND
Proteins		
Vitamins		
Carbohydrates		
Fats		
Minerals		

			Grades
Demonstration	10	Make butter from cream and serve on bread to children in class. Permit each child a chance to shake the jar containing the cream.	P
	11	Make giant paintings of favorite fruits or vegetables on paper bags. Cut holes for the head and arms and have children wear these bags while they tell pupils in other classes what they like about these fruits and vegetables.	P
	12	With the help of parents or teachers, prepare and serve a variety of nutritious breakfasts.	P, I
	13	With parents, plan, prepare, and serve a meal that contains foods from a foreign country.	I, U
	14	Children participate in the planning and preparation of nutritious foods for class or school parties. Avoid the usual cakes, candies, and soft drinks, substituting such items as fruit, fruit juices, popcorn, and nuts.	I, U
	15	Pupil committee tries to improve the attractiveness of the cafeteria through the use of posters, table settings, and flowers.	I, U
	16	Demonstrate ways to test foods for content.	I, U

Starch—Soften, crush, and dissolve foods in water. Place in a test tube with some water and add a drop of iodine (1% solution). If solution turns blue, starch is present.

Fat—Place foods on pieces of paper. Remove foods and place papers on radiator to heat. Fatty foods will leave grease spots.

Protein—Burn foods in direct flame of Bunsen burner. Protein foods (raw, lean meat; cheese; dried beans) will emit odor of burning feathers. May need to burn a feather first so that pupils recognize odor.

NUTRITION—cont'd

Grades

Minerals—Burn various foods on a small asbestos or metal plate. High mineral content foods (dried milk, beans, peas, and egg yolk) will leave a gray ash containing one or more minerals such as calcium. Nonmineral foods such as sugar will leave only a small residue of black carbon.

Water—Expose fruits, leafy vegetables, and other foods containing high water content to air and they become shriveled after a while. They may be weighed before and after dehydration to determine the amount of water lost.

Discussion

17 Have children read the cafeteria lunch menu each day and compare this with the balanced food chart found on the bulletin board. On their return from lunch, pupils discuss the meal.   I

18 Discuss and help plan a school lunch menu.   I, U

19 Discuss a well-balanced lunch in class and select menus to show foods containing the necessary vitamins and minerals needed for growth. Pupils discuss items purchased in cafeteria and best ways to spend money to obtain proper foods.   I, U

20 Obesity, weight reducing, and vitamin pills.   U

21 The kinds and purposes of foods necessary for growth, as well as the deficiency diseases.   U

22 Participate as a member of a school health advisory committee to help solve school nutrition problems.   U

Dramatization

23 Dramatize visits to the dairy, grocery store, and food markets by constructing a store having shelves filled with empty food cans, boxes, and other such items. Also play house and dramatize foods eaten for breakfast, lunch, and dinner.   P

24 Children prepare and participate in plays and radio and TV broadcasts presenting various aspects of nutrition.   P, I, U

Drawings

25 Have children draw pictures of foods using a worksheet like the one below.   P

MILK	ORANGE JUICE	BUTTER
BREAD	CELERY	MEAT
EGGS	APPLE	CARROTS

NUTRITION—cont'd

		Grades
Excursions	**26** Visit the dairy, grocery store, and local food markets to observe the availability and storage of different foods.	P
	27 Visit the school lunch room to observe foods being prepared for the noon meal.	P, I
	28 Observe the sanitary methods used in the preparation, serving, and storage of foods in a restaurant or in the school cafeteria.	I, U
	29 Visit milk or food processing plants.	I, U
Exhibit	**30** Prepare a display or exhibit of well-balanced breakfasts, lunches, and dinners using real foods or food models.	P, I, U
	31 Have a "Food Fair" during which children display various kinds of foods, adequate lunches, dinners, and breakfasts, and appropriate snack-time foods. Pupils may construct murals, bulletin board displays, write-ups for the newspaper, and invitations to parents.	I, U
	32 Set up a nutrition corner displaying pamphlets, books, magazines, and other materials for pupil reference and use during the nutrition unit.	I, U
Experiment	**33** Place grass seed in a sponge, add some water, and watch the sprouts grow.	P, I
	34 Participate in the white rat experiment (see p. 241) to learn the importance of food for life and growth.	P, I
	35 Soak a corn seed in water overnight, remove the bran coat, and then discuss the significance of this outer coat to the white part underneath.	I, U
	36 Soak a small uncooked chicken bone in vinegar for 3 days. The mineral matter will dissolve and the bone will lose its strength and firmness so that it can be easily bent. This experiment demonstrates the presence of minerals (especially calcium and phosphorus) in bones and points out the importance of minerals in the diet.	I, U
Finger play	**37** Prepare finger play, such as:	P

TUNE: *Mulberry Bush*
This is the way we drink our milk,
Drink our milk, drink our milk,
This is the way we drink our milk,
Every night and morning.

This is the way it makes us grow,
Makes us grow, makes us grow.
This is the way it makes us grow,
Every single day.

Flannelboard	**38** Read the following poem and have children (as many as possible) place the appropriate foods mentioned on the board.	P

Three little pigs and their dinners

There were three little pigs so happy and gay,
As each started to go his way one day.
Said the first little pig, in his house of straw,
"Now I can eat all the candy I want, hurrah."
So he filled his tummy with candy and cake,
'Till it began to ache and ache.
"Oh I wish I had listened to Mommy," he said,
As he rolled over and over in his bed.

NUTRITION—cont'd

The second little pig in his house of twigs,
Said, "Now I have no Mommy to make me eat figs."
So he had doughnuts, popsicles, and root beer.
Soon he yelled loud, "Oh dear! Oh dear!
My tooth is aching, my tummy's in pain.
I'll never do that, no never again."

The third little pig, remembering what his Mommy said,
Had meat, fresh vegetables, milk, and bread.
He ate oranges and apples, singing their praise,
As he felt peppy and strong all of his days.
"I'm always healthy, happy, and strong.
I get my sleep and nothing goes wrong.

MARY STULTZ

		Grades
39	Place the following food pictures on a flannelboard and have children prepare three different breakfasts: fruit, whole wheat bread, cocoa, eggs, nuts, bacon, milk, and cereal.	P, I
40	Have food models available and permit children to show the foods they ate for breakfast, lunch, dinner, and snack time, and also the foods they should eat for breakfast, lunch, dinner, and snack time.	P, I
41	Use food models to illustrate the basic four foods, as well as a balanced breakfast, lunch, and dinner.	I, U
42	Pictures from magazines are brought to class and children cut out good food items. Pupils paste these foods on cardboard plates and post them.	P
43	Pupils prepare lists of foods they like and dislike and make comparisons with the basic four food groups.	I, U
44	Children write a brief summary paragraph or two in answer to the question, "What are the proper kinds of foods to eat, and why must we eat them?"	P, I
45	Serve as a class committee member to meet with the school lunch manager to learn how nutritious lunches are prepared and report findings in an oral or written report to the entire class.	I, U
46	Pupils write letters of request to various companies for available nutrition materials for use in class.	I, U
47	Prepare magazine articles regarding school lunch menus, weight reduction, and other important phases of nutrition for publication in the school newspaper.	U
48	Analyze weight-reducing procedures advertised in newspapers and magazines.	U
49	Analyze several newspaper or magazine advertisements about foods and food products.	U
50	Pupils prepare lists of food fallacies and do research to discover why these are considered to be such.	U
51	Students prepare notebooks of food pictures cut out of newspapers and magazines and grouped according to the basic four food groups.	P
52	Students identify one favorite food and determine the nutrients, caloric value, and contributions to health.	I, U

Individual and group reports *(margin label, aligned with items 43–52)*

		NUTRITION—cont'd	

Grades

Mobile   **53** Make a food mobile illustrating individual foods found in the basic four food groups.   P, I

   54 Teacher prepares a large block (at least 12 inches square) and places pictures of the basic four food groups on each side. The block is hung as a mobile during the time that nutrition is being discussed. Manila cardboard can also be used to construct the block because it can be folded and stored more easily.   P, I

Model   **55** Prepare food models from clay, sawdust mixtures, cardboard, newspaper clippings, and other materials to be used for exhibit purposes or in the discussion on nutrition.   P, I

   56 Prepare papier-mâché fruits and vegetables using real foods as forms. These items can be used in dramatic play and in the discussion of nutrition.   P, I

Panel   **57** Participate in a panel discussion of the problem "Diet and its relationship to weight control."   U

Poem   **58** Create original poems about nutrition, such as the following: P

> There was an old woman
> Who lived in a shoe.
> She had so many children
> But she knew what to do.
> She fed them milk, fruit,
> And vegetable greens.
> So they were the best children
> You have ever seen.

> Iggildy, piggildy, wiggildy, doo!
> I'm Mrs. Carrot, How do you do!
> I'm lean and crisp,
> I come in a bunch.
> Eat me and see that I'm so good to munch.
> I'm good for teeth.
> I make them chew.
> I make them exercise.
> That's what I do.
> I'm good for eyes to see things, too!

> Oodle, doodle, humpty dumpty!
> I'm white and smooth and never lumpy.
> Drinking me keeps you in trim.
> Drink me well 'cause I'm filled to the brim.
> Strong bones and teeth is what I give.
> Drinking me makes you really live!
> My vitamins make skin smooth as silk.
> You should know me,
> I'm Mr. Milk.

NUTRITION—cont'd

Grades

Puppets

59 Make puppets from construction paper and tongue blades (Fig. 12-20). The puppet heads should be about 12 inches high with the following rhymes written on their backs:

Celery: "I'm Mr. Celery
So much fun to eat
Serve me at your snacktime
Then you'll want no sweet."

Apple: "I'm Ms. Apple.
A juicy, swooshy bite
Eat me every day
To keep your teeth just right."

Orange: "I'm Madam Orange
The sunshine color you see
I protect you from illness
Because I give you vitamin C."

Milk: I'm your nice, sweet milk
I'll make your bones and teeth grow strong.
Drink and drink and drink some more
Then you'll be healthy your whole life long."

Carrot: "I'm Ms. Carrot
So much fun to eat.
I go crunch, crunch, crunch, crunch
Between your strong, white teeth."

60 Have a puppet show centered around a boy visited by Mr. Candy and Ms. Pop, who persuade him to eat these items as snacks instead of oranges and other fruits. Later the fruit (Ms. Orange) and vegetables (Ms. Carrot and Mr. Celery) come along and persuade the boy to try them as snack foods.

P, I

61 Use puppets or marionettes made in class to dramatize nutrition concepts, such as drinking milk daily, eating fruits and vegetables, and the importance of a good breakfast.

P, I

P

FIG. 12-20

NUTRITION—cont'd

		Grades
Riddle	62 Have children write such riddles as the following:	P, I

You find me in the garden,
I'm orange with long green hair,
You might find me on your table
So look for me there.
Who am I?

		Grades
Scrapbook	63 Locate pictures and information in magazines, newspapers, and pamphlets for making different kinds of sandwiches and preparing lunch boxes more attractively and put them into a booklet to be taken home.	P, I, U
	64 Prepare scrapbooks using pictures from magazines and other sources of such foods as fruits, vegetables, cheese, milk, butter, eggs, meat, fish, and poultry. Also organize these items into nutritious breakfasts, lunches, dinners, and snack foods.	P, I, U
Shadow box	65 Make shadow boxes depicting the basic four food groups, as well as nutritious breakfasts, lunches, and dinners.	P
Speakers	66 Invite such resource people to class as nutritionists, school lunch managers, and others to discuss various aspects of nutrition.	U
Stories, songs, and rhymes	67 Write stories, songs, rhymes, and plays about nutrition.	P, I
Survey	68 Survey the number of children in class who eat breakfast, as well as the nature of the food consumed.	I, U
	69 Survey the number of children purchasing lunches at school and compare this figure with the number who bring their lunches to school.	I, U
	70 Conduct a 1- to 3-day survey of snack foods eaten by pupils.	I, U
	71 Participate in a 3-day diet survey.	I, U
	72 Survey the number of children who eat candy or soft drinks at lunch time, as well as the amounts consumed.	I, U
Tasting party	73 Have a bunny party in which children make head bands with paper ears and all eat raw green vegetables and carrots.	P
	74 Participate in the eating of nutritious snack foods by having milk, fruit, fruit juices, nuts, celery, and carrot sticks instead of cake, candy, and soft drinks.	P, I, U
	75 Plan, prepare, and serve nutritious food items for parties and social gatherings at school.	U
Vegetable garden	76 Grow such vegetables as lettuce, tomatoes, and carrots to provide knowledge of some of the foods needed for growth and development.	P, I

REST AND SLEEP

		Grades
Bulletin board	1 Display pictures that children bring to class or draw showing sleep, work, play, and relaxation.	P, I
	2 Display humorous illustrations of the basic rules of sleep and rest.	P, I
Chart	3 Construct a clock chart that shows children how to budget their time to get adequate amounts of rest, sleep, and exercise.	P, I, U
Demonstration	4 Demonstrate a variety of exercises that can help one to relax.	P, I, U

REST AND SLEEP—cont'd

			Grades
Discussion	5	Collect, show, and discuss pictures of animals at sleep and rest.	P
	6	Have children suggest ways to rest and relax and list these on the blackboard: warm bath, lying down, sit with head on desk, listening to music.	P
	7	Importance of sleep and rest and the amount needed.	P, I
	8	Rest, relaxation, and music.	P, I
	9	Children plan the work, play, and rest period for the day.	P, I
	10	Discuss the following questions in class: What happens when we sleep? When did you get up this morning? Did you sleep well? Did you feel rested? What time did you go to bed last night?	P, I
	11	Discuss the best conditions for sleeping and include comments about air, bed, and the room itself.	P, I, U
	12	Discuss the meaning of the terms *relaxation* and *tension*. Demonstrate by having the pupils flex muscles in their bodies and then relax them.	I, U
	13	The causes of fatigue, the signs of fatigue, what to do when fatigued, and the effects of overfatigue.	I, U
	14	Sleep and rest in terms of their value; how one feels and acts when sufficiently rested; and the need for balance between sleep, rest, and exercise.	I, U
	15	Why we tire; how rest affects posture, work, and play; and how anxiety, fear, anger, and eating before bedtime may affect sleep.	I, U
Dramatization	16	Children play house and devote part of their play to stressing sleep and rest.	P
	17	Prepare a play emphasizing desirable habits of sleep and rest to be presented in class, to a school assembly, or to a parent group.	I
Drawings	18	Draw pictures about sleep, rest, and relaxation.	P, I
Experience chart	19	Prepare an experience chart or record of important points about sleep and rest.	P
Experiment	20	Tie a weighted string near the tip of the left third finger of a pupil volunteer. Have the pupil raise and lower his/her finger as long as possible. Allow the child to rest for a minute and then repeat the procedure. Try this experiment using different fingers on both hands. The results show that exercise is fatiguing and there is need for rest and relaxation.	P, I, U
Finger plays	21	Have children participate in finger plays.	P, I

Rest and listen

I like to rest and listen.
Let me listen while I rest.
My eyes are closed so I can't see.
I'll listen while you count for me.
Sh—whisper, count to ten . . .
Now listen while I rest again.

Time for us to take a rest.
Lock the door up tight (lock lips).
Pull the little window shades (close eyes)
We'll play that it is night.

REST AND SLEEP—cont'd

Finger plays—cont'd

Let's play rag doll
Let's play rag doll.
Don't make a sound.
Fling your arms and bodies
Loosely around.
Fling your hands!
Fling your feet!
Let your head go free!
Be the raggediest rag doll
You ever did see.

Grades

Individual and group reports	22 Pupils prepare oral and written reports on rest, sleep, fatigue, and relaxation.	I, U
	23 Write a story on the three R's: rest, relaxation, and recreation.	I, U
Music	24 Play restful and relaxing music in class.	P, I, U

Brahms' Lullaby
Clair de Lune, Debussy
Air from Suite No. 3 in D major, Bach
The Swan from Carnival of the Animals, Saint-Saens
The Lake from Adventures in a Perambulator, Carpenter
White Peacock, Griffes

Poems	25 Children listen to, participate in the reading of, and act out poems on sleep, rest, and relaxation.	P, I, U

I am a limp rag doll,
I have no bones,
My feet are flat and still,
My hands are in my lap,
My head is limp,
Now my head rests on my knees
And my hands hang at my sides.

SARAH T. BARROWS

Close your eyes, head drops down
Face is smooth, not a frown
Roll to left, head is a ball
Roll to right, now sit tall
Lift your chin, look at me
Deep, deep breath, one, two, three
Big, big smile, hands in lap
Make believe you just had a nap
Now you're rested from your play
Time to work again today.

I went into a circus town
And met a funny Bunny Clown,
He winked his eye, he shook his head,
"This is splendid exercise," he said.
He shook his head, he shook his feet,
He wobbled, bobbled, down the street,
He moved his jaw both up and down
This funny little Bunny Clown.

He played that he was a lazy man
And then sat down like a Raggedy Ann.
His head fell down and his arms fell, too,
And he went to sleep for an hour or two.

REST AND SLEEP—cont'd

The stretching game

Link your thumbs;
Raise your arms
Straight up and past your ears,
Stretch and pull;
Pull and stretch;
Try to touch the sky.
Pull and stretch;
Stretch and pull;
Pull—pull—pull!
Drop your arms, now sigh.

FRANCES C. HUNTER

			Grades
Posters	26	Make posters or pictures illustrating activities conducive to play, sleep, and relaxation.	P
Puppets	27	Make two puppets and call them "Sleepy Head" and "Wide Awake." Have children dramatize aspects of rest and sleep.	P, I
	28	Make paper-bag puppets and dramatize a problem, such as a boy who wants to stay up past his bedtime to watch TV.	P, I
Scrapbook	29	Prepare scrapbooks of pictures showing restful and relaxing activities.	P, I
Stories	30	Read and create stories about rest, sleep, and relaxation.	P, I

SAFETY

Bicycle safety			**Grades**
Bulletin board	1	Display children's drawings on bicycle safety.	P, I, U
	2	Display bicycle safety posters and other printed materials available from the American Bicycle Institute and such organizations.	P, I, U
	3	A committee of pupils prepares a bulletin board display showing an outline of a bicycle labeled with its main parts and the safety rules (Fig. 12-21).	I, U
Chart	4	Children prepare a chart listing bicycle safety rules.	P, I, U
Checklist	5	Pupils prepare a checklist for use in the inspection of the mechanical safety of bicycles. The assistance of a bicycle repair person may be necessary.	I, U
	6	Organize a bicycle club in school.	I, U
Demonstration	7	Children demonstrate the following procedures correctly: getting on a bicycle, getting off a bicycle, guiding a bicycle, applying the brake, and stopping and parking the bicycle.	P, I, U
	8	Pupils demonstrate and practice the proper hand signals when riding bicycles.	P, I, U

SAFETY—cont'd

CHECK YOUR BIKE FOR SAFE OPERATION

SADDLE
Adjust frequently for comfort and growth. Tighten saddle and seat post nuts securely, leaving at least 2½ inches of seat post down in the frame.

FENDERS
Be sure they are undamaged and securely fastened.

COASTER BRAKES AND HAND BRAKES
Check before your first ride. Must brake evenly every time, no slippage. The purchaser should periodically inspect and maintain brakes. The coaster brake arm must be securely fastened to the frame.

CHAIN
Chain should be checked frequently for damage and stretch, and be readjusted if necessary. It should be lubricated frequently with light oil.

PEDALS
This bicycle is equipped with reflectorized pedals for added safety in night riding. It is imperative that the shoulder of the pedal axle be securely tightened against the crank arm. If pedals become worn or damaged, replace them with reflectorized pedals.

BELL OR HORN
Be sure it works properly, loud and clear.

LIGHTS AND REFLECTORS
This bicycle is equipped with reflectorized pedals and other reflective materials. If these materials are damaged or lost, replace them immediately for your own safety. Lights and reflectors should be visible at dusk and at night; headlights from 500 feet, rear reflector from 300 feet. Be sure reflectors are state approved.

HANDLEBARS AND GRIPS
Handlebar should be adjusted frequently for comfort and growth. Keep at least 2½ inches of handlebar stem down in the frame, then tighten it securely. Handlebar grips should fit snugly, and worn ones replaced.

TIRES
Should be inspected frequently for wear and leaks. Remove imbedded stones, nails, glass, cinders, etc. Keep inflated to the correct pressure which is stamped on the sidewall of the tire.

WHEELS
Should rotate smoothly without wobbling from side to side. If necessary, they should be realigned. Axle nuts should be kept tight.

SPOKES
Replace broken ones promptly. Keep them tight.

HAVE YOUR BICYCLE INSPECTED TWICE A YEAR BY A COMPETENT PERSON

FIG. 12-21. Bicycle safety check. *(Courtesy the Bicycle Institute of America, Inc., New York.)*

			Grades
Demonstration—cont'd	9	Demonstrate the mechanical inspection of a safe bicycle in class. It is advisable to bring a bicycle into the room.	P, I, U
	10	Have a demonstration of minor bicycle repairs. It may be necessary to invite a bicycle repair person to class.	I, U
	11	Conduct a bicycle field day in which pupils participate in a variety of activities that show their ability and skill to ride bicycles safely. Automobile clubs and other organizations in the community often will provide assistance with this program.	I, U
	12	Pupils prepare a demonstration of bicycle safety to be presented to a school assembly.	I, U
Discussion	13	The motor vehicle laws and regulations, in terms of licensing of bicycles, the need to comply with rules, proper hand signals, parking, and others.	P, I, U
	14	Safety factors involved in riding a bicycle to school.	P, I, U
	15	Pupils bring newspaper and magazine articles about bicycle safety or accidents to class.	I, U
	16	Pupils discuss the causes of bicycle accidents and how to prevent them. This could lead to a series of unanswered questions and start the problem-solving approach to bicycle safety.	I, U
Dramatization	17	Children dramatize riding a bicycle and demonstrate the necessary safe practices.	P, I, U
Excursion	18	Visit a bicycle repair shop to observe how bicycles are repaired.	I, U

SAFETY—cont'd

		Grades
Experience chart	19 Prepare an experience chart or record of bicycle safety rules.	P
Guest speaker	20 Invite a police officer to class to discuss bicycle safety traffic rules.	P, I, U
Individual and group reports	21 Prepare oral and written reports on the safest way to ride bicycles to and from school.	I, U
	22 Prepare oral and written reports on bicycle safety.	I, U
	23 Prepare school newspaper articles titled "Bicycle safety tips."	I, U
	24 Write a group letter to the police department or some other organization requesting a speaker to discuss bicycle safety.	I, U
	25 Children prepare a code of safety for bicycle riders. This can be posted on the bulletin board or may be printed in the school newspaper.	I, U
	26 Children write to the Bicycle Institute of America or other organizations for bicycle safety materials.	I, U
	27 Pupils prepare reports on the yearly accidents occurring on bicycles in the nation, state, county, and city.	U
Interview	28 Interview a police officer or some other authority on bicycle safety.	I, U
Scrapbook	29 Prepare a scrapbook containing newspaper and magazine articles, pictures, stories, and other obtainable materials on bicycle safety.	P, I, U
Self-test	30 Prepare a self-test or pretest on bicycle traffic safety.	I, U

Sample questions	YES	NO
1. A bicycle can be ridden on the sidewalk in a business area.	☐	☐
2. A bicycle rider should obey all traffic signs, lights, and devices.	☐	☐
3. Pedestrians do not have the right-of-way in crosswalks.	☐	☐
4. You should walk your bicycle across heavily traveled streets.	☐	☐
5. Night riding without a light and reflector is unsafe.	☐	☐
6. It is safe and proper to carry a passenger on a bicycle.	☐	☐
7. Hitching to a moving truck is safe if you are careful.	☐	☐
8. It is best to ride three abreast when riding in a group.	☐	☐
9. You should give hand signals when turning at all times.	☐	☐
10. On a country road you should ride on the left side of the road.	☐	☐

		Grades
Survey	31 Pupils conduct a survey of bicycle traffic violations noted on the way to and from school.	I, U

Bus safety

		Grades
Bulletin board	1 Display pictures, drawings, slogans, cartoons, and posters about bus safety.	P, I, U
	2 Make a bus out of construction paper and display this along with appropriate captions about bus safety.	P, I, U
Demonstration	3 With a small toy truck and blocks demonstrate why it is necessary to be seated at all times in the school bus. Show how blocks will fall when a sudden stop is necessary.	P, I
	4 Have children practice bus loading and unloading and discuss safe behavior while riding.	P, I, U
Discussion	5 The need to cooperate with the bus driver when riding the school bus.	P, I, U

SAFETY—cont'd

		Grades
Discussion—cont'd	6 Discuss bus safety with children preparing a list of safe behavior rules.	P, I, U
Dramatization	7 Arrange chairs in classroom to represent a school bus. Have children act out the right way and the wrong way to get on and off the bus and practice safe bus rules.	P, I
Excursion	8 Visit a bus and have the driver discuss safe behavior while boarding and riding.	P, I
Experience chart	9 Prepare an experience chart or record of safe procedures on the bus.	P
Guest speaker	10 Invite the bus driver to discuss bus safety.	P, I
Mural	11 Prepare a mural depicting safety on the bus.	P, I
Scrapbook	12 Construct a scrapbook of pupil drawings about bus safety.	P, I
Songs and poems	13 Compose songs and poems about bus safety.	P, I

Disaster safety

Bulletin board	1 Display pictures, drawings, or diagrams of procedures to follow in the event of an atomic attack.	P, I, U
	2 Prepare an illustrated display of foods suitable for storing for emergency use.	P, I, U
Chart	3 Prepare a wall chart for each classroom showing the floor plans, exits and entrances to the building, and the shortest route to the nearest shelter.	P, I, U
Demonstration	4 The signals in schools that signify alerts or attack and practice identification.	P, I, U
	5 Demonstrate and practice ways to protect the eyes, ears, nose, and mouth when under simulated attack.	P, I, U
	6 Demonstrate and practice thorough washing of hands, nails, face, and hair to decontaminate these areas.	P, I, U
	7 Demonstrate and practice emergency drills for evacuation or seeking cover.	P, I, U
	8 Have pupil committees prepare to demonstrate decontamination and other emergency procedures to children in school or to the community.	I, U
	9 Food pollution through the use of simple fungi and bacteriological experiments.	I, U
	10 How and where to store foods safely at home during an attack.	I, U
	11 How to preserve perishable foods without refrigeration.	I, U
	12 How to properly dispose of polluted food.	I, U
	13 Demonstrate and display an appropriate first-aid kit for civil disasters.	I, U
	14 How to preserve and package foods for emergencies.	I, U
	15 First-aid procedures after civil disasters.	I, U
Discussion	16 What children may do (activities) while waiting in a shelter at school until the all-clear signal is sounded.	P, I, U
	17 The procedures to follow if caught outdoors during an attack or if an alert is on.	P, I, U
	18 The location of emergency shelters in the school and community.	P, I, U
	19 The meaning of civil defense and why it is necessary.	P, I, U
	20 The nature of radiation and its effect on human beings.	I, U

SAFETY—cont'd

			Grades
	21	The hazards from atomic, biological, and chemical warfares.	I, U
	22	The procedures to follow if one has survived an atomic attack.	I, U
	23	The problems of emotions, panics, and other behaviors that will occur during an atomic catastrophe.	I, U
	24	First-aid procedures necessary in civil disasters.	I, U
	25	The contamination of food and water and ways to protect these items.	I, U
Dramatization	26	Dramatize proper conduct during disasters.	P, I, U
Exhibit	27	Display pamphlets and other printed materials for pupil reference and use.	I, U
Guest speakers	28	Invite civil defense and Red Cross speakers to discuss aspects of atomic, biological, chemical, or other civil disasters.	I, U
Individual and group reports	29	Have individual or group oral or written reports on the civil defense recommendations for the protection of people in the event of atomic, biological, or chemical warfare.	I, U
	30	Pupils write articles for the local newspaper or school paper on how individuals can protect themselves at home, at school, or when outdoors during an atomic attack.	U
Interview	31	Interview civil defense authorities and others about the feasibility of building home shelters or community shelters.	I, U
	32	Pupils interview local health officers and medical personnel about the availability of services and hospital facilities in the event of civil disasters.	U
	33	Pupils interview the health officer or a representative from the civil defense office on that person's role in civil defense.	U
Survey	34	Survey the school and community to locate the designated shelter areas.	I, U

Farm safety

Bulletin board	1	Children obtain pictures or make drawings of tools and machinery found on the farm, such as tractors, cotton pickers, cotton trailers, harvesters, plows, and discs, and place caption "Dangerous equipment" below. Pictures may be obtained from pamphlets available from farm machinery companies or from farm organizations.	P, I, U
Discussion	2	Safe practices when riding on trucks and other farm machinery.	P, I, U
	3	The hazards of insect stings, poisonous sprays, canals, irrigation ditches, tools, and other unsafe places and equipment on the farm.	P, I, U
	4	The hazards of sharp implements such as pitchforks, hoes, saws, and axes used on the farm.	P, I, U
	5	Safety around horses, bulls, and other farm animals.	P, I, U
Experience chart or record	6	Children help prepare an experience chart or record on farm safety rules.	P
Exhibit	7	Display a variety of sharp implements used in farm work and discuss the dangers of their improper use.	P, I, U
Individual and group reports	8	Children prepare oral and written reports on farm safety.	I, U

SAFETY—cont'd

Fire safety   Grades

Bulletin board   1 Prepare an illustrated bulletin board display about fire prevention using   P, I, U
                    construction paper, real clothing materials, or crayons.

                  2 Display pictures or news items about fires in the community.   P, I, U

                  3 Use pictures and drawings to display the varieties of types of fire   I, U
                    extinguishers.

                  4 Display pictures of "drop and roll" and crawling in smoke-filled room.   P, I, U

                  5 Pictorially illustrate the action to be taken when fires occur or smoke   P, I
                    appears at home and include escape plan and other procedures.

Chart   6 Prepare a list of illustrated fire safety rules.   P, I

                  7 Make an illustrated chart listing the common causes of fires in the   P, I, U
                    home.

                  8 Make an illustrated chart of the fire exits in school.   P, I, U

Demonstration   9 Light two candles and fan one of them to show how moving air causes   P, I
                    a flame to burn more vigorously.

                 10 Sound the fire alarm bell and have children practice responding to it   P, I, U
                    for a fire drill.

                 11 The way to report a fire using an alarm box and the telephone.   P, I, U

                 12 Ways of putting out fires using a variety of fire extinguishers.   P, I, U

                 13 How to put out a fire when someone's clothing is ablaze.   P, I, U

                 14 How to use matches safely—use only safety matches and strike match   P, I, U
                    with the cover closed; dispose of burned matches by breaking them
                    and placing in a glass or tin container.

                 15 Drop and roll and crawling low in smoke-filled room procedures.   P, I, U

                 16 Demonstrate the making of a fire extinguisher by putting some vinegar   P, I, U
                    in a bottle and adding some baking soda. (Wrap the soda in a tissue
                    before adding it to the vinegar. This will delay the formation of the
                    carbon dioxide gas.) Put a rubber stopper and a pipet in the bottle,
                    turn it upside down and pour the fluid into a pail or sink.

                 17 The combustibility of a variety of materials such as asbestos, glass,   P, I, U
                    paper, water, cotton, cloth, wood, kerosene, and various types of cloth-
                    ing. Also discuss spontaneous combustion.

                 18 Place a piece of cardboard against a small light bulb and show the   P, I
                    brown spot that occurs. Explain in terms of the fire triangle.

                 19 Teacher lights a candle in class, and pupils watch it burn. A glass is   P, I, U
                    placed over the candle, and children attempt to explain, in terms of
                    the triangle of fire, why the flame was extinguished.

Discussion   20 Fire safety rules and reasons for fire drills.   P, I

                 21 Beneficial and hazardous effects of fire.   P, I

                 22 Fire hazards on special occasions, such as Christmas and the Fourth   P, I, U
                    of July.

                 23 Discuss and practice fire drills in school.   P, I, U

                 24 Discuss these questions: What causes fires? How do fires start? What   P, I, U
                    materials burn? Where should matches be kept? What should you do
                    in case of fire? How should you put out a picnic fire? How can fires
                    be prevented?

SAFETY—cont'd

		Grades
	25 The value of the home inspections conducted by firemen. Introduce common electrical terms, such as wire, plug, socket, bulb, fuse, and fuse box.	I, U
	26 Ways to prevent fires by good housekeeping procedures, proper disposal of rubbish and ashes, safe storage of fuel, correct installation and care of stoves, electric equipment, and furnaces.	I, U
	27 The types of fires and how they may be extinguished.	I, U
	28 Pupils participate as members of the fire-safety patrol to inform other pupils about fire prevention.	I, U
	29 Baby-sitting.	I, U
	30 Smoke detectors.	P, I, U
	31 Fire escape plans from homes and other buildings.	P, I, U
	32 First-aid procedures for burns.	P, I, U
	33 Hazards and use of electricity and flammable materials.	I, U
	34 Identity and proper storage of flammable liquids.	P, I, U
	35 Fires reported in newspapers and magazines in terms of causes and prevention.	I, U
	36 To whom and how to report fires and smoke discovered.	P, I
	37 Combustibility and flammability of various types of clothing and other substances.	I, U
	38 Importance of drop and roll and crawling low procedures.	P, I, U
	39 False alarms.	I, U
	40 Ways to call fire department.	P, I, U
Dramatization	41 Build a fire engine using large blocks, cardboard boxes, and other items. Children participate in dramatic play by having a corner in the classroom as a firehouse. Pupils bring their toy telephones to practice reporting fires.	P
	42 Dramatize the procedures to follow when reporting a fire by telephone.	P, I, U
	43 Dramatize fire safety through sociodramas, puppet shows, and plays.	P, I, U
Drawings	44 Children make drawings of ways to prevent fires, escape from fires, and signal when fire is discovered.	P, I
	45 Draw pictures of wires, plugs, sockets, electric appliances, and other items with descriptions placed below telling of the safe ways to use these items.	I, U
Excursion	46 Visit the firehouse.	P, I, U
	47 Children walk around the school to locate fire hazards or become familiar with the locations of extinguishers, exits, and alarm boxes.	P, I, U
	48 Visit a fireboat.	
Exhibit	49 Invite the fire department to display fire-fighting equipment and its uses.	P, I, U
	50 Display a variety of combustible materials, such as paper, wood, cloth, gasoline, and kerosene.	P, I, U
	51 Display books, magazines, pamphlets, and stories about fire safety for pupil use.	P, I, U

SAFETY—cont'd

		Grades
Exhibit—cont'd	52 Show pictures and materials of fire hazards, such as overload of electric circuits, trash accumulation, frayed electric wires, and gasoline storage containers.	P, I, U
Experience chart or record	53 Prepare an experience chart or record about fire safety.	P
Experiment	54 Place a lighted candle on a table and let the class watch it burn. Cover the candle with a clear glass so that no air can enter. Have pupils note what happens to the candle—it goes out when the oxygen supply has been used. Relate this to extinguishing fires.	P, I, U
Flip chart	55 Prepare a series of illustrated flip charts for a discussion about fire safety. Include answers to these questions: How is fire helpful? What are the causes of fire? How many fires occur in our community? How can we prevent fires?	P, I
Games	56 Make crossword puzzles, riddles, and other games about fire prevention and fire safety.	P, I, U
Guest speaker	57 Invite a fire fighter to discuss fire safety.	P, I, U
	58 Invite the fire chief from your local fire department to discuss the junior fire marshall program and to encourage children to participate.	I
	59 Request the local fire department to conduct a demonstration of the types of fire extinguishers and smoke detectors.	U
	60 Invite a member of the National Board of Fire Underwriters Laboratory to discuss the work of this organization in fire safety.	U
Individual and group reports	61 Write stories about their experiences in fire safety.	P, I
	62 Write to insurance companies and others concerned with fire safety and request materials for display and class reading.	I, U
	63 Prepare oral or written reports on the causes, effects, and prevention of fires.	I, U
	64 Write articles for the school newspaper about fire safety.	I, U
	65 Students prepare reports on baby-sitting and fire safety.	I, U
Inspection	66 Prepare checklist to search for fire hazards in home or school.	I, U
Map	67 Prepare a map of your community identifying the locations of firehouses, hydrants, alarm boxes, and other fire safety features.	I, U
	68 Students prepare home escape-from-fire plans in consultation with parents.	P, I
Models	69 Construct a fire alarm box, a firehouse, and fire prevention equipment for use in dramatic play.	P
	70 Make fire fighter hats out of construction paper.	P, I
	71 Draw or build a home that is free of fire hazards.	I, U
Mural	72 Prepare a mural of ways to prevent fires.	P, I
Poems and songs	73 Create and learn poems, songs, jingles, and stories about fire safety.	P, I
Posters	74 Conduct a contest for the best school poster on fire safety.	I, U
Scrapbook	75 Pupils prepare scrapbooks containing pictures, photos, stories, poems, newspaper articles, and written reports about fires and fire prevention.	P, I, U

SAFETY—cont'd

		Grades
Self-test	**76** Give the following self-test:	I, U

Fire safety

Circle the correct answers to the right. If you do not know the answer, circle the letter "D."

1. A grease fire may be put out by pouring water on it.	T	F	D
2. One should run to extinguish flames when clothes are on fire.	T	F	D
3. A frayed wire on an electric appliance is a dangerous fire hazard.	T	F	D
4. Fire drills are not necessary at schools.	T	F	D
5. It is safe to run a lamp cord under a rug.	T	F	D
6. The leading causes of fire are matches and smoking.	T	F	D
7. A penny is a good substitute for a blown-out fuse.	T	F	D
8. "EXIT" on a door means the door leads to the outside.	T	F	D
9. A wood fire may be put out by pouring water on it.	T	F	D
10. Gasoline can be stored safely in glass bottles.	T	F	D
11. Oily rags can catch fire without a match.	T	F	D
12. One should always close the cover of a safety match book before striking a match.	T	F	D

		Grades
Show and tell	**77** Children tell of their experiences with fire, fire engines, and fire fighters.	P
	78 Children identify names, addresses, and home telephone numbers.	P
Survey	**79** Pupils make survey forms to check their homes for fire hazards.	P, I, U
Television box	**80** Students make a movie with a title such as "The day Mary's house burned." Pupils draw pictures of the discovery of the fire and what they did.	P
Word lists	**81** Prepare a list of new words learned about fire prevention.	P, I, U

First aid

		Grades
Bulletin board	**1** Show pictures and drawings that display first-aid procedures to be followed at school.	P, I, U
	2 Display pictures or drawings of poisonous snakes, insects, and plants.	P, I, U
Demonstration	**3** Have nurse or other person demonstrate how to cleanse a wound with soap and water, apply a sterile dressing and bandage, and stop a nosebleed and other bleeding.	P, I, U
	4 Demonstrate the correct procedure for removing foreign objects from the eye.	I, U
	5 Provide for a demonstration of the mouth-to-mouth procedure of artificial respiration.	I, U
Discussion	**6** What to do when injured at school, home, or when away from home.	P, I, U
	7 First-aid procedures for sunburn, chapped skin, poison oak or ivy, and insect bites and stings.	P, I, U
	8 Discuss reasons for cleansing wounds and applying sterile dressings and bandages.	P, I, U
	9 First-aid procedures for minor cuts, burns, and bruises.	P, I, U

SAFETY—cont'd

			Grades
Discussion—cont'd	10	Dog bites and the necessary first-aid procedures, as well as other action that must be taken.	P, I, U
	11	First-aid procedures for bone fractures.	I, U
	12	The general first-aid procedures when accidents occur.	I, U
Dramatization	13	Children play doctor or nurse attending a child who has been injured.	P
	14	Dramatize the reporting of an accident at school, home, and elsewhere.	P, I
	15	The procedure to follow in an emergency or when someone is injured.	P, I, U
	16	Dramatize a series of injuries and then permit the class to try to determine the first-aid procedures to be followed: A student is using a penknife at school to whittle on some wood and cuts his/her hand; a student is running his/her hand along a wooden bench that is full of splinters and gets some in his/her hand; a student is tackled playing touch football and falls, striking his/her wrist on the ground.	I, U
Drawings	17	Pupils prepare drawings of first aid being administered to injured children.	P, I
Exhibit	18	Display a variety of poisonous substances or containers that hold such materials.	P, I
	19	Display the contents of a simple first-aid kit. Nurse may be helpful in determining items to be included.	I, U
	20	Display an assortment of materials, such as dressings, bandages, triangular bandages, and splints used in first aid.	I, U
Experience chart or record	21	Construct an experience chart or record that describes what to do when injured at school.	P
Guest speaker	22	Invite the school nurse to come to class to discuss first-aid procedures.	P, I, U
Individual and group reports	23	Children prepare reports on first-aid procedures for snake bites, epileptic seizures, frostbite, and fractures.	I, U
	24	Children prepare a letter inviting a member of the Red Cross to come to class to discuss first aid.	I, U
Problem solving	25	Present a series of first-aid problems to individuals or committees and let them try to solve them. Such problems might include:	U
		What would you do if a person cut his/her finger while preparing dinner? What would you do if your sister swallowed a poison, such as ammonia? What would you do if a pupil at school fell from the horizontal bar that is 7 feet high?	
Scrapbook	26	Make scrapbooks containing stories, pictures, magazine articles, and drawings about first aid.	I, U
Self-test	27	Prepare a self-test for use in the discussion on first aid.	I, U
Show and tell	28	Children tell of what they experienced when they were injured.	P

Home safety

Bulletin board	1	Display pictures and magazine and newspaper articles on home accidents and safety.	P, I, U
	2	Pupils construct for display a graph or pie-shaped chart showing the numbers and types of home accidents.	U
Discussion	3	Children's prepared lists of hazardous conditions in and around the home.	P, I

SAFETY—cont'd

		Grades
	4 Student-planned "pick-up" day at home to remove hazards.	P, I
	5 Children's observations of safe and unsafe practices in the home and elsewhere.	P, I
	6 The causes and possible ways to prevent the accidents reported in newspaper articles brought to class by students.	I, U
	7 The safe handling of blasting caps and the procedures to follow when they are found.	I, U
	8 How to turn off the electricity and the gas at home.	U
	9 Prepare a list of responsibilities of baby-sitters and discuss the safety problems that sitters may have to handle.	U
Dramatization	10 Children act out such situations as a stranger offering a ride, a cross dog barring the sidewalk, and one child double-daring another to do something reckless. Ask pupils to consider these questions: "What would you do?" and "Would you be acting safely?"	P, I
	11 Dramatize an accident in the home, such as slipping on a scatter rug that has no rubber backing, and discuss how this could have been prevented.	I, U
	12 Prepare a play on home safety for presentation to a parent group or to a school assembly.	I, U
Drawings	13 Following a discussion on safe play areas at home, children draw pictures of where they play at home.	P
	14 Following a unit on home safety, each child draws pictures of what he/she does at home to make it a safer place.	P
Exhibit	15 Children bring some of the dangerous objects found in their back yards for display.	P, I
	16 Children construct a medicine cabinet using cardboard boxes and construction paper and have all items properly labeled.	P, I
	17 Prepare an exhibit of hazardous objects or materials found in the home such as metal toys with sharp edges, sharp knives improperly stored, rugs without rubber backing, and oily rags improperly stored.	P, I, U
	18 Display pamphlets, booklets, and other resource materials on home safety for pupils' use.	I, U
	19 Display poisonous substances found in the home, such as ammonia, disinfectants, drugs, chocolate laxatives, moth balls, and crayons.	I, U
Experience chart or record	20 Prepare an experience chart on home safety containing such activities as walking carefully on polished floors, picking up toys when finished with them, and not playing with matches.	P
Flannelboard	21 Prepare home safety stories and use a flannelboard to illustrate them.	P
Guest speaker	22 Invite a representative from the National Safety Council or the local safety council to come to class to discuss home safety.	I, U
Individual and group reports	23 Pupils use drawings or pictures to illustrate daily activities that will keep themselves safe.	I, U
	24 Collect newspaper articles about accidents in the home and categorize them by types. Committees then do research and write reports about how they could have been prevented.	I, U
Model	25 Make a container for father's used razor blades.	P

SAFETY—cont'd

			Grades
Model—cont'd	26	Pupils construct a cross section of a house out of cardboard or wood and illustrate the possible hazardous places within.	I, U
Mural	27	Make a large cooperative mural of safe play areas in the neighborhood.	P, I
Newspaper	28	Pupils prepare a home safety newspaper to be published periodically containing stories about safety in the home.	I, U
Panel	29	Have a panel discussion on the topic, "Making a safe home."	I, U
Posters	30	Make posters showing how to correct hazardous conditions found in the home, such as not touching radio or electric light cords when bathing, proper position of cooking utensils on stove with handles turned in, and using a stepladder rather than a chair to stand on.	I, U
Scrapbook	31	Children prepare a scrapbook with pictures, stories, and newspaper articles on "Safety at home."	P, I, U
Show and tell	32	Children tell about home accidents.	P
Songs and poems	33	Create home safety songs and poems.	P
Survey	34	Survey the neighborhood and prepare a report on the safe and unsafe places to play.	I, U
	35	Conduct a survey of home hazards using a checklist prepared by children. Discuss how these problems can be changed. Emphasize specific areas such as unlighted, cluttered stairs; unscreened fireplaces; electric outlets and wiring; and proper place to store garden tools, matches, nails, pins, and sewing needles.	I, U
Telephone card	36	Make a card to be hung by the telephone with the number of the fire and police departments, an ambulance, the family doctor, the nearest relative, and also the home address.	P, I
Telephone number	37	Children dial home telephone number and give the last name of parent, address, and identity of road and street landmarks.	P, I
Pedestrian safety			
Bulletin board	1	Prepare a display of student drawings about pedestrian safety.	P, I, U
	2	Develop pedestrian safety slogans for use on the bulletin board such as "Courtesy is safety," "Cross at the crosswalks," and "Wait for the traffic signal before crossing streets."	P, I
	3	Make a series of charts or graphs for display showing the number and kinds of pedestrian accidents.	U
Chart	4	Prepare a chart that lists the pedestrian safety rules.	P, I
Demonstration	5	Demonstrate and practice the proper way to cross streets.	P, I
	6	Prepare a table simulating a street corner using small cars, bicycles, policeman, and traffic lights and demonstrate safe pedestrian practices.	P, I
	7	Darken room and have students dressed in various colored clothes walk in front of the room. Be sure to have someone wearing white among these students. Children discuss which colors were more easily seen.	P, I, U
	8	In a darkened room have two lighted flashlights representing auto headlights. Have a student with dark clothes and one with white clothes walk in front of the lights to show the difference in the reflection of light.	P, I, U

SAFETY—cont'd

			Grades
Discussion	9	The importance of knowing names, addresses, and telephone numbers.	P
	10	What action to take if a stranger invites you to take a ride in an automobile.	P, I
	11	The school safety patrol and its role in helping children cross streets safely.	P, I
Dramatization	12	Children bring small toy cars, trucks, and buses for use in dramatic play about pedestrian safety.	P
	13	Using a large space in the classroom or on the playground, lay out an intersection with strips of tape or chalk, including crosswalks, and have children cross the street properly. Prepare a number of crossing signal models, such as a traffic light with appropriate color, a walk-wait signal, and a stop sign.	P
Drawings	14	Children make drawings about pedestrian safety.	P, I
	15	Children draw pictures of how they come to school, pointing out safe practices.	P
Excursion	16	Visit the street corner nearest the school to see the traffic signals, the police officer, the yellow crossing lines, and other safety features.	P
Exhibit	17	Display a variety of traffic signs and discuss their meanings for traffic and pedestrian safety.	I, U
Experience chart and record	18	Prepare an experience chart or record of safety pedestrian rules that may include:	P

> Red means stop.
> Yellow means wait.
> Green means go.
> Cross at the crosswalks.

			Grades
Flannelboard	19	Prepare illustrations to tell a story of pedestrian safety with emphasis on the danger of playing between parked cars.	P, I
Game	20	Write safety rules on strips of tagboard and cut them in half to form a simple puzzle. Children try to match the cut pieces and locate the correct safety rules.	P, I
Guest speaker	21	Invite a police officer to discuss pedestrian and traffic safety.	P, I, U
	22	Invite a member of the school safety patrol to discuss correct ways to cross streets.	P, I
Individual and group report	23	Record the number and type of pedestrian accidents listed in local newspapers for a designated period.	I, U
	24	Write letters to the National Safety Council, automobile clubs, and other community organizations requesting material on pedestrian safety for use in class.	I, U
	25	Pupils prepare oral or written reports on the number, kinds, and causes of pedestrian accidents.	U
Interview	26	Pupils interview a traffic police officer and a representative of the automobile club about pedestrian accidents and how to prevent them.	I, U
Map	27	Prepare a large map showing the route each child takes to school and discuss the safest ways to come to school.	P, I
Model	28	Make a traffic signal box with red, green, and yellow lights or signals for use in dramatic play.	P

SAFETY—cont'd

		Grades
Poems	**29** Children create and learn poems about pedestrian safety, such as the following:	P

> Red says stop,
> Green says go.
> Yellow says wait,
> You'd better go slow.
> When I reach a crossing place,
> To left and right I turn my face.
> I walk, not run, across the street
> And use my head to guide my feet.
>
> Stop, look, and listen
> Before you cross the street.
> Use your eyes, use your ears
> Before you use your feet.

Posters	**30** Prepare posters and enter them in the school contest on pedestrian safety.	I, U
Problem solving	**31** Have children discuss this problem: "You come to a street corner that you must cross, but there is no signal. How will you get across?"	P, I
Puppets	**32** Make puppets and dramatize ways to be a safe pedestrian.	P
Quiz	**33** Have children write on a piece of paper the five numbers listed below and place yes or no answers beside the appropriate number to the statements listed.	P

1. We should cross streets at crosswalks.
2. We should cross streets when the traffic light is green.
3. We should look one way when crossing streets.
4. We should always go with the traffic when walking on roadways.
5. We know the yellow light at a crosswalk means wait.

| Riddle | **34** Children make up riddles, such as the following: | P |

> It stands near the corner.
> It turns red and green.
> It helps keep us safe.
> What is it?

Scrapbook	**35** Make illustrated scrapbooks with pedestrian safety rules, slogans, rhymes, and limericks.	P, I, U
	36 Prepare a scrapbook of pictures and drawings showing safety as a pedestrian.	P, I
Self-test	**37** Pupils take following self-test.	I, U

SAFETY—cont'd

Grades

Do you
	YES	NO
1. Cross streets only at intersections or marked crosswalks?	☐	☐
2. Look left and right before crossing streets, making sure that the entire crossing can be made safely?	☐	☐
3. Cross only on green light or "go" signals?	☐	☐
4. Obey directions of safety patrols or officers?	☐	☐
5. Walk on the left side facing traffic if walking on roadway and give way to approaching vehicles?	☐	☐
6. Wear white at night or carry a light?	☐	☐
7. Always get into and out of a vehicle on the side nearest the curb?	☐	☐
8. Give the motorist the right of way where there are no signals?	☐	☐
9. Stay out of streets when playing?	☐	☐
10. Watch for oncoming traffic when catching or leaving a bus?	☐	☐

Score ("yes" answers)

9-10—You may live to a ripe old age.

6-8—You may expect to get hurt before long.

5 or less—Stay in your own yard; you're living on borrowed time.

			Grades
Show and tell	38	Children tell about pedestrian hazards they have seen.	P
Television	39	Make a shadow box or TV box and have students prepare a series of drawings about pedestrian safety. Include such illustrations as wearing white at night, crossing at street corners, and waiting for the green light.	P

Recreation safety

Bulletin board	1	Prepare displays of pictures and drawings of water skiing, hunting, camping, picnicking, fishing, skating, hiking, and vacation safety.	P, I, U
	2	Display posters or drawings showing the correct and incorrect ways to get in and out of rowboats, canoes, and motorboats.	P, I, U
Chart	3	Pupils prepare and complete charts of summertime safety for reference and use at home during vacation.	I, U

Summertime safety

My summer activities:

1. _____

   _____

2. _____

   _____

3. _____

   _____

4. _____

   _____

SAFETY—cont'd

			Grades

Chart—cont'd

What could hurt me:

1. _____
   _____

2. _____
   _____

3. _____
   _____

4. _____
   _____

How to keep safe:

1. _____
   _____

2. _____
   _____

3. _____
   _____

4. _____
   _____

Method	No.	Activity	Grades
Demonstration	4	Have the Red Cross conduct a demonstration of swimming, boating, and beach safety at one of the local swimming pools, lakes, or rivers.	P, I, U
Discussion	5	Safety on special occasions, such as Halloween and the Fourth of July.	P, I, U
	6	The people who can help when you are injured or lost.	P, I, U
	7	Safety on picnics and outings.	P, I, U
	8	Show pupils pictures of recreational equipment, such as a canoe, gun, skate, sled, ski, baseball bat, and fishhook, and have them tell of a good safety practice when using these items.	P, I, U
	9	Safe and unsafe features of swimming in lakes, rivers, oceans, canals, and other places. Learn how to choose a safe swimming area.	I, U
	10	The laws with which pupils should be familiar when hunting, fishing, and camping.	I, U
	11	Methods of protection while participating in various sports, such as football, baseball, basketball, and skiing.	I, U
	12	Safety in skin and scuba diving.	I, U
	13	Safe hunting procedures.	U
Dramatization	14	Children participate in dramatic play of safe practices while camping or picnicking.	P
	15	Prepare and present a skit on snow safety to an assembly, or a parent group, or broadcast it over the local radio station.	I, U
	16	Pupils write a play ("Comedy of Errors") on how not to go on a camping trip.	I, U
Drawings	17	Make drawings of safe practices while boating, swimming, skiing, playing in the snow or at the beach.	P, I, U
Exhibit	18	Display the items of a "Lost" kit that may be usable when camping or out in the woods including such things as a single-edge razor blade, fishhooks, fish line and wet flies, pencil and notebook, Band-Aids, soap and disinfectant, compass, sugar lumps, strong string (shoe laces), and matches water-proofed with paraffin. Seal the contents in a can and attach with a belt strap.	P, I, U

SAFETY—cont'd

		Grades
	19 Display such hazardous objects as fishhooks, darts, sharp-pointed sticks, and blasting caps.	P, I, U
	20 Display the appropriate clothing to wear in various outdoor activities, such as hiking, camping, hunting, skiing, and boating.	P, I, U
	21 Display the equipment needed for skin and scuba diving and discuss safety features.	I, U
	22 Display safety items that give protection in various sports: football—mouth protectors; baseball—mask; and skiing—safety binders.	I, U
Experience chart or record	23 Make an experience chart or record about safe procedures on vacations, when swimming, and at other times.	P
Game	24 Play the game "Little child lost." The teacher is a police officer and a student is lost. Have children determine what they would do, or should do, if this happens to them.	P
	25 Children collect pictures from magazines and newspapers of safe and unsafe ways of playing. Place all of these in a box and permit each child to select one item and tell whether it is a safe or unsafe procedure.	P, I, U
Guest speaker	26 Invite a member of the Red Cross or the school nurse to discuss first-aid procedures for possible recreation emergencies, such as sunburn, poisonous plants and insects, and blisters.	P, I, U
	27 Have a forest ranger discuss safe procedures in parks and playgrounds.	P, I, U
	28 Have a representative from the Red Cross or a skin and scuba diving club discuss the safety aspects of this sport.	I, U
	29 Invite guest speakers to discuss safety in such activities as football, basketball, skiing, tennis, and swimming.	I, U
	30 Have a member of the local rifle club demonstrate and discuss safety while hunting or the safe handling of guns.	U
Individual and group reports	31 Pupils prepare oral and written reports on the safety rules when camping, boating, hiking, fishing, swimming, hunting, skiing, and roller or ice skating.	I, U
	32 Pupils write a report of their favorite recreational activities and include the safety rules that should be observed when participating.	I, U
Map	33 Prepare a map showing the safe swimming area in the immediate vicinity and within a comfortable driving distance from the local community.	I, U
Mural	34 Make a mural of safe places and safe ways to play while skiing, boating, swimming, hiking, skating, and others.	P, I, U
Puppet	35 Prepare a puppet show or dramatization of a safe camping or hiking trip.	P, I
Scrapbooks	36 Pupils prepare scrapbooks containing pictures, newspaper and magazine articles, stories, and other items on safety categorized into such areas as fishing, camping, swimming, boating, hunting, skiing, and skating.	I, U
School safety		
Bulletin board	1 Prepare a display of pictures and drawings showing safety at school.	P, I, U
Cartoon	2 Conduct a school safety cartoon or slogan contest.	I, U

SAFETY—cont'd

		Grades
Chart	3 Pupils prepare a chart or graph of the nature, number, and location of accidents that occur in school.	I, U
Demonstration	4 The safe use of tools, blocks, and other equipment.	P, I
	5 The safe way to use stairways, drinking fountains, and school equipment.	P, I
	6 The safe way to use playground apparatus and equipment, such as slides, swings, bats, and tetherballs.	P, I
Discussion	7 School safety helpers, such as the teacher, nurse, custodian, and bus driver.	P
	8 The dangers of throwing sticks, climbing fences, throwing balls improperly, and running in the halls or crowded areas.	P, I
	9 The proper use of fountain pens, scissors, and other implements in class, as well as the proper way to open doors and walk in the corridors.	P, I
	10 Prepare a list of safety rules for the classroom and the playground that may include:	P, I

> I walk in the halls.
> I use the slides properly.
> I use scissors and pencils carefully.
> I do not push when in line.
> I do not throw rocks or other objects.

		Grades
	11 What to do when injured at school.	P, I, U
	12 School and playground hazards and accidents.	P, I, U
Dramatization	13 Make puppets and dramatize safety practices at school.	P
	14 Dramatize safety precautions when playing softball, lining up in the cafeteria, waiting for the bus, and other situations.	P, I, U
Drawings	15 Make drawings of play areas and equipment and place captions below about school safety.	P, I
Excursion	16 Walk around the school and locate hazards to safety.	P, I
Exhibit	17 Children prepare drawings on safety in school, such as keeping feet under tables and desks, not pulling chairs away from others, and the correct way to use the drinking fountain.	P, I
Experience chart or record	18 Prepare an experience chart or record of safe practices in school.	P
Flannelboard	19 Make two children out of construction paper (or make drawings) and call them "Safety Sam" and "Silly Billy." Tell a story about school safety including these two characters and use drawings to illustrate their activities.	P, I

> Safety Sam:
> Waits in line
> Stops the swing and gets off
> Uses pencils properly
>
> Silly Billy:
> Pushes in line
> Jumps off the swing
> Jabs pencils in his hand

SAFETY—cont'd

		Grades
Guest speaker	**20** Invite a physical education teacher or the supervisor of physical education to discuss and demonstrate safety on the playground.	P, I, U
Handbook	**21** A committee of pupils prepares an illustrated handbook of safe practices at school for distribution to all students.	I, U
Individual and group reports	**22** Pupils or pupil committees prepare articles for the school newspaper on school safety.	I, U
	23 Pupils prepare written reports on the causes of school accidents and ways to prevent them.	I, U
Interview	**24** A committee of pupils interviews the school nurse to find out how accidents occur in the school. After reporting their findings in class, they formulate a plan of prevention.	I, U
Map	**25** Prepare a composite map of the neighborhood indicating the location of the traffic lights, stop signs, police officers, and sidewalks. Have students draw the safest way home using colored crayons or yarn. Children may also prepare individual maps to be taken home to parents.	P, I
	26 Draw map of the school grounds and illustrate safe and unsafe places to play.	I, U
	27 Plot locations of accidents on map of school and school grounds.	I, U
	28 Teacher prepares map of school showing drinking fountains, bicycle racks, incinerators, and other places. Place on bulletin board and have children mark the hazardous places in school and locate accidents that occur.	P, I
Panel	**29** Have panel discussion on "Safety at school."	I, U
Problem solving	**30** Discuss solutions to these safety problems:	P, I
	A student runs from the cafeteria with an ice cream stick in his/her mouth. Two groups walking in the corridor meet at a corner. One student opens a door and bumps two students standing in the corridor. A student throws his/her bat while playing in a softball game. A student steps in front of another student who is using the swing.	
	31 Form a school safety committee to locate hazardous school areas and plan ways to prevent accidents.	I, U
Questionnaire	**32** Prepare a "Do you remember?" questionnaire as a concluding activity to the unit on school safety. Include 15 to 20 questions to be answered verbally by yes or no, such as, "Do I always walk down the halls and stairways properly?"	P, I
Songs and poems	**33** Create songs, poems, stories, and drawings about school safety.	P
Survey	**34** Children conduct a hazard hunt on school property and safely remove such objects as glass, rocks, wire, tacks, and nails.	P, I
	35 Children are "safety detectives" and locate examples of safety at school.	P, I
	36 Pupils prepare a safety checklist and then survey the school for hazards.	I, U

		TOBACCO★	

			Grades
Buzz group	1	Conduct a buzz group discussion on the question, "Why should young people not use tobacco?"	U
Chart	2	Pupils prepare charts for bulletin board displays regarding the rise in death rates of major diseases associated with smoking; comparison of overall death rates of smokers and nonsmokers; location of disorders associated with smoking on an outline figure of the human body; and computation of the cost of smoking one to two packages of cigarettes a day or a week for 1 year and listing of other uses of the same amount of money.	I, U
Debate	3	Have a debate on the use of tobacco by teenagers. Try to answer the questions: "Should teenagers chew tobacco or smoke? Should tobacco advertising in newspapers and magazines be controlled?"	U
Demonstration	4	Prepare materials as shown in Fig. 12-22. Open and close pinch clamp (acts as siphon—water may need to be replaced several times) to stimulate puffing on cigarette and observe (a) smoke collecting, (b) color of water after shaking flask, and (c) residue on walls of flask. Later discuss relationships to lung tissue in persons who smoke. Place pieces of cotton in glass tube between cigarette and flask without stopping up tube. After smoking several cigarettes (use siphon action previously mentioned), remove cotton and examine. Wipe tar-stained cotton on growing plants and observe results (abnormal growths will appear).	I, U
	5	Blow cigarette smoke through a clean handkerchief or paper tissue with and without inhaling. Observe difference in amount of residue and relate to lung tissue.	I, U
	6	Place a drop of solution containing paramecia on a microscopic slide and observe movement under the low-power lens of a microscope. Blow smoke on the slide and observe the effect on the paramecia.	I, U
	7	Wipe a cotton pellet that has been saturated with tobacco tars on the tongue of a live frog and note the frog's temporary collapse.	I, U
	8	Make a nicotine insecticide by soaking cotton pellets from a smoking machine or cigarette tobacco in water. Test and use as a spray on insects.	I, U
	9	Prepare a smoking machine using materials shown in Fig. 12-23. Insert loosely packed cotton into the tubing and put a cigarette into the open end of tubing. Press firmly on the plastic container to force air out before lighting the cigarette and then proceed with slow and regular pumping action. Later, cotton can be withdrawn from tubing to show the accumulation of tar.	I, U
	10	Prepare a smoking machine using materials shown in Fig. 12-24. Light the cigarette and pump the vacuum so as to draw smoke from cigarette into gallon jar and water until the cigarette is burned completely. Use additional cigarettes until tars can be seen in the water and around the jar. Cotton can be inserted in tubing behind the cigarette and examined later for tars.	I, U

★Check the local American Lung Association or the American Cancer Society for resources and material aids.

Two-holed
rubber
stopper

FIG. 12-22. Smoking machine demonstration.

			Grades
Discussion	11	The nature of tobacco smoke.	I, U
	12	The physiological effects of tobacco on the human body.	I, U
	13	The relationship of the use of tobacco to lung cancer.	I, U
	14	Analyze the claims of several tobacco advertisements.	I, U
	15	Why people smoke.	I, U
	16	Laws related to smoking.	I, U
Dramatization	17	Prepare a skit illustrating social pressures used by students to get others to smoke. Follow with a discussion regarding actions pupils should take to handle such situations.	U
Exhibit	18	Display a variety of brands and kinds of cigarettes. Break open several and show the types of filter tips.	I, U
	19	Display magazines, pamphlets, and other materials for student reference and use.	I, U
	20	Display newspaper and magazine articles on the use of tobacco.	I, U
	21	Display a variety of advertisements found in newspapers and magazines.	I, U

TOBACCO—cont'd

FIG. 12-23. Smoking machine demonstration.

FIG. 12-24. Smoking machine demonstration.

			Grades
Exhibit—cont'd	22	Display a variety of charts and graphs available from the American Cancer Society on the extent and effect of smoking.	U
	23	Obtain samples of lungs of smoker and nonsmoker or photographs from the American Cancer Society.	I, U
Experiment	24	Obtain some nicotine and dissolve it in water in a fish bowl. Place a tadpole in the bowl and observe the results.	I, U
Graph	25	Pupils prepare graphs showing the incidence of heart disease, lung cancer, and emphysema among smokers and nonsmokers, as well as the costs of smoking cigarettes yearly.	U
Guest speaker	26	Invite a physician to discuss and answer questions about the effect of tobacco on health.	I, U
Individual and group reports	27	Pupils investigate the laws regarding the sale of tobacco to minors.	U
	28	Pupils prepare oral and written reports on recent magazine articles about tobacco.	I, U

TOBACCO—cont'd

		Grades
	29 Pupils prepare oral and written reports on emphysema, chronic bronchitis, lung cancer, effectiveness of filter-tipped cigarettes, and number of cigarettes sold.	I, U
	30 Students prepare individual notebooks on tobacco and health, including analysis of advertising, magazine article summaries, research data, and pictures.	I, U
Interview	31 Interview the local health officer for information about the incidence of lung cancer in the community.	U
	32 A committee of children interviews one or more physicians about the effect of tobacco on health.	U
	33 Ask people who smoke and do not smoke for advice on their decision to smoke or not to smoke.	U
Newspaper	34 Prepare articles for the school newspaper as part of an antismoking or an antichewing campaign.	U
Parents	35 Involve parents in an antismoking campaign program with students writing letters against smoking, distributing pamphlets, or inviting them to see a film at school.	I, U
Self-test	36 Conduct a self-test on tobacco.	I, U

What do you know about smoking?

Circle the correct answers to the right. If you do not know the answer, circle the letter "D."

1.	Smoking reduces the appetite.	T	F	D
2.	Smoking irritates the throat.	T	F	D
3.	Inhaling causes a smoker to absorb more nicotine.	T	F	D
4.	Smoking may become a habit.	T	F	D
5.	Teenagers often start smoking because they want to act like adults.	T	F	D
6.	Some people smoke to relieve tension.	T	F	D
7.	Smoke from tobacco may be annoying and unpleasant to other persons.	T	F	D
8.	Smoking can cause lung cancer.	T	F	D
9.	Filter-tipped cigarettes prevent the absorption of nicotine into the body.	T	F	D
10.	The use of tobacco causes a shortness of breath.	T	F	D

		Grades
Survey	37 A committee of pupils conducts an opinion survey of parents, friends, doctors, coaches, and teachers on the use of tobacco by teenagers.	U
	38 Conduct a survey of the tobacco using habits of pupils in the class. Have pupils post results on the bulletin board in the form of a bar graph.	U

SUMMARY

Methods and techniques of teaching health are important in the instruction program that seeks to develop health practices and attitudes based on scientific information. It is also important for the teacher to utilize a variety of methods because different approaches will appeal to the particular learning style of different children. Teachers who are familiar with the variety of activities described in this chapter and are competent in the selection of appropriate activities with content can provide effective health education programs for their students.

Selecting and using good instructional aids for teaching health and evaluating outcomes are closely associated with methods and techniques. The next two chapters deal specifically with instructional aids and evaluation. Teachers should consider all three chapters in planning their programs. Many of the teaching ideas contained in this chapter are a composite of techniques and instructional aids and in some cases could also be used as evaluative techniques.

QUESTIONS FOR DISCUSSION

1. What is the role of the teacher in the learning process in health education?
2. What are the meanings of the terms *method* and *technique?*
3. What factors related to learning must receive teacher consideration?
4. What are the types of methods that contribute to effective health teaching and what are illustrations of each to health education?
5. What are the advantages and disadvantages of the various types of teaching methods that may be used in the health instruction program?
6. What guidelines help the teacher determine the methods of health teaching to be used in the primary, intermediate, and upper grades?
7. What is meant by the term *incidents* or *incidental teaching* in health education? Provide illustrations.
8. What are the limitations and possible problems in the use of incidents in health teaching?
9. How should the textbook be used when teaching health?
10. How can instructional materials be used effectively with methods in health teaching?
11. What are several ways students may be used in peer education programs?
12. What are the relationships between the objectives of health education and the techniques in teaching?
13. What factors should receive consideration when selecting activities and experiences for health teaching?
14. What are several activities or experiences suitable for health teaching in the primary, intermediate, and upper grades?
15. What are several health areas in which bulletin boards may be used in health teaching?
16. What are several demonstrations suitable for the primary, intermediate, and upper grades when teaching health?
17. In what grades are the use of buzz groups and self-tests probably most appropriate?
18. What are several experiments suitable for teaching fire safety, dental health, nutrition, and communicable disease control?
19. What are several illustrations of dramatic play that are usable in health teaching?
20. What are some examples of the use of the flannelboard in the health instruction program?
21. How can models, charts, and graphs be specifically used in the teaching of health?

SELECTED REFERENCES

American School Health Association: How to plan and present a school-community health fair, Journal of School Health **45:** Dec., 1975.

Banks, M.E.: Gifted children benefit from health classes accelerated to their needs, Journal of School Health **53:** Aug., 1983.

Canfield, J., and Wells, H.C.: One-hundred ways to enhance self-concept in the classroom, Englewood Cliffs, N.J., 1976, Prentice-Hall, Inc.

Clark, K.M.: A multimedia approach to mental health, School Health Review **3:** March/April, 1972.

Cornacchia, H.J., Smith, D.E., and Bentel, D.J.: Drugs in the classroom: a conceptual model for school programs, ed. 2, St. Louis, 1978, The C.V. Mosby Co.

Costa, A.L., editor: Developing minds: a resource book for teaching thinking, Alexandria, Va., 1985, The Association for Supervision and Curriculum Development.

Crosby, R.: Self-concept development, Journal of School Health **52:** Sept., 1982.

Dinkmeyer, D., and Ogburn, K.D.: Psychologists' priorities: premium on developing understanding of self and others, Psychology in the Schools **11:** Jan., 1974.

Frager, A.M.: Toward improved instruction in hearing health at the elementary school level, Journal of School Health **56:** May, 1986.

Horowitz, L.G.: The self-care motivation model: theory and practice in healthy human development, Journal of School Health **55:** Feb., 1985.

Jaycox, S., et al.: Theory-based health education activities for third to sixth grade children, Journal of School Health **53:** Dec., 1983.

Kellam, S.G., et al.: Mental health and going to school, Chicago, 1975, University of Chicago Press.

Kittleson, M.J., and Ragon, B.M.: Project panther[2], Health Education, Dec., 1984/Jan., 1985.

McGuire, R.: Flintstones and Snoopy join the antismoking campaign, School Health Review 3: March/April, 1972.

Merki, M., and Merki, D.: Breaking down barriers in the classroom, Health Education, Sept./Oct., 1982.

Moody, L.E., and Laurent, M.: Promoting health through the use of storytelling, Health Education, Jan./Feb., 1984.

National Clearing House for Smoking and Health: Smoking and health experiments, demonstrations and exhibits, 1968, U.S. Department of Health, Education, and Welfare, Public Health Service.

Perry, C., Mullis, R.M., and Maile, M.C.: Modifying the eating behavior of young children, Journal of School Health 55: Dec., 1985.

Petosa, R.: Enhancing the health competence of school-age children through behavioral self-management skills, Journal of School Health 56: Aug., 1986.

Pfeffer, J.: Youth scene theater: health education comes alive in rural Maryland, Journal of School Health 56: Aug., 1986.

Richardson, G.E., Burns, A., and Falcone, J.: Environmental health simulations: island city and production, Health Education, Oct./Nov., 1986.

Simon, S.B., Howe, L.W., and Kirschenbaum, H.: Value clarification: a handbook of practical strategies for teachers and students, New York, 1972, Hart Publishing Co., Inc.

Steinhausen, G.W.: Peer education programs: a look nationally, Health Education, Nov./Dec., 1983.

Talabere, L.R., and Beyrer, M.K.: Health education: perspectives in poetry, Health Education, Oct./Nov., 1986.

Turner, S.B., and Connor, M.J.E.: The Brooklyn Center, Minnesota, student health fair: an impetus for learning, Journal of School Health 54: Nov., 1984.

Wolff, M.A.: According to whom? Helping students analyze contrasting views of reality, Educational Leadership 44: Oct., 1986.

CHAPTER

13

INSTRUCTIONAL AIDS FOR HEALTH TEACHING

If the only tool you have is a hammer, you tend to see every problem as a nail.

ABRAHAM MASLOW

KEY CONCEPT: Achievement of favorable health attitudes and health behaviors can be aided through the selection and use of appropriate teaching aids.

The quality and value of health instruction depends largely on the classroom teacher's effective use of appropriate methods, techniques, and strategies and the careful selection of the best available teaching aids. The teacher faces a challenging task in the selection and use of instructional aids for health education.

Health instruction must be sensitive to the latest and most reliable research and information from the broad spectrum of the biological, social, and physical sciences. Unlike some other areas of the elementary school curriculum, content and concepts in health and safety often change markedly and abruptly with new developments in medicine, public health, dentistry, nutrition, pharmacology, physiology, psychology, physical fitness, first aid and emergency care, and many other areas.

Therefore the classroom teacher—involved in a diverse range of subject matter areas—must keep abreast of the significant and applicable contributions of all those fields that bear on personal, family, and community health. To do this, the teacher needs to know where to locate scientifically accurate information and appealing teaching aids.

Resources and instructional aids are what the teacher makes of them. The best materials may be of little value when used improperly or ineffectively.

WHAT ARE INSTRUCTIONAL AIDS IN HEALTH EDUCATION?

Instructional aids are those materials used to enhance pupil learning. They are meant to complement effective teaching. Everything in the pupils' environment that contributes in any degree to learning may be considered an aid. Defined in these broad terms, instructional aids include all items that teachers and pupils use, such as bulletin boards, cartoons, charts, pictures and photographs, maps, objects, specimens, models, posters, textbooks, workbooks, programmed instruction guides, newspaper and magazine articles, pamphlets, films, filmstrips, computer software, videotapes, tape recordings, records, songs, radio and TV programs, slides, transparencies, and exhibits. Pencils, paper, chalk, chalkboards, and so on are also in reality instructional aids, but they will not be discussed here.

Aids to learning are used for a variety of purposes, but in general they serve as (1) sensory experiences that provide greater understanding of abstract thoughts and ideas, making them concrete and specific, and (2) important motivational devices.

Bulletin boards are an effective way to present information using cartoons, charts, graphs, maps, posters, and other illustrative materials. Teachers should constantly be alert for potential bulletin board material relating to health and safety; it may appear in newspapers, magazines, pamphlets, and other printed materials. Students can actively participate in locating and preparing suitable material for the bulletin board.

Cartoons relating to a wide range of current problems in child health and safety can be produced by the students or selected from newspapers and magazines. Cartoons often provide the qualities of humor and relevance that can motivate pupils toward improved attitudes and behaviors (Fig. 13-1). Teachers should take care that the humor does not overshadow the message presented.

"I don't care if it does run up the light bill . . . brush them!"

FIG. 13-1. *(Copyright 1969 by Consumers Union of United States, Inc., Mount Vernon, NY 10550. Reprinted by permission from Consumer Reports, March 1969.)*

Charts, graphs, maps, posters, and *data* (Fig. 13-2) for these visual aids are readily available from numerous sources or can be prepared by students, teachers, or both. They should not be too involved or complicated; they should represent one or a few basic ideas or concepts that can be readily perceived and understood by pupils.

Objects, specimens, and *models* may be animate or inanimate. Hamsters may be used in classroom diet studies. On occasion children may bring a pet to class and talk about caring for its health and safety. Specimens, such as lung tissue (smoker and nonsmoker) or animal organs, can provide realism in certain learning situations. Anatomy models—a torso, ear, eye, or brain—can help students better understand the remarkable interrelationships of body organs and systems in maintaining good health.

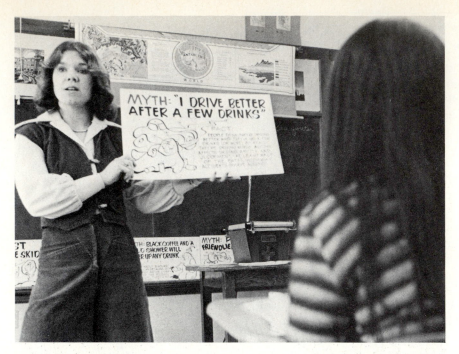

FIG. 13–2. Posters are usable in health teaching. *(Courtesy Mary Wilbert Smith, Educational Service District #121, Seattle, Wash.)*

Textbooks are available and serve as basic reference sources for both pupil and teacher. These aids are discussed in greater detail later in this chapter.

Newspaper items, magazine articles, pamphlets, books, and *other printed material* (Figs. 13-3 and 13-4)—including popular paperbacks and reference books—offer good sources of information for the teacher and students in connection with research projects, class discussion, bulletin board material, and related assignments. Care should be taken to assure that these sources are up to date and scientifically sound.

Poems are generally more effective with younger children. Even with children in the lower grades, the message should be clear and precise, not vague and trite.

Filmstrips, films, videotapes, transparencies, and *slides* are available in many topical areas. Most are commercially produced, though pupils and teachers can prepare some of their own. See the section on student- and teacher-prepared instructional aids (p. 343) for additional details.

Tape recordings are generally available in two forms: cassettes and reel-to-reel tapes. The cassette is by far the more popular and easier to handle for use in schools. Tapes are available with prepared audio, or they can be purchased blank. Prepared tapes often accompany some other material, such as a model or filmstrip. Student- and/or teacher-prepared tapes can add much excitement to health learning. Even young students can learn to make their own recordings using a cassette. In addition, the audio portions of radio and TV programs and films can be recorded for use in the classroom. Resource people can be interviewed using tape recordings for enrichment of classroom studies.

Music, records, and *songs* appeal to children. Music can aid in relaxation, the lyrics of a catchy tune can assist in conveying health content, and songs can be a fun way of learning.

FIG. 13–3. Students use magazine materials to learn health concepts. *(Courtesy Mary Wilbert Smith, Educational Service District #121, Seattle, Wash.)*

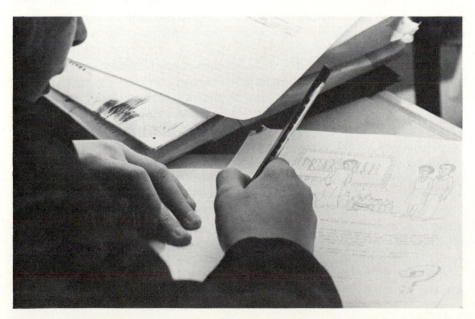

FIG. 13–4. Duplicated materials aid students in learning about drugs through independent study. *(Courtesy Mary Wilbert Smith, Educational Service District #121, Seattle, Wash.)*

TV and *radio,* both at school and in the home, offer many opportunities for timely and worthwhile health education. Specials on TV and radio deal with the health and safety problems of children and adults. Problems are usually accurately presented and analyzed by the networks and many local stations. These two all-pervasive media also provide health news items and public service announcements, the latter usually bringing a message from an official or voluntary health agency or a professional society within the health professions.

Even commercials on TV and radio can be used as teaching aids. Students can discuss the questions of the validity and reality of commercials promoting products and services for weight reduction and skin problems, the nutritional value of foods, eye care, toy safety, alcoholic beverages, motor vehicles (including motor bikes and mopeds), and other health-related topics.

Multimedia kits for teaching about specific health topics are now purchased and used by many schools. They generally are made up of all the material aids a teacher will need to teach some specific health concepts or content. A simple kit might include a set of filmstrips, a record or a cassette, and a teacher's guide. More complex kits also include 16-mm films, puppets, games, worksheets, posters, and other "hands-on" items. Good kits are extremely helpful because all the materials needed to teach the unit are located in one place, which saves the teacher much valuable time.

Exhibits may be the result of a pupil project or they may be bought, rented, or obtained free from commercial sources, health departments, voluntary health agencies, agricultural extension services, military organizations, and professional—medical, dental, or nursing—societies. Exhibits should be timely and attractive, should offer a clear message, and should not be left on display for too long. They may serve in three ways: (1) motivation of students, (2) peer education, and (3) parent education.

Computers are rapidly being accepted as classroom teaching aids. Health-related computer programs ("software") are available for purchase. One example of such a program is "Grab a Byte," a computer program in nutrition for grades 6, 7, and 8, produced by the Washington State Dairy Council and the Seattle Pacific Science Center. There are three separate programs within this packet:

Restaurant: Students enter their own height, weight, and age into the computer. From an accompanying menu they then choose a variety of foods to create a meal. The computer responds by displaying the nutritional value of the chosen meal based on calories, proteins, vitamins, and so on.

Grab a Grape: Students choose from six nutritional categories to be quizzed at three levels of difficulty. Categories include food facts, weight management, and food and sports, among others.

Nutrition Sleuth: The student becomes "Inspector Good Diet" and is given a clue to solve a nutrition mystery. An incorrect response results in a new clue. The score is displayed as each new nutrition concept is presented.

A major problem with computers in the classroom is nonstandardized equipment. A package programmed for use with computer brand *A* cannot directly be used in computer brands *B, C,* or *D.* To overcome this problem, teachers can learn to develop their own programs. Some major computer retail outlets offer free or inexpensive courses to prospective purchasers, and colleges and universities have training available. Fortunately, recent increases in the amount of software available for all major computer systems, accompanied by improvement in quality and content, has alleviated the problem somewhat.

The computer possibilities for innovative health teaching that will motivate students is extremely exciting. However, since recent research indicates that when left on their own, boys tend to use computers more often than girls in the school setting, teachers must be alert to scheduling equal computer time for all of the students.

HOW SHOULD INSTRUCTIONAL AIDS BE USED?

Teachers should give consideration to certain basic procedures when they use instructional aids if they are to obtain the best results. The following factors must receive consideration: (1) the selection of proper aids, (2) the availabilty of items, (3) adequate preparation for use, and (4) evaluation.

Guiding principles

The following suggestions will help guide the teacher in the proper use of instructional aids:

1. The teacher must clearly know how a particular learning aid fits into a specific situation. Instructional aids are not meant to do the teaching for the teacher. They should be used to provide greater meaning to the lesson.

2. Audiovisual materials should always be previewed by the teacher before use in class.

3. Teachers should have aids readily accessible when the lesson starts. It is disconcerting for a class to have to wait for the teacher to locate materials that have been misplaced. When this occurs, continuity and interest in the lesson are often lost.

4. If a number of different instructional aids are to be used, it may be advisable to use them one at a time in sequence. More than one item can be displayed at a time when it is necessary to show relationships with graphs or charts. When used in a logical sequence, instructional aids should complement each other.

5. Evaluation should be made each time instructional aids are used. This need not be a cumbersome process. Teacher observations of pupil attention, interest, opinions, and other subjective feedback are often adequate ways of obtaining clues to the effectiveness of a particular learning aid. Questions can be asked to ascertain if students understand the main points represented, if the aids show the relationships to material already introduced, and if the aids helped achieve the objectives of the lesson.

Selection of instructional aids

The variety of materials available in health instruction and the many uses for these materials require the need for careful selection by the teacher. Each type of aid has a particular function, that is, each aid usually can be used to the best advantage with some particular type of presentation. Some examples of this follow:

1. If an object or its parts are to be named, selected, or manipulated, have the object or a model of it for students to view and use; objects can include items such as actual food, food containers, animal organs, microscopes and slides, bicycles, seat belts, stethoscopes, and sphygmomanometers.

2. If an object is inaccessible, perhaps it can be adequately represented by still pictures. A series of still pictures can capture an event. They can be used in station work or on bulletin boards for students to work with in small groups or independently.

3. Films and videotapes are appropriate when motion and time-space relationships are important, such as when learning about the circulatory and other body systems, environmental concepts, and consumer health issues. Films are also effective in depicting social interaction and behavioral concepts.

Another important point in the proper selection of any audiovisual aid is its suitability and appropriateness for the age, maturity, family and community background, and experience of the children with whom it is to be used. A teaching aid is most valuable when it meets these criteria. Consequently, if an aid is unsuited to the level of maturity, background, experience, interest, or needs of a particular group, it cannot provide the maximum impact. If an aid is too advanced or difficult for the group, it may be frustrating. If it is below the maturity level of a group, it may stifle interest.

Availability of instructional aids

Teachers must plan well in advance of the need for instructional aids to be assured of availability at the time needed. It may take 6 to 8 weeks or longer to reserve films, cassettes, books, or other audiovisual materials from the health resource center, building library, local community health agency, or other source. Planning generally ensures the availability of the desired teaching aids and allows time for preview and examination before classroom use. In addition, should teachers find an item cannot be obtained on the desired date or dates, they have sufficient time to change their teaching schedule, locate substitute materials, or prepare teacher-made aids.

Preparation for use of instructional aids

Adequate preparation by both the teacher and the pupils is necessary for instructional aids to be used effectively. One undesirable tendency in the use of instructional aids is to use them without attempting to ensure that the pupils derive the greatest benefit from their use. Films and TV have often been used more for entertainment than for their contribution to learning. This does not mean to imply that aids should not be entertaining. It does mean that aids cannot be justified in health education solely on the basis of their entertainment value.

With some visual aids (motion pictures, videotapes, slides, and filmstrips) lesson plans and teachers' guides are supplied. In most cases, though, it is necessary for teachers to adapt these lessons or guides based on their knowledge of the students' needs.

Proper preparation by both teacher and pupils helps avoid passive receptivity on the part of the children. The teacher should clearly articulate to the students the learning objectives to be derived from using material aids. Thus the learners know what is expected of them, what to examine the material for, and how the experience relates to their study.

A preplanned question- and answer-period should follow the use of most material aids. This can be done orally or in writing, individually or in groups, and can be led by either the teacher or student(s). Questions similar to the following can help the teacher assess student understanding and perceptions. "What were some of the important things you learned from this film?" "How do you think the young girl felt when her dog died?" "How do you think the young boy felt when he learned his family was moving to the city?" "If you were going to make a film about this topic, what would you do differently?" "Were there things you didn't understand about the film?" "What were they?"

An important teaching technique is to use the material more than once. For example, a film might be introduced and shown to the students. Following a discussion in which students articulate what they observed, heard, and learned, the same film is shown again. Before the second viewing the teacher can suggest certain key points students should look and listen for to clarify discrepancies expressed during the discussion and alert them to detect significant facts that were apparently missed or misunderstood during the first viewing. The second viewing should also be followed by a question- and answer-session or assignment.

Effective use of instructional aids can improve learning, but aids should not limit the degree of creativity and ingenuity of the teacher or limit student interaction.

Evaluation of instructional aids

Instructional aids in health education need to be evaluated to determine (1) their value in the educational process, and (2) their contribution to the achievement of the instructional goals.

Objective evaluation of instructional aids is difficult for the classroom teacher because assessments are complex and time consuming, and reliable and valid instruments are not available. However, subjective measurements can serve as indicators of the value of the aids being used.

The following are suggestions for general questions to be asked to determine the effectiveness of instructional aids:

How well do the materials used contribute to the students' achievement of the objectives?

Are the materials appealing to the students as evidenced by class interest and attention?

What changes in the materials are needed to make them more appealing to students and to more effectively achieve the instructional objectives?

Are arrangements for the use of the materials convenient?

Is the content presented accurate?

Are the materials suitable for grade level, maturity, and experience of students?

Are there sexual, racial, or other biases in the material?

Are the costs reasonable?

What is the value of the material in terms of effort and time in preparation and expense?

In some cases, the answers to these questions will be all the teacher needs to decide whether to use a particular material aid. Other situations may require a more extensive evaluation. Samples of specific evaluation forms for a variety of learning materials including textbooks, films, resource speakers, and others are given in Chapter 14 and Appendix I.

WHERE CAN TEACHERS FIND INSTRUCTIONAL AIDS?

Instructional aids for teaching health may be found within the school building or district, county or regional educational entities, and organizations outside the school. In schools, the sources include textbooks, libraries/learning resource centers, and individuals. Outside of schools, material may be obtained from health film centers, professional journals, popular magazines, state departments, the federal government, state and national organizations, clearinghouses, professional organizations, and agencies, and commercial businesses.

Materials found within the school

School textbooks. Textbooks on health and safety are available for all grade levels in the schools. Several commercial publishers offer series of textbooks that range from grades K through 8. Numerous schools throughout the country now provide one or more of the health series to encourage systematic progression of learning, beginning with the primary grades and progressing through the upper elementary grades.

Although the quality of elementary school health textbooks has improved greatly, the textbooks still have obvious limitations. First, it is impossible for authors and publishers to keep the contents up to date because of the lag between writing, publishing, and delivering a textbook. The amount of health research and information generated annually is staggering, and it is impossible to incorporate this knowledge into the textbook publishing process in a timely manner.

Second, textbook publishers must give major consideration to including only topics that will be acceptable to screening committees in populous states with statewide textbook adoption lists. Thus topics that might be of great interest to students may be downplayed or omitted for economic reasons. Some publishers now offer supplemental booklets on topics considered important but too controversial to include in the textbook itself.

Finally, the readability of the text will probably be too easy for some students and too difficult for others in the same classroom. Thus some learners may be bored while others are frustrated.

Given these limitations, textbooks can still be a valuable aid in teaching health. They contain much good information in a concise, well-ordered form. A good text can serve as the base for an enriched exploration of health topics, but it should be supplemented by appropriate aids as discussed in this chapter. In addition, it can provide an inexperienced teacher of health education with a secure starting point.

There are five major advantages to using a good health textbook:

1. It gives an accurate presentation of essential facts.
2. It presents an orderly and comprehensible arrangement of the material.
3. It furnishes a common core of content for the class.
4. It contains such teaching and learning aids as references, questions, summaries, reviews, exercises, pictures, maps, and diagrams.
5. It saves time.

TEXTBOOK SERIES FOR ELEMENTARY SCHOOLS. The textbook series are generally accompanied by a teacher's manual either bound with the text or as a separate booklet. Some publishers provide free and inexpensive materials for health education, including charts that outline the concepts to be taught at the various grade levels.

Health and safety textbooks for elementary schools can be obtained from the following sources:

Scott, Foresman & Co.
1900 E. Lake Ave.
Glenview, IL 60025
(312) 729-3000

> 1986 edition of *Health for Life:* volumes available for kindergarten through grade 8.

Laidlaw Brothers
Thatcher & Madison
River Forest, IL 60305
(312) 366-5320

> 1983 edition of *Good Health For Better Living:* volumes available for kindergarten through grade 8 (current program: "Healthful Living"):
> Kindergarten—*Study Prints*
> Grade 1—*Your Health*
> Grade 2—*Being Healthy*
> Grade 3—*Your Health and You*
> Grade 4—*Keeping Healthy*
> Grade 5—*Growing up Healthy*
> Grade 6—*Health for Living*
> Grade 7—*A Healthier You*
> Grade 8—*Your Health and Your Future*

Steck-Vaughn Co.
Box 2028
Austin, TX 78768
(512) 476-6721

> 1983 edition of *Choosing Good Health:* volumes available for kindergarten through grade 8.

Harcourt Brace Jovanovich, Inc.
5 Sampson Street
Saddlebrook, NJ 07667
(212) 308-7263

> 1978 edition of *Health Decisions for Growth:* volumes available for grades 1, 2, and 3. 1983 edition of *Health Decisions for Growth:* volumes available for grades 4, 5, and 6:
> Grade 1—*As You Grow*
> Grade 2—*You Make Choices*
> Grade 3—*At Your Best*
> Grade 4—*You Learn and Change*
> Grade 5—*Balance in Your Life*
> Grade 6—*Toward Your Future*
> 1983 edition of *HBJ Health Program:* volumes available for grades 4 through 8.

Charles E. Merrill Publishing Co.
1300 Alum Creek Dr.
Columbus, OH 43216
(614) 258-8441

> 1984 edition of *Health Focus on You:* volumes available for grades K through 8.

Libraries/learning resource centers. The school library is an excellent first place to look for good teaching aids other than textbooks. In many schools, libraries also serve as learning resource centers where a variety of teaching aids such as filmstrips, flat pictures, small kits, and other materials may be found. In some districts, a separate audiovisual center has been established that should be explored for health materials. Teachers should develop a close working relationship with the librarians and learning resource center staff.

Fiction and *nonfiction books* relating to numerous pertinent health topics can be found in the school library. Such books provide a meaningful and appropriate medium for integrating health learning with reading skills. A limited list of health-related library books, categorized by subject area with appropriate grade levels, may be found in Appendix E. Annotations are included to illustrate the possibilities of expanding and individualizing the health instruction program through the use of library books.

Encyclopedias and *almanacs* offer an interesting variety of health information that can serve as a valuable resource for integrating and correlating health studies with language skills, mathematics, and research. A sampling of topics contained in these reference materials includes census data; U.S. health expenditures; statistics about the handicapped; health costs per capita; information on heart disease including warning signs and risk factors; cardiovascular disease statistical summaries (charts and graphs); suicide rates; and data on fires, accidents, agriculture, air pollution, first aid, nutrition, and many other subjects. Also, most almanacs have a chronology of the year's events, which includes many health-related items. Reference books like these can be valuable, quick, and easy sources of information for students and teachers.

Newspapers often carry special articles by health authorities and science writers and often include daily news items on health and safety. The content is generally accurate but may at times be sensationalized. Newspaper articles can provide current information for bulletin board displays and help pupils develop the ability to critically analyze material.

A major advantage of using the various current materials in health education is that, from an early age, children may be taught to become discriminating and careful in their evaluation of reports that may be sensational, unsubstantiated, or inadequately documented.

Individuals. The *school nurse* can be an invaluable help in locating good teaching aids. Most school nurses are extremely interested in health education and willing to assist the classroom teacher in a supportive and competent manner.

Building principals, district health coordinators, and curriculum generalists are addi-

tional resource people the teacher can consult to locate appropriate sources of instructional material. Many building principals will also help the teacher find ways to offset the cost of health materials.

One should also check with *other teachers* in the building or district who conduct classes at the same grade level. Most teachers are willing to share not only materials and sources, but also teaching/learning activities and teaching ideas.

Materials located outside the school environment

Health film centers. There are many films, videotapes, and filmstrips available from a variety of sources outside the school setting. No attempt has been made in this section to identify specific audiovisual aids by title, description, or grade level because distributors continually withdraw old offerings and add new ones to keep their lists current. Therefore listed next will be the major central sources of these teaching aids. Teachers should check local units for assistance.

College and university film libraries generally have good films on health and safety. Check with the film librarian or the library nearest to you.

Departments of health at city, county, or state levels usually maintain a health film library. Many of these relate to the health problems of elementary students. Write or call for a film catalog.

Voluntary health agencies produce and distribute excellent films usually dealing with those health problems or diseases with which the agency is mainly concerned. Consult your local telephone directory or that of the major city in your state for information on the locations of the leading voluntary agencies. Write or call for a film catalog.

Commercial organizations and firms prepare and distribute films on health and safety. They also provide catalogs of health films that may be found in the school library or obtained by writing directly to the organization.

State departments of education may maintain a film library. However, since their interest is

Journal of School Health

AMERICAN JOURNAL OF

Public Health

FDA CONSUMER

AMERICAN HEALTH

Consumer Reports

FIG. 13-5. Health source journals.

in both elementary and secondary schools, it is important to check carefully to determine the grade level for which a particular film is designed.

Professional organizations of local and state medical or dental societies have films suitable for showing to nonprofessional young people. Telephone directories will help in locating these organizations.

In addition to these centralized general sources, there are many commercial film and videotape distributors. Building librarians and learning resource specialists receive catalogs and other descriptive pamphlets from distributors and producers on a regular basis. Often, films can either be rented or purchased.

Professional journals. Health education professional journals (Fig. 13-5) found in many college, university, and public libraries, are another source of information on teaching aids. Note that some of the information about aids in these journals is carried in paid advertisements, whereas other aids are examined by authorities and appear in the materials review sections. Professional journals contain many reports and studies of value in the instruction program. They also include information on children's health problems, as well as content information. Some of these journals include the following:

Health Education
The Journal of School Health
Journal of Nutrition Education
American Journal of Public Health
New England Journal of Medicine
Journal of the American Medical Association
Science
Health Values
Scientific American
FDA Consumer
American Health (general public)

Popular magazines. Popular magazines often provide well-written, authoritative articles on new developments in health. These articles must be carefully evaluated for scientific accuracy.

State departments. Local, county, and state health departments often have education sections staffed by individuals willing to help classroom teachers obtain good materials. State departments of education and the state library system may also be tapped for sources of information. The teacher is advised to be specific in making requests.

Federal government. The federal government is valuable as a source of free or inexpensive materials. Some telephone directories contain information on federal bookstores and specific regional federal offices. Assistance in obtaining federal publications can usually be obtained from the home office of one's senator or representative. Inquiries and orders can also be made directly by writing the Superintendent of Documents, U.S. Government Printing Office, Washington, D.C., 20402.

State and national organizations. Many national public and private orgnizations with health improvement goals provide suitable materials for teacher and student use. In some instances the national organizations have state or local affiliates, such as The American Heart Association, The American Cancer Society, and the March of Dimes Birth Defects Foundation. When a teacher is aware of a state or local affiliate, all requests for material should first be sent to that unit. A list of some of the national organizations that provide free and low-cost health education material is found in Appendix F.

Clearinghouses. The growth of interest in health during the past decade is reflected in the increasing number of clearinghouses of information related to various health topics. A listing of the various clearinghouses is found in Appendix G.

TEACHER- AND STUDENT-PREPARED INSTRUCTIONAL AIDS

Technological advances have opened the doors for teachers to develop their creativity even further and instill new excitement and meaning into their health instruction programs. Audio cassettes, videotapes, classroom computers, 35-mm and Polaroid cameras, and super

FIG. 13-6. Identification of emotions using "Feelings Wheel." *(Courtesy Mary Wilbert Smith, Educational Service District #121, Seattle, Wash.)*

8-mm cameras with or without sound are some of the equipment that teachers and pupils can easily operate. This equipment also provides an opportunity for cross-grade teaching with older students working on productions with younger students.

Having students role play saying no when offered an alcoholic beverage is a fairly common classroom activity. Recording the role playing on film or videotape brings a whole new dimension to the learning process. Often when students role play in front of the class, they are nervous and do not recall what happened. What they say and do cannot be reflected upon or recalled. Use of a recorder enables pupils to see and hear how they responded. It provides an excellent opportunity to discuss the experience with the pupils, analyze what actually occurred, and explore other effective options.

Pedestrian, bicycle, and motor vehicle passenger safety practices and procedures are often discussed in elementary health lessons. A teacher- or student-made super 8-mm film of actual safety hazards and positive preventive actions in the students' school and community environments can add realism and new meaning to the study. A "home-made" slide presentation with teacher or student narrative is another creative alternative to the presentation of this information.

Teacher-created slides and other materials can be used in testing. A hazardous situation depicted on the screen can be the focus for the questions, "What problems do you see?" "What would you do in this situation?" and "If you saw a younger child here what would you do or what would you tell him or her?"

Photographs, flat pictures (Fig. 13-6), and slides are among the least expensive instructional materials that can be created. Quality pictures can help learning be more interesting and effective. An appropriately selected picture will help a student (1) view more clearly a complex relationship, (2) recall a concrete or specific situation, (3) grasp the appearance of a reality, (4) easily understand an important concept, and (5) come up with questions that will often lead far beyond the immediate purpose of the photographs.

Whether photographs contribute to learning depends on how the teacher structures the learning situation. As in reading, pupils need to have their attention directed to things they can expect to find in photographs. Students must be helped to see rather than merely left to look. Carefully planned questions such as the following must be prepared by the teacher: "What do you see in this picture?" "What is the baby trying to reach?" "Is this a safe place to be?" "What do you see that makes you think it is safe?" and "What do you see that makes you think this person is lost?"

The teacher is also responsible for structuring the situation to ensure the attainment of specific outcomes. It is possible to use photographs and get responses ranging from a simple recitation of facts to complex and creative thinking. Photographs can be mounted on bulletin boards with names or written descriptions covered by flaps of paper. After a student identifies the picture, he/she lifts the flap to check the answer. Students can identify pictures they have not seen before that illustrate the idea or concept under study. They can describe what they see in the photograph along with the application of their own creative thoughts about the concept.

Flat pictures can either be held up for the entire class to see or mounted on a bulletin board for viewing individually and at greater length by students. They can be placed at a specific class station where students are asked to arrange them in a logical order to show cause-and-effect relationships or changes in sequence. Pictures dealing with the specific topics can be mixed with irrelevant pictures, and students can be challenged to select the pertinent pictures (see Fig. 13-3).

Students may be asked to list appropriate questions about a picture or series of pictures. Photographs can also be used to test students' understanding of relationships and major concepts.

These questions can serve in the selection of photographs appropriate for specific classroom instruction:

Is the photograph clear and forceful?

Is the detail clear and large enough for study?

Is the photograph large enough for group study or should it be used by one individual at a time?

Is the photograph interesting?

Does the photograph have a definite center of interest?

Does the photograph direct attention to the most significant facts rather than to unimportant details?

Is the photograph authentic?

Does the photograph cover information that the students need?

Does the photograph answer questions or explain or clarify concepts?

A filmstrip can be made without expensive photographic equipment from a roll of 35-mm clear or white movie leader and magic markers or a variety of colored, felt-tipped pens. The leader usually comes in 50-foot rolls and can be purchased at a nominal cost from most photography equipment stores.

A story line, theme, or sequence of events should be developed before the preparation of the filmstrip. Students can then draw or write directly on the leader with the colored markers. Each picture should be about 1 inch by 1 inch in size. A commercially made filmstrip should be available for comparison to ensure that all characters are drawn in the proper direction. (The tops and bottoms of each picture should be adjacent to each other.) The finished product can be shown through a regular 35-mm filmstrip projector.

Films can now be made with relative ease and minimal cost because of technologic advances in the equipment and processing of super 8-mm film and videotape equipment. This provides an opportunity for the elementary school health teacher to develop and maintain an inexpensive film library related specifically to the health curriculum.

Some suggestions for teacher and student films and videotapes include the following:

Identify the purpose and the objective of the film.

Limit subject matter to one major idea or concept or a few closely related concepts. The focus should be on the major purpose of the lesson.

Involve subject matter or techniques that cannot be covered in the normal classroom setting in other ways.

Develop a storyboard before filming to ensure a logical sequence of action.

Confine the length of the film to 4 to 6 minutes, although the actual presentation of the film might take longer if the teacher elects to make selective stops during viewing for special emphasis.

Videotaping has many advantages over filming and since most schools have access to the equipment, teachers should be encouraged to use it for enhancing learning in health. Although the following pointers relate specifically to videotaping, many of them are also useful when using 8-mm film.

The video cassette recorder, camera, and monitor are relatively easy pieces of equipment to use, and they are invaluable for providing students fairly immediate feedback of their performance or production. When using this equipment, one should keep in mind the following tips.*

1. Know the equipment. Take time beforehand to become familiar with all of the equipment. Do not waste valuable time during class trying to figure out the various functions of the machinery.

2. Let students adapt. Have the camera and monitor on when students enter the room. In this way the students can get the initial shyness,

curiosity, and playfulness out of their systems and be more prepared to role play in front of the camera later in the lesson.

3. Do not backlight. Students will not show up on film well with backlighting, so try to set up the camera with light coming in from the front or side, rather than from a window behind the students.

4. Tape only after practice. The idea behind videotaping is to make the students look good and enable them to see themselves looking good. Therefore tape only after the student is able to respond appropriately to your cues. It may be that at first a student can master only a memorized sentence, (for example, "What are we going to do there?") rather than an entire sequence of responses. Videotape that sentence and let the student see a successful, albeit limited, performance. Also, shut the monitor off when taping. Watching themselves being taped can prove distracting to students.

5. Play back only successful tapes. Do not play back mistakes. The class's amusement may be a student's embarrassment.

6. Start with the camera far away, then move in gradually. The videotape process may intimidate a student, so be as unobtrusive as possible. You can move closer after the class begins to disregard the camera.

7. Keep the camera on target. There will be times when a student will stand from a sitting position or move from a standing position (for example, when the response calls for the student to leave the situation). Follow the student's face with the camera. Do not get caught focusing on an empty chair or a student's knees.

8. Tape shy students from the side. There may be some students who cannot get accustomed to the camera; film these students from the side. Similarly, there may be students who positively do not want the class to see them on camera. Approach these students as the class is letting out and offer to show them the tape privately. Use extra reinforcement (for example, [student's name], I think you'll be surprised at how good you look. Why don't you let me show you?).

9. Be mobile. See if you can obtain a porta-

*Modified from Here's looking at you, 2000, teacher's guide, Seattle, 1986, The Comprehensive Health Education Foundation. By permission.

pack or equipment that will allow you to tape in locations other than the classroom, (for example, hallways, playground). Not only will students enjoy the activity more, but they will be more able to transfer learning to situations approximating "real life."

Puppets are excellent teaching aids. There are many types of puppets that children and teachers can make out of inexpensive materials and odds and ends. Paper plates mounted on wooden tongue depressors, tongue depressors with facial features drawn directly on them, paper bag puppets, and hand puppets made from old stockings with buttons, yarn, and felt sewn for eyes, mouth, nose and hair are among the various kinds.

Puppets do not have to be elaborately made for children to love and identify with them. With skillful guidance by the teacher, puppets can be used to help students resolve many situations and problems on the playground, deal with feelings of rejection, learn about ways to treat others, deal with someone who cheats or bullies, learn how to say no to pressure from other children, and learn positive ways to express feelings.

SELECTED PROBLEMS WITH INSTRUCTIONAL AIDS
Eliminating bias in the selection and use of instructional aids

For years little attention was paid to the hidden messages in many educational materials. Most prominent among these were messages of sexism, ageism, and racism. Although the reasons are complex, girls were generally portrayed as passive and boys as assertive and adventuresome. Boys became doctors, fire fighters, scientists, and police officers, whereas girls became nurses and mothers. With rare exceptions, senior citizens, blacks, native Americans, Asians, Latinos, and those of other cultures and races either did not exist in these materials or were presented in demeaning ways.

Because of a raised consciousness of these matters, there is no longer any need to tolerate the use of biased materials by any teacher except in a study of bias. The following criteria are listed as illustrative of the kind of considerations the teacher should use to detect bias when reviewing material aids for health instruction.*

1. Check the illustrations.
    Look for stereotypes.
    Look for tokenism.
    Who's doing what?
2. Check the storyline.
    What is the main message?
    Are one group's standards projected as the ideal?
    How are problems presented and resolved?
    Could the story be told if the sex roles were reversed?
3. Examine the lifestyles presented.
    Are negative value judgments implied?
    Do the lifestyles reflect reality.
4. Examine the relationships between people.
    Who has the power?
    Who is portrayed in supporting, subservient roles?
    How are family relationships depicted?
5. Note the "heroes."
    Whose interest is a particular hero really serving.
6. Consider the effects on a child's self-image.
    Are norms established that limit any child's aspirations or self-concept?
    Does the material reinforce or counteract positive associations with the color white and negative associations with the color black?
    Who performs all the brave and heroic deeds?
7. Watch for loaded words.
    Are there words or phrases that have offensive overtones?
    The generic use of the word *man* was accepted in the past; its use in this way today is outmoded.

---

*Adapted from Guidelines for selecting bias-free textbooks and storybooks, New York, no date given, Council on Interracial Books for Children.

Determining readability of written materials

The reading level of a written material indicates the approximate *reading grade level* a student must have attained to be able to read the material successfully. Reading level is an important factor in determining whether written materials are appropriate for the grade levels at which they may be introduced. Within any given elementary school classroom, the wide variance in student reading ability results in pupils being assigned to reading groups according to their skill. Reading specialists sometimes help with this, but the good teacher is able to analyze printed health education materials to determine those items appropriate for students' reading ability in groups or individually.

There are several systems used for determining the readability level of written materials. The Fry Readability Formula (Fig. 13-7) is one of the most widely used instruments for measuring readability. Others include the SMOG, New Hampshire, LORGE, SPACHE, Dale-Chall, and CLOZE. Although readability scores arrived at through any of these procedures must be considered approximations, they are a great asset in analyzing pamphlets, magazine articles, texts, and other written materials.

Other factors than readability level, however, should also be considered by teachers when selecting reading material for students. The appeal of the format and student interest in the topic are major determinants as to whether students will read material. The teacher should also consider nonverbal qualities, such as the use of space, graphs, illustrations, and color when selecting reading material.

Sponsored materials

Many groups and individuals offer educational materials for classroom use. Much of this material is good and can be used to supplement, broaden and enrich the content found in the regular text and reference books. Such material is valuable to the health program in that it can provide students with a variety of points of view on important problems and issues. It also usually represents the special interest of the sponsoring organization; therefore it is referred to as *sponsored material*. The list in Appendix F is illustrative of sources of sponsored material.

The introduction of sponsored materials into the classroom must be done with a certain degree of caution. All materials must be carefully evaluated by the teacher with assistance from other personnel such as the nurse and principal. One of the first things a teacher new to a district should learn is the policy and procedures relating to the use of sponsored materials.

The following questions can serve as general guidelines for deciding whether to use sponsored materials in the classroom:

1. Is the content accurate?
2. Is the material helpful in achieving the goals and objectives set up for a particular lesson, unit, or course?
3. Can the material be used without obligating the school to an individual or group in any way?
4. Is the material free of obtrusive or objectionable advertising?
5. Does the material promote or support the point of view of a special interest group? If so, are classroom materials available to present other points of view?

When in doubt as to whether to use sponsored material, teachers should try to view the entire lesson from the perspective of the students. Teachers should determine all the messages the students will receive from the questionable material and the context in which it will be presented. They should also consider the possibilities for modifying the materials. If the content is accurate and important to the lesson, but there is an excess of advertising, the advertising should be physically eliminated.

Games for health education

Using games as educational tools is a practice that has been on the rise in recent years. There

GRAPH FOR ESTIMATING READABILITY —EXTENDED

by Edward Fry, Rutgers University Reading Center, New Brunswick, N.J. 08904

DIRECTIONS: Randomly select 3 one hundred word passages from a book or an article. Plot average number of syllables and average number of sentences per 100 words on graph to determine the grade level of the material. Choose more passages per book if great variability is observed and conclude that the book has uneven readability. Few books will fall in gray area but when they do grade level scores are invalid.

Count proper nouns, numerals and initializations as words. Count a syllable for each symbol. For example, "1945" is 1 word and 4 syllables and "IRA" is 1 word and 3 syllables.

EXAMPLE:

	SYLLABLES	SENTENCES
1st Hundred Words	124	6.6
2nd Hundred Words	141	5.5
3rd Hundred Words	158	6.8
AVERAGE	141	6.3

READABILITY 7th GRADE (see dot plotted on graph)

For further information and validity data see the Journal of Reading December, 1977.

FIG. 13-7. Fry Readability Graph. *(Courtesy Edward Fry, Rutgers University.)*

Continued.

EXPANDED DIRECTIONS FOR WORKING READABILITY GRAPH

1. Randomly select three (3) sample passages and count out exactly 100 words beginning with the beginning of a sentence. Do count proper nouns, initializations, and numerals.

2. Count the number of sentences in the hundred words estimating length of the fraction of the last sentence to the nearest 1/10th.

3. Count the total number of syllables in the 100-word passage. If you don't have a hand counter available, an easy way is to simply put a mark above every syllable over one in each word, then when you get to the end of the passage, count the number of marks and add 100. Small calculators can also be used as counters by pushing numeral "1", then push the "+" sign for each word or syllable when counting.

4. Enter graph with <u>average</u> sentence length and <u>average</u> number of syllables; plot dot where the two lines intersect. Area where dot is plotted will give you the approximate grade level.

5. If a great deal of variability is found in syllable count or sentence count, putting more samples into the average is desirable.

6. A word is defined as a group of symbols with a space on either side; thus, "Joe," "IRA," "1945," and "&" are each one word.

7. A syllable is defined as a phonetic syllable. Generally, there are as many syllables as vowel sounds. For example, "stopped" is one syllable and "wanted" is two syllables. When counting syllables for numerals and initializations, count one syllable for each symbol. For example, "1945" is 4 syllables and "IRA" is 3 syllables, and "&" is 1 syllable.

FOOTNOTE: This "extended graph" does not outmode or render the earlier (1968) version inoperative or inaccurate; it is an extension.

FIG. 13-7, cont'd. Fry Readability Graph. *(Courtesy Edward Fry, Rutgers University.)*

are many educational games now on the commercial market, and some businesses offer schools free or inexpensive games related to their products. The games most notable among these deal with nutrition. Product-related games must be carefully analyzed by the teacher. Often they teach nothing, or they teach misconceptions, about health.

Some games promoted as educational aids in reality promote (directly or indirectly) a particular product or brand line. Many games are not adequately field tested or evaluated. Competitive games may encourage winning the game rather than learning. Teachers should critically evaluate any educational health games before trying them with students.

Before deciding to use any specific game for teaching health, the teacher should give consideration to these questions:

1. Is the game appropriate for the age group?
2. What is the primary function of the game? (What is it to do or represent?)
3. How will the game help students reach the health objectives of the particular lesson or unit?
4. Is the emphasis of the game on learning or winning?
5. What kinds of decisions must the players make? (Pure guesses, chance, logical or evaluative decisions, and so on.)
6. Are the anticipated results worth the class time invested?
7. Does the game directly or subtly promote a special interest or product?
8. What are the potential side effects of the game?

Factors of effective use of TV

The teaching effectiveness of instructional TV programs designed for classroom use and programs designed for general viewing is well documented by over 20 years of research. A critical factor in what a child will learn from TV is the presence of a mentor (teacher or parent) who shares the viewing and discusses what is seen with the child. Among the variables that account for successful learning from TV are those listed here.*

Characteristics of effective instructional TV programs. Significant gains in student achievement can take place with TV programs having these characteristics:

Key concepts are repeated in a variety of ways.

Use is made of animation, novelty, variety, and simple visuals.

The program entertains and informs.

A trained communicator is used to present information.

There are opportunities for students to participate in a learning activity, either in response to information presented in the program or as part of a game presented by the program.

The length of the program is matched to the attention span of the intended audience.

The principles of effective audiovisual presentation are followed.

Characteristics of effective instructional TV viewing. Achievement gains from viewing TV occur when teachers do the following:

Prepare students to receive information to be presented by the TV program

Provide reinforcing discussions and activities following viewing

Provide corrective feedback to students in follow-up discussions between students and teachers based on what students reveal they have understood from the program

Provide students with feedback on their achievement as a result of viewing

The use of TV as an instructional aid also provides an excellent opportunity for parent-teacher cooperation. It provides a convenient and important activity for home and school team teaching. It is the teacher's responsibility to initiate these activities with parents and to provide them with clear guidelines for their involvement.

---

*Adapted from Television in the classroom: what the research says, Olympia, Wash., 1981, State Superintendent of Public Instruction.

SUMMARY

Properly selected and applied instructional aids combined with skilled teaching bring excitement and fun to health learning. The interest of the general population in health has resulted in an abundance of information and materials about health-related topics. This abundance of instructional aids has increased the importance of wisdom and discretion in selecting and using health materials.

Elementary school teachers of health should know the proper and most effective uses of the various forms of instructional aids, where to find them (both within the school and from outside sources), and how to create their own aids when appropriate. Teachers also need to find access to scientifically valid health information through libraries, colleges and universities; state and federal offices; professional journals; and the mass media.

There are problems associated with many instructional aids. Teachers need to know how to identify and eliminate sexism, racism, and ageism in instructional materials; determine the readability of written materials; and analyze commercial or special-interest messages in sponsored materials.

Identification and selection of instructional aids for health teaching is an important responsibility for the elementary school teacher. The school nurse, librarian, learning resource staff, principal, and district health coordinator or curriculum director are key resource people who can help the teacher in locating, selecting, using, and evaluating instructional materials.

QUESTIONS FOR DISCUSSION

1. What are the two main purposes served by instructional aids?
2. Identify some specific kinds of instructional aids and give examples of how they can be used to enhance health teaching.
3. What are the four major factors to consider when using instructional aids? Elaborate on each factor.
4. Explain the statement, "Subjective measurements can serve as indicators of the value of instructional aids."
5. What are the pros and cons concerning the use of textbooks for health instruction?
6. Identify the different kinds of instructional aids for health teaching that can be found in the school library.
7. What sources of instructional aids for health, besides the school library, are available for teachers?
8. What are sponsored materials for health education? How can they be used? Identify any concerns the teacher should be aware of before using sponsored material.
9. Identify and describe the kinds of inexpensive instructional aids that can be made by teachers and students.
10. Describe the major teacher considerations when videotaping students.
11. What are the key considerations for getting the maximum benefit from the utilization of popular TV as a teaching aid in health instruction?

SELECTED REFERENCES

Beyrer, M.K., Nolte, A.E., and Solleder, M.K.: A directory of selected references and resources in health instruction, ed. 3, Atlanta, Ga., 1983, U.S. Department of Health and Human Services, Center for Health Promotion and Education.

Children's books about special children, Childhood Education **57**:March/April, 1981.

Cornacchia, H.J., Smith, D.E., and Bentel, D.J.: Drugs in the classroom: a conceptual model for school programs, ed. 2, St. Louis, 1978, The C.V. Mosby Co.

Dawson, M.E., and Gay, G., editors: Guidelines for avoiding biases and stereotypes in instructional television, Bloomington, Ind., 1978, Agency for Instructional Television.

Dubois, P.A., and Schubert, J.G.: Do your school policies provide equal access to computers? Are you sure? Educational Leadership **43**:March, 1986.

Elementary school library collection: a guide to books and other media, ed. 13, Greensboro, N.C., 1982 Bro-Dart Foundation.

Elementary teachers guide to free curriculum materials, Randolph, Wis., published annually, Educators Progress Service, Inc.

Eta Sigma Gamma: Selected sources of instructional materials: a national directory of sources of instructional materials in health education, patient education, and safety education, Muncie, Ind., 1980, Eta Sigma Gamma.

Guidelines for selecting bias-free textbooks and storybooks, New York, Council on Interracial Books For Children.

Handbook I: Guidelines for the development of instructional materials selection policies, Olympia, Wash., revised 1985, Superintendent of Public Instruction.

Handbook II: Textbook selection criteria, Olympia, Wash., 1981, Superintendent of Public Instruction.

Here's looking at you, 2000, teacher's guide, Seattle, 1986, The Comprehensive Health Education Foundation.

Hopkins, L.B.: The best of book bonanza, New York, 1979, Holt, Rhinehart & Winston.

Human Interaction Research Institute in collaboration with National Institute of Mental Health: Information resources and how to use them, Rockville, Md., 1975, The National Institute of Mental Health.

Kemp, J.E.: Planning and producing audiovisual materials, ed. 4, New York, 1980, Harper & Row, Publishers, Inc.

Lockheed, M.E., and Frakt, S.B.: Sex Equity: increasing girls' use of computers, The Computing Teacher, April, 1984.

Moursund, D.: Teacher's guide to computers in the elementary school, LaGrande, Ore., 1980, International Council for Computers in Education and Eastern Oregon State College.

Muther, C.: What every textbook evaluator should know, Educational Leadership **42**:April, 1985.

National Information Center for Educational Media: Computerized up-to-date references on films, Los Angeles, University of Southern California.

Schloss, P.J., and Milliren, A.P.: Learning aids: teacher-made instructional devices, Springfield, Ill., 1975, Charles C Thomas, Publisher.

Standards for evaluation of instructional materials with respect to social content, Sacramento, Ca., 1986, California State Department of Education.

Television in the classroom: what the research says . . . , Olympia, Wash., 1981, State Superintendent of Public Instruction.

Thomas, J.L., editor: Nonprint in the secondary curriculum: readings for reference, Littleton, Colo., 1982, Libraries Unlimited, Inc.

PART

VI

EVALUATION

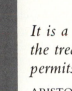

CHAPTER

14

EVALUATING THE SCHOOL HEALTH PROGRAM

It is a mark of the trained mind never to expect more precision in the treatment of any subject than the nature of that subject permits.

ARISTOTLE

KEY CONCEPT: The school health program needs periodic assessment with teachers primarily responsible for the instruction phase.

Evaluation has always been important to teachers. Conscientious teachers want and need to know the effect of their teaching on pupils. These understandings are important so that teachers may continually strive to improve. In health education they are especially significant in determining the impact of instructional programs on the lives of students. According to Hochbaum,* "The task of health education is to equip people intellectually and emotionally to make sound decisions on matters affecting their health, safety, and welfare." The process used

to determine the achievement of this task is referred to as *evaluation*.

School health programs continue to receive little or no evaluation attention. Health education in particular has not received much consideration in this regard. One reason for this neglect has been that authorities have had to concentrate their efforts in gaining acceptance of the need for the establishment of health instruction programs in schools. Also, the evaluation process is more complex in health education than in many other educational areas because of the difficulties faced in trying to determine improvement in students' health behavior. Some pupil health attitudes and practices may be immediately observable, whereas others may not

---

*Hochbaum, G.M.: Measurement of effectiveness of health education activities, International Journal of Health Education 14:April/June, 1971.

be noted for months or years after the instructional program is completed. These delayed changes may be the result of the additive effects of reinforcing information, new life situations, psychological maturation, or changed environments.

In recent years, not only has the quantity of research in school health increased, but the quality of these studies has also improved. However, it is important to note that the vast majority of school health evaluation studies reported in the literature are conducted by graduate students and university researchers, not classroom practitioners. If a school district desires a serious, meaningful evaluation of its health program, it should consider contracting with a credible university person for advice, guidance, and other services required for such an evaluation.

At this point it is important to reemphasize that this book is written for the classroom teacher. This chapter is limited to those things that are reasonable expectations for teacher understanding and practical evaluation techniques that can be readily used. Individuals desiring in-depth information on program evaluation in health education should obtain the following resources:

Green, L.W., and Lewis, F.M.: Measurement and evaluation in health education and health promotion, 1986, Mayfield Publishing Company, 285 Hamilton Ave., Palo Alto, Ca., 94301

Journal of School Health, **55**(8):Oct., 1985, P.O. Box 708, Kent, Oh., 44240

Health Education, **15**(4): 1900 Association Drive, Reston, Va., 22091

This chapter is designed to provide understandings about evaluation as applied to the total school health program and to offer practical suggestions that teachers may find useful in their classrooms and schools. This coverage is not meant to be all inclusive because of the complexity of the problem and the limited information available. It includes the four major components of the health program—instruction, services, environment, and coordination—with primary emphasis on instruction.

WHAT IS EVALUATION?

Evaluation is a process of comparing the worth or value of something with a given purpose or objective. This definition contains the three necessary parts of an evaluation: (1) a comparison, (2) a thing or object of interest, and (3) a standard (purpose or objective). The word is often erroneously used synonymously with the term *measurement*. Measurement is the part of evaluation that deals with quantitative results. It is the assignment of numbers to objects, events, or people. It answers the questions: "How much?" "Is there a health instruction curriculum?" "How much time is devoted to health instruction at each grade level?" "How many teaching aids are available?" "How many nurses are employed per 1,000 students?" The more important questions that must be answered include, "How good and of what value is the school health program?" "What impact does it have on the lives of elementary school children?" "How does it help children live in a healthful manner?" "Are all students with health problems identified, and are school programs adjusted to their needs?" "Are teaching materials current and useful?"

Evaluation must be concerned with both quantitative (How much?) and qualitative (How good?) information. Quantitative data refer to such information as the test scores of pupils, the number of nurses employed, and the number of meals served in the school lunch program. Qualitative data provide such understandings as the effectiveness of the program on children in terms of school adjustments and correction of health problems, nurse efficiency, nutritional value of meals in the school lunch or breakfast program, and the extent of behavioral change in pupils.

The technique used to gather information for assessment purposes may provide objective or subjective evidence. Objective data are obtained through such methods as surveys, checklists, inventories, and examinations given before and after programs have started, which are then organized and statistically analyzed. Subjective data are derived from the observations and opinions of teachers and others. Conclusions are drawn from these observations.

Evaluation is both a process and a product. It is not only a means to an end but an end in itself. It must concern itself with the procedures used to achieve the objectives of the program and with the methods used to reach these goals. For example, the teaching/learning activities and the teaching aids used are interrelated with the pupil behaviors sought by the teacher in the instructional program. These activities serve as the means to the end (pupil behaviors). If they are inappropriate or ineffective, they may not adequately contribute to the objective of helping pupils live in a healthful manner.

Evaluation is a continuous process. It may involve planned and organized efforts using procedures to gather objective evidence, or it may be day-to-day assessment by teachers to obtain subjective information through observations. Evaluation is an integral part of teaching that is in need of emphasis equal to that for the other phases of the health instruction program.

WHY EVALUATION IN SCHOOL HEALTH?

At this point there is need to review the *reasons for evaluating* the school health program.

First, it is sound practice to continually assess the achievement of objectives in the instructional, services, and environmental aspects of the program to assure that it keeps up with new developments in education and the health services.

Second, there is the responsibility or accountability to measure, evaluate, and report on policies, procedures, and learning outcomes to pupils, parents, school health coordinators, and other concerned persons.

Third, evaluation is an essential part of good teaching. Whereas testing and other evaluative techniques may be overdone in some classes, they are part and parcel of the teaching/learning process. Both teacher and pupil can function more efficiently when they are periodically apprised of where they are, where they are going, and how much progress they have made.

Fourth, health services help identify children who are experiencing problems that affect learning, motivation, and discipline. A periodic evaluation of the health services program is essential to ensure that the program is functioning properly and benefiting the maximum number of students on a cost-effective basis.

Fifth, the school environment must be regularly evaluated to be certain controls that maximize teaching and learning effectiveness and minimize environment-related stress are maintained. An evaluation of the school environment should include the structure of daily activity and the mechanics associated with the physical environment.

The *specific uses of evaluation* in school health instruction include the following:

1. To use as a diagnostic device. Tests can be given at the beginning of a subject or unit of study for this purpose. Both teacher and pupil benefit from knowing what they know (and, perhaps more importantly, what they do not know), how they feel, and what they do with respect to certain health and safety problems.

2. To determine progress toward objectives and to appraise the changes in understandings, attitudes, and practices that result from learning experiences in health education. In this way pupil progress may be directly assessed—though it should be kept in mind that important changes in attitude and behavior often may not occur or show for months or years.

3. To motivate pupils by stimulating their curiosity about specific health issues. The teacher can then observe the way they react to such problems in thought and practice.

4. To identify students who may be in need of special health guidance or counseling.

5. To provide data useful in the continual revision of course and curriculum content. Testing affords an objective approach to curriculum improvement in terms of meeting pupil needs.

6. To provide a basis for grading. The results of sound tests will help provide information for grading and reports of pupils' progress.

7. To provide a basis for meaningful parent education and involvement during parent-teacher conferences. Discussing student progress in health studies lends itself to reinforcing parental responsibility for student health and allows the opportunity for the parent to share observed student health attitudes and practices in the nonschool setting.

8. To provide information useful in program planning. Results of student interest tests and achievement tests can help determine appropriate grade level placement for content and time allotments in the total curriculum.

9. To improve instruction by providing feedback on teaching methods and instructional aids.

10. To develop good public relations for the health instruction program. Students and parents alike tend to place a higher value on those subjects or courses in which students are tested and assigned a grade. Also, reports of status and progress in specific units of study help communicate the idea that modern health education is significantly more comprehensive and sophisticated than the old "narrow-gauge" hygiene course that was centered around anatomy and physiology.

WHAT IS TO BE EVALUATED?

The total school health program should be subject to evaluation. This includes the major components of instruction, services, and environment and the coordination of the program. The combined impact on health behavior of these components, as shown below, indicates the importance of their assessment.

$$
\text{Coordination} \rightarrow
\begin{array}{c}
\nearrow \text{Health Services} \\
\updownarrow \\
\text{Health Instruction} \\
\updownarrow \\
\searrow \text{Healthful Environment}
\end{array}
\left.\begin{array}{c} \\ \\ \\ \\ \\ \end{array}\right\}
\begin{array}{c}
\text{Health} \\
\text{Behavior}
\end{array}
$$

Appendix H contains a good checklist of evaluative criteria for a total program. The suggested evaluation is to a degree both quantitative and qualitative.

Teachers should not be threatened by evaluation. If they feel the need for assistance, there is always someone in the school or school district who can help.

This section deals primarily with evaluation of the elementary health instruction program since this is the major purpose of the text. However, attention is given to the health services, environment, and coordination because classroom teachers should be prepared to assist in the evaluation of these components.

School health services

On the surface, evaluation of the school health services program may seem to be a rather simple matter of marking yes or no on a checklist. Is the service available or is it not? Checklists for evaluating school health services do help and are a legitimate part of any such assessment. However, they reveal nothing about the quality of service actually available. It is not as important for students, teachers, and parents to know how many nurses are employed or contracted for by the district as it is for them to know how often nurses are available to the district, and whether the nurses are capable of contributing to the elementary school health program. Since there are no mandated standards for school health services, one may anticipate a wide divergence in the quantity and quality of programs in local school districts. Appendix H provides one of the better checklists available for evaluating school health services programs.

Checklists for school health services usually include questions relating to health examinations; emergency care; screening tests for vision, hearing, and growth; dental inspections or examinations; immunizations; teacher observation of pupil health; first aid; and follow-up programs. Although a checklist may be useful in describing the scope of services available, it does not help in understanding the teacher's role. Most of the actual services are provided by the nurse or other qualified health professionals. There are, however, four important areas in which teachers have considerable responsibility: (1) observation for health problems, (2) emergency care, (3) follow-up programs, and (4) educational programs that complement some of the health services.

1. *Teacher observation* for student health problems is a major responsibility requiring conscientious effort. Few teachers are actually trained to identify children with possible vision, hearing, or postural problems. Lice and ringworm may be easier to spot, but identifying those problems still requires some training and experience. Problems relating to physical, sexual, and mental abuse are often more difficult to observe, as are those concerning drug and alcohol abuse. The teacher should ask, "If observation for health problems is one of my duties, who trains me, or how am I to gain the necessary skill?"

2. *Emergency care* is a matter all teachers have to face sometime in their career. The situation may involve a simple bruise, a seizure, broken bone, or an appendicitis attack. If the nurse is not in the building all day, is there someone else qualified to handle emergency care? Who? Is there a clearly written emergency care policy and procedure for district personnel? Has it been approved by appropriate medical and emergency care personnel? Is the teacher expected to give immediate care at the emergency site? If so, will the district provide periodic in-service training for teachers in first aid and emergency skills?

3. *Follow-up programs,* in this context, refer to what happens to the child with an identifiable health problem. It may include referral, treatment, and reentry into the school program. It is important that the teacher be kept informed as to the status of the child to plan for a smooth reentry to the classroom. The nurse can play a helpful role in this situation by carefully instructing the teacher on what to expect from the child and by providing clues for teacher observation to ensure that any signs of remission are noted and quickly reported. Follow-up programs are extremely difficult without the service of a school nurse.

4. *Educational programs* should relate to many of the health services provided to children. Basic visual, hearing, and growth and weight screenings offer excellent opportunities to teach about sight, sound, and the body. Too often these opportunities are missed and chil-

dren go from year to year never knowing what their vision test results were or what having 20/20 vision means. Nor do these children realize that someday they must assume full responsibility for their own health checkups. This is another area in which nurse and teacher should collaborate.

A thoughtful review of the school health services program should lead one to conclude that the nurse is the key element to a good program. An evaluative checklist can show on paper that a program exists, but it is usually the nurse who brings life, depth, and quality to the services. In assessing a school health services program, the key questions to be asked are: "How often is the nurse in the building?" "What is the role of the nurse?" "How much support does he or she receive?" The answers to these three questions will provide a better evaluation of the school health services program than any checklist.

The scope of school health services, including basic policies and procedures, should be written and made available to all school employees. Teachers must understand their role in relation to student health problems. They should be familiar with what services are available, where and how to make referrals, and the proper procedures to follow.

Healthful school environment

Many health factors of the school environment are relatively easy to evaluate with a checklist that includes some of these questions: "Is the water supply inspected regularly?" "Does the sewage system function properly and meet state standards?" "Is there an automatic fire alarm system, and is it checked regularly?" "Is playground equipment in good repair, organized for maximum safety, and regularly checked?" "Does the classroom lighting meet acceptable standards?" "Are heat and ventilation systems functioning properly?" Appendix H provides an illustrative instrument that may be used to assess the school environment.

There are other factors that have a more subtle effect on the school environment. One example is personal space. Students, especially older children, have need for personal space, as well as space for social interaction. Personal space can include a desk for younger students in a self-contained classroom or a locker for older students. It can also include areas such as courtyards where students can find solitude or spend quiet time during breaks or recess. This factor can have a significant impact on the emotional environment of the school and classroom. Noise, color, texture, and odor are other subtle features of a healthy school environment that must receive consideration.

The teacher is the most critical environmental factor in the emotional setting of the school. The climate in the classroom that provides security for children, the opportunity for freedom of student expression, and the fair and just treatment of all students are factors that must constantly be assessed by teachers. Sound teacher health behaviors in regard to rest, nutrition, exercise, and personal habits are necessary for optimal functioning. Teachers may need to prepare a self-inventory for their own personal use.

Coordination

Coordination refers to the planned interrelation of health instruction, services, and environment. It refers to the consistency with which each of the three components of the health program is performed throughout the district. The degree of coordination of the health program depends to a large extent on the size of the district.

The following are some of the basic criteria to consider when assessing coordination of the school health program:

1. The school district has a planned health education program with identified objectives and scope and sequence of instruction for each grade level.

2. Responsibilities are defined for all persons involved in the health program (principals, teachers, school nurses, and others).

3. The district has assigned personnel to provide leadership for the implementation and maintenance of a comprehensive health education program and has provided the necessary resources.

Additional criteria are listed in Appendix H under "Administration."

EVALUATING THE HEALTH INSTRUCTION PROGRAM

The health instruction program can be assessed in terms of the process used and the product (impact on students). Each of these categories can in turn be assessed both quantitatively and qualitatively. *Process evaluation* includes teaching aids and teaching strategies and techniques. It may also cover a variety of other areas, such as adequacy of objectives and content in meeting student needs and interests, the curriculum guide, appropriate grade level for topics, and content and teaching aids. *Product evaluation* refers generally to the effect of the program on students in terms of the extent to which the stated knowledges, attitudes, and practice objectives have been achieved.

Should teachers desire to conduct a brief but limited quantitative assessment of the instructional program, Appendix H contains a section that will be useful. This checklist also includes some qualitative assessment material.

This section of the text limits its coverage of instructional program evaluation to those short-term aspects that are feasible for teacher implementation. These aspects include student achievement and progress, instructional aids, and instructional methods.

Techniques used in evaluation

The techniques used in evaluation may also be referred to as instruments, devices, procedures, and strategies. Those that may be appropriate for the teacher to use in the classroom include (1) paper-and-pencil procedures—self-appraisal, peer appraisal, questionnaires, checklists, tests, surveys, anecdotal records, samples of pupils' work (projects, reports), and rating scales—and (2) observations of pupils by teachers and parents.

Teachers who plan to use paper-and-pencil

tests should conduct both pretests and posttests. Without pretests to enable the teacher to make a comparison of learning achievements, there is no way to determine whether the knowledges, attitudes, and practices reflected in posttests existed before the instructional program or whether they can be attributed to the educational activities themselves. The teacher should realize that administering a pretest becomes part of the instructional program, as it will be a learning experience for the students. Thus student gains on a posttest may be partially a result of the fact that they have taken the pretest.

In grades K through 2, paper-and-pencil devices may be used, but they will have to be presented in pictorial form. Also, with the help of parent information received from conferences and other sources, teachers may have to rely to a greater extent on observations of pupils' behavior and emotional expressions.

Evaluating student achievement and progress

How can a teacher know whether pupils have been affected by the health instruction program if no effort is made to determine what they have learned? The need for clear and concise cognitive, affective, and action domain objectives for accurately assessing pupil achievement must be reemphasized. The taxonomy of objectives by Bloom and others shown in Chapter 11 provides the information that will aid in the preparation of these objectives. When written out in this fashion, they give direction to the evaluation process.

Measuring health knowledge. Health knowledge is the easiest of objectives to measure. However, teachers will need to determine the type and frequency of devices to use depending on the length of the health instruction program and the amount of time available for evaluation. Teachers can select the strategies that are appropriate for their classrooms from those presented next.

TEACHER-PREPARED PAPER-AND-PENCIL PROCEDURES. Paper-and-pencil procedures are the most universal means of collecting evidence related to health knowledge. They may take the form of tests, self-appraisals, or peer appraisals.

Tests. The two kinds of paper-and-pencil tests most often prepared by teachers are the objective test and the written essay or subjective test. Objective test items may be placed in the two broad categories of *recognition* and *recall*. The recognition type of test item requires that the pupil recognize and select the correct answer, which is shown among other, incorrect answers in the test item. The recall type of test item requires that the pupil supply the correct answer, which has been omitted from the test item.

There are several variations of the recognition test item. Some of these include true-false, multiple choice, and matching. In measuring for health knowledge, it is recommended that the teacher use a variety of recognition test items rather than rely on one type. The purpose of this is to help offset the limitations involved in the various recognition items.

The true-false test item may have little diagnostic value since a correct response may be merely an indication that the pupil guessed correctly in selecting the answer. When true-false items are used, extreme care should be taken in constructing the false items so they will not leave a fixed false idea with pupils, particularly slow-learning pupils. Teachers should keep the following criteria in mind when developing or reviewing true-false questions:

1. Are statements true or false without additional qualifications?
2. Are statements expressed simply and clearly?
3. Are items relatively short and restricted to one central idea?
4. Are statements ambiguous?
5. Do statements contain determiners? False statements—only, never, all, always, none, every, no; true statements—usually, several, sometimes, constantly, often.

The *multiple-choice item,* when carefully prepared, can be thought provoking. It is an excellent way of determining whether pupils have achieved the desired health knowledge and information. In the multiple-choice test item, there are usually three to five possible responses. Five responses are preferred because as the number of possible answers is increased the possibility of guessing the correct answer is reduced. Points to consider when developing or reviewing multiple-choice questions include the following:

1. Are there four or five distractors with only one answer?
2. Are the distractors reasonably plausible?
3. Is there grammatical consistency?
4. Does the introduction contain clues?
5. Are choices of answers brief?
6. Are ambiguities eliminated?

The matching test item, when properly constructed, can be useful in measuring achievement and educative growth. Matching test items have the obvious limitation of being the type of items used for the collection of mere factual information. The following four questions can serve as guides in creating or reviewing matching type questions:

1. Are lists of comparative items as homogeneous as possible?
2. Are some items included that cannot be matched?
3. Can questions be easily scored?
4. Are lists of responses relatively short?

The completion test item requires the pupil to supply the correct answer in the form of a recall or fill-in item. This test item places a premium on rote memorization of health facts. A limitation is that the test item may be such that more than one correct answer can be given. For example, in a recall test such as "Exercise generally shows an increase in _____ development," both "muscular" and "organic" are correct answers. On the other hand, a recall item such as "_____ makes up the greatest part of the body," has only one possible correct answer, which is "water." When there is a possibility of more than one correct answer, the teacher should include each in the test scoring key.

These three points will help the teacher develop or select good completion-type items:

1. Make certain that only one response is correct.
2. Do not put in so many blanks that the question loses meaning.

3. Do not permit the syntax of the statement or the length of the blank to give a hint as to the answer.

Perhaps the greatest limiting factor among the preceding types of tests is that they all prohibit the students from expressing all their knowledge about the topic. Therefore other types of appraisals are also recommended to provide a well-rounded picture of how well students are progressing in their health education.

Essay. The written essay or *subjective test* of health knowledge, although somewhat lacking in objectivity, helps gain evidence of achievement and educative growth that often cannot be measured through the purely objective test. For example, the teacher can formulate questions in such a way as to provide for better problem-solving situations than are usually possible in straight objective tests. The teacher may ask pupils to write a summary of what has been learned through the study of a certain health unit. If this procedure is undertaken, the teacher should analyze the summaries to determine how closely they are related to the objectives of the unit. In this way the teacher should be able to ascertain to a reasonable degree whether pupils have gained insight into the understanding and concepts that formed the basis for the unit objectives. To realize the optimal benefit from essay-type questions, the following points are suggested.

1. Questions should be clearly and carefully constructed.
2. Written instructions for answering should be clear and explicit.

Self-appraisals. Merely asking pupils to indicate what they have learned by giving them a blank sheet of paper so they can present their anonymous comments often provides valuable clues to evaluative information.

Peer appraisals. The technique of having other students assess the learnings of their classmates has advantages if selectively used by teachers. Careful planning is necessary if this technique is to be successful because pupils need to clearly understand the purpose and the procedure.

ORAL QUESTIONING. When used, oral questioning necessitates that the teacher devise a technique suitable for keeping satisfactory records. Otherwise there will be no documentary evidence of growth when final evaluations and appraisals are made. Some teachers find it desirable and helpful to keep a log in which results of oral questioning can be quickly recorded.

Oral inquiry may be formal or informal in nature. In any event, questions should be such that the teacher can actually determine whether pupils are accumulating satisfactory health knowledge. Because of this, certain types of questions usually should be avoided. For example, questions that require only a yes or no answer may have little value because the pupil will have a 50% chance of guessing the correct answer. On the other hand, questions necessitating critical thinking and judgment can be phrased in such a way that the teacher shoud be able to immediately detect evidence of accurate health knowledge. One of the main disadvantages that teachers have found in using the oral questioning technique is that it may be difficult to appraise the achievement of all pupils if classes are large. The chief advantage of this means of measurement is that the teacher may obtain a more valid estimate of the individual's learning, especially for those students who experience difficulty with written tests.

DEMONSTRATIONS. Measurement of health knowledge through demonstrations can be carried out by either teacher demonstrations or pupil demonstrations. When the teacher demonstrates, the pupils are required to identify those things that are demonstrated. When pupils perform a demonstration, they show the health knowledge they have gained, as well as their interest in the topic.

The efficacy of this approach to health knowledge measurement is obvious; it tests pupil knowledge in a lifelike situation that could be carried over and applied in a practical way, such as helping in the selection of nutritious foods while shopping with the family.

Asking pupils to demonstrate certain procedures that were developed in a health unit is a valid way of measuring health knowledge. The chief disadvantage of this technique is the amount of time required. Measurement of health knowledge through pupil demonstration may provide for a better indication of educative growth in those pupils who do not express themselves well on written tests.

PUPIL PROJECTS. Appraisal of learning in terms of health knowledge need not always take the form of testing. For example, the teacher can evaluate scrapbooks, notebooks, special projects, and other materials prepared by pupils. This can be done for the purpose of determining whether pupils have gained insight into certain health concepts necessary for the satisfactory preparation of these materials.

TEACHER OBSERVATION. One of the best techniques in health appraisal, teacher observation, can also be a primary measure in the assessment of pupils' progress. Teachers know their pupils. They see them day in and day out. They are in a good position to judge pupil learnings. Since parents also observe their children, communication between teachers and parents is most helpful in evaluating pupil progress.

STANDARDIZED TESTS. There are a number of standardized tests used to gather information regarding health knowledge. The standardized test is one that has been previously administered to a large number of pupils to establish norms for specific grade levels or combinations of grade levels.

One of the major problems of using standardized tests is that they often lack curricular validity. Since many test items do not relate to the objectives, content, and learning activities of the local school health instruction program, they lack relevance.

Appraising health attitudes. Assessment of pupils' attitudes toward health is difficult, and it is almost impossible to obtain objective information. Attitudes are concerned with one's feelings, emotions, beliefs, and values, which are often reflected in behavior. Observations of pupils' actions may provide clues to their feelings and emotions. However, attitudes are elusive and may change with the time of the day or the environment or situation. Some pupils may not wish to reveal their true feelings because of their home situations or other conditions. Therefore

STUDENT FIRE SAFETY ATTITUDES

Please circle the numbers to the right that best express your feelings about each of the following statements:

	Strongly agree	Agree	Don't care	Disagree	Strongly disagree
1. The stop, drop, and roll procedure should be used when clothes are on fire.	5	4	3	2	1
2. In smoke-filled rooms people should crawl low to get out.	5	4	3	2	1
3. Fire drills at school are important.	5	4	3	2	1
4. Smoke detectors are needed in homes.	5	4	3	2	1
5. Fire and smoke discovered should be promptly reported to fire departments.	5	4	3	2	1
6. Fire fighters are community protectors.	5	4	3	2	1
7. Home escape plans are necessary in case of fire.	5	4	3	2	1
8. Fire burns may be dangerous to people.	5	4	3	2	1
9. Fire inspection of buildings should take place on occasions.	5	4	3	2	1
10. Improper storage of flammable materials is hazardous.	5	4	3	2	1
11. Matches, flammable substances, and electrical appliances should be used safely.	5	4	3	2	1
12. Lightning may cause fires.	5	4	3	2	1
13. Overloaded electrical circuits are hazardous.	5	4	3	2	1
14. Baby-sitter fire safety plans protect individuals.	5	4	3	2	1
15. Electrical equipment that has been tested for fire and safety hazards should be used.	5	4	3	2	1

FIG. 14-1. Student fire safety attitudes.

pupil replies may be unreliable, and the information received from whatever technique used by teachers is suspect and should be kept in proper perspective. These data should serve only as indicators of student attitudes. The chances of obtaining more reliable general information may be increased when attitudes are obtained from an entire class rather than from individual students. Thus procedures should be completed anonymously by students; names should not be required on any paper-and-pencil devices used to assess attitudes.

There are a variety of techniques that classroom teachers may use to assess attitudes. The paper-and-pencil inventory using a Likert-type scale, as shown in Fig. 14-1, is one example. A series of sentence completions on the subject of mental health is another example.

I am happiest when I _____ .

I feel best when people _____ .

The thing I want most _____ .

I feel important when _____ .

I'd like my friends to _____ .

Other techniques that have been tried with some degree of success include students' completions of unfinished stories about health situations and anonymous pupil self-appraisals of their feelings. Sometimes informal pupil conferences and conversations can reflect health attitudes.

Self-confidence survey

Check box to the right of each statement that best indicates how you view yourself.

	NO				YES
	1	2	3	4	5
Am easily upset emotionally	☐	☐	☐	☐	☐
Dislike meeting people	☐	☐	☐	☐	☐
Find criticism hard to take	☐	☐	☐	☐	☐
Have trouble solving problems	☐	☐	☐	☐	☐
Feel inferior most of the time	☐	☐	☐	☐	☐
Will not try anything if it means failure	☐	☐	☐	☐	☐

Perhaps the simplest and most practical strategy is the use of teacher observations. For example, teachers can observe (1) pupils' eating habits in the school cafeteria with regard to food preferences, (2) students freely asking questions informally before and after class about particular health topics covered, and (3) children's safety behavior on playgrounds, to and from school, and during fire drills.

The unreliability of the evidence from the attitude procedures described does not mean they should not be used. Attitudes are closely related to behaviors, and they must be assessed despite the limitations of procedures that only provide indications of pupils' feelings and emotions. Objective data may be obtained if teachers keep anecdotal records of pupils' emotions and comments and periodically analyze them for attitudinal changes. In addition, attitudes can often by validated through conversations with parents and other teachers.

Assessing health practices. Health practices may be more difficult to assess than attitudes. Most health behaviors are not observable in the classroom because they take place in the home or in the community. Also, many may not emerge for months or years after pupils have completed their schooling. Therefore most of the information collected may have to be subjective in nature.

The procedures to use for health practices evaluation include paper-and-pencil devices, such as questionnaires and checklists, informal conferences and discussions with pupils and parents, and teacher observation. Paper-and-pencil checklists, such as the one illustrated for grades 5 through 8, have limitations because the information received may not be reliable. If students are permitted to complete these forms anonymously, the chances for truthful information are increased.

Informal conferences and discussions with children, parents, and other school personnel may provide indications that pupils are brushing and flossing teeth, eating nutritious foods, and being safe pedestrians.

In assessing health practices, teachers will probably have to rely mainly on their own observations and those of others. Reports may come from nurses, physicians, parents, and

```
                    AUDIOVISUAL EVALUATION FORM

   Film                 Filmstrip                 Other

   Title:

   Length:

   Year produced:

   Color        B&W

   Description of content:




   Intended teaching purpose(s):




   Main ideas and/or skills presented:




   Production rating                        Encircle
   Photography                          Good        Bad
   Sound                                Good        Bad
   Vocabulary                           Good        Bad
   Acting                               Good        Bad

   Contents rating
   Accurate and authentic               Yes         No
   Correlated with curriculum           Yes         No
   Presents needed facts                Yes         No
   Stimulates pupil activity            Yes         No
   Void of racial, ethnic, sex bias     Yes         No

   Types of learning                    Check
   Developing concepts

   Values clarification

   Critical thinking

   Behavior modification

   List particular strengths or weaknesses:
```

FIG. 14-2. Audiovisual evaluation form.

school personnel that will provide indications of the extent of behavioral changes or behaviors. Teachers may wish to prepare a parent inventory to be taken home by students before and after a particular health unit. Although this procedure is not completely reliable, it can provide supportive information to teacher observations.

Teacher evaluation of health practices must involve a variety of the strategies presented here to validate the pupil behavior indicators that have been observed.

Evaluating health instruction material aids

Instructional material aids generally refer to such items as textbooks, films, cassettes, slides, still pictures, and other things that are helpful in the teaching process. In those instances when they are used for individual instruction, cassettes and programmed learning materials may in themselves serve as the basic program.

The selection of materials for use in health education should be done on a systemized basis with thoroughness and awareness of need. Materials should not be selected before objectives and content have been determined.

Health teaching aids should be evaluated on a regular basis, before and after the selection process. Educators should use existing devices for evaluation or create their own. The information collected should be kept on file for reference as needed. Fig. 14-2 illustrates a sample audiovisual evaluation form. Appendix I contains a more detailed instrument that teachers may find more useful. These procedures may be modified to meet specific teacher needs. Teachers may also observe student reactions to material aids in terms of interest and motivation to obtain a rapid assessment.

Teaching aids should be free of sexual, racial, ethnic, and other biases. Suggestions and criteria for assessing such matters may be found in Chapter 13 and Appendix I.

Resource speakers are considered a type of instructional aid and should be evaluated. These questions are useful in the assessment process:

1. Was the presentation biased or slanted?
2. Was the presentation appropriate for the age level addressed?
3. Was the presenter well organized?
4. What objectives were met by the presentation?

Students should be asked to respond to the question, "What did you learn from this person?"

Teachers should be cautioned to inform building principals in advance when planning to use an outside resource person. Teachers waive their right of administrative support if problems occur with a resource speaker and the principal was not notified *before the event*.

Evaluating health instruction methods

The methods teachers use in the classroom are fundamental to the successful achievement of the established objectives in health education, as in other subject areas. Therefore teachers must continually assess the procedures they use.

One phase of methods evaluation involves the selection of appropriate teaching procedures before instruction starts. Information found in Chapter 12 provides guideline questions that are helpful.

These five rather simple techniques can help in assessing the effectiveness of health instruction methods:

1. Teachers observe pupils' reactions and check their own internal feelings of effectiveness. Experienced teachers know when instruction is going well and when a method or activity is going flat.

2. Teachers ask students to respond orally or in writing to these questions:

"What did you learn today about *(topic)*?"
"How did you feel when we used *(method/ activity)*?"
"If you were going to teach today's lesson to your friends, how would you do it?"

3. Use a tape recorder to capture the dialog and tone of the class during the lesson. Analyze the tape.

4. Videotape the lesson if feasible. Analyze the tape.

5. Ask the principal, nurse, coordinator, or another teacher to attend class to evaluate a specific lesson or lessons.

Student grades in health instruction

Pupils and parents alike show great interest in report cards. Pupils generally like to be rated in comparison with their classmates and with their own previous marks. The typical elementary school child expects to get a report on status and progress. Often, the report card provides parents with their only information about what is taught in the school. It can reflect school philosophy and serve as an important medium for communication with the public. Although many elementary schools use the letter system (A-B-C-D-F) for reporting pupil progress and performance, the trend toward more functional and descriptive methods continues.

Many elementary schools today attempt to assess a pupil's progress in the light of that pupil's capacities and abilities. Such an approach usually means that a pupil is marked as O for making outstanding progress, S for making satisfactory progress, and U for making unsatisfactory progress. The emphasis is on the progress, or educational growth, of each child as an individual. At the elementary school level, progress reports are usually supplemented by parent-teacher conferences. These conferences should bring about a sharing and comparing of knowledge and observation that contributes to a better understanding of the child's performance in school.

The parent-teacher conference should use the report card simply as a point of departure for analyzing the pupil's strong and weak points. Usually, if parents are objective, they can provide the teacher with significant information on a child's health attitudes and practices in and around the home. Skilled teachers make the most of these all-too-brief conferences.

Principles of grading pupils. There is no single best way to assign grades in health instruction at all grade levels. These are some basic principles teachers can use to assure that grading is fair for all students.

1. Grades should reflect *actual class achievement*. Factors such as neatness, spelling, handwriting, and absence do not reflect on achievement in health learning and therefore should not be considered as criteria for grading. However, teachers should encourage and strive for quality of performance.

2. Grades should *not* be used for disciplinary or manipulatory purposes. Such practice detracts from the importance of health learning.

3. Students should be well acquainted with the grading method to be used by the teacher.

4. Pupils should have access to their grade progress throughout the study of health. They should be provided guidance in ways to improve their standing at any time.

Basis for grading. Teachers should collect sufficient data of student achievement to permit valid judgments to be made. *It is better to use several kinds of indicators of progress rather than one*. Remember, individuals learn in different ways and react to measuring techniques differently. Some students can express themselves and are articulate orally but have little success on written examinations.

Grades should be based on a combination of performances including the following:
Daily recitations and oral presentations
Homework
Written assignments or graphics
Examinations and quizzes
Extra credit opportunities
Pupil self-evaluation

Obviously, some of these activities are too advanced for young children, but many can be modified to provide for a combination of performances. Primary grade students can do daily recitations and simple oral reports. They can also draw or cut pictures from magazines to illustrate health learnings, and they can be given simple oral examinations.

Problems in grading. Grades in health education should be based on pupil achievement in terms of knowledge gained, projects and activities completed, and general quality of work performed. Health attitudes and practices, however important in terms of objectives, are virtually impossible to use for grading purposes. Doing so can result in external motivation, untruthfulness, and other problems. Also, determining specific student progress is difficult.

For some pupils, grades become the end purpose of study. These pupils become preoccupied with the process of memorizing the subject matter and consider the grade the end result. They do not apply their knowledge to personal decisions that will positively affect their health.

Teachers can also create problems in grading. Some use grades for disciplinary or motivational purposes when other methods fail. Others lack objective, clearly defined criteria for assigning grades. Some teachers tend to grade students with whom they work well higher than the student's achievement warrants.

Occasionally, personality conflicts between a pupil and teacher can cause the pupil to be penalized when grades are assigned. The problems of discipline and personality conflict must be dealt with as separate issues.

Many of these problems can be avoided if the teacher is organized, has a well-planned grading system that allows for individual differences, and communicates the proper perspective of grades in the educational process to pupils and parents alike.

WHO EVALUATES?

The answer to the question, "Who evaluates?" is based on the answer to the question, "What is to be evaluated?" This chapter deals with evaluating the total school health program. The elementary teacher should not be expected to evaluate the total health program. This is a major undertaking for which the responsibility should be shared by school administrators, board members, district health or curriculum specialists, teachers, nurses, parents, and in some instances, health professionals from the community, local university, and state departments of education.

The teacher is the key person in the evaluation of the instructional program in the classroom. Evaluation of the instructional program includes content, methods, materials, and student progress evaluations. Assistance in this evaluation may come from the principal, nurse, librarian, district health or curriculum specialist, parents, and students.

Effective evaluation is not easy, but it is necessary and can be rewarding. It can result in a teacher feeling like a significant contributor in the development of student, as well as personal, health behavior. Positive community public relations can result when teachers demonstrate pride in their school health programs. More importantly, evaluation enables students to receive improved health instruction and helps them learn to make intelligent decisions about lifestyles that will affect their health.

SUMMARY

Evaluation is a way to determine the worth or value of something. In school health there is need to determine the effectiveness, in terms of process and product, of the total program and its components. These include instruction, services, environment, and coordination.

The teacher has an important role in evaluation. It is limited in terms of the total program, as well as in terms of the services, environment, and coordination aspects. However, the teacher has a major responsibility for determining the impact of the health instruction program on students.

Evaluation of health knowledge objectives can be achieved relatively easily and effectively. However, assessment of health attitudes and practices is more complex and difficult. Teacher observations can be used as indicators of success despite their subjectiveness. They can be organized to provide objective and fairly reliable data.

Grades are valuable in the health instruction program because they provide student motivation and parent information. They should be based on student achievement. Student attitudes and practices are virtually impossible to grade and therefore should not be a part of the grading system.

QUESTIONS FOR DISCUSSION

1. What is the difference between measurement and evaluation?
2. Why is evaluation important to the school health program?
3. What use can parent-teacher conferences be in assessing pupil learning in health?
4. What are some of the basic points to consider when evaluating instructional aids for health?
5. If you could only evaluate one portion of the school health services, which would you select? Why?
6. What are the most effective kinds of recall and recognition items for a health test? To what extent would you use such items? Why?
7. What are the specific uses of evaluation in health? Which of these do you consider most important? Why?
8. How are behavioral objectives related to the evaluative procedures and techniques a teacher uses?
9. Can a student's health values be realistically and reliably evaluated? Defend your answer.
10. Why is it important to periodically evaluate teaching methods in health?
11. What is your opinion about grading in elementary health education?
12. Who is responsible for evaluation of health education?

SELECTED REFERENCES

Baranowski, T.: Methodologic issues in self-report of health behavior, Journal of School Health 55:May, 1985.

Brooks, C.H., and Howard, D.J.: Evaluation of an activity-centered health curriculum: assessment of cognitive knowledge, Journal of School Health 52:Nov., 1982.

California State Department of Education: Elementary school health education program inventory, Sacramento, Ca., 1977, The Department.

Charles, C.M.: Individualizing instruction, ed. 2, St. Louis, 1980, The C.V. Mosby Co.

Christenson, P.D.: An evaluation of quantitative and qualitative assessment techniques on the impact of the SERR Curriculum, Journal of School Health 55:May, 1985.

Foder, J.T., and Dalis, G.T.: Health instruction: theory and application, ed. 3, Philadelphia, 1981, Lea & Febiger.

Frazer, G.H., Kush, R., and Richardson, C.E.: Research questions in health education: a professional evaluation, Journal of School Health 54:May, 1984.

Green, L.W., and Gordon, N.P.: Productive research design for health education investigations, Health Education 13:May/June, 1982.

Green, L.W., and Lewis, F.M.: Measurement and evaluation in health education and health promotion, Palo Alto, Ca., 1986, Mayfield Publishing Company.

Gunn, W.J., Iverson, D.C., and Katz, M.: Design of the school health education evaluation, Journal of School Health 55:Oct., 1985.

Henerson, M.E., Morris, L.L., and Fitz-Gibbon, C.T.: How to measure attitudes, Beverly Hills, Ca., 1978, Sage Publications, Inc.

Hochbaum, G.M.: Measurement of effectiveness of health education activities, International Journal of Health Education 14:April/June, 1971.

Iverson, D.C.: Issues related to designing and conducting school health education research, Health Education 15:Sept./Oct., 1983.

King, K., Taylor, M.E., and Dignan, M.P.: Health education evaluation, Health Education 13:Sept./Oct., 1982.

Kolbe, L.J., and Iverson, D.C.: Research in school health education: a needs assessment, Health Education 11:Jan./Feb., 1980.

Morris, L.L., and Fitz-Gibbon, C.T.: Evaluator's handbook, Beverly Hills, Ca., 1978, Sage Publications, Inc.

Olsen, L.K., et al.: Development and application of student test used in the school health education evaluation, Journal of School Health 55:Oct., 1985.

Parcel, G.S.: Theoretical models for application in school health education research, Health Education 15:Sept./Oct., 1983.

Pine, P.: Critical issues report: promoting health education in schools—problems and solutions, American Association of School Administrators, 1985.

Pikulski, J.J., and Shanaban, T., editors: Approaches to the informal evaluation of reading, Newark, Delaware, 1982, International Reading Association.

Sanders, N.M.: Classroom questions: what kinds? New York, 1966, Harper & Row, Publishers, Inc.

Schinke, S.P., and Gilchrist, L.D.: Primary prevention of tobacco smoking, Journal of School Health 53:Sept., 1983.

Stiggins, R.J.: Evaluating students by classroom observation: watching students grow, National Education Association, 1984.

Appendixes

APPENDIX

A

AIDS: PRESCHOOL AND SCHOOL ISSUES*

JEFFREY L. BLACK

ABSTRACT: *This paper reviews the epidemiological, clinical, and public health aspects of Acquired Immunodeficiency Syndrome (AIDS) in the pediatric population. Evidence establishing modes of transmission is emphasized. Guidelines are presented to assist school staff in the educational management of children infected with the AIDS virus.* (J Sch Health **56**(3):93-95, 1986)

Since Acquired Immunodeficiency Syndrome (AIDS) was described in 1981, about 200 cases have been reported in children and adolescents 18 years of age or younger in the United States.[1] This number constitutes less than 2% of all AIDS cases. Most pediatric AIDS patients have been preschool children who die before they begin school.

The past year has been characterized by public hysteria about AIDS. Particularly disturbing are the stories of discrimination, including denial of normal educational services to school-age children because of the syndrome. The hysteria results partially from the perception that little is known about AIDS, when in reality, the syndrome has been remarkably well characterized in a brief four-year span.

*This article is the official position statement of the American School Health Association relative to AIDS and school children. Jeffrey L. Black, M.D., Assistant Clinical Professor of Pediatrics, Department of Pediatrics, University of California, San Diego, 225 Dickinson St., San Diego, CA 92103.

ETIOLOGY, EPIDEMIOLOGY, AND CLINICAL COURSE

Recent evidence strongly implicates a virus as the cause of AIDS. Because the virus primarily infects the blood cell derived from the thymus that is responsible for cellular immunity, it is called human T-lymphotrophic retrovirus III (HTLV-III).[2] The AIDS virus preferentially infects a subset of T-lymphocytes, known as helper T cells, which play a central role in the immune response.

Infection with HTLV-III is associated with a variable suppression of immune function and a broad clinical spectrum. Four-six weeks after exposure, some individuals develop an antibody indicating infection.[3] About 10% of patients who develop antibody eventually progress to end stage disease. After exposure, an extended asymptomatic period of incubation exists with a median of eight months in infants and 28 months in adolescents and adults.[4] Early symptoms,

375

called AIDS-Related Complex (ARC), include generalized swelling of lymph nodes, chronic diarrhea, weight loss, enlarged liver and spleen, and fevers. During a period of months to years, some but not all individuals progress to AIDS with the development of cancers and infections that predominately affect immunodeficient individuals. Patients who meet the diagnostic criteria for the AIDS state of HTLV-III infection generally do not survive. Mortality in excess of 80% within three years has been reported.

In adults and adolescents, more than 95% of cases have occurred in persons belonging to six high-risk groups. These groups are bisexual or homosexual men, intravenous (IV) drug abusers, Haitians, hemophiliacs, other persons receiving blood or blood products, and sexual partners of infected persons. This epidemiological evidence indicates that, in adults and adolescents, AIDS is transmitted through both heterosexual and homosexual contact, by sharing needles, or through blood product transfusions.

In younger children, the two risk factors associated primarily with infection are receiving blood or blood products and birth to a mother who has AIDS, is a member of a high-risk group, or has a sexual partner in a high-risk group. The route of transmission in those children born to high-risk parents is unknown, but data suggest that the infection may be acquired in utero.[5]

Between 5% to 10% of cases fall into the "other/no risk" category. This category includes persons who died or were otherwise lost to follow-up and persons who refused to be interviewed. Some individuals also in this category do not admit to homosexual or IV drug contact or are unaware that their sexual partners were in high-risk groups. The percentage of cases in this category has not changed over time so AIDS is not spreading beyond the limits of risk groups defined by blood or sexual exposure.

HTLV-III has been isolated from blood, semen, saliva, and tears, but transmission has not been documented from saliva and tears. It is expected that the virus will be isolated in other body fluids that contain blood. About 75% of persons with positive antibody to HTLV-III have the virus in their body fluids. The virus is present in the body fluids of asymptomatic as well as symptomatic individuals.[6]

Inestimable opportunities have existed for household contact with saliva and other body fluids of more than 500,000 persons estimated to be infected with the HTLV-III virus, especially during the asymptomatic period when the disease is not suspected. *No evidence exists* of person-to-person transmission through the air or by casual contact. No documented cases have occurred in individuals who only were household (nonsexual, nonchildbirth) contacts of AIDS patients. This fact has been verified through blood testing for antibody evidence of infection.[7]

Educational personnel can be reassured by evidence from health care workers with occupational exposure to AIDS patients.[8] Despite numerous reports of accidental exposure to potentially infectious material from AIDS patients, only needlestick injury rarely has led to a documented transmission of AIDS virus.

DIAGNOSIS AND MEDICAL MANAGEMENT

Establishing a diagnosis of AIDS during childhood requires that criteria for inclusion are fulfilled and that other disorders of immune function can be excluded. Based on clinical signs and symptoms, a case is defined as having an opportunistic infection or malignancy, indicating an underlying cellular immunodeficiency.[9] Other causes of immunodeficiency such as congenital immunodeficiencies, congenital infections, medications, lymphoreticular malignancy, and starvation must be ruled out. With recent data implicating a human retrovirus as the etiologic agent causing AIDS, direct cultures and serologic tests for antibody against this agent are additional methods for diagnosis. Because this definition requires the presence of an opportunistic infection or malignancy, the most severe cases of AIDS retrovirus infection are reported to the Centers for Disease Control, Atlanta (CDC).

The current management of children with AIDS is aimed at prevention and early treatment of opportunistic infections and malignancies to which they are susceptible.[10] This approach may prolong survival but, as yet, no effective specific treatment to eradicate the HTLV-III infection or reverse the immunologic abnormalities has been found. A number of antiviral drugs and agents directed at augmenting immune function are under investigation and efforts to produce an immunization to prevent HTLV-III infection are under way. The ability of the virus to spontaneously change its structure has made vaccine development very difficult. Other live-virus vaccines are strictly contraindicated in children with AIDS as they are for other types of immunodeficiency.

SCHOOL ATTENDANCE AND GENERAL PRECAUTIONS

No identified U.S. cases of HTLV-III infection are known to have been transmitted in school, day care, or other casual person-to-person contact. For epidemiologic purposes, the potential for casual transmission from adults and school-age children infected with the HTLV-III is comparable. Abundant evidence indicates that casual person-to-person contact as would occur among school-age children does not transmit the HTLV-III. Opportunistic infections of AIDS patients should pose no risk to their immunologically normal classmates.

Studies of the risk of transmission through contact between younger preschool children and neurologically handicapped children who lack control of their body secretions are limited. When compared with the larger number of cases in adults, relatively few cases of HTLV-III infection exist in pre-school or neurodevelopmentally delayed children. Based on experience with other communicable diseases, a theoretical potential for transmission would be greatest among these children. Any possible transmission most likely would involve exposure of open skin lesions or mucous membranes, to blood, and to other body fluids of an infected person.

Attendance in classroom programs is not recommended for young preschool children with AIDS because the oral behavior and incontinence of toddlers would be expected to increase the theoretical risk of transmission. These children should be provided an appropriate education in a nonclassroom setting. Admission to the classroom should be individualized primarily according to the child's achievement of bowel and bladder control and tendency to bite.

With few exceptions, older children should be educated in the usual manner. In general, school-age children with AIDS should be allowed to attend school if they are continent, have no open or oozing lesions, and behave acceptably (they do not bite). HTLV-III infection may result in immunodeficiency. Immunodepressed children are at greater risk of suffering severe complications from certain other infections. Assessment of the risk to the immunodepressed child is best made by the child's physician. The child's physician should consider removing the immunocompromised child from school during epidemics of infection such as measles or chickenpox. Each child with AIDS should be considered on an individual basis with the child's personal physician continually evaluating the risks of infectious disease transmission and acquisition. The slight possibility of an isolated episode of incontinence in a toilet-trained child or the small risk that a nonaggressive child might bite someone should not be grounds for limiting school attendance.

Though no cases have been attributed to nonsexual, nonchildbirth/pregnancy, or nonparental contact with body secretions, precautions should be directed at reducing exposure to the body fluids of children with AIDS.[11] Other children should not have oral contact with their eating utensils, toothbrushes, or other objects that were placed in the mouth. Any blood or body-fluid soaked item should be placed in a leak-proof bag. Any open lesions on the infected person should be covered. A bleach solution (10:1 ratio of water to bleach) should be used to clean all spills of blood or other body fluids. Gloves should be worn by those with cuts or open skin lesions while cleaning these spills, treating any open lesions, or during other direct contact with the body fluids of children with AIDS. Thorough handwashing also should be practiced. Because infections other than AIDS might be transmitted by blood or body fluids of any individual, the previously mentioned precautions should apply regardless of whether or not children with AIDS are involved.

LEGAL AND ETHICAL ISSUES

Hepatitis B virus infection serves as a precedent, both for mode of transmission and for legal action regarding exclusion from school, of children carrying an agent that had not been proven transmissable in that setting. In 1977, some New York City parents became concerned about the placement of mentally handicapped hepatitis B carriers in classrooms. Responding to public pressure, the New York City Board of Education excluded 49 carriers from school in 1978 and made alternative arrangements for their education. A federal court struck down the separation of carriers from susceptible classmates because such action violated the carriers right to a "least restrictive environment" as stated in Public Law 94-142.[12] An appellate court sustained the decision on the basis of discrimination against the handicapped.

No scientific reason exists for school personnel to be excused from educational involvement with otherwise normal school-age children with AIDS. Those who believe they are at risk for infection because of their own immune status should be encouraged to discuss their work responsibilities with their personal physician. If the physician determines that there are certain assignments that the employee should not accept, this fact should be communicated in writing to the employing department for appropriate action. In cases in which employees refuse to perform their duties, the issue is an ethical, legal, and administrative problem that must be handled on an individual basis.

The diagnosis of AIDS evokes fear of contagion from some who come in contact with the patient. A potential exists for social isolation. School personnel should respect the need for confidentiality and the right of privacy in these cases. The number of school personnel who are aware of the child's condition should be kept at the minimum needed to assure proper care of the child, such as the principal, school nurse, and the child's teacher, and to detect situations where the potential for transmission may increase, such as frequent biting.

HEALTH EDUCATION AND COUNSELING

High school students have been found to have very limited knowledge about AIDS. Most information they have received has been from superficial, inadequate, and sometimes incorrect reports in the mass media.[13] School courses on sexuality and drug abuse should include instruction about AIDS. An alteration in sexual practices, including a reduction in the number of sexual partners and participation by adolescents in drug rehabilitation programs, would help to reduce cases. Also important is to use birth control to prevent congenital cases.

Children at high risk for AIDS virus infection may have other social problems in addition to the ones associated with AIDS. School staff should be sensitive to the indication of emotional maladjustment in these children and facilitate appropriate mental health interventions. Students with AIDS will need ongoing supportive counseling and health education. Their psychosocial burden should be minimized by providing an educational experience that is as close to normal as possible.

CONCLUSION

The AIDS issue challenges the health education resources of school health professionals. Fear and misinformation about the transmission of AIDS is rampant in the general population. In response to public pressure, some school boards have ignored medical facts and adopted restrictive policies. Teachers have threatened work stoppages and parents have boycotted schools to block admission of AIDS-afflicted students. Students also lack sufficient knowledge about this sexually transmitted disease.

Informed school health personnel can play an important role in correcting misconceptions about HTLV-III infection. Heightened public interest in children with AIDS provides the impetus for school-based programs of community education. Accurate knowledge and appropriate beliefs about the disease can be promoted through in-service instruction for school staff and appropriate health education curricula for students. The periodic provision of the latest scientific information to members of school boards and administrations could promote medically sound policy decisions.

For more information about AIDS, the author suggests that interested persons obtain copies of *Morbidity and Mortality Weekly Report,* published by CDC, which regularly contains epidemiologic updates and infection control guidelines.

REFERENCES

1. Education and foster care of children infected with human T-lymphotrophic virus type III/lymphadenopathy-associated virus, *MMWR* 34:517-521, 1985.
2. Gallo, R.C., Salahuddin, S.Z., Popovic, M., et al.: Frequent detection and isolation of cytopathic retroviruses (HTLV-III) from patients with AIDS and at risk for AIDS, *Science* **224**:500-503, 1984.
3. Antibodies to retrovirus etiologically associated with Acquired Immunodeficiency Syndrome (AIDS) in populations with increased incidences of the syndrome, *MMWR* 33:377-379, 1984.
4. Rogers, M.F.: AIDS in children: a review of the clinical, epidemiologic, and public health aspects, *Pediatr Infect Dis* 4:230-236, 1985.
5. Cowan, M.J., Hellman, D., Chudwin, D., et al.: Maternal transmission of Acquired Immunodeficiency Syndrome, *Pediatrics* **73**:382-386, 1984.
6. Salahuddin, S.Z., Groppman, J.E., Markham, P.D., et al.: HTLV-III in symptom-free seronegative persons, *Lancet* **2**:1418-1420, 1984.
7. Kaplan, J.E.: Evidence against transmission of human T-lymphotrophic virus/lymphadenopathy associated virus (HTLV-III/LAV) in families of children with the Acquired Immunodeficiency Syndrome, *Pediatr Infect Dis* 4:468-471, 1985.
8. Hirsch, M.S., Wormser, G.P., Schooley, R.T., et al.: Risk of nosocomial infection with human T-cell lymphotrophic virus III (HTLV-III), *N Engl J Med* **382**:1-4, 1985.
9. Revision of the case definition of Acquired Immunodeficiency Syndrome for national reporting—United States, *MMWR* 34:373-374, 1985.
10. Ammann, A.J., and Shannon, K.: Recognition of Acquired Immune Deficiency Syndrome (AIDS) in children, *Pediatr in Rev* 7:101-107, 1985.
11. Conte, J.E., Hadley, W.K., and Sande, M.: Infection control guidelines for patients with Acquired Immunodeficiency Syndrome (AIDS), *N Engl J Med* **309**:704-744, 1983.
12. *New York State Association for Retarded Children, Inc, et al. v Carey,* 466F2d479.
13. Price, J.H., Desmond, S., and Kukulka, G.: High school students' perceptions and misperceptions of AIDS, *J Sch Health* **55**(3):107-109, 1985.

APPENDIX

B

PARTIAL HEALTH UNITS

The illustrative partial units in this Appendix cover a broad approach to pupil health interests and needs. Topical health areas included are: community, consumer, dental, disease control, drugs (including alcohol and tobacco), fitness, family, mental, nutrition, safety and first aid, and vision and hearing. This material follows the basic principles identified in Chapter 11.

Teachers can select or modify the material contained herein for use with students when developing health units. Content is presented in outline form to provide the teacher a time-saving format. More detailed knowledge can be ob-

tained from a variety of sources to ensure current and accurate content (see Chapter 13 and Appendixes E, F, and G). Teaching activities to achieve selected objectives can be chosen from the examples in Chapter 12 or from other sources after the unit framework (teacher scope and sequence) has been constructed from the material in this Appendix.

Every effort has been made to present this resource material in a manner that will be useful to teachers regardless of how many times they change grade level teaching assignments.

COMMUNITY HEALTH UNIT

Outline of content

Physiological

Definitions: public health (community health), preventive medicine, preventive health care, immunity, screening tests

Community health problems: communicable diseases (sexually transmitted disease, tuberculosis, upper respiratory infections, hepatitis, measles, German measles, polio, rabies, tetanus, typhoid, mononucleosis, food infections); noncommunicable diseases (heart and circulatory disorders, cancers and leukemias, emphysema and chronic bronchitis, diabetes, arthritis, allergies, ulcers, skin conditions); blindness and other eye defects; dental problems; maternal and child health; mental health; suicide; drug abuse, including alcohol and tobacco; accidents; malnutrition; pollution, accidental pollution

380

Psychological

Why public health? lack of public understanding of purposes and activities of community health personnel and organizations; improvement of individual, family, and group health; preventive approach; need for group efforts to prevent or correct certain health and accident problems

Social

Public health organizations: U.S. Public Health Service; state health department; local health department; World Health Organization; The American Heart Association; The American Cancer Society, Inc.; The American Lung Association; The National Society to Prevent Blindness; The National Association for Mental Health, Inc.; The National Foundation; The National Association of Hearing and Speech Agencies; National Clearinghouse for Drug Abuse Information; The Planned Parenthood Federation of America, Inc.; The American Social Health Association; The American National Red Cross; The American Diabetes Association, Inc.; National Sickle Cell Anemia Research Foundation; Muscular Dystrophy Association of America, Inc.; The National Safety Council

Community health programs and activities: prevention and control of diseases (communicable and chronic); infant and maternal deaths; malnutrition; mental illness; drug abuse; accidents; dental and oral defects; hearing problems; blindness and vision disorders; suicide; accidental poisoning; environmental pollution

Public health personnel: increasing need for community health personnel; career opportunities in public health (health educator, public health physician, public health dentist, public health nurse, sanitarian, environmental specialist, safety consultant, mental health counselor, hospital administrator, school nurse, and dental hygienist)

Professional societies: medical society, dental society, osteopathic association, optometric association

Spiritual

Values: value of public health in protecting, maintaining, and improving human health

Moral issues: Should citizens contribute money voluntarily to private agencies and through taxes to official organizations for the support of community health programs? Is each individual responsible for the health and safety of others?

Concepts

Concept	Application of health definition
1 Public health programs protect, maintain, and improve the health of people in a community through group effort.	Social-spiritual
2 As members of the community, children and youths are entitled to public health services and resources.	Social-spiritual
3 Public health agencies and organizations function at the local, state, national, and international level.	Social
4 Community health programs are carried out by official and voluntary organizations.	Social-spiritual
5 All citizens can help improve individual, family, and community health by supporting the work of health departments and health agencies.	Social-spiritual-psychological
6 Community health organizations conduct preventive and control programs for diseases, infant and maternal deaths, malnutrition, mental illness, drug abuse, accidents, blindness and other visual defects, hearing problems, dental neglect, poisoning, and environmental problems.	Physical-social
7 Public health departments generally are not adequately supported by tax funds.	Social

Concepts—cont'd

Concept	Application of health definition
8 Through careers in the health sciences, many individuals contribute to the health of the community.	Social-spiritual-psychological
9 The school health program is part of the overall community health program.	Social

Objectives for grades K–3

Domain	Objectives for students	Basic concepts
Cognitive	1. Explains the general purpose of public health	1
	2. Identifies several local health agencies	3, 4
	3. Explains why public health services should be available to everyone	1, 2, 6
	4. Lists reasons why people should support community health programs	5, 7
Affective	1. Displays interest in learning more about health departments and agencies	3, 4, 6
	2. Asks questions about who pays for community health programs	5, 7
	3. Asks questions about the work of physicians, school nurses, dentists, public health workers, and other people concerned with community health	2, 5, 8
	4. Shows interest in the value of group effort in preventing and solving certain health problems	1, 5, 6
Action	1. Cooperates with teachers, school nurses, and others involved in the school health program	2, 5
	2. Assists wherever possible with school or community health efforts	2, 5

Objectives for grades 4–6

Domain	Objectives for students	Basic concepts
Cognitive	1. Lists the major purposes of health departments	1
	2. Cites examples of public health organizations and agencies	3, 4
	3. Explains chief differences between official and voluntary health agencies	4
	4. Understands the importance of school health and other community programs concerned with child health	2
	5. Explains the need for community support of public health programs	5, 7
	6. Cites examples of health careers	8
	7. Lists health problems that may be prevented or solved by community health programs	6
Affective	1. Displays interest in the basic philosophy of public health	1
	2. Asks questions about the different programs and aims of official and voluntary health agencies	3, 4
	3. Accepts the need for community health programs and personnel	1, 2, 5
	4. Appreciates the need for financial and other public support of community health programs	1, 5, 7
	5. Shows interest in and concern for major community health problems	5, 6
	6. Displays interest in career possibilities in public health work	8
Action	1. Seeks reliable sources of information regarding community health programs	2, 5, 6
	2. Visits the health department and other local agencies when recommended as part of a community health project	2, 5, 6
	3. Cooperates with school health projects	2, 9

Objectives for grades 7-8

Domain	Objectives for students	Basic concepts
Cognitive	1. Discusses the importance of public health for all communities	1
	2. Lists reasons why community health programs are especially important for children and youth	2
	3. Explains the nature and functions of health departments at the local, state, national, and international levels	3
	4. Explains differences between official and voluntary agencies with regard to personnel, financing, relative emphasis on services, research, and education	4, 5, 7
	5. Compares the need for the group approach with that of private medical and dental care	1, 6, 8
	6. Cites the reasons for public support of community health programs	5, 7
	7. Identifies major health agencies in the community by purpose, activities, and location	3, 4
	8. Explains the three basic phases of the school health program	9
Affective	1. Appreciates the social values of community health programs	1, 5
	2. Shows interest in the quality of local community health services	2, 5, 7
	3. Asks questions about the most pressing needs in public health at the local, state, national, and world levels	3, 6, 7
	4. Appreciates the purposes of the school health program	9
	5. Offers opinions on the responsibility of government to provide effective public health programs for all citizens	1, 3, 7
	6. Displays interest in differences between official and voluntary health agencies	4, 5
	7. Inquires about public health career opportunities	8
	8. Shows concern for the quality of the school health program	9
Action	1. Cooperates whenever possible with special projects of the health department or voluntary agencies	2, 4-6
	2. Talks with parents about the values of a good community health program	1, 3, 5-7
	3. Takes part in school health projects	2, 9
	4. Seeks information on needed legislation for the improvement of local, state, and federal public health programs	1, 4, 5, 7
	5. Seeks information on educational requirements and opportunities in one or more public health careers	8

CONSUMER HEALTH UNIT★

Outline of content

Psychological

Definitions: consumer health (economics of health), health products, health services, self-diagnosis, self-medication, prevention, effects of health products, nature of various health examinations, medical care, health insurance

---

★See also Cornacchia, H.J., and Barrett, S.: Consumer health: a guide to intelligent decisions, ed. 3, St. Louis, 1985, Time Mirror/Mosby College Publishing.

Outline of content—cont'd

Psychological

Why consumer health? self-diagnosis and self-medication; advertising inducement; spiraling costs; misinformation and lack of information; vast amount of scientific information; preventive medicine concept

Why do people purchase health products and services? self-diagnosis and self-medication; less expensive treatment; improvement of health status; advertising; the need for help; condition minor in nature; ignorance of hazards; lack of information; religious beliefs; friend or peer recommendations

Why do people go to quacks? lonely; refusal of physician to listen to problem; hopeless case for treatment or cure; mysticism; the desire for pleasant, easy cure; physician's limitation in dealing with problem; psychological problems

Budgeting for health care: estimate of yearly costs of products and services; insurance; emergencies

How to act as an intelligent health consumer: skeptical; critical and analytical of what is read, seen, or heard regardless of source; initiator of investigation; identification of quacks and quackery, fads and frauds, or suspicious of same; knowledge about when to call or visit doctor, dentist, or other health professionals; knowledge about how to select a doctor, dentist, and other health professionals; knowledge of what to expect from a physician, dentist, and other health professionals, and also what is expected by these individuals of patient; application of sound criteria in purchase of health products or services; reading of labels; knowledge of where to seek, how to obtain, and how to seek reliable health information; initiative taken to go to protection agencies and organizations for help

Social

Health products

Arthritis—cures, devices

Athletics and fitness—drugs, vitamins, weight reduction, mechanical aids, spot reducers, vibrator machines, isometric versus isotonic exercises

Cancer—Krebiozen, Laetrile, Hoxsey treatments and cures

Cosmetics—deodorants, hormone creams, and wrinkle removers

Dental—toothpaste, toothbrushes, Water Pik, and others

Drugs—use and misuse, aspirin, over-the-counter, and others

Hearing—hearing aids, mail order of aids

Mechanical—bust developers, rupture devices, silicones, vibrators, seawater

Nutrition—vitamins, food additives, weight control diets, organic and natural foods

Tobacco—smoking cures and filters

Vision—glasses by mail, sunglasses, and contact lenses

Others—cough and cold remedies, laxatives, preparations for hemorrhoids, skin blemish removers, allergic conditions, bad breath, hair restorers, and impotency cures

Health services

Health examinations—what, when, who does, frequency, and cost

Types of health specialists

Physicians—general practitioners, internal medicine, pediatrics, or surgery

Dentists—general practice, orthodontics, oral surgery, and others

Psychologists—general, clinical, and family counselor

Also podiatrists, pharmacists, optometrists, osteopaths, and nurses

Hospitals and clinics—types, licensing, standards

Health insurance—types, services, costs

Criteria for selection of health specialists—license to practice, preparation and training, member of local health profession society in good standing, night calls, discussion of fees in advance, opinion of others, hospital affiliation

When to call health specialist—complaint or symptoms too severe to be endured; persistence for more than few days; symptoms' repeated return; accident

Role of business in health products: self-control versus governmental control; psychology of selling; mass communication media; analysis of advertising

Protection of the consumer

  Agencies and organizations

    Government—FDA, FTC, U.S. Postal Service, health departments

    Professional—AMA, ADA, American Pharmaceutical Association

    Voluntary—cancer, arthritis, heart, lung, Better Business Bureau

  Laws—federal Food, Drug and Cosmetic Act; advertising limitations; labeling of products

  Education—formal and informal, sources of information from family, friends, and school

Sources of reliable health information: reputable individuals, such as physicians or dentists; also scientific books, magazines, and publications; questions such as, "What is reputation, training, and experience of authors and sources?" "Is there a profit motive involved in the writing?" "Are the data accurate and up to date?" "What do other sources say about the topic or material?"

Quacks and quackery

  Definition—boastful pretender to medical skills; a charlatan; ignorant or dishonest practitioner

  Motivational factors—money, power, prestige

  Identifying factors—disregard or misinterpretation of scientific evidence; acceptance of money for worthless or questionable treatments, products, or services

  Why some quack cures work? spontaneous remission of some diseases, placebo effect, psychosomatic effect of encouragement of patient

Spiritual

Values: differing healing philosophies or cult values—medicine, osteopathy, acupuncture, herbalists, faith healers, Christian Science, Jehovah's Witnesses, and others

  What is the effect of differing values on the selection, purchase, and use of health products and services?

Moral issues: Is an ethical code needed in advertising, in the business world? Is an ethical code needed in medicine, dentistry, and the health professions? What should be the relationship between medical practitioners and patients?

Concepts

Concept	Application of health definition
1 Health products and health services may have beneficial and harmful effects on individuals.	Physiological
2 Self-diagnosis and self-medication and the use of quacks and quackery may be hazardous and costly to individuals.	
3 Individuals purchase and use health products and services for a variety of reasons.	Psychological
4 Wise decisions regarding the selection, purchase, and use of health products and services necessitate individuals acting as "intelligent health consumers."	
5 The use of scientific information is necessary for the effective evaluation, selection, purchase, and use of health products and services.	
6 Appraisal, selection, purchase, and use of health products and services are influenced by past experiences and the environment.	Social
7 There are reliable and unreliable sources of health information.	
8 The community provides a variety of organizations, agencies, and laws to protect the health consumer.	

Concepts—cont'd

Concept	Application of health definition
9 Individuals differing in values and philosophies regarding the healing and health treatment of individuals influence the selection, purchase, and use of health products and services.	Spiritual
10 Ethical considerations are involved in the selling of health products and the rendering of health services.	

Objectives for grades K-3

Domain	Objectives for students	Basic concepts
Cognitive	1. Identifies people who can help promote and protect one's health	8
	2. Identifies people who can help when injured or ill or who prescribe medicines	8
	3. Explains the reasons for caution when taking medicines	1, 2, 4
	4. Lists the reasons adults should help supervise the taking of medicines	1, 4, 8
	5. Concludes that medicines may be necessary at times for health	1, 4, 7
	6. Explains the effect of mass media on the purchase and use of health products	3-6, 8
	7. Identifies a variety of sources of health information	4, 5, 7
Affective	1. Asks questions about the hazards involved in taking medicines without adult supervision	1, 4, 8
	2. Is attentive to the discussion regarding the dangers involved in the consumption of unfamiliar food and liquids	1, 3
	3. Supports the need for medicines when prescribed by physicians	1, 2, 4, 8
	4. Is attentive to discussion about the various people who can help when a person is ill or injured	8
	5. Displays interest in the effect of the mass media on the purchase and use of health products	3-6, 8
Action (observable)	1. Informs parents, teachers, and others when injured or not well	8
	2. Demonstrates skill in analyzing mass media advertising	3, 4, 7, 8
	3. Seeks health information from a variety of sources	4, 5, 7
(nonobservable or delayed)	4. Refrains from taking medicine without adult supervision	1, 4, 8
	5. Refrains from consuming unknown foods and liquids	1, 2, 4

Objectives for grades 4-6

Domain	Objectives for students	Basic concepts
Cognitive	1. List the hazards of self-diagnosis and self-medication	2
	2. Identifies reliable sources of health information	7
	3. Explains factors that affect the reliability of health information	4, 5, 7
	4. Lists the types of mass media that may have an influence on the purchase and use of health products and health services	6
	5. Is able to apply criteria in analyzing labels and advertisements of various kinds	1, 3, 6, 8
	6. Explains the influences of friends and family on the plans to purchase and use health products and health services	6, 8
	7. Identifies a variety of health products that are used in self-treatment and explains problems related to their use	1, 2, 8

	8. Discriminates between reliable and unreliable health information and advertising	7
	9. Cites examples of agencies and organizations that protect the consumer	8
Affective	1. Displays interest in the need for reliable sources of health information	5, 7
	2. Asks questions in regard to the hazards of self-diagnosis and self-medication	1, 2
	3. Accepts the need for establishing criteria for use in the selection of health products and health services	4, 5, 7
	4. Is aware of the significance of the influence of religious beliefs, customs, superstitions, fads, and family on consumer health purchasing	3, 6, 9
Action (observable)	1. Seeks reliable sources of health information when necessary	5, 7
	2. Seeks appropriate health services personnel when injured or ill	8
	3. Can analyze labels and advertisements using established criteria	3, 4, 8
(nonobservable or delayed)	4. Avoids self-diagnosis and self-treatment	2
	5. Uses established criteria when making decisions to purchase and use health products	4, 5, 7

Objectives for grades 7–8

Domain	Objectives for students	Basic concepts
Cognitive	1. Identifies a variety of health products available and explains their effects on individuals	1
	2. Recalls the laws that attempt to protect the health consumer	8
	3. Explains quacks and quackery and their effects on people	1-4
	4. Describes the nature, frequency, cost, and significance of health examinations	2, 4, 8
	5. Identifies the various types of health specialists and services available to help individuals	2, 4, 8
	6. Compares the healing or health treatment philosophies or cults found in society	6, 8, 9
	7. Identifies the criteria to follow to become an "intelligent health consumer"	4
	8. Compares the role of a variety of community organizations and agencies in protecting the health consumer	8
	9. Identifies the reasons why individuals purchase and use a variety of health products and services	3
	10. Explains the reasons supporting a code of ethics for business establishments making health products available and for those rendering health services	10
Affective	1. Accepts the need for reliable sources of health information	4, 5, 7
	2. Displays interest in the need for skepticism in consumer health	4
	3. Supports the need for laws and community organization and agencies to protect the people in consumer health	8
	4. Is supportive of the need to understand quacks and quackery	1, 2, 4, 5, 7
	5. Is attentive to the need for health examinations	1, 8
	6. Listens to the discussion regarding the types of health specialists available	2, 8
	7. Asks questions about the different healing and health treatment philosophies	6, 9
	8. Displays interest in the need for the application of a code of ethics in the business world for manufacturers, advertisers of health products, and those rendering health services	10

Objectives for grades 7-8—cont'd

Domain	Objectives for students	Basic concepts
Action (observable)	1. Seeks reliable sources of health information	4, 5, 7
	2. Is skeptical regarding health information from advertising and other sources until it can be verified	4, 5, 7
(nonobservable or delayed)	3. Uses the criteria for an "intelligent health consumer" when considering the purchase or use of health products and health services	4
	4. Seeks the help of community agencies and organizations when information or assistance is needed in regard to health products and health services	8
	5. Refrains from the purchase and use of health products that are detrimental to one's health	1, 2

DENTAL HEALTH UNIT

Outline of content

Physiological

Structure and functions of teeth

Structure—divisions—crown (top), neck, root (base); layers—enamel, dentin, cementum, pulp

Types and numbers of teeth—primary (deciduous), twenty (incisors, cuspids, molars); permanent, thirty-two (eight incisors, four cuspids, eight bicuspids, twelve molars)

Functions—chewing; speech; appearance; primary hold spaces for permanent teeth

Diseases and disorders

Dental caries—tooth decay

Causes—bacteria plus sugars = acid = decay; pathway—enamel, dentin, pulp; plaque—gluey, gelatinlike substance adhering to teeth where bacteria collect and act on food

Contributing factors—heredity, tooth structure, saliva, bacteria, sugar

Periodontal diseases

Gingivitis—inflammation of gums; pyorrhea—advanced gingivitis involving gums and bone

Symptoms—"pink" toothbrush from bleeding gums; red, swollen, tender, gums

Causes—irritation from dental calculus that results from substances secreted by bacteria in plaque; sharp edges of badly decayed teeth, worn-out fillings rubbing on gums; malocclusion, poor nutrition, systemic diseases

Prevalence—major cause for tooth loss over 35 years

Malocclusion—improper bite; effects—interferes with chewing, speech, and appearance; harder to clean

Causes—heredity, acquired factors—pressures on teeth including thumb sucking, mouth breathing, tongue twisting, lip sucking, and sleeping habits

Stains—(1) extrinsic—food pigments, tobacco and caffeine, metallic dusts; green stain in children— bacteria, fungi plus inorganic elements (calcium); (2) intrinsic—within tooth structure; caused by pigments in blood; imperfect tooth development

Abscess—infection affecting blood, lymph vessels, and nerves in pulp; caused by neglect of decay

Halitosis—bad breath; caused by poor dental hygiene, carious teeth, unclean mouth, periodontal disease, pyorrhea, infection, possible gastrointestinal problems, and others

Plaque—sticky, almost colorless layer of organized microcolonies of bacteria in a gelatinous substance; clings to teeth, especially near gum line

Calculus—calcified (hardened) plaque, also known as tartar; mineral deposits around gum lines that harden and are removed only by scaling

Nutrition

Need for balanced diet from basic four food groups; excess vitamins and minerals (calcium and phosphorus) not generally needed

Good "snack" food—no or minimal sugar and refined sugars: (1) potato chips, corn chips, popcorn, nuts, cheese, hard boiled eggs, raw fruits and vegetables, unsweetened fruit juices, milk; (2) detergent foods (cleanse teeth and provide exercise), raw vegetables—carrots, celery, green peppers, cauliflower, radishes; raw fruits—apples, oranges

Poor "snack" foods—candy, pastry, cookies, chocolate milk, sweetened beverages, syrups, jellies, and carbohydrate foods that are sticky and cling to teeth

Psychological

Why oral health? proper tooth functioning necessary for chewing; speech; affects appearance, acceptance and rejection by peers; prevents diseases and disorders

Care of teeth and proper oral hygiene by individual

Toothbrushing—clean teeth and mouth; eliminate food particles; remove plaque; massage; prevent stains and calculus, when to brush, after eating; if not, "swish and swallow"

Toothbrush—rinse and let dry in sunlight; selection—three to four rows of bristles in straight line

Mouthwash—removes excess particles; can do with water; commercial products not effective in removing film, neutralizing acids, curing halitosis, or preventing decay; temporarily freshens and sweetens mouth; may mask disease

Flossing for plaque control with waxed or unwaxed floss between the teeth

Dentifrice—no best kind; possibly one with fluoride

Fluorides—possible use in toothpastes or powders, in tablet form, in bottle water

Periodic dental visits

Proper nutrition

Avoidance of injuries and accidents—follow safe practices; avoid detrimental habits—thumbsucking, tongue-thrusting, chewing hard objects

Social

Problem: 90% or more of all children and youths need better oral health

Care of teeth

By dentist who examines mouth for diseases and disorders, fills cavities, provides bridges and crowns, applies topical application of fluoride, cleans and polishes teeth, replaces missing teeth, teaches dental hygiene, helps with orthodontia, and uses x-ray films, different types of fillings—silver amalgam, gold, porcelain—mouth mirror and explorer, scaler, drill, and other equipment; when to visit dentist—preferably twice yearly

By community through fluoridation of water supply (1 ppm); sodium fluoride is a chemical that becomes part of the tooth and strengthens it against decay; applied by topical application, in water, and by taking pills; favorable claims—inexpensive; reduces tooth decay significantly; reaches all people; reduces costs of repairs; unfavorable claims—forces people to drink fluoridated water against their will; dangerous to health; type of socialized medicine

Types of dentists—general practice, orthodontia, prosthetics, periodontia, pedodontia, oral surgery, and endodontia

How to select dentist—call local dental society for three names; call reputable hospital and ask chief of dental services for suggestions; see if dentist is member of local dental society; does postgraduate work; attends clinics and does not advertise; ask family dentist in previous community; call nearby dental school; check neighbors who are satisfied with dentist

Effects of mass media including advertising on dental health products and services

Dental health insurance

Costs of products and services for dental care

Outline of content—cont'd

Spiritual

Values: importance of dental health to self-identity; self-esteem

Moral issue: fluoridation of water supply; responsibility of individual and community (including schools) to help needy students without funds obtain dental health products and services

Concepts

Concept	Application of health definition
1 Positive oral health and oral health neglect have differing effects on individuals.	Physiological
2 Most dental diseases and disorders are preventable and treatable.	
3 Differing motivations influence decisions regarding dental health.	Psychological
4 A variety of environmental factors are important contributing causes of dental diseases and disorders and influence the purchase and use of dental health products and services.	Social
5 The community has a responsibility in the control and prevention of oral health diseases and disorders.	
6 All individuals are affected by dental health neglect.	
7 Community resources are available to assist individuals with oral health problems in varying kinds and amounts	
8 Dental health is affected by an individual's values.	Spiritual
9 Fluoridation of the water supply is a moral issue.	
10 Dental health services and products should be available to, or provided for, all individuals.	

Objectives for grades K–3

Domain	Objectives for students	Basic concepts
Cognitive	1. Explains ways to clean teeth, as well as when this action should take place	1, 2
	2. Recalls foods that help in promoting dental health	1, 2
	3. Identifies the different teeth and their functions	2
	4. Lists ways to prevent tooth decay or other disorders	1, 2, 4, 7
	5. Explains the proper way to brush teeth	1, 2
	6. States the practices that may be harmful to oral health	4
	7. Identifies the reasons why the dentist or dental hygienist can help individuals	2, 7
	8. Explains the procedures to follow in preparing an inexpensive dentifrice	2
	9. Explains the proper way to floss the teeth	1, 2
Affective	1. Displays interest in brushing teeth properly	1, 2
	2. Listens carefully to the ways to prevent tooth decay and other disorders	2, 4
	3. Asks questions about teeth and their functions	2
	4. Brings pictures to class, or is attentive to discussion of foods that may be helpful and detrimental to dental health	1, 2, 4
	5. Talks about the need for daily health care	1, 2, 6
	6. Accepts the dentist or dental hygienist as a friend	2, 7

Action		Basic concepts
(observable)	1. "Swishes and swallows" when brushing the teeth is not possible	1, 2
(nonobservable)	2. Prepares an inexpensive dentifrice in the classroom	2
	3. Eats nutritious foods, including "snack" foods	1, 2
	4. Attempts to refrain from harmful dental health practices	
(nonobservable, or	5. Brushes teeth properly after eating when possible	1, 2, 4
delayed)	6. Attempts to floss teeth once daily	1, 2, 4
	7. Uses own toothbrush and gives it proper care	1, 2, 4
	8. Visits the dentist periodically	2, 7

Objectives for grades 4-6

Domain	Objectives for students	Basic concepts
Cognitive	1. Explains the type, structure, functions, growth, and development of teeth	1, 2
	2. Identifies ways in which oral health influences appearance and social relationships	3, 4
	3. Summarizes the procedures to follow for dental health	2, 5, 7
	4. Lists the factors that control and prevent tooth decay	2, 5, 7
	5. Recalls the diseases and disorders that occur from oral health neglect	1, 4, 6
	6. Explains the causes of tooth decay	1, 2, 4
	7. Identifies the reasons for topical application of fluorides to the teeth	1, 2, 6
	8. Recites the services that a dentist can render to an individual	5, 7
	9. Demonstrates the proper way to floss teeth	1, 2
Affective	1. Accepts the responsibility for personal dental health care	1, 3, 6-8
	2. Talks about the need for dental care including periodic dental visits	1, 2, 7, 8
	3. Displays interest in wanting to learn more about the role of nutrition in dental health	1, 2, 4
	4. Listens to discussion about the importance of the individual's oral health	2, 6, 8
	5. Reaches the conclusion that dental health plays a role in the social acceptance and self-esteem of individuals	2, 4, 8
	6. Supports the need for flossing teeth as an important preventive dental health procedure	1, 2, 6
Action	1. "Swishes and swallows" when brushing is not possible	2
(observable and nonobservable)	2. Refrains from using teeth in hazardous ways	1, 2
	3. Eats nutritious foods and especially detergent foods	1, 2, 4
	4. Limits the consumption of sweets	1, 2, 4
(nonobservable, or delayed)	5. Attempts to floss teeth daily	1, 2
	6. Brushes teeth properly after eating when possible	1, 2
	7. Visits the dentist periodically	1, 2, 7
	8. Uses care in the treatment and storage of the toothbrush	2

Objectives for grades 7-8

Domain	Objectives for students	Basic concepts
Cognitive	1. Compares the claims made for and against fluoridation	5, 9
	2. Compares advertising claims of the product effectiveness on dental health	4
	3. Identifies the community resources available to assist in dental health care	7
	4. Explains the use of x-ray films in the dental care process	1, 2, 7
	5. Lists the importance of teeth to appearance, speech, and digestion	1, 3

Objectives for grades 7-8—cont'd

Domain	Objectives for students	Basic concepts
Cognitive—cont'd	6. Lists the variety of dental specialists and the kinds of services they render	7
	7. Compares the costs of dental services with and without proper dental care	4, 7
	8. Identifies sources of reliable and current scientific dental health information	4, 5, 7
Affective	1. Talks about fluoridation of the water supply as a moral issue	9, 10
	2. Displays interest in learning about dental health and its relations to social acceptance and appearance	3
	3. Asks questions regarding the costs of dental services with and without preventive dental care	4, 7
	4. Discusses the place of dental health in an individual's values	8
	5. Is attentive to information presented about the variety of dental specialists and auxiliary dental personnel available in the community	4, 7
	6. Asks questions about the benefits and hazards in the use of x-ray films by dentists	1, 2, 7
Action (observable and non-observable)	1. Is able to differentiate between reliable and unreliable dental health information	4, 7
(nonobservable, or delayed)	2. Supports community efforts to fluoridate the water supply	5, 6, 9, 10
	3. Supports community efforts to make dental health services and products available to needy students	6, 10
	4. Is able to make wise decisions regarding personal dental health care	3, 4, 8

DISEASE CONTROL UNIT

Outline of content

Physiological

Definitions: disease, communicable disease, noncommunicable or chronic disease, host (focus), avenue, susceptible, acute, chronic, antigen, antibody, immunity, pathogen, vaccine, serum, antibiotic, resistance, epidemic

Types

Communicable—respiratory—colds, bronchitis, pneumonia, influenza; tuberculosis, "strep" throat; infectious hepatitis; mononucleosis; skin diseases; sexually transmitted diseases; gastrointestinal—food poisoning; childhood—measles, mumps, smallpox, chickenpox, and poliomyelitis

Causes—microorganisms—bacteria (sexually transmitted diseases, tetanus, tuberculosis, "strep" throat); viruses (colds, infectious hepatitis); fungi (ringworm); protozoa (dysentery, malaria); parasites (worms)

Contributing causes—heredity; lack of sanitary procedures; individual susceptibility; lack of nutritious food; and exposure

Modes of transmission: air, food, water, direct contact, insects, and animals

Portals of entry—mouth, nose, breaks in skin, and other body openings

Disease process—fever, pain, infection, redness, loss of weight, bleeding, shortness of breath, and other signs and symptoms

Body defenses—skin and mucous membranes; fever; white blood cells; antibodies

Noncommunicable—heart, cancer, allergy, arthritis, diabetes, mental illness, and acne

   Contributing causes—heredity; food; dysfunctioning of body organs; irritations; pressures; and a variety of other environmental factors

   Effects—damage, destruction, and altered function of cells, tissues, organs, and systems; illness; disability; death

   Prevention and treatment—individual—isolation, health habits; community—control of environment through laws and regulations; immunization; sanitation; water and food controls; drugs and medicines; surgery; radiation; and medical help

Psychological

Effect of diseases and disorders on mental and emotional health: adjustment of self and others; success in social world

Importance of early diagnosis and treatment

Individual responsibility in disease control

Fear of disease, disability, and death

Disease and death in the family

Social

School and community responsibilities for prevention and control

Control procedures: laws and regulations; sanitary procedures; immunizations; availability of health department services; adequate supply of physicians and hospital and clinic facilities

Sources of help: physicians; health departments; voluntary health agencies

Spiritual

Values: appreciation of healthy body; differing religious and healing philosophies toward disease

Moral issues: ethics of disease prevention and treatment on the part of individuals and the community; attitudes toward people with disease; appreciation of healing arts; concern for others

Concepts

Concept	Application of health definition
1 Diseases can cause disability, temporary or permanent, and sometimes death.	Physical-social-spiritual
2 Communicable diseases are caused by germs and may be transmitted directly or indirectly from an infected person, or host, to someone who is not immune.	Physical-social
3 For a communicable disease to spread, there must be a host (focus of infection), an avenue or means of transmission, and a susceptible person.	Physical-social
4 Noncommunicable—sometimes called chronic—diseases are caused by hereditary factors, metabolic disorders, aging, diet, stresses, and unknown influences.	Physical
5 Acute diseases are of short duration; chronic diseases are long-lasting.	Physical
6 Elementary-school pupils should be routinely immunized against measles, polio, German measles, diphtheria, whooping cough, and tetanus.	Physical-social
7 Parents are responsible for having their children properly immunized.	Social-spiritual
8 Communicable diseases are often spread in elementary schools because of inadequate control measures at home and in school.	Physical-social-spiritual
9 Diseases occur more often among poor children and contribute to lower learning achievement for all elementary pupils.	Social-spiritual
10 Adequate medical care and public health services are necessary for control of disease in a community.	Social-spiritual

Objectives for grades K–3

Domain	Objectives for students	Basic concepts
Cognitive	1. Tells why it is important to avoid disease	1, 9
	2. Explains the reasons for covering coughs and sneezes in the classroom	2, 3, 8
	3. Lists the ways a communicable disease may be spread	2, 3, 8
	4. Identifies some communicable diseases fairly common among children	2, 3, 8
	5. Tells why it is necessary to be immunized against certain diseases	2, 3, 6
Affective	1. Displays interest in preventing and controlling disease	1, 8
	2. Asks questions about different kinds of diseases	2, 4
	3. Is aware of spread of "catching diseases" among children	2, 3, 6, 8
	4. Accepts the value of immunizations	3, 6
	5. Appreciates the effect of illness on learning	9
Action	1. Covers coughs and sneezes and follows other sanitary practices in school	2, 8
	2. Cooperates in school or community immunization program	6, 7
	3. Remains at home when ill with a communicable disease	8
	4. Talks about reasons why poor people are sick more often than others	9

Objectives for grades 4–6

Domain	Objectives for students	Basic concepts
Cognitive	1. Lists the major disease causes of death for all Americans and for children of elementary school age	1
	2. Explains the differences between communicable and chronic diseases	1-5
	3. Cites the differences between a vaccine and a serum	2, 6
	4. Compares acute diseases with chronic diseases	5
	5. Gives reasons for higher rates of disease among poverty groups	4, 7, 9, 10
	6. Lists the communicable diseases against which elementary pupils should be immunized	6
	7. Explains causes, prevention, and medical care for major chronic diseases	1, 4, 10
Affective	1. Is attentive to information presented on methods for individuals, families, and communities to control diseases	1, 3, 4, 9, 10
	2. Accepts the responsibility for taking steps to avoid spreading disease to others	3, 6, 8
	3. Appreciates the responsibility of parents to have children immunized against certain diseases	6, 7
	4. Supports local, state, and federal efforts to control communicable and chronic diseases	1, 10
	5. Displays interest in government plans for health care of older people and other Americans	1, 9, 10
Action	1. Follows personal and family practices to prevent disease	1, 8
	2. Seeks medical care when symptoms of illness are present	1, 10
	3. Cooperates with school policy by keeping immunizations up to date and staying home when ill	3, 6, 8, 10
	4. Reports symptoms of illness to parents, teacher, or school nurse	3, 8, 10

Objectives for grades 7–8★

Domain	Objectives for students	Basic concepts
Cognitive	1. Explains specific causes, preventive measures, and community control of heart diseases, cancers, stroke, and other major diseases	1, 4, 9, 10
	2. Cites differences between communicable and noncommunicable and acute and chronic diseases	1, 2, 4, 5
	3. Lists recent medical and health science advances that have helped control disease	1, 10
	4. Illustrates ways that individuals, families, and communities can help control disease	1, 8, 10
Affective	1. Appreciates the fact that some diseases can be controlled more easily than others	1, 4, 5, 10
	2. Displays interest in plans to provide better medical and hospital care for all Americans	1, 9, 10
	3. Realizes the importance of immunizations for self-protection and the protection of others	3, 6, 7
	4. Supports government and other research efforts to improve preventive and control measures for disease	1, 10
	5. Accepts responsibility for having periodic medical checkups	1, 10
Action	1. Has regular medical checkups	1, 10
	2. Has all routinely recommended immunizations	3, 6, 8
	3. Participates in personal and family practices to prevent disease	1, 8
	4. Avoids smoking, drinking, drug use, and other practices that may cause illness	1, 9
	5. Avoids or minimizes physical, chemical, or emotional stresses that may cause disease	1, 4

DRUG UNIT (INCLUDING ALCOHOL AND TOBACCO)

Outline of content

Pharmacological

Definitions: drug; drug use, misuse, and abuse; addiction; dependency; habituation; tolerance; toxicity; slang terms; tobacco; alcohol; alcoholic beverages; alcoholism

Alcohol synonyms: ethyl alcohol, ethanol

Identification of abused drugs: technical help needed

Classification of drugs:

  Legal and illegal

    Legal—over the counter and prescription

    Illegal—marijuana, heroin, cocaine and others

  Pharmacological

    Stimulants—amphetamines, tobacco, coffee, cocaine

    Depressants (sedatives-hypnotics)—alcohol, barbiturates, inhalants, marijuana

    Psychedelics—LSD, psilocybin, peyote, STP

    Narcotics—heroin, morphine, opium, codeine, methadone

★Special attention may be given to heart disease and risk-taking factors and cancer.

Outline of content—cont'd

Pharmacological—cont'd

Tranquilizers—Thorazine, **Compazine**, Serpasil

Over-the-counter—aspirin, **antihistamines**, cough medicines, diet pills, sleeping pills

Common or trade name **(brand) and** generic (chemical) identity

Alcoholic beverages: distilled spirits (40% to 50%)—whiskey, brandy, scotch, gin, vodka; wine (12% to 20%); beer (4%)

Tobacco: cigars, cigarettes, pipes, chewing tobacco

Physiological

The nervous system

Drug effects: dependent on dose response, biologic variability, potency, tolerance, body size

Medical uses: dependent on drug used

Abuse potential: physical and psychological dependence, tolerance

Alcohol:

Short-term effects: intoxication, reaction time slowed, released inhibitions and relaxation at low doses, dulling effects at high doses; also, absorption, metabolism, excretion, brain effects

Long-term effects: alcoholism, liver malfunction, brain damage

Tobacco:

Short-term effects: stimulation, irritation of mucous membrane, improvement in short-term performance, chronic use affects interchange of O_2, CO, CO_2

Long-term effects: lung cancer, emphysema, heart disease, and other circulatory disorders

Duration of action: dependent on drug used

Method of administration: pills, capsules, injections, sniffing, liquid, smoking, chewing

Benefits:

Alcohol: antiseptic, diet stimulation (small amounts), tonic when prescribed by physicians

Tobacco: stimulation

Psychological

Why people use, misuse, and abuse drugs: curiosity; personal conflicts—insecurity, escape, boredom, rebelliousness; kicks; peer pressures; search for identity-adulthood; rejection of culture including schools; TV; commercial exploitation

Why people don't use: alcohol—religion, no wish to impair physical/mental health, do not like taste, personal convictions against use; tobacco—odor, cost

Characteristics of potential drug abusers: high-risk youths are those with behavioral problems at school with mild conduct disorders; lack of self-confidence; maybe self-centered and self-indulgent

Alternatives to drugs: athletics and recreational activities; counseling and group therapy in personal development; improved communications; social service participation; political service activities; intellectual motivation—reading discussion, creative games; participation in creative art activities; philosophic discussions on ethics, morality, values; spiritual involvement; survival training

Social

Patterns of drug use and abuse: classification of users and abusers

Nature and extent of drug use and abuse: legal and illegal; youth (alcohol—60% to 90%; tobacco—40% to 60%), adults

Factors affecting drug use and abuse

Conflicts in reality—escape, values

Economics—business and communication media

Social and political climate

Youth lifestyles—counter-culture, youth identity, adolescent revolt

Role of home, school, community: prevention, control, treatment, and rehabilitation
Rehabilitation and treatment: multimodality concept
  Crisis intervention
  Detoxification
  Aftercare
    Pharmaceutical—cyclazocine, methadone
    Psychiatric—individual counseling in psychiatric hospital
    Psychosocial—check for local programs
    Religious—Teen Challenge, AA
Courts and the law: laws; enforcement procedures and problems; criminal justice process
Community resources: federal, state, and local governmental agencies—FTC, FDA, DOE, NIAAA, NIDA; private sources; mass media and the business world; education; laws and enforcement; facilities—crisis centers, clinics, hotlines, ongoing groups, self-help groups; drug abuse council or committee
Identification of drug abusers
  Observations of signs and symptoms
    General and specific—change in attendance, discipline, and performance; unusual activity or inactivity; deterioration of personal appearance and health habits; unpredictable outbreaks of temper
    Characteristics of potential users
    Tell-tale evidence
  Peer identification, self-identification, clinical test

Spiritual

Values: developing a value system; self-identity and self-concept
Moral issues: implications of use and abuse of drugs on self, home, and community; drug use by students and adults; commercial interests; the mass media; the sale of drugs; the justice of laws controlling drugs; individual and community responsibilities for drug abusers; the job market for rehabilitated drug abusers or drug abusers in industry

Concepts

Concept	Application of health definition
1 Drugs differ in kind and degree; they have multiple uses with a variety of effects on individuals.	Pharmacological
2 Proper use of drugs may be beneficial to individuals, the family, and the community.	
3 Improper use of drugs may result in health and safety problems to individuals, the family, and the community.	
4 Numerous factors and forces influence the availability, as well as the use and misuse of legal and illegal drugs by individuals and the community.	Psychological-social
5 The individual, the family, and the community have interrelated and reciprocal responsibilities to help control the availability, prevent the misuse and abuse, and assist individuals who become misusers and abusers of drugs in society.	Social
6 The use and misuse of drugs by individuals involve moral principles and issues and are related to one's sense of values, as well as to the humane and just treatment of all people in society.	Spiritual

Objectives for grades K-3

Domain	Objectives for students	Basic concepts
Cognitive	1. Identifies drugs commonly used	1
	2. Illustrates ways common drugs are used by individuals	1
	3. Lists beneficial effects of drugs	2
	4. Identifies substances that can be harmful or misused	3
	5. Lists responsible people who can help when medicines are needed	2, 3
	6. Explains why medicines should be taken under supervision of parent as prescribed or recommended by a physician or dentist	4
	7. States conditions under which individuals show lack of responsibility when using medicine	5
	8. Cites ways in which individual shows respect for drugs	5
Affective	1. Is aware of differences between alcohol and other drugs and of their usage by individuals	1, 4
	2. Displays interest in learning about the beneficial, as well as harmful, effects of drugs	2, 3
	3. Desires to use drugs in useful and responsible ways	4, 5
	4. Shows interest in discovering people who can help when medicines are needed	5
Action (nonobservable, or delayed)	1. Uses only substances that aid in proper responsible supervision	3
	2. Takes medicines and drugs only under responsible supervision	3
	3. Refuses to accept substances from strangers	3-5
	4. Limits or refrains from use of drugs, except medicines prescribed and recommended, until adulthood	2, 6

Objectives for grades 4-6
(introduce alcohol/tobacco at this level)

Domain	Objectives for students	Basic concepts
Cognitive	1. Identifies varieties of drugs used by individuals	1
	2. Lists reasons for drugs in society	3
	3. Explains medical uses of commonly used drugs	2
	4. Explains physiological effects of some of the commonly used drugs	1
	5. Lists reasons persons react differently to chemicals contained in drugs	1
	6. Cites examples of misuse and abuse of drugs	3, 4
	7. Identifies difficulties or possible problems from misuse and abuse of drugs	3
	8. Explains why misuse and abuse of drugs may start early in life	4
	9. Lists ways society tries to protect individuals from abuse of drugs	4
	10. Identifies ways to protect self against misuse and abuse of drugs	3, 4
	11. Analyzes information about drugs on TV, in newspapers and magazines	4, 5
Affective	1. Displays interest in learning about varieties of drugs and their effects on the body	1-3
	2. Asks questions about problems involved with misuse or abuse of drugs	3, 5
	3. Seeks further information about community efforts to help people who misuse and abuse drugs	5
	4. Discusses ways to protect self against misuse and abuse of drugs	5, 6
	5. Expresses desire to use drugs responsibly and usefully	2, 6

Action (nonobserv- able, or delayed)	1. Uses only substances that aid in proper growth and development	2
	2. Takes medicine and drugs only under responsible supervision	3
	3. Limits or refrains from use of drugs, except medicines prescribed or recommended, until grown up	3
	4. Refuses to use illegal drugs	3, 6
	5. Starts to develop own practices and habit patterns to protect self against abuse of drugs	3, 4

Objectives for grades 7–8
(including alcohol and tobacco)

Domain	Objectives for students	Basic concepts
Cognitive	1. Recalls varieties of drugs used by people	1
	2. Describes how medicines can be used to benefit individual	2
	3. Lists variety of individual and social factors that influence misuse and abuse of drugs	4
	4. Interprets role of business and advertising in sale of drugs	4, 5
	5. Identifies differing effects of variety of drugs on the body	1, 4
	6. Compares benefits of smoking, drinking, and using drugs with possible detrimental effects	2, 3
	7. Identifies reasons why people do and do not use, misuse, and abuse drugs	4
	8. Illustrates ways to cope with social and emotional pressures of life other than through use of drugs	4, 5
	9. States procedures used by communities to control availability, sale, and use of drugs	5
	10. Discusses need for development of a value system	6
	11. Recalls signs and symptoms of drug misusers and abusers	1
Affective	1. Is attentive to information presented on varieties of drugs used by people, their benefits, their hazards, and their differing physiological effects	1-3
	2. Shows interest in comparisons of benefits and detrimental effects of alcohol, tobacco, and drugs on individuals and society	2, 3
	3. Gives opinions regarding role of business and advertising in sale and availability of drugs	2, 3, 5
	4. Asks questions about alternatives to drug use	4, 5
	5. Displays interest in developing a value system	6
	6. Is aware and discusses long-term results from frequent and regular misuse and abuse of drugs	4, 5
Action (nonobserv- able, or delayed)	1. Make judgments about drugs and drug users after reviewing all aspects of problem	4-6
	2. Seeks to discover one's own identity and purposes in life	6
	3. Participates in a school-education-information program	5
	4. Seeks help from school personnel if having a drug problem	4, 5
	5. Refrains from regular use of drugs that may lead to dependency, disease, or disability	3-6
	6. Avoids use of drugs that may affect ability to think clearly and react normally	3-6
	7. Refuses to use illegal drugs	3-6

FITNESS

Outline of content

Physiological

Definitions: physical fitness, physiology, physiology of exercise, body mechanics, muscular system, cardiovascular system, strength, speed, endurance, posture, rest, sleep

Exercise

Muscles—types—skeletal (external body control), heart, and smooth (internal organs—blood vessels, glands, others)

Characteristic—contractility when stimulated by nerves

Skeletal muscles:

Structure—attached to bones of body

Locations—back, chest, abdominal wall, arms and legs

Functions—movement of body (exercise), maintenance of posture, production of body heat

Kinds of exercise—many forms; light or heavy, including walking, running, bicycling, hiking, sports, recreational activities

Effects—muscle tone, strength, size and control of skeletal muscles; aid in individual's meeting demands of daily activity; help in creation of reserves for emergencies and safety; aid in cardiovascular, respiratory, and nervous system functioning; improvement of posture; stamina, endurance; relief from tension; fun and pleasure; aid in mental health; control of body weight; one factor involved in heart disease

Rest, relaxation, and sleep

Requirements—need for a balance of work, play, rest, relaxation, and sleep daily; sleep requirements—8 to 10 hours daily for children and adolescents

Fatigue—types—physical, mental, or emotional

Causes—intense or prolonged physical activity; psychologic factors—nervousness, boredom, worry, tensions and stress, emotions, noise; infections and disease conditions

Effects—less attention, drowsy, irritability, lowered resistance to fatigue, less alert to possible hazards—more accident prone, less ability to perform effectively

Procedures for relaxation—sleep, rest, exercise, change of activity, music, art, and other pleasurable activities

Body control

Dependent on proper exercise; practice of bodily movements; adequate rest, relaxation, and sleep; nutrition; and other environmental factors

Poor posture because of lack of, or improper, exercise, rest, and sleep; poor habits of sitting, standing, reclining, or walking; improper nutrition; ill-fitting clothes and shoes

Psychological

Importance of relaxation in helping endure stress

Importance of exercise, rest, and sleep to the individual

Selection of activities to fulfill individual needs

Competition and its psychological effects on children and youth

Games and sports and their provision for success experiences and self-reliance opportunities

Social

Role of school, home, and community: providing facilities and opportunities for exercise, rest, and relaxation

School curriculum: its inclusion of an education program to help students with postural or exercise problems or to fulfill pupil needs

Social interaction: through games, sport, dance, or other forms of exercise and activity; improvement of teacher-pupil relationships

Spiritual

Values: appreciation of physical fitness, rest, sleep, relaxation, and posture to health and effective living; appreciation of differing attitudes of individuals toward exercise and physical activity

Moral issues: fair play and good sportsmanship in games and sports

Concepts

	Concept	Application of health definition
1	Physical fitness is one aspect of total health and requires regular vigorous exercise.	Physical
2	Regular exercise produces good muscle tone and efficient circulation and helps maintain desirable body weight.	Physical-social
3	Everyone needs a balance of exercise and rest for optimal health.	Physical-psychological
4	Sports and dance provide opportunity for healthful exercise and pleasant social interaction.	Physical-social-psychological
5	Sound body dynamics improves efficiency and appearance.	Physical-social-psychological

Objectives for grades K-3

Domain	Objectives for students	Basic concepts
Cognitive	1. Tells why exercise, rest, and relaxation are important for good health	1-4
	2. Identifies ways to relax	3
	3. Recalls pleasant experiences in games or dance activities	4
	4. Identifies the values of good posture and sound body mechanics	5
	5. Explains the importance of rest, relaxation, and sleep to optimal health	3
Affective	1. Appreciates value of exercise, rest, and relaxation in maintaining good health and growth	1, 2
	2. Desires to learn and play games regularly	1, 2, 4
	3. Shows interest in individual and group games and dances	1, 2, 4
	4. Shows interest in using own body most efficiently	5
	5. Is aware of the daily need for rest, relaxation, and sleep	3
Action	1. Takes an active part in games and dances at school and after school	1, 2, 4
	2. Practices good body dynamics in daily activities	5
	3. Sleeps 8 to 10 hours each night and rests occasionally during the day	3
	4. Demonstrates good sportsmanship and a spirit of cooperation in games and dances	4

Objectives for grades 4–6

Domain	Objectives for students	Basic concepts
Cognitive	1. Explains physiological reasons for regular, vigorous exercise	1, 2
	2. Understands emotional health values of sports and dance	4
	3. Can demonstrate the basics of functional body movement	5
	4. Lists reasons for adequate rest, relaxation, and sleep	3
	5. Identifies ways to relax at home and school	3
Affective	1. Appreciates the values of physical fitness as a part of total good health	1, 2, 4
	2. Asks questions about the physiological and mental benefits of exercise	1, 2, 4
	3. Desires to learn more about basic skills, strategy, and rules of sports	4
	4. Is attentive to information on the importance of rest, relaxation, and sleep	3
	5. Appreciates the aesthetic and physiological values of efficient body movement	5
Action	1. Takes an active part in games and dance activities at school	1, 2, 4
	2. Participates in sports after school and on weekends	1, 2, 4
	3. Sleeps 8 to 10 hours each night and rests when fatigued during the day	3
	4. Demonstrates good sportsmanship in sports and dance activities	4
	5. Practices good body dynamics in daily activities	5
	6. Takes time daily to participate in some type of relaxation activity	3

Objectives for grades 7–8

Domain	Objectives for students	Basic concepts
Cognitive	1. Explains specific changes in muscular and circulatory systems during exercise	1, 2
	2. Describes mental health values of sports and dance	4
	3. Understands the kinesiology of fundamental body movements as in standing, sitting, walking, lifting, pushing, and pulling	5
	4. Cites the physical and mental values of proper sleep, relaxation, and rest	3
	5. Lists health values of regular exercise	1, 2, 4
Affective	1. Believes that physical fitness is one of the values in the good life	1-5
	2. Appreciates the physiological and emotional values of regular exercise	1, 2, 4
	3. Desires to learn more about basic skills, strategy, and rules of sports	4
	4. Appreciates the physical and mental values of adequate rest, relaxation, and sleep	3
	5. Believes that one's appearance and efficiency are enhanced by sound body dynamics	5
Action	1. Participates regularly in sports, dance, or other forms of physical exercise	1, 2, 4
	2. Sleeps 8 to 10 hours each night and rests when fatigued during the day	3
	3. Demonstrates cooperation, leadership, and good sportsmanship in sports or dance activities	4
	4. Maintains desirable muscle development and figure control through exercise	1, 2
	5. Follows principles of sound body dynamics in daily activities	5
	6. Relaxes daily using a satisfactory method	

FAMILY HEALTH UNIT

Outline of content

Physiological

Life: purpose and order, a life cycle or pattern of growth, all living things from living things

Characteristics—a beginning, changes, and death; reproduction; need for food, water, air, protection; movement; response to light, sound, cold, pain, danger

Differences—form, structure, functions, life cycle, pattern of growth, dependency and needs, methods of reproduction

Types—plant, animal, and human; plant reproduction—budding, runners, seeds, pollination; animal reproduction—asexually—cell division or fission; sexually—internally with males and females, and externally as in some fish that lay eggs

Human life: human being—unique; rational; decision maker; possessor of freedom, self-awareness, consciousness, and dignity; controller of actions; similarities and differences—heredity, race, size, intellect, ethnic background

Human growth and development

Definitions—"growing up," puberty, maturity

Puberty—special growth stage reaching physical adulthood; girls reach this stage 1½ years earlier than boys

Maturity—growth stage in which the person is more cooperative; has positive sex attitudes; is not easily hurt; is not dominated by moods; is able to meet problems constructively; is able to meet responsibilities; is able to make wise decisions

Cause—action of endocrine glands and their hormones

Results—a variety of physical, emotional, and social changes

Physical—size and shape changes; appearance of secondary sex characteristics; boys—muscle development; hair on face, chest, and pubic areas; seminal emissions; appearance of sex drive; girls—hair under arms and pubic areas; breasts, widening of hips; menstrual cycle; appearance of sex drive

Emotional—physical attraction; fears and emotions with possible moodiness

Social—increase in boy-girl relations; need for friends

Role of heredity—physical characteristics; chromosomes and genes

Human reproduction

Start of life—union of male (sperm) and female (ovum) cells; need for father and mother

Reproductive organs

Male—external—penis, scrotum, testicles; internal—urethra, bladder, prostate, seminal vesicles, vas deferens, epididymis

Female—external—labia majora and minora, urethral opening, clitoris, vaginal opening, hymen; internal—vagina, cervix, uterus, oviduct, ovaries, urethra, bladder

Other concepts—fertilization, conception, implantation, fetus growth, birth, menstruation, birth control, pubic hair

Psychological

Understanding self: strengths and weaknesses; personality; worth; ability to succeed, but ability to accept failure; understanding and control of emotions; experience of joy through self-fulfillment; wholesome relations with others; decision making by problem solving process; good use of abilities

Sex drive—normal reaction; perpetuation of population; provides pleasure

Outline of content—cont'd

Psychological—cont'd

Sex behavior in adolescence—interest in one's body and sex normal; questions of sex before marriage; sex deviation—homosexuality, exhibitionism, rape

Factors influencing sex drive—biological makeup; early childhood experiences; parental attitudes; environmental influences

Purpose of family—satisfaction of physical and psychological needs; stability and security important for good mental health; guidance of individuals to adulthood

Social

The family

Nature—size; structure, or composition; culture or ethnic; religion; changes

Types—two parents; one parent; no parents, guardian; stepparents; mixed ethnic

Needs—physical, psychological, and emotional

Functions—different roles because of different types of families and geographical location, but inclusion of sharing and transmission of feelings, ideas, heritage, and income; security by fulfilling needs; aid in education; growth and development; affection, worthy use of leisure time

Role of individual family members—assumption of responsibilities; cooperation in functioning of home; respect of others' rights; consideration; acceptance of differences; trying to understand members; not making unreasonable demands; working together; helping in different ways including financial support; use of constructive ways to solve differences

Status in family of oldest child—only child; only boy in group of girls; only girl in group of boys

Family influence on ability of members to make adjustments in society dependent on—cultural background of parents; family dwelling and location; health practices of members; economic status; type of structure; values

Problems and conflicts—parents; siblings; grandparents; money; use of car; discourtesy; failure to assume responsibilities at home, school, or elsewhere; use of drugs; choice and selection of friends; use of time

Boy-girl relations

Development—building of friendships; popularity; qualities boys and girls are seeking

Purpose—sense of belonging; affection; getting along with opposite sex; enjoyment; learning of social behavior

Dating—types; purposes; responsibilities; choosing a date; dating behavior and society's moral code; drinking and drugs

Steady dating—why; advantages and disadvantages; parents' attitudes and reactions

Values of sex in marriage—legal; emotional; social; medical; spiritual

Family planning

Love

Spiritual

Values: finding a purpose and meaningfulness in life; a philosophy of life; importance of friendships; interpersonal relationships with adults and peers; influence on personality development; relation to acquisition and use of money

Moral issues: premarital sex; failure to assume home responsibilities; relations with others, including parents

Concepts

	Concept	Application of health definition
1	All living things come from living things.	Physiological
2	Individuals in some ways are like all individuals, in some ways like some individuals, and in some ways like no other individual.	
3	The sex drive and reproduction are normal functions of humans.	Psychological
4	Maturity is dependent on a variety of physical, social, and emotional factors.	
5	The family, with its unique features that are subject to change, is the basic unit in American society.	Social
6	Individuals influence and are influenced by the family and its members.	
7	Boy-girl relationships are important preludes to family life and family relations.	
8	Values and moral issues affect attitudes and behaviors regarding the family and sex.	Spiritual

Objectives for grades K–3

Domain		Objectives for students	Basic concepts
Cognitive	1.	Identifies the differences that exist between boys and girls	2
	2.	Concludes the human baby grows and develops inside the mother	1, 2
	3.	Recites the correct vocabulary for body parts and body functions	1, 2
	4.	Lists the responsibilities to be completed at home and at school	5, 6
	5.	Explains how humans reproduce	1
	6.	Compares how families differ in their composition and functions	5
	7.	Recalls that living things come from living things	1
	8.	Explains the way parents and family members help individuals	4-6, 8
	9.	Identifies the rights of others in need of respect	2, 4-8
	10.	Describes the role and responsibilities of family members	5
Affective	1.	Displays interest in learning about the differences between boys and girls	2
	2.	Asks questions about the growth of the baby inside the mother	1, 2
	3.	Is interested in wanting to learn the correct vocabulary for body parts and body functions	1, 2
	4.	Believes there are responsibilities individuals must give their attention to at school and at home	5, 6
	5.	Is attentive to the discussion regarding human reproduction	1, 2
	6.	Talks about the differing compositions and functions of families	5, 6
	7.	Accepts the conclusion that living things come from living things	1
	8.	Believes that parents and family members may be helpful to individuals	4-6, 8
	9.	Is supportive of the need to respect the rights of others	2, 5-8
	10.	Is attentive to the discussion about the role and responsibilities of family members	5
Action (observable) (observable and non-observable)	1.	Uses the correct vocabulary for body parts and functions	1, 2
	2.	Assumes responsibilities at school and at home	5, 6
	3.	Tries to respect the rights of others, including their right to privacy	5, 6

Objectives for grades 4-6

Domain	Objectives for students	Basic concepts
Cognitive	1. Identifies the responsibilities that need attention as a family member	5, 6
	2. Lists the rights of others in need of respect	2, 4-8
	3. Is familiar with the terminology used in describing the human reproductive process	1
	4. Summarizes the meaning of puberty and its effect on growth and development	1-4
	5. Explains the responsibilities of all members of a family	5, 6
	6. Recalls that sex is a basic life function	1-4
	7. Identifies the role of heredity in the growth and development of individuals	2-4, 7
	8. Lists the variety of characteristics displayed by the family	5, 6
Affective	1. Believes that it is necessary as a family member to assume home responsibilities	5, 6
	2. Supports the concept that the rights of others must be respected	2, 4-8
	3. Is interested in learning the terminology necessary to describe the human reproductive process	1
	4. Listens to the discussion about puberty and its effect on growth and development	1-4
	5. Displays interest in the responsibilities of all family members	5, 6
	6. Accepts sex as a basic life function	1-3
	7. Asks questions regarding the role of heredity on the growth and development of individuals	1, 2, 4
	8. Accepts the basic life function of menstruation as an important phenomenon	2, 3
	9. Believes it is necessary to cooperate with other family members to achieve a happy family unit	5, 6
	10. Is aware that families display a variety of characteristics	5
Action (observable, nonobservable, or delayed)	1. Assumes responsibilities at home as a family member	5, 6
	2. Tries to cooperate with family members to achieve a happy family unit	5, 6
	3. Makes efforts to consistently respect the rights of others	2, 4-8
(observable)	4. Is able to discuss human reproduction without embarrassment using appropriate terminology	1

Objectives for grades 7-8

Domain	Objectives for students	Basic concepts
Cognitive	1. Explains the sex drive and its effect on individuals	1-4, 7
	2. Identifies factors that may influence one's sex drive	3, 4, 6-8
	3. Differentiates between physical, emotional, and social maturity	4
	4. Summarizes the human reproductive process from conception through birth	1-3
	5. Concludes that the family is the basic unit of American society and is familiar with its changing roles	5

	6. Identifies the importance of boy-girl relationships and the qualities boys and girls seek in one another	7
	7. Prepares criteria for behavior on dates	3, 4, 7, 8
	8. Compares the advantages and disadvantages of steady dating	7, 8
	9. Discusses sexual behavior in adolescence and before marriage	3-5, 8
	10. Explains the meaning of love	7
	11. Identifies the social, economic, and cultural influences on family life	5, 6, 8
	12. Selects values or a value system having meaning in life	8
	13. Is familiar with the problem solving process to help make decisions about the family and sex behavior	4, 5, 8
	14. Concludes there are moral issues involved in premarital sex, acceptance of responsibilities in the home, and others	3-5, 8
	15. Describes the concept and purpose of family planning	3-5, 7, 8
Affective	1. Accepts sex as a natural drive and function of individuals that is accompanied by related responsibilities	1-4, 7
	2. Believes that maturity in life is essential for successful living	4
	3. Displays interest in the human reproductive process from conception through birth	1-3
	4. Is sensitive to the acceptance of the family as the basic unit of American society and its changing roles	5
	5. Is aware of the need to develop boy-girl relationships and procedures for building friendships	7
	6. Asks questions regarding the advantages and disadvantages of steady dating	7, 8
	7. Is interested in discussing and preparing criteria for behavior on dates	3, 4, 7, 8
	8. Displays a readiness to want to discuss sexual behavior in adolescence and before marriage	3, 4, 7, 8
	9. Accepts the meaning of love to be more inclusive than physical attraction	7
	10. Is aware of the variety of social, economic, and cultural influences on family life	5, 6
	11. Believes that individuals need to determine the values that help them develop a philosophy of life	8
	12. Supports the problem solving process as a useful method in making decisions about sex and family behavior	4, 6
	13. Is sensitive to the moral issues involved in premarital sex relations, acceptance of responsibilities in the home, and others	3-5, 8
	14. Is aware of the importance of family planning	3-5, 7, 8
Action (observable and non-observable or delayed) (nonobservable or delayed)	1. Attempts to act as a physically, emotionally, and socially mature individual	4
	2. Tries to become a contributing and effective member of the family	5, 6
	3. Demonstrates the ability to achieve a balance between expression, behavior, and the sex drive	1-4, 7, 8
	4. Develops wholesome relationships with members of the opposite sex	7
	5. Behaves in socially accepted ways with members of the opposite sex	7
	6. Attempts to develop values or a value system that will give life meaningfulness	8
	7. Uses the problem solving process to help make decisions about the family and sex behavior	3, 4, 6

MENTAL HEALTH UNIT

Outline of content

Physiological

Definitions: mental health—adjustment to self and society; faces realities of life; functions effectively
Mental illness—varying degrees of emotional disturbance; in severe forms—psychoses, neuroses, personality disorders

Growth and development of individual: factors influencing
Heredity—nervous system and endocrine glands; effect on thinking, feeling, acting
Environment—economically rich or deprived; stresses and pressure of parents, peers, or teacher; physical atmosphere—housing, climate
Interrelationship of biological and environmental influences—heredity sets limits; environment determines level of attainment; stress situations may cause biological reactions and anxiety; pleasant environment brings feelings of calmness and tranquility

Psychological

Mentally healthy individual: pursuer of reasonable goals; self-respect; knowledge of being liked and loved; sense of security; ability to think and act rationally; distinguishes between facts and feelings; maintenance of integrity in work and play; ability to work in group; respect for rights of others; faces realities of life; acceptance of responsibilities

Needs of individuals: physical—food, air, water, rest and sleep, housing, clothing, freedom from disease
Psychological—affection, security, acceptance as an individual, achievement, independence, authority, self-respect, success

Mature personality: a clear self-concept*
Definition of personality—involving total physical, social, mental, and emotional aspects of individual including interests, size, shape, dress; the way the individual walks, talks, thinks, feels; ability to get along with people
Understanding of own strengths, weaknesses, and academic, intellectual, and physical potentials
Understanding of emotions' role in development
Types—anger, fear, love, hate, jealousy, happiness, prejudice, sorrow, joy
Effects—helpful or harmful
Relief from effects by talk with someone, play, work, hobbies
Influence on personal health—sleep and rest; eating; posture; physical activity
Control—sense of humor; ability to accept criticism, disappointment, failure, and unhappiness in normal fashion
Understanding of the physical growth changes taking place

Ability to make adjustments, develop coping skills
Solving of problems and making decisions after weighing alternatives and consequences about study, work, sex, parent relations, peer relations
Establishment of realistic goals within potentials; achievable to reduce stress
Assumption and carrying out of responsibilities at home, school, and community

---

*Stenner and Katzenmeyer (see Chapter 11 References) claim that children during the early school years who have positive self-concepts are confident of their ability to meet everyday problems and demands and are at ease in their relationships with other people. These children tend to be independent and reliable and are relatively free from anxiety, nervousness, excessive worry, tiredness, and loneliness. They are seldom considered behavior problems. They tend to be above average in reading and mathematics. They view school as a happy, worthwhile place.

Ability to handle stress

    Nature—tensions or pressures build attempting to carry out responsibilities, achieve goals, or solve problems resulting in anxieties, fears, worries and other emotional responses; degree dependent on factors involved

    Causes—competition, desire to succeed, failure, sibling rivalry, parental expectations, school demands

    Values and limits—some individuals work better under slight stress; may be motivational; may interfere with normal response

    Relief from—modification of goals; activity change; balance of work and play; assumption of responsibilities; talking it out; taking one thing at a time; working off

    Risk taking—positive and negative; includes financial gambles, risks of bodily harm and physical injury, ethical, self-esteem, and social risks

    Coping with death and dying; bereavement and grief

Adjustment mechanisms: result from inability to adequately solve problems; individual resorts to other procedures to gain satisfaction, such as rationalization, projection, identification; misuse results in maladjusted behavior

Causes of mental illness: multiplicity of complex environmental factors

    Physical and chemical—infections, nutritional deficiencies, accidents, gland deficiencies, alcohol, anemia, physical defects

    Psychological—social relations, love and marriage, family conflicts, sibling conflicts, sex adjustments, religious conflicts, parental attitudes and personality, school and peer experiences

Emotional maladjustment or mental illness: mental illness is a matter of degree and kind; for some individuals, mild emotional disturbances; for others, severe mental health problems manifested in a variety of symptomatic behaviors

Death: meaningfulness and relation to birth and life, individuals, animals, and pets; bereavement and grief—stages of grief, need for others, need to be alone, helping others grieve; coping mechanisms—denial, anger, bargaining, depression, acceptance; feelings—perception of death; suicide—causes, signs, and symptoms

Social

Building of satisfying human relations: effective interaction with adults, peers, and opposite sex

    Acquisition and retention of friends; sharing possessions and time; development of trust and fair play; respect of people as individuals; willingness to work with people; courteous and considerate; ability to give, as well as to take

    Choice of friends: need to establish criteria

    Influence of people: rewards; threats; authority; expertness

    Warm, safe, and secure home and school climate

    Alternative lifestyles

    Successful group functioning involving respect and acceptance of all members; participation of all members; acceptance of responsibilities by each member; need for authority; a must to have constructive ways to resolve differences

Recognition of worth: realization that all individuals have differing human worths; ability to give consideration to rights of others; value of individual differences including race, religion, or ethnic origin

Community resource available to help with problems: school—nurse, teacher, counselor; home—parents; church—clergymen; community—physicians, psychiatrists, organizations and agencies, public health departments

Death: death rituals and funerals—cultural and ethnic differences; communication with terminally ill; costs; suicide—sources of help

Outline of content—cont'd

Spiritual

Values: the individual needs to attempt to define own values or value system; the individual's acceptance of differing values and value system of others

Moral issue: basic principles to use in the development and retention of relationships with others; recognition that all individuals should receive equal and just treatment regardless of socioeconomic status, religious, cultural, or ethnic backgrounds

Concepts

Concept	Application of health definition
1 Mental health is influenced by biological and environmental factors.	Physiological
2 Each individual is like all others, like some others, and like no others.	
3 Understanding and acceptance of the concept of one's self is important in mental health.	Psychological
4 All individuals have dignity and worth.	
5 Individuals should be able to face the realities of life with emotional maturity.	
6 Stress can be beneficial and detrimental to individuals.	
7 The ability to get along with others is important in mental health.	Social
8 The community has a variety of sources available to help individuals with mental and emotional problems and difficulties.	
9 Values help provide meaningfulness to life.	Spiritual

Objectives for grades K-3

Domain	Objectives for students	Basic concepts
Cognitive	1. Explains the reasons why sharing and taking turns are necessary	7
	2. Lists ways to respect the feelings, rights, and property of individuals	4, 7
	3. Lists ways of making and keeping friends	7
	4. Identifies basic emotions	5-7
	5. Discusses ways emotions may be helpful and harmful and their effects on personal worth	5-7
	6. Recalls possible ways to sublimate or control emotional reactions	1, 3, 5-7
	7. Recites ways to assume responsibilities in school and at home	7
	8. Identifies ways to have success and be independent at school	3, 5
	9. Explains ways to prevent hurting someone or causing hard feelings	1, 4, 5, 7
	10. Explains life and death in terms of loss of pets and animals	5
Affective	1. Is interested in sharing and taking turns	7
	2. Talks about the feelings, rights, and property of individuals	4, 7
	3. Is attentive to discussion regarding emotions and their effects on individuals	1, 5-7
	4. Asks questions regarding ways to prevent hurting people or causing hard feelings	1, 4, 5, 7
	5. Accepts the need for successful and independent school experiences	3, 4
	6. Displays interest in wanting and learning how to make and retain friends	7
	7. Supports the need to assume responsibilities in school and at home	7
	8. Realizes that living things must die	5

Action	1. Participates in sharing and taking turns	7
(observable,	2. Experiences success and independence in a variety of ways in school	3, 4
nonob-	3. Is able to acquire friends and maintain them	4, 7
servable,	4. Respects the feelings, rights, and property of others	4, 7
and de-	5. Attempts to control emotions	1, 5-7
layed)	6. Is able to express feelings in a mature fashion	1, 5-7
	7. Refrains from behavior that will hurt someone or cause hard feelings	1, 4, 5
	8. Assumes responsibilities expected in school and at home	7

Objectives for grades 4-6

Domain	Objectives for students	Basic concepts
Cognitive	1. Identifies adults who are receptive to talking over problems	8
	2. Identifies adults who are available to help with problems	8
	3. Lists the rules necessary for classroom behavior	1, 7
	4. Identifies the characteristics in which individuals are alike, different, or unique	1, 2
	5. Identifies goals that are within the possibility of achievement by the individual	3, 5
	6. Describes ways emotions can be controlled	1, 3, 5-7
	7. Explains the reasons for treating all individuals with dignity and respect	4
	8. Discusses the biological and environmental factors affecting mental health	1
	9. Lists situations when stress may occur and discusses helpfulness or harmfulness	1, 6
	10. Recalls the scientific principles needed to solve problems	5
	11. Illustrates ways to be able to work productively as an individual in small groups	3, 4, 7
	12. Recalls a variety of interesting leisure time activities	1, 3, 8
	13. Identifies ways individuals try to adjust to demands of daily living	5
	14. Explains the role of the brain, nervous system, and endocrine glands in mental health	7
	15. Explains risk-taking behavior	6
	16. Discusses life and death, meaning and causes	5
Affective	1. Believes a variety of individuals are willing and available to help solve problems	8
	2. Accepts the realization that there are adults willing to help students with problems	8
	3. Is attentive to the preparation of rules for classroom behavior	1, 7
	4. Talks about the significance of establishing realistic goals	3, 5
	5. Displays interest in characteristics that identify individuals as alike, different, or unique persons	1, 2
	6. Believes emotions need to be controlled	1, 3, 5-7
	7. Is attentive to the importance of treating all individuals with dignity and respect	4
	8. Asks questions regarding the biological and environmental factors affecting mental health	1
	9. Believes stress situations may be helpful and harmful	1, 6
	10. Supports the need to try to solve problems using scientific principles	5
	11. Displays interest in being able to work productively as an individual and in small groups	3, 4, 7

Objectives for grades 4-6

Domain	Objectives for students	Basic concepts
Affective— cont'd	12. Enjoys and is interested in participating in a variety of leisure time activities	1, 3, 8
	13. Believes that risk-taking behavior may be hazardous	6
	14. Realizes that grief is part of life	5
Action (observable, nonob-servable, and de-layed)	1. Participates in the formulation of rules for classroom behavior	1, 7
	2. Seeks help when facing unsolvable problems	8
	3. Talks over problems with trusted adults	8
	4. Attempts to establish realistic goals	3, 5
	5. Treats all individuals with dignity and respect	4
	6. Attempts to control emotions	1, 3, 5, 7
	7. Attempts to avoid or reduce stressful situations	1, 6
	8. Tries to solve problems using scientific principles	5
	9. Is able to work productively as an individual and in groups	3, 4, 7
	10. Participates in a variety of interesting leisure time activities	1, 3, 8

Objectives for grades 7-8

Domain	Objectives for students	Basic concepts
Cognitive	1. Describes the values believed to be important to self	9
	2. Explains the interrelationships between biological and environmental influences on mental health	1
	3. Identifies the characteristics of the mentally healthy individual	3, 5
	4. States the strengths, weaknesses, and potential abilities of the self	1, 2, 3
	5. Describes the growth and developmental changes taking place in the individual	1, 2
	6. Concludes an individual's personality is comprised of a variety of components and is unique	2
	7. Discusses the procedures necessary and problems faced in attempting to improve relationships with parents and teachers	7
	8. Compares the helpful and harmful aspects of friends and friendships	7
	9. Explains the scientific principles usable in solving problems	5
	10. Translates all the evidence needed to make decisions	5
	11. Interprets the effect of peer pressures on individual behavior	6
	12. Indicates ways stress produced by peer pressures can be handled	6
	13. Identifies the types and symptoms of maladjustive behavior and the community sources and services available	1, 8
	14. Discusses positive and negative aspects of risk-taking behavior	6
	15. Identifies awareness of death and life	5
	16. Lists ways to cope with death of family member or friend	5
	17. Analyzes suicide in terms of causes, signs and symptoms, and sources of help	5
Affective	1. Believes that establishing values or a value system is necessary to find meaningfulness in life	9
	2. Is attentive to discussion about the interrelationships between biological and environmental influences on mental health	1
	3. Displays interest in the characteristics of the mentally healthy individual	3, 5
	4. Is supportive of the need to constantly improve individual abilities	2, 3, 5

5. Asks questions regarding the growth and developmental changes that take place in the individual   1, 2

6. Is interested in identifying own personality; characteristics and uniqueness   2, 3

7. Believes that parent and teacher relationships are important   7

8. Accepts the fact that friends can be helpful, as well as harmful, to individuals   5, 7

9. Supports the need to solve problems using scientific principles   5

10. Listens to the idea that decisions cannot be made without careful consideration   5

11. Displays interest in learning the effect of peer pressures on behavior   2, 3, 5, 6

12. Believes that stress created by peers may not always be beneficial   6

13. Asks questions regarding the types and symptoms of maladjustive behavior and the treatment sources and services available in the community   1, 8

14. Realizes the positive and negative aspects of risk-taking behavior   6

15. Asks questions regarding funerals, rituals, and bereavement   5

16. Is attentive to discussion about euthanasia   5

Action
(observable, nonobservable, and delayed)

1. Tries to develop a set of values or a value system   3-5

2. Attempts to improve the strengths, weaknesses, and potential abilities of the self   7

3. Endeavors to improve parent and teacher relationships   2, 5, 7

4. Chooses friends after careful consideration of a variety of factors

5. Solves problems using scientific principles   5

6. Tries to make decisions after viewing all the alternatives and consequences   5

7. Attempts not to be unduly influenced by stress created by peers   2, 3, 5, 6

8. Seeks help when maladjustive symptoms of a persistent nature appear   8

9. Attempts to help others in times of death of loved ones   5

NUTRITION UNIT

Outline of content

Physiological

Definitions: food, nutrition, calorie

Purposes of food: energy, tissue building, protection and maintenance of bodily functions

Nutrients needed: reasons; good sources of proteins and fats; daily recommended allowances by age, sex, size, activity

Food needed: basic four food groups; daily recommended allowances by age, sex, activity

Planning for meals or sample meals: breakfast, lunch, dinner, snacks, camping, picnics, sports, children, elderly, pregnancy, parties

Diet and weight control: desirable weights—age, sex, size; identification of overweight and obesity; food intake; role of exercise; reducing fads and fallacies; sources of help; reliable and unreliable sources of information

Body processing of foods: digestion; absorption; use

Effects on the body: performance—mental, nervous stability, motor, disease; body structure and size—teeth, bones, soft tissues; length of life; energy needs—internal and external body activities

Disorders and diseases: appendicitis, constipation, allergies, diabetes, cancer, food poisoning, heart disease (genetic and environmental risk factors)

Outline of content—cont'd

Psychological

Food = Power: security; prestige and status; symbol of hospitality and friendship
Effect and outlet for emotions: joy, sorrow, conflict, comfort, fear, worry, anxiety
Motivations for modifying food habits
   Specific—weight reduction; weight control; lower blood pressure; pregnancy; sports; looks and personality; old age
   General—good health; longer life

Social

Eating patterns and preferences: influencing factors including cultural, ethnic, religious, racial, and social customs and traditions—Italian, Mexican, Asian, native American, black; economic factors; age, sex, size; sensory reactions to food—texture, color, odor, taste, looks; social climate and atmosphere including companionship; education influences—TV, radio, newspapers, magazines, school, family, community, friends, neighbors
Sanitation and safety: home, school, community (restaurants); laws; protective agencies
Preparation, processing, preservation, and storage: procedures—canning, frozen, dehydrated, powdered, refrigerated, pasteurized, irradiated, adulterated
Consumer protection: laws—additives, advertising, safety, adulteration, pasteurization, sanitation, food production, processing; agencies—FDA, FTC, health departments
Fads and fallacies: misconceptions, weight control, "soul," natural and organic foods
Selection and purchase of foods: wise economic expenditures
Problems of hunger in society: role of individual and community

Spiritual

Values: value of food in human life; importance of food for health of individuals
Moral issues: Does society have the obligation to feed the hungry and the poor? Should the hungry and the poor receive food? How should people treat individuals who are hungry and in need of food?

Concepts

Concept	Application of health definition
1 Foods differ in kind, sources, and nutritive value and serve a variety of purposes for individuals.	Physiological
2 Individuals require the same nutrients but in varying amounts throughout life.	
3 The selection of nutritious foods contained in a balanced diet are necessary for the proper growth, good health, and everyday functioning of the individual.	
4 Lack of nutritious food resulting from a variety of factors may be detrimental to the health of individuals.	
5 Differing motivations influence the types and amounts of food consumed by individuals.	Psychological
6 Foods help satisfy the emotional needs of individuals.	
7 Cultural, social, economic, and educational factors affect an individual's food selections.	Social
8 Production, processing, storage, preparation, and dispensing of foods influence their nutritional value, safety, and consumption.	

9 The social atmosphere present at meals, or when food is consumed, may have positive or negative effects on individuals.

10 Food should be made available to all individuals regardless of their cul-   Spiritual
tural, social, economic, or educational status.

Objectives for grades K-3

Domain	Objectives for students	Basic concepts
Cognitive	1. Identifies the basic four food groups	1-3
	2. Recalls the importance of milk in the daily diet	1-3
	3. Explains the purposes of food and relates to the basic four food groups	1, 3
	4. Lists nutritious snack foods	3
	5. Is able to plan simple nutritious breakfasts, lunches, and dinners from the basic four food groups	1, 3
	6. Recalls the sources of foods from plants and animals	1
	7. Explains the reasons for sanitary practices in the preparing, serving, and eating of foods	9
	8. Identifies the cultural and social differences in foods consumed by people	8
Affective	1. Is attentive to discussions about the basic four food groups	1, 3
	2. Displays interest in eating a variety of foods	1, 3
	3. Raises questions regarding the sources of food from plants and animals	1
	4. Accepts the importance of tasting new and different foods	1, 3
	5. Listens to the discussion for socially acceptable behavior at mealtime	10
	6. Talks about cultural and social differences in foods consumed by people	8
Action (observable)	1. Eats breakfast before attending school or while at school	3
	2. Eats nutritious snack foods	1, 3
	3. Acts in a socially acceptable manner at mealtime	10
	4. Follows sanitary practices in the preparing, handling, and eating of foods	9
(nonobservable and delayed)	5. Eats well-balanced meals selected from the basic four food groups	1, 3
	6. Demonstrates willingness to try and eat a variety of foods, including new ones	1, 3
	7. Takes only the amount of food that can be eaten	8

Objectives for grades 4-6

Domain	Objectives for students	Basic concepts
Cognitive	1. Recalls the basic four food groups	1-3
	2. Identifies the nutrients found in foods, as well as the foods in which they are found	1
	3. Is able to plan nutritious meals with some degree of efficiency	1, 3
	4. Identifies the reasons why individuals need the same nutrients but in varying amounts throughout life	2
	5. Recalls how the body processes foods in terms of digestion, absorption, and use	2, 3
	6. Compares the foods and eating practices of various community, ethnic, religious, racial and cultural groups of people to the basic four food groups	7
	7. Explains the relationships of poorly balanced diets and lack of food to diseases and disorders	4
	8. Lists factors that affect choices of foods by individuals	5

Objectives for grades 4-6—cont'd

Domain	Objectives for students	Basic concepts
Cognitive—cont'd	9. Compares the nutritive values of highly advertised foods to the basic four food groups and to the nutrients needed by individuals	1, 2, 7
	10. Identifies reliable sources of nutrition information	7
Affective	1. Listens to discussions about the importance of nutritious foods for growth and health	1-3
	2. Displays interest in the selection of nutritious foods	1, 3
	3. Accepts the fact that new and different foods can add interest to eating	1-3
	4. Questions the value of highly advertised foods	1, 3
	5. Reacts to class discussions by raising questions regarding how foods satisfy differing emotional needs of individuals	6
	6. Raises questions regarding reasons individuals require different types and amounts of food	2
	7. Displays interest in learning more about the relationships of food to disease and disorders	4
	8. Is attentive to discussions regarding the cultural and ethnic patterns and eating practices of individuals	7
	9. Supports the need to locate and use reliable sources of nutrition information	7
Action (observable)	1. Eats nutritious foods at mealtime and at snacktime	1, 3
	2. Eats breakfast before attending school or while at school	3
	3. Follows sanitary practices in the preparation, serving, storing, and eating of food	8
(nonobservable, or delayed)	4. Eats a variety of foods and is willing to try new ones	1, 3
	5. Uses reliable sources for nutrition information	7

Objectives for grades 7-8

Domain	Objectives for students	Basic concepts
Cognitive	1. Explains how it is possible to obtain all the essential nutrients by eating a balanced diet selected from a variety of foods	1, 3
	2. Describes diseases and disorders that may be associated with nutritional practices	4
	3. Lists the dangers to growth, health, and body functioning through the consumption of improper foods or poor eating habits	4
	4. Identifies the differing motivations that bring about changes in food consumption habits, such as sports, weight control, length of life	5
	5. Analyzes TV and other commercials about food and their nutritive value	1, 3, 5, 7
	6. Identifies federal, state, and local agencies and their functions in the control of the purity and quality of foods	8
	7. Explains how weight can be controlled in many individuals through proper diet and exercise	2
	8. Summarizes the current food fads and misconceptions	5, 7
	9. Illustrates the differing effects of food and lack of food on the body	4
	10. Compares the cultural or ethnic food patterns of community groups with the basic four food groups	1, 7

	11. Concludes that all people need food and that efforts should be made to assure that it is available when needed	10
	12. Examines food consumption at breakfast, lunch, dinner, and snacktime and compares with basic four food groups	1, 3
	13. Identifies the genetic and environmental risk factors related to heart disease	4
	14. Lists reliable sources of nutrition information	7
Affective	1. Displays interest in attempting to help individuals in need of food	10
	2. Accepts the importance of weight control through proper diet and exercise	2
	3. Accepts and understands the cultural and ethnic differences in foods consumed by individuals	7
	4. Asks questions in regard to agencies and their functions that have responsiblity for the control of the purity and quality of foods	8
	5. Is attentive to discussions regarding current food fads and misconceptions	5, 7
	6. Displays interest in the differing motivations for food habits	5
	7. Talks about food as a socializing agent by participating in discussions	7, 9
	8. Is supportive of the concept that a balanced diet selected from a variety of foods is necessary for proper growth and health	1, 3
	9. Believes that advertising about foods and food products must be carefully analyzed in terms of nutritional value	1, 3, 5, 7
	10. Realizes the role of nutrition as a risk factor in heart disease	4
	11. Accepts the importance of the use of reliable sources of nutrition information	7
Action (observable) (nonobservable, or delayed)	1. Eats breakfast before attending school or while at school	3
	2. Eats nutritious foods at mealtime and snacktime	1, 3
	3. Periodically provides assistance by helping needy individuals obtain food	10
	4. Attempts to keep weight and intake of foods under control through the wise selection and consumption of nutritious items	2, 3
	5. Refrains, or attempts to encourage parents to refrain, from purchasing highly advertised foods unless they have been analyzed for nutritional value	1, 3, 5, 7
	6. Reduces intake of foods related to heart disease	4
	7. Uses reliable sources of nutrition information	7

SAFETY AND FIRST AID UNIT*

Outline of content

Physiological

Definitions: injury, sudden illness, hemorrhage, respiration, concussion, fracture, shock, abrasion, laceration, resuscitation, burn classifications, poisons, sprains, strain, contusion, heat stroke and heat exhaustion, defensive driving

Effects of accidents: disability and death

Areas: home; school; community; fire and electric; bicycle; farm; sports and recreation; firearms; winter and summer

---

*Also see Chapter 7.

Outline of content—cont'd

Psychological

Individual responsibility for safety
Accident proneness
Emotional factors in accidents and emergencies
Alcohol and other drugs in accidents
Emotional effects of accidents and emergencies on first aiders
Emotional influence in shock
Attitude toward mouth-to-mouth resuscitation
Importance of safe practices

Social

Accident costs in money, disability, and death responsibility: safe construction of motor vehicles, highways and information signs, toys, household appliances, farm and ranch equipment, houses and hotels, schools, business and industrial plants, children's clothing, and industrial equipment
Dangerous strangers and dangerous acquaintances
Responsibility for community emergency care programs
Sources of aid in accidents and emergencies

Spiritual

Values: importance of safety and health for all
Moral issues: protection of life and health of others in school, home, and other places; responsibility of individual and community to prevent accidents and provide emergency care

Concepts

Concept	Application of health definition
1 Accident hazards and unsafe conditions exist in all environments.	Physical
2 An individual's safety depends on own ability to adjust to own environment.	Physical
3 Accidents are the leading cause of death and injury among elementary-school pupils.	Physical
4 Combinations of factors and forces contribute to the occurrence of accidents.	Psychological-social
5 Individuals, families, and community groups should be prepared to act effectively in the event of injury or sudden illness.	Social
6 Everyone has an obligation to reduce accident hazards in the environment.	Social
7 Safety and emergency care procedures are based on appreciation of the value and quality of life.	Spiritual
8 Risk-taking behavior is the result of a variety of motivations.	Psychological-social

Objectives for grades K–3

Domain	Objectives for students	Basic concepts
Cognitive	1. Identifies accident hazards in own immediate environment	1, 2, 6
	2. Explains the reasons for protecting people from accidents	1-3
	3. Lists ways of avoiding accidents	2, 4
	4. Cites examples of disrespect for safety procedures in motor vehicle, home, school, and public activities	4, 6, 7

	5. Explains why first aid is important	5, 7
	6. Identifies ways to care for minor injuries	5, 7
	7. Cites best methods for getting help in emergencies	5, 7
	8. Lists most common kinds of accidents among kindergarten to third grade pupils	3, 4
Affective	1. Asks questions about hazards in the environment	1, 2, 6
	2. Shows interest in the causes of accidents	2, 4, 6
	3. Reacts to class discussions on loss of life and health by accidents	2, 3, 6
	4. Expresses a desire to do something about the accident problem	1, 3, 6
	5. Is attentive to information presented on simple first-aid measures and procedures for obtaining expert assistance	5, 7
	6. Displays interest in helping others who may be sick or hurt	5, 7
Action	1. Follows safe practices in classroom, lunchroom, hallways, and playground	1-6
	2. Acts in a safe manner enroute to and from school—in bus or car, as pedestrian, or cycling	1-4, 6
	3. Seeks aid from school personnel for injury or sudden illness	5
	4. Helps other pupils when they are hurt or sick	5, 7
	5. Improves safe practices at home and in the immediate environment	1-4, 6
	6. Provides care for minor injuries	5

Objectives for grades 4-6

Domain	Objectives for students	Basic concepts
Cognitive	1. Identifies the four classes of accidents: motor vehicle, home, public, and occupational	1, 2
	2. Lists new environmental accident hazards resulting from technological advances	1, 2, 4
	3. Explains ways to reduce potential for accidents	1, 2, 4, 6
	4. Tells how mental upsets may help cause accidents	1, 4
	5. Lists the steps in first aid to help someone who has been injured or becomes ill	5, 7
	6. Explains the most common emergency care procedures	5
Affective	1. Asks questions about specific potential causes for various types of accidents	1-4, 6
	2. Shows interest in environmental improvement to remove hazards	1-4, 6
	3. Displays an appreciation of the accident toll on children, youth, and adults	3, 7
	4. Is aware of the indifference and ignorance of the public with regard to safety	2, 4, 7
	5. Inquires about ways to improve safety conditions in and around the school	1, 3, 6, 7
	6. Expresses desire to become competent in first-aid methods	5, 7
	7. Shows concern for need to improve emergency care programs	5, 7
Action	1. Acts in a safe manner in school and in the community	1-4, 6
	2. Starts to develop habits of helping others in preventing accidents	3, 6, 7
	3. Assists safety patrol or other school personnel when occasion arises	3, 6, 7
	4. Seeks information on underlying causes of accidents	4, 6
	5. Administers first aid for minor injuries	5, 7
	6. Secures information on the community's emergency aid program	5, 7

Objectives for grades 7-8

Domain	Objectives for students	Basic concepts
Cognitive	1. Lists deaths and injuries by age groups for the four major classes of accidents	1, 2
	2. Explains the ways in which modern environment can threaten own safety	1, 2, 4, 7
	3. Contrasts of pleasures and dangers of motorcycling, aquatic sports (scuba and skin diving, surfing, and water skiing), snow skiing, and other locally popular sport activities	1, 4, 6
	4. Identifies reliable sources of safety information	1, 3, 6
	5. Identifies safety organizations at the national, state, and local level	1, 6
	6. Explains and illustrates specific major first-aid procedures	5
	7. Lists reasons for needed improvements in community emergency care programs	5, 7
	8. Lists school and community resources that can render assistance in emergencies	5
Affective	1. Displays interest in doing own part to reduce hazards	2, 6
	2. Accepts the need for improving environmental conditions and human behavior	1, 2, 4, 6, 7
	3. Supports the concept that safety is everyone's responsibility	6, 7
	4. Believes that improved safety measures could reduce deaths and injuries among elementary-age children and youth	2, 3, 7
	5. Supports the work of the National Safety Council and other organizations in accident prevention	6, 7
	6. Is aware of the need for better first-aid training for youth and adults	5, 7
	7. Believes that there is an immediate need to improve community programs for emergency care	5, 7
	8. Realizes there are school and community resources that provide assistance in emergencies	5
Action	1. Attempts to act in a consistently safe manner under all conditions	1, 2, 6
	2. Shows leadership in helping others avoid accidents	2, 3, 6
	3. Demonstrates acceptance of the values of safe behavior	2, 7
	4. Seeks solutions to accident problems in a scientific manner	2, 4, 6
	5. Demonstrates leadership in school, home, or community emergency care program	1, 5, 7
	6. Uses school and community resources in emergencies	5-7
	7. Effectively carries out sound first-aid measures if and when an emergency occurs	5, 7

SAFETY-FIRE UNIT*

Outline of content

Physiological

Effects

 Harmful—3 million fires; 300,000 injuries (50,000 hospitalized); 8,800 deaths; $4 billion property damage yearly

 Beneficial—warmth, cook food, manufacture products, scientific research, others

Leading causes of fire: electrical, smoking and matches, heating and cooking equipment, incendiary, children and matches, open flames, flammable liquids, lightning, chimneys and flues, spontaneous ignition

Types of fires: slow-burning, flash, explosion

Classes of fires: combustibles (A); flammable liquids, grease, and oil (B); electrical (C); metals (D)

Fire essentials: heat, fuel, oxygen

Where fires start in homes in rank order: living room, den or family room, basement, kitchen, bedroom, bathroom

Fabric flammability: cotton, linen, and silk burn more easily; tight-weave materials and those treated with flame-resistant substance and also nylon, acrylic, or polyester materials are more difficult to ignite; nylon, and so on, when ignited melts and causes severe burns

Control of fires: remove fuel (turn off electricity, dispose of wood, trash, and so forth), remove heat (cool), remove oxygen (smother)

Psychological

Risk-taking behavior hazards: injuries, deaths, property damage

Prevention behaviors

 Before fires occur

  Public places—hotels, theaters, restaurants, and others—identify escape exits and plan for escape; schools—participate in fire drills

  Homes

   Escape plans, periodic inspection of hazards, installation of smoke and flame detectors

   Safety procedures

    General—good housekeeping—trash removal, as well as clutter in basements, attics, and other places; safe storage of flammable materials; remove damaged wires

    Specific

     Matches—close matchbook before striking, extinguish completely, do not play with

     Outside fires—burn trash only when permitted, do not burn unless with adult, do not use flammable liquid to start and rekindle, among others

     Lightning—stay indoors in storms; be away from metal objects, such as wire fences; if outside avoid trees and small sheds, get away from water

     Flammable liquids—do not use for home dry cleaning

     Electrical appliances—turn off when not in use, do not use if fuse blown, keep away from objects that can burn, inspect regularly

     Electricity—do not overload circuits, remove broken or bare wires, replace blown fuses

     Clothing—wear sturdy jeans, tight-fitting jerseys, blouses without frills, jersey pajamas, tight-fitting or short-sleeve clothes

---

* National Fire Protection Association developed and launched this fire prevention and safety program in American schools in 1979. To date, 73 lives have been saved in the United States as a result.

Outline of content—cont'd

Psychological—cont'd

  Baby-sitter—know all exits, escape plan, emergency telephone number; do not leave children alone

  Holidays—do not use fireworks, use flashlight rather than candles on Halloween, do not use paper decorations, keep Christmas trees and hannukah bushes moist and in water and turn off lights when not at home or nearby

 After fires occur

  General—survival, escape, alarm, rescue, first aid

  Specific

   Home or building—follow escape plan

   Report of fire—telephone, alarm box

   When trapped—*crawl low* and get out of room, check door before opening and if hot fill cracks, signal for help in window with light-colored cloth or use telephone

   First aid—burns, asphyxiation, summon medical aid

   Clothing—drop to ground and roll

Social

Fire department: sole responsibility to fight fires, services usually available 24 hours daily, telephones readily available

Fire alarm boxes: purpose to summon fire fighters quickly, false alarms delay saving of lives and property

Fire codes, regulations, and laws

Spiritual

Values: importance of fire prevention and safety to prevent injuries and death and protect property

Moral issue: protection of people and property is a responsibility of all individuals

Concepts

Concept	Application of health definition
1 Fire has both beneficial and harmful effects.	Physical
2 Risk-taking behavior is the result of a variety of motivations.	Psychological
3 Individuals, families, and communities can prevent fires, save lives, and prevent injury and loss of property.	Psychological-social
4 Fire fighters are friends and necessary community helpers who render necessary services.	Social
5 Fire codes, regulations, and laws are necessary for the protection of individuals and property	Social
6 Individuals have responsibility to protect their own lives and property, as well as their neighbors'.	Spiritual

Objectives for grades K-3

Domain	Objectives for students	Basic concepts
Cognitive	1. Identifies the benefits and harmful effects of fire	1-3, 6
	2. Describes the actions to take in a fire drill	3-6
	3. Demonstrates the proper stop, drop, and roll technique when clothes are on fire	3, 6
	4. Describes the crawling low method to exit from a smoke-filled room	3, 6

5.	Lists the procedures to follow when smoke or fire is discovered in a building	3, 6
6.	Explains the reasons for reporting fire and smoke conditions immediately	1, 3, 4, 6
7.	States reason to look for two exits from every building	1, 3, 5, 6
8.	Lists the dangers of playing with or using matches improperly	1-3, 6
9.	Recalls the dangers and safety procedures around heat-producing appliances	1-3, 6
10.	Lists the types of electrical hazards in homes	1, 3, 5, 6
11.	Recites the need for fire-safe holidays	1-3, 6
12.	Recalls the way combustibles can be ignited	1-3, 6

Affective

1.	Values fire and smoke drills as necessary for fire safety	3, 5, 6
2.	Supports the need to use the stop, drop, and roll technique when clothes are on fire	3, 6
3.	Is interested in learning the crawling low procedure to exit from a smoke-filled room	3, 6
4.	Values the need for prompt action when smoke or fire is discovered	1, 3, 4, 6
5.	Realizes why fire and smoke conditions should be reported immediately	1, 3, 6
6.	Realizes the importance of identifying and being able to locate two exits at all times	3, 6
7.	Wishes to protect self and others from the hazards of improper use of matches	1-3, 6
8.	Is interested in learning about fire safety around lighted stoves, heaters, and small appliances	1-3, 6
9.	Wishes to keep family members fire safe when camping, picnicking, or cooking outdoors	1-3, 5, 6
10.	Recognizes that electrical hazards may result in fire, injury, death, and loss of property	1-3, 6
11.	Believes in identifying and removing fire hazards	1, 3, 4, 6
12.	Supports the need for fire-safe holidays	1-3, 6
13.	Realizes the hazard of inserting objects into electrical outlets	3, 6

Action
(observable
and non-
observ-
able)

1.	Participates in fire and smoke drills at schools	3, 5, 6
2.	Participates in the planning of a home evacuation plan	3, 4, 6
3.	Immediately reports fire, heat, or smoke conditions to a responsible adult	3, 4, 6
4.	Refrains from playing with or improperly using matches in home, school, or outdoors	1-3, 6
5.	Refrains from playing near stoves, heaters, or fireplaces	1-3, 6
6.	Reports electrical hazards to responsible adults	1, 3, 4, 6
7.	Is able to crawl low to exit from a smoke-filled room	3, 6
8.	Prepares evacuation plan for multistoried building when necessary	3, 6
9.	Applies cold water to minor burns if no adult is present	3, 6
10.	Seeks help for severe burns	3, 6
11.	Practices and encourages family members to practice fire safety when camping, picnicking, or cooking outdoors	1-3, 5, 6
12.	Practices and encourages fire safety on holidays and special occasions	1, 3, 6

Objectives for grades 4–6

Domain	Objectives for students	Basic concepts
Cognitive	1. Describes the actions to take in fire drills	3-6
	2. Demonstrates the proper way to stop, drop, and roll when clothes are on fire	3, 6
	3. Identifies hazardous types of clothing	3, 6
	4. States reason for crawling low in a smoke-filled room	1, 3
	5. Lists procedures to follow when smoke or fire is discovered	1, 3, 4, 6
	6. Explains reasons for reporting fire and smoke conditions immediately	1, 3, 4, 6
	7. Describes the purpose of two exits from buildings	3, 4, 6
	8. Identifies the first-aid procedures for burns	3, 6
	9. Explains the procedures for fire safety when serving as a baby-sitter	1, 3, 6
	10. States the reasons for remaining clear of fire fighters while fires are in progress	4
	11. Recites the reasons for refusing to turn in false fire alarms	2, 4
	12. Lists the dangers of playing with or using matches improperly	1-3, 6
	13. Identifies fire safety behavior around lighted stoves, heaters, and small appliances	1-3, 6
	14. Recalls how to store flammable liquids safely	1-3, 5, 6
	15. Explains the ways to extinguish outdoor fires	1, 3, 6
	16. Identifies the types of electrical hazards in homes	3, 6
	17. States the reasons for conducting periodic home hazard inspections	2, 3, 6
	18. Recalls the need to use gasoline in well-ventilated places outside of buildings	2, 3, 6
Affective	1. Values fire and smoke drills for fire safety	3-6
	2. Values the need to use the stop, drop, and roll technique when clothes are on fire	3, 6
	3. Is interested in learning the crawling low technique to exit a smoke-filled room	3, 6
	4. Realizes the importance for prompt action when smoke or fire is discovered	1-4, 6
	5. Appreciates the importance of locating two exits from buildings	3, 4, 6
	6. Realizes the need for immediate attention to burns	3, 6
	7. Supports the need to refrain from interfering with fire fighters while fires are in progress	4
	8. Believes that false fire alarms are dangerous	4
	9. Wishes to protect self and others from the misuse of matches and lighted objects	1-3, 6
	10. Realizes the hazards of lighted stoves, heaters, and small appliances	1-3, 6
	11. Recognizes the hazards of improperly stored flammable liquids	1-3, 5, 6
	12. Supports the need to extinguish outdoor fires properly	1, 3, 5, 6
	13. Believes in the importance of the use of nonflammable substances inside homes and buildings	1-3, 6
Action (observable) (observable and non-observable)	1. Helps teachers conduct fire drills	3, 6
	2. Helps family in the preparation and the following of a home evacuation plan	3, 6
	3. Immediately reports fire, heat, or smoke observed to a responsible adult after leaving a building	1, 3, 4, 6

	4. Refrains from improperly using matches and helps store them properly	1-3, 6
	5. Practices and encourages others to practice fire safety when outdoors	1-3, 5, 6
	6. Assists in regular inspection of buildings and grounds	3, 6
(nonobserv-able)	7. Performs accurately the stop, drop, and roll technique when clothes are on fire	3, 6
	8. Properly performs the crawling procedure to exit a smoke-filled room	1, 3, 6
	9. Establishes an evacuation plan in case of fire in a multistoried building	3, 5, 6
	10. Applies cold water to a minor burn if no adult is present or seeks help with a severe burn	3, 6
	11. Aids fire fighters on arrival regarding location of fire and whether persons are in building	4, 5
	12. Refrains from turning in false fire alarms	4, 5
	13. Helps maintain storage of flammable liquids in proper containers	1-3, 5, 6
	14. Encourages safe smoking habits in buildings, outdoors, and other places	2, 3, 6
	15. Persuades others to use gasoline and other volatile substances in well-ventilated places	1-3, 6

Objectives for grades 7–8

Domain	Objectives for students	Basic concepts
Cognitive	1. Identifies reasons for fire drills	3-6
	2. Demonstrates proper technique for stop, drop, and roll technique to use when clothes are on fire	3, 6
	3. Identifies reason to crawl low to exit from smoke-filled room	1, 3, 6
	4. Lists procedures to follow when smoke or fire is discovered	1, 3, 4, 6
	5. Explains reasons for reporting fire and smoke conditions immediately when discovered	1, 3, 4, 6
	6. Demonstrates first aid for use with burn victims	3, 6
	7. Describes procedure to plan a baby-sitter safety plan	3, 6
	8. States the importance of remaining clear of fire fighters while fires are in progress	4
	9. Lists the hazards of false fire alarms	4
	10. Lists the hazards of the improper use of matches	1-3, 6
	11. Recalls the dangers and safety procedures when around cooking, heating, and other heat-producing appliances	1-3, 6
	12. Describes the flammability dangers from volatile substances	1-3, 6
	13. Identifies the safety procedures for use in outdoor fires	1-3, 5, 6
	14. Explains the purposes of fuses and the safe way to replace them	1, 3, 6
	15. Lists procedures used in the regular inspection of buildings for fire hazards	3, 6
	16. Lists the procedures to follow for fire-safe holidays	3, 6
	17. Recalls the need for safe smoking habits in buildings, outdoors, and in automobiles	1, 3, 5, 6
	18. Explains the types, costs, and operation of fire and smoke detectors	3, 5, 6
	19. Describes the significance of the use of the UL label on electrical appliances and equipment	3, 5, 6
	20. States the reason for licensed or certified personnel performing electrical repairs and maintenance	3, 5, 6

Objectives for grades 7-8—cont'd

Domain	Objectives for students	Basic concepts
Affective	1. Supports the need for fire drills and accepts responsibility for sharing in their conduct	3-6
	2. Values the need to use the stop, drop, and roll technique when clothing is on fire	3, 6
	3. Is interested in learning the crawling low method to exit from a smoke-filled building	3, 6
	4. Values the need for prompt action when smoke or fire is discovered	1, 3, 4, 6
	5. Is interested in learning the first aid for burn victims	3, 6
	6. Believes it is necessary to help children escape from fire when serving as a baby-sitter	3, 6
	7. Supports the need to refrain from interfering with fire fighters while fires are in progress	4
	8. Believes that false fire alarms should not be turned in	4
	9. Realizes the importance of using matches safely	1-3, 6
	10. Willingly accepts the responsibility to protect children when around heat-producing equipment	1-3, 6
	11. Recognizes the hazards of improperly used and stored flammable liquids	1-3, 6
	12. Desires to practice fire safety outdoors	2, 3, 5, 6
	13. Realizes the need for fuses and circuit breakers to protect from electrical overloads	3, 5, 6
	14. Values the importance of periodic building inspections for fire hazards	3, 6
	15. Supports the need for fire-safe holidays and special occasions	3, 5, 6
	16. Recognizes the high risk of smoking in bed and the improper disposal of smoking materials	2, 3, 6
	17. Supports the need for fire and smoke detectors	3, 5, 6
	18. Is interested in learning the importance of the UL label	3, 5, 6
	19. Recognizes the need for the repair and maintenance of electrical equipment by licensed or certified personnel	3, 5, 6
	20. Is aware that lightning may cause fires and personal injury	1, 3, 5, 6
Action (observable) (observable and non-observable) (nonobservable)	1. Willingly participates in fire and smoke drills at school and assumes responsibility to help conduct same	3-6
	2. Participates in helping family and others develop and follow a home escape plan	3, 6 / 3, 5, 6
	3. Prepares fire evacuation plan for use in multistoried building	3, 6
	4. Conducts or assists in periodic building fire safety inspections	3, 6
	5. Performs stop, drop, and roll technique to use when clothes are on fire	
	6. Performs crawling low procedure to exit from smoke-filled room	3, 6
	7. Immediately reports observed fire, heat, or smoke after leaving a building to responsible adult or fire department	1, 3, 4, 6
	8. Administers first aid for minor burns and shock and seeks medical help for major burns	3, 6
	9. Plans safety procedures with parents when baby-sitting	3, 6
	10. Assists fire fighters regarding location of fires and persons in burning buildings	3, 4, 6
	11. Refrains from turning in false fire alarms	3, 4, 6
	12. Refrains and discourages others from the improper use of matches	1-3, 6

13. Helps keep children away from heat-producing equipment and appliances   3, 6
14. Aids in the proper use and storage of flammable liquids   1, 3, 6
15. Assists with the removal of electrical hazards in the home   3, 6
16. Encourages safe smoking habits in buildings, outdoors, and automobiles   1, 3, 6
17. Persuades others to install fire and smoke detectors and to purchase electrical equipment with the UL label   1, 3, 5, 6
18. Encourages adults to install lightning protection on buildings where appropriate   1, 3, 6

VISION AND HEARING UNIT

Outline of content

Physiological

Definitions: hyperopia, myopia, astigmatism, amblyopia, glaucoma, color blindness, night blindness, strabismus, conjunctivitis, ophthalmologist, optometrist, optician, otitis media, otitis externa, conduction deafness, nerve deafness

Structure and function of eyes and ears

 Eye structure—cornea, iris, lens, retina, optic nerve

 Eye function—vision, appearance

 Ear structure—outer ear, middle ear, inner ear, auditory nerve

 Ear function—hearing

Refractive errors; eye diseases and ear disorders

Signs and symptoms of problems (see Appendix J)

Psychological

Emotional problems: caused by strabismus, nearsightedness and farsightedness, partial or complete blindness, partial or complete deafness, learning difficulties

Purposes of testing and care of vision and hearing

Social

Selection of eye specialist

Selection of physician for earache or hearing problem

Choice of glasses, contact lenses, or hearing aid if needed

Periodic eye and ear examinations or screening tests—types, frequency

Spiritual

Values: importance of eye and ear health to self-image

Moral issues: provision of eye and ear care by government funding or private sources; protection of workers' vision and hearing in certain industries; attitudes toward blind and deaf people; responsibility to help blind and deaf persons

Concepts

Concept	Application of health definition
1 Vision and hearing are the two most important senses for life and health.	Physical
2 Vision should be clear, sharp, and bright, with good distinction of color.	Physical
3 Common eye disorders include nearsightedness, farsightedness, and astigmatism.	Physical

Concepts—cont'd

Concept	Application of health definition
4 One in five elementary pupils has a visual problem requiring professional care.	Physical-social
5 Visual disorders may cause learning difficulties or psychological problems.	Psychological-social
6 Good hearing depends on efficient function of the outer, middle, and inner ear, as well as the auditory nerve.	Physical
7 Most hearing loss in childhood is a result of middle ear infection.	Physical
8 Nerve deafness may be caused by long-term exposure to loud noise, birth defects, certain diseases or medicines, head injury, or heredity.	Physical-social
9 One in twenty elementary school pupils has a hearing problem requiring professional care.	Physical-social
10 Hearing disorders may cause learning difficulties or psychological problems.	Psychological-social
11 During the elementary school years, parents have the primary responsibility for correction of hearing or vision problems in pupils.	Spiritual
12 Prompt professional care can correct or improve most disorders of vision and hearing.	Physical-spiritual

Objectives for grades K-3

Domain	Objectives for students	Basic concepts
Cognitive	1. Tells why good eyesight and hearing are important	1
	2. Explains the reasons for having vision and hearing tests	2-4, 7, 9, 12
	3. Identifies the main parts of the eye and ear	1, 2, 6
	4. Lists ways that good sight and hearing can help learning	5, 10
	5. Discusses factors that may impair vision or hearing	3, 7, 8
	6. Recalls any experiences of visual difficulty or earache	3, 7
Affective	1. Is aware of the importance of good vision and hearing	1
	2. Accepts the need for vision and hearing tests	4, 9, 12
	3. Displays interests in how the eyes and ears function	2, 6
	4. Listens carefully to the ways to protect vision and hearing	1, 5, 10
	5. Shows interest in finding professional specialists in eye and ear health	11, 12
Action	1. Participates cooperatively when vision or hearing tests are given at school	4, 5, 9, 10
	2. Tells about any personal seeing or hearing difficulty	4, 9, 12
	3. Uses textbooks and other printed materials in a proper, efficient manner	2, 5
	4. Does not habitually ask the teacher or others to repeat themselves	6, 10

Objectives for grades 4-6

Domain	Objectives for students	Basic concepts
Cognitive	1. Explains the basic structure and function of eyes and ears	1, 2, 6
	2. Identifies ways to protect vision and hearing	1, 3, 7, 8
	3. Cites major causes of visual and hearing disorders	3, 4, 7-9
	4. Illustrates how middle ear infection can cause hearing loss	6, 7
	5. Describes effect of glare on visual acuity and eye fatigue	2
	6. Explains important effects of color blindness and night blindness	1, 2
	7. Explains the importance of regular eye and ear checkups and follow-up for corrections	4, 9, 11, 12

Affective	1. Understands and appreciates the critical value of good vision and hearing	1, 5, 6
	2. Accepts responsibility along with parents for care of eyes and ears	1, 4, 9, 11, 12
	3. Displays interest in the effects of heredity on eye and ear disorders	3, 8
	4. Appreciates the role of teachers, school nurses, and health specialists in the prevention and correction of eye and ear defects	4, 5, 9-12
	5. Believes that healthy vision and hearing are necessary for a good education	5, 10
Action	1. Takes an active, cooperative part when vision or hearing tests are given at school	4, 5, 9, 10
	2. Protects own eyes and avoids endangering the eyes of others in sports and other physical activities	1
	3. Reports any personal problem of seeing or hearing to the teacher, school nurse, or other professional person	4, 9, 12
	4. Avoids probing ears with sharp objects, looking directly at sun, or other practices that can be harmful	1
	5. Does not habitually ask the teacher or others to repeat themselves	6, 10
	6. Avoids exposure to excessively loud rock music or other high-decibel noise	1, 8

Objectives for grades 7-8

Domain	Objectives for students	Basic concepts
Cognitive	1. Explains major errors of refraction in terms of altered structure and function and professional care	3, 12
	2. Cites causes, prevention, and reasons for professional care of middle ear infection	7, 12
	3. Lists types of environmental noise that can damage hearing	8
	4. Analyzes differences between and among ophthalmologists, optometrists, and opticians	12
	5. Describes possible effects on studying and learning of eye and ear disorders	5, 10
	6. Describes possible emotional effects of eye and ear disorders	5, 10
	7. Compares advantages and disadvantages of glasses and contact lenses	12
	8. Cites dangers of delayed treatment for amblyopia (lazy eye) and glaucoma	12
Affective	1. Understands and appreciates the critical value of good vision and hearing	1, 5, 6
	2. Accepts responsibility for protecting and caring for own eyes and ears	1, 4, 9
	3. Recognizes the responsibility of parents to seek professional care for children with eye or ear problems	1, 4, 9, 11
	4. Inquires about the relative merits of various types of eye and ear specialists	4, 9, 12
	5. Discusses the problems of providing medical care for the poor who have eye or ear problems	1, 12
	6. Recognizes and appreciates the growing problem of noise pollution in the environment	1, 8
Action	1. Takes an active, cooperative part when vision or hearing tests are given	4, 5, 9, 10
	2. Protects own eyes and avoids endangering the eyes of others in sports, laboratory work, and other physical activities	1
	3. Is able to make wise decisions regarding personal eye and ear care	1
	4. Supports school and community efforts to protect and improve eye and ear health	1, 4, 9, 11, 12
	5. Seeks reliable information on eye and ear health	1, 3, 7, 8
	6. Consistently wears glasses or hearing aid if prescribed	1, 5, 10
	7. Avoids exposure to excessively loud rock music or other high decibel noise	1, 8

APPENDIX C

EDUCATION FOR HEALTH IN THE SCHOOL COMMUNITY SETTING

A POSITION PAPER*

The school is a community in which most individuals spend at least 12 years of their lives, and more if they have the advantages of early childhood programs, college education, and continuing education for adults. The health of our school-age youth will determine to a great extent the quality of life each will have during the growing and developing years and on throughout the life cycle. Their capacity to function as health-educated adults will in turn help each to realize the fullest potential for self, family, and the various communities of which each individual will be a part.

The American Public Health Association (APHA) believes that health education should be a continuing process, from conception to death, and that such education must be comprehensive, coordinated, and integrated in all community planning for health.

The school as a social structure provides an educational setting in which the total health of

the child during the impressionable years is of priority concern. No other community setting even approximates the magnitude of the grades K to 12 school educational enterprise, with an enrollment in 1973-1974 of 45.5 million in nearly 17,000 school districts comprising more than 115,000 schools with some 2.1 million teachers. This is to say nothing of the administrative, supervisory, and service manpower required to maintain these institutions. In addition, more than 40% of children aged 3 to 5 are enrolled in early childhood education programs. Thus it seems that school should be regarded as a social unit providing a focal point to which health planning for all other community settings should relate.

Schools provide an environment conducive to developing skills and competencies that will help the individual confront and examine a complexity of social and cultural forces, persuasive influences, and ever-expanding options as these affect health behavior. Today's health problems do not lend themselves to yesterday's solutions. Specificity of cause is multiple rather than singular. The individual must assume increasing responsibility for solutions to major public health problems and consequently must be educated to do so.

---

*Adapted from Governing Council of the American Public Health Association: Education for health in the school community setting; a position paper, New Orleans, Oct. 23, 1974, The Council, A "position paper" is defined as a major exposition of the Association's viewpoint on broad issues affecting the public's health.

Education for and about health is not synonymous with information. Education is concerned with behavior—a composite of what an individual knows, senses, and values, and of what one does and practices. Factual data are but temporary assumptions to be used and cast aside as new information emerges. Health facts unrenewed can become a liability rather than an asset. The health-educated citizen is one who possesses resources and abilities that will last throughout a lifetime, such as critical thinking, problem-solving, valuing, self-discipline, and self-direction, and that will lead to a sense of responsibility for community and world concerns.

The school curriculum offers an opportunity to view health issues in an integrated context. It is designed to help the learner gain insights about the personal, social, environmental, political, and cultural implications of each issue. Planning for health care delivery, for example, is not simply a matter of providing for manpower, services, and facilities. These things must be considered in concert with housing, employment, transportation, cultural beliefs and values, and the rights and dignity of the persons involved. Nor will nutritional practices be improved substantially by programs based on groupings, labeling, or issuing stamps, because food practices and eating patterns are equally influenced by how, when, where, why, and with whom one eats.

APHA is concerned about the traditional crisis approach to health care. The expense involved in treatment, rehabilitation, recuperation, and restoration to health has sent medical costs soaring. More facilities, services, and manpower to staff the facilities and to provide the services appear to be the nation's leading priorities. The alternative is a redirection of the nation's health goals toward a primary preventive—and constructive—approach to health, through education for every individual.

Because of vested interests, political pressures, mass media sensationalism, and health agency structures with categorical interests, health education programs in schools are compelled to deal with a multitude of separate health issues, with only a few of these given priority at any given time. Too often programs developed to deal with crucial issues are eliminated although the problems remain because another crisis emerges calling for more new crash programs. A revolving critical issue syndrome has been the result, with the same problems considered crucial a decade or more ago emerging once again. Focusing on selected categorical issues has potential value if time, energy, personnel, and money are available to sustain the emphasis and expand such efforts into an integrated and viable health education framework. A broad concept of healthful living that has consideration for psychosocial dimensions should be the basis for health education.

APHA is encouraged by recent developments in an increasing number of states that attest to recognition of the significance of a comprehensive health education program in grades K to 12. Also encouraging are the exemplary programs being established in many school districts and the expressed intention of the federal government to implement an action plan for "better health through education."

Therefore the American Public Health Association supports the concept of a national commitment to a comprehensive, sequential program of health education for all students in the nation's schools, kindergarten through the twelfth grade. The Association will exert leadership through its sections and affiliates to assure the following for health education:

1. Time in the curriculum commensurate with other subject areas.
2. Professionally qualified teachers and supervisors of health education.
3. Innovative instructional materials and appropriate teaching facilities.
4. Increased financial support at the local, state, and national levels to upgrade the quantity and quality of health education.
5. A teaching/learning environment in which opportunities for safe and optimal living exist, and one in which a well-organized and complete health service is functioning.

APPENDIX D

SOURCES OF SELECTED ELEMENTARY HEALTH EDUCATION PROGRAMS AVAILABLE IN SCHOOLS*

Actions for Health
Charles E. Lewis, M.D.
Professor of Medicine
Department of Medicine
School of Medicine
University of California
Los Angeles, CA 90024
(213) 825-6709

Adolescent Smoking and Alcohol Project (ASAP)
Carol Pittman
Supervisor of Health Programs
N.E. Florida Educational Consortium
PO Box 198
Bostwick, FL 32007
(904) 328-8811

Assisting Adolescents in Personal Decision Making through Health Education
Milton Schmidt
Director, Instructional Services
Cherry Creek School District #5
Holly Ridge Center
3301 South Monaco Boulevard
Denver, CO 80222
(303) 757-6201

Beverly Public Schools Health Education Curriculum
Thomas J. Durkin, Ed.D.
Health Resource Specialist
Beverly Public Schools
4 Colon Street
Beverly, MA 10915
(617) 927-5651

Blast Off to Health
Judith Miller
Project Director
Hibbing Senior High School
Hibbing, MN 55746
(218) 263-4850

---

*Adapted from U.S. Department of Health and Human Services, Centers for Disease Control, Center for Health Promotion and Education: A compendium of exemplary school health education classroom programs and teaching/learning resources, Atlanta, 1984.

Caspar Alcohol Education Program
Lena DiCicco
Director, Caspar, Inc.
Alcohol Education Program
226 Highland Avenue
Somerville, MA 02143
(617) 623-2080

Chicago Heart Health Curriculum Program
Albert Sunseri, Ph.D.
Co-Investigator, Chicago Heart Health
  Curriculum Program
Chicago Heart Association
20 North Wacker Drive
Chicago, IL 60606
(312)346-4675

Clayton County Puppet Show Someone to Talk to
Kathryn Flanagan
Clayton County Department of Family and Children
  Services
129 King Street
Jonesboro, GA 30236
(404) 478-0295

Cohasset Comprehensive Health Education
Michael Gill
Cohasset High School
143 Pond Street
Cohasset, MA 02025
(617) 383-6107

Community Alcohol and Smoking Prevention
Elaine Bartelt
Apalachee Community Mental Health Services, Inc.
PO Box 1782
Tallahassee, FL 32302
(904) 487-2930

**Conceptual Approach to Functional Health
  Education**
Fredna Cross
Coordinator of Health, Safety, and Physical Education
Meridian Public Schools
PO Box 31
Meridian, MS 39301
(601) 483-6271

DARTE: Drug Abuse Reduction through Education
Kenneth Kaminsky
Director, DARTE
33500 Van Borm Road
Wayne, MI 48184
(313) 467-1368

The Doofus Stories
Carol Bershad
Learning for Life Project Director
Management Sciences for Health
165 Allandale Road
Boston, MA 02130
(617) 524-7799

An Early Start to Good Health
Jerry Maburn
American Cancer Society
777 Third Avenue
New York, NY 10017
(212) 371-2900

Epilepsy School Alert
Ann Scherer
Director, Public Information & Education
Epilepsy Foundation of America
4351 Garden City Drive
Landover, MD 20785
(301) 638-5229

The Eyes Have it
Lydia Maguire
Director of Public Relations
National Society to Prevent Blindness
79 Madison Avenue
New York, NY 10016
(212) 684-3505

**Family Life Sex Education Comprehensive
  Curriculum Guide**
Sara Traphagen
Planned Parenthood Association of Humboldt County
2316 Harrison Ave
Eureka, CA 95501
(707) 442-2961

Food: Your Choice
Richard J. Walther, M.P.H.
Program Consultant
National Dairy Council
6300 North River Road
Rosemont, IL 60018
(312) 696-1020

Getting to Know Me
Consultant, Health Education
State Department of Education
Len B. Jordan Building
Boise, ID 83720
(208) 334-2281

Growing Healthy
(see: School Health Curriculum Project, and Primary
  Grades Health Curriculum Project)

Have a Healthy Heart
Sherry Avena
Program Developer
4095 173rd Pl., S.E.
Bellevue, WA 98008
(206) 746-0331

**Hazelwood School District Comprehensive
  School Health Education Program**
Karen Helms
Physical Education, Health, & Safety Consultant
Hazelwood School District
15955 New Halls Ferry Road
Florissant, MO 63031
(314) 921-4450

Health Activities Project
David R. Butler
Director, HAP K-3
Lawrence Hall of Science
University of California
Berkeley, CA 94720
(415) 642-3679

Health Course of Study
Richard J. Webster
Consultant of Health & PE
Rochester Public Schools
Coffman Building
Rochester, MN 55901
(507) 285-8558

**Health Education Curriculum United Way
  Health Foundation**
Margaret Kirkpatrick
Director, United Way Health Foundation
618 Second Street, N.W.
Canton, OH 44703
(216) 455-0378 or 455-4547

Health Education Risk Reduction
John Tapscott
National Council on Alcoholism and Other
  Drug Dependencies
706 Fleming Building
Des Moines, IA 50309
(515) 244-2297

**Health Skills for Life: Health Education
  Project (HEP)**
James A. Terhune
Health Skills for Life
20 E. 13th Avenue
Eugene, OR 97401
(503) 687-3561 or 484-2601

**"Here's Looking at You, 2000" Alcohol and
  Drug Education Project**
Roberts, Fitzmahan and Associates
9131 California Ave. S.W.
Seattle, WA 98136
(206) 932-8409

Healthy Mothers, Healthy Babies
Robert Goldberg
March of Dimes Birth Defects Foundation
1275 Mamaroneck Avenue
White Plains, NY 10605
(914) 428-7100 x261

I Do Declare: I Am Aware
Horace W. Moore
Director, Youth Services
American Red Cross
17th and D Streets, N.W.
Washington, DC 20006
(202) 857-3604

Inside-Out
Bob Fox
Associate Executive Director
Agency for Instructional Television
Box A
Bloomington, IN 47402
(812) 339-2203

"It's Up to You"
Marcia W. Hunker
96 Green Street
Brattleboro, VT 05301
(802) 257-7144 or 722-4338

Jamestown Elementary Nutrition Curriculum
Kathryn Richards
Project Director
PO Box 269
Jamestown, ND 58401

Jefferson County Schools Human Sexuality Strand of Health Education Program
Don Shaw
Coordinator of Health
Jefferson County Schools
1209 Quail
Lakewood, CO 80215
(303) 231-2387

Know Your Body
Linda Barrett, Coordinator
Educational Intervention
American Health Foundation
320 East 43rd Street
New York, NY 10017
(212) 953-1900

Kokomo Health Crisis Education Project
Bill Keaffaber
Project Coordinator
Health Crisis Education Project
100 West Lincoln Road
Kokomo, IN 46901
(317) 453-5400

Learn Not to Burn
National Fire Protection Association
Batterymarch Park
Quincy, MA 02269
(619) 770-3000

Lincoln School Health Education Program
Dean A. Austin, Ph.D.
Consultant for H & PE
Lincoln Public Schools
PO Box 82889
Lincoln, NE 68501
(402) 473-0263

Long Beach Health Education Program
Sandra French
Consultant, Health Education, Long Beach Unified
  School District
710 Locust Avenue
Long Beach, CA 90813
(213) 436-9931

The Magic of Sight
Lydia Maguire, Director of Public Relations
National Society to Prevent Blindness
79 Madison Avenue
New York, NY 10016
(212) 684-3505

Me/Me Drug Prevention Education Program
Artie Kearney, Ph.D.
Me/Me Incorporated
400 South Linwood Avenue
Appleton, WI 54911
(414) 735-0114

Multidisciplinary Health Education Project
Annette Jacobson, Curriculum Consultant
Grants Pass School District
223 S.E. "M" Street
Grants Pass, OR 97526
(503) 479-2628

North Clackamas School District Health Education Program
John Chamberlin
Director of Instructional Development
North Clackamas School District #12
1905 S.E. Oak Group Blvd.
Milwaukie, OR 97222
(503) 653-3831

Nutrition Density Nutrition Education Curriculum
F. Greg Robinson
Utah State University Foundation
UMC 93
Logan, UT 84322
(801) 750-2603 or 753-7340

Nutrition Education and Training (NET) Program
Harold Armstrong
Ohio Department of Education
65 South Front Street
Columbus, OH 43215
(614) 466-8251

Ombudsman: A Classroom Community
Kathy Manners
Dissemination Coordinator
Charlotte Drug Education
1416 E. Morehead Street
Charlotte, NC 28204
(704) 374-3211

An Option to See
Lydia Maguire
Director of Public Relations
National Society to Prevent Blindness
79 Madison Avenue
New York, NY 10016
(212) 684-3505

**Primary Grades Health Curriculum Project
Growing Healthy**
Roger Schmidt
American Lung Association
1740 W. Broadway
New York, NY 10019
(212) 245-8000

**Project Charlie (Chemical Abuse Resolution Lies in
Education)**
Jeannie Ryan
Storefront Youth Action
5701 Normandale Road
Adina, MN 55424
(612) 925-9706

Project CHEK
Wanda Jubb
Michigan Department of Education
Box 30008
Lansing, MI 48909
(517) 373-1484

**Project Healthpact (Participatory and Assertive
Consumer Training)**
Judith B. Igoe
University of Colorado
School of Nursing
4200 East 9th Avenue
Denver, CO 80262
(303) 394-7435

Project Prevention
Howard Gonser
Project Director
Chenowith School District No. 9
3632 West 10th Street
The Dalles, OR 97058
(503) 296-6141

Putting Your Heart into the Curriculum
Arleta Estes
American Heart Association
7320 Greenville
Dallas, TX 75231
(214) 750-5497

Racine School Health Education Project
Grace C. Piskula
Director, Health/Safety/Physical Education
Racine Unified School District
2220 Northwestern Avenue
Racine, WI 53404
(414) 631-7071

RIPPLES
Bob Fox
Associate Executive Director
Agency for Instructional Televison
Box A
Bloomington, IN 47402
(812) 339-2203

The School Health Education Program
Dr. Valorie E. Nybo
Executive Director, Health Programing, Inc.
59 Court Street
Augusta, ME 04330
(207) 622-3170

Seekonk School Health Education Program
Robert Frazer
Supervisor of Health Education
Seekonk High School
Seekonk, MA 02771
(617) 336-7273

Seymour Safely Vision Education Program
Harold Zimm
Director, Communications Division
American Optometric Association
243 North Lindbergh Boulevard
St. Louis, MO 63141
(314) 991-4100

**Smoking and Alcohol Prevention Program for
Children and Adolescents**
Fred M. Bates
San Diego Unified School District
4100 Normal Street
San Diego, CA 92103
(619) 293-8603 or 8096

Snooper
Cindy Howard
Public Relations Officer
Blue Cross/Blue Shield
PO Box 1911
Wilmington, DE 19899
(302) 421-3000

The Sunflower Project
Donna Osness, Ed.D.
Director of Health Education & Health Services
Mohawk Instructional Center
6649 Lamar
Shawnee Mission, KS 66202
(913) 384-6800, ext. 226

3R'S and HBP
School Program Coordinator
American Heart Association, Georgia Affiliate
Box 13589
Atlanta, GA 30324
(404) 261-2260

What Makes Me Tick
Edith P. Vincent
Health Education/Services
Department of Public Instruction
PO Box 1402
Dover, DE 19901
(302) 736-4601

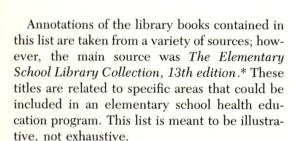

APPENDIX
E

A SAMPLE OF HEALTH EDUCATION FICTION AND NONFICTION BOOKS

Annotations of the library books contained in this list are taken from a variety of sources; however, the main source was *The Elementary School Library Collection, 13th edition*.* These titles are related to specific areas that could be included in an elementary school health education program. This list is meant to be illustrative, not exhaustive.

The list has been organized by topic areas, with books listed alphabetically by authors. Approximations of reading levels are included by the following code: P, primary; I, intermediate; U, upper.

AGING

GAUCH, PATRICIA, Grandpa and Me, Coward, 1972. (I)
  Beautifully illustrated portrayal of grandfather and grandson in a vacation setting. Older man is strong, active, and caring. Fiction.

---

*Winkel, L., et al., editors: The elementary school library collection, a guide to books and other media, ed. 13, Williamsport, Pa., 1981, Bro-Dart Foundation.

GOFFSTEIN, M.B., Fish for Supper, Dial, 1976. (P)
  Independent older woman catches, cleans, and cooks her own fish in this simple, well-illustrated book for very young children. Fiction.

HEIN, LUCILLE, My Very Special Friend, Judson, 1974. (I-U)
  Sensitive relationship between a young girl and her elderly, yet active and creative, great-grandmother. Fiction.

KIRK, BARBARA, Grandpa, Me and Our House in the Tree, Macmillan, 1978. (I)
  After there is a debilitating illness, grandfather and grandson must restructure their formerly physically active relationship. Sensitive portrayal of the needs of both. Fiction.

LASKY, KATHRYN, I Have Four Names for My Grandfather, Little, Brown & Co., (P)
  Grandfather and grandson are photographed in both active and passive situations. Especially good presentation of communication across generations. Nonfiction.

MACLACHLAN, PATRICIA, Through Grandpa's Eyes, Harper & Row, 1980. (P)
  John loves to visit his blind Grandpa who teaches him how to "see" through touch, sound, and smell. A tender story with poetic illustrations. Fiction.

438

MATHIS, SHARON BELL, Hundred Penny Box, Viking, 1975 (Newberry Honor Book). (I)

When Michael's 100-year-old, Great-Great-Aunt Dew comes to live with them, she brings along an old, beat-up box, with as many pennies as her age in it. He loves to hear the tales she tells about the year she got each penny, while he counts out the pennies. A warm story of the love between old age and youth. Fiction.

MATHIS, SHARON BELL, Hundred Penny Box (phonodisc), Newberry Award Records/Random House School Division, 1977, 2s 12-inch, 33 rpm. Also available as cassette. Includes teacher's guide. (I)

Adapted from the Newberry Honor Book of the same title, this rendition is set against a background of song and provides an extra dimension of real interest for the book. Guide provides discussion on "Aging in the United States" and other data helpful for the teacher. Fiction.

MAXER, NORMA FOX, Figure of Speech, Delacorte, 1973 (I)

Thirteen-year-old Jenny has always found it difficult to relate to anyone in her family except Grandpa. But her parents refer to the 83-year-old man as "failing," and she overhears them say that "everyone passes away," and "his time is coming." That night they find that Grandpa has pinned a note to the bulletin board saying, "I ain't going to pass away. I'm goin' to die. My time ain't going to come. I'll be dead." Jenny and Grandpa share together his attempt to salvage the last shreds of his dignity in a touching and also realistic tale. Fiction.

SKORPEN, LIESEL, Mandy's Grandmother, Dial, 1975. (P)

Unconventional Mandy meets conventional grandmother. Each comes to appreciate the other, and they develop a warm and loving relationship. Fiction.

WHITMAN, SALLY, A Special Trade, Harper & Row, 1978. (I-U)

At first an elderly man and a young girl are presented with the man as the initiator—caring, helping, teaching. After there is a serious illness, roles change, but the relationship remains strong and mutual. Fiction.

WILLIAMS, BARBARA, Kevin's Grandma, Dutton, 1975. (P)

Two boys compare grandmothers. One is conventional, yet interesting and self-sufficient. The other is outrageous, delightfully eccentric, and not quite believable. Fiction.

ALCOHOL

FITZMAHAN, DON, The Roller Coaster, Comprehensive Health Education Foundation, Seattle, Wa., 1986 (I)

This beautifully illustrated book describes the impact an alcoholic mother has on her family. It is a positive story that provides specific ideas on how family members can cope with the problem and maintain their own sense of wellness. Fiction.

FORRAI, MARIA S., Look at Alcoholism, Larner, 1977 (Larner Awareness series). (I-U)

The graphic photographs clearly depict the problems of alcohol abuse to any student regardless of reading level. The accompanying minimal text will encourage classroom discussion. Nonfiction.

MAZER, HARRY, War on Villa Street, Delacorte, 1978. (I-U)

Willis Pierce is an eighth-grade boy with an alcoholic father and an overworked mother. A lonely and unhappy boy, repeated threats and beatings by a bully and his gang only increase his frustration. But Willis, while sensitive, is not a quitter. Tutoring a sixteen-year-old retarded boy in athletic skills while daring to compete in track himself, he gains in confidence. This memorable portrait of adolescence is very popular with young readers. Fiction.

NEVEILLE, EMILY CHENEY, Garden of Broken Glass, Delacorte, 1975. (I-U)

Brian, his sister, and their mother who drinks to the point of alcoholism; fat Martha, Dwayne, and his parents who force him to keep a straight and narrow path . . . these are the friends whose life in a black ghetto is described by a Newberry Prize Winner with perception and understanding. Fiction.

SEIXAS, JUDITH S., Alcohol—What It Is, What It Does, Greenwillow, 1977 (Greenwillow read-along books). (I)

Through bright cartoon illustrations, facts about alcohol; what it is, where it can be found, and its effects on the mind and body are introduced. Straightforward information with no sermonizing in an easy-to-read format. Nonfiction.

SEIXAS, JUDITH S., Living With a Parent Who Drinks Too Much, Greenwillow, 1979. (I-U)

Explains what it is like to live with a parent who drinks too much by describing alcoholism, behavior of alcoholics, and problems the family faces. Suggests ways to cope with medical emergencies for the alcoholic and counseling help for the child. Nonfiction.

SILVERSTEIN, ALVIN, and SILVERSTEIN, VIRGINIA B., Alcoholism, Lippincott, 1975. (U)

After learning the medical and historical facts about drinking, the authors hope readers will be able to make an intelligent decision about drinking. In a clear, concise text these reknowned authors discuss all major aspects of alcohol use and abuse, causes and treatment of alcoholism, teenage drinking, and living with an alcoholic parent. Nonfiction.

ANATOMY AND PHYSIOLOGY

ALLISON, LINDA, Blood and Guts; a Working Guide to Your Own Insides, Little, Brown & Co., 1976. (I)

A refreshing and fun look at the parts of the human body. They are all described in text and stories, and there are experiments and projects explained to discover how our parts function. Many humorous cartoons illustrate the experiments and descriptions. A real up-tempo book that will appeal to many students. Nonfiction.

BRANDRETH, BYLES, This Is Your Body, Sterling, 1979. (U)

Approaches the study of structure and function of the body in an entertaining, yet accurate, manner. The 26 chapters are alphabetically arranged, offering one or more projects to be completed by an individual. Can be used by single student or as support material in health or anatomy class. Nonfiction.

BRENNER, BARBARA, Bodies, Dutton, 1973. (P)

Everyone has a body and here in vital, vibrant photos showing bodies of many shapes and sizes you can see how one works and what it can do. Nonfiction.

CURTIS, DR. ROBERT H., Medical Talk for Beginners, Messner, 1976. (U)

When new vocabulary pops up, steer older readers to this book. It is an attractively designed dictionary of medical terms from abdomen to x-ray. Nonfiction.

GLEMAN, RIATA GOLDEN, and BUXBAUM, SUSAN KOVACS, Ouch? All About Cuts and Hurts, Harcourt, 1977. (P-I)

The volume is organized alphabetically and is a simple introduction to what happens to the body when common injuries occur, such as black-and-blue marks, bumps, cuts, nosebleeds, stitches, and scars, and how the body reacts to repair such damage. Nonfiction.

GROSS, RUTH BELOV, Book About Your Skeleton, Hastings House. In Canada, Sounders of Toronto, 1979 (A Science starter book). (P)

This lucid explanation of the bone structure of the body includes the various functions of bones and the skeleton. Two complete skeletons are shown at the end, labeled with common and scientific names. Nonfiction.

KAUFMAN, JOE, How We Are Born, How We Grow, How Our Bodies Work . . . and How We Learn, Webster, 1975. (I-U)

Contains a treasure lode of information for children of all ages. An attractive, oversized volume designed to give girls and boys a true understanding of their bodies. It answers many questions children might pose. For example: What makes you yawn when you are sleepy? Where do tears come from? Why does your body shiver when you are cold? Colorful illustrations help illuminate human processes such as birth, sight, digestion, dreaming, learning, and memory. Younger students will glean a great deal just by thumbing through the pages; older students can use the text for reference. Nonfiction.

KLEIN, AARON E., You and Your Body; a Book of Experiments to Perform on Yourself, Doubleday, 1977. (I)

A different approach to the study of human physiology through a series of quick and easy experiments that do not require any complicated equipment. The directions are clear and concise, and the experiments can be performed by individuals, small groups, or an entire class. Nonfiction.

McGUIRE, LESLIE, Susan Perl's Human Body Book, Platt & Munk, 1977. (A Cricket book). (P-I)

Simple, direct answers for a multiplicity of questions about the human body, such as What holds the body up? and What happens to food after it is eaten? are complimented by delightful, whimsical pictures. A different book to share with younger children. Nonfiction.

SHOWERS, PAUL, A Drop of Blood, Crowell, 1967. (P)

Explains what blood is, how it works for our bodies, and why it is important to us. Nonfiction.

SHOWERS, PAUL, Your Skin and Mine, Crowell, 1967. (P)

This book encourages readers to make and examine fingerprints. It is also available in Spanish, as *Tu Piel y la Mia*. Nonfiction.

SILVERSTEIN, ALVIN, and SILVERSTEIN, VIRGINIA B., Skeletal System; Frameworks for Life, Prentice-Hall, 1972. (U)

Analyzes the structure and function of the human skeletal system and compares it with that of other animals. Excellent and informative text includes terminology and definitions for intermediate readers. Can be used for classroom projects, individual study, enjoyable reading by those who wish to know more about the human body. Nonfiction.

THOMPSON, STEPHANIE, Know Your Human Body, Rand McNally, 1977. (I-U)

Each chapter consists of only two pages but explains in detail every aspect of the human body, using large, clear diagrams. A quiz with the answers and a page of suggested projects are also included. Nonfiction.

TULLY, MARIANE, Facts About the Human Body, Watts, 1977. (I-U)

Unusual information is offered in this question-and-answer book about various parts of the human body. Authors have used actual questions from students and have responded with direct answers. Unfamiliar words printed in boldface type are all found in the glossary in the back of the book. Nonfiction.

DEATH

CARRICK, CAROL, Accident, Clarion, 1976. (P-I)

Christopher and his dog Badger walk along the road to meet his father and mother, but when a truck comes along, Badger starts to cross the road and is killed. Christopher is grief stricken, and it is only when he and his father search for a stone marker for Badger's grave that he can express his grief. Fiction.

MANN, PEGGY, There Are Two Kinds of Terrible, Doubleday, 1977. (P)

Robbie breaks his arm on the last day of school and has to spend summer with a big cast on it. He thinks that is terrible, but then he discovers that there are two kinds of terrible—regular terrible that can happen to anyone and you can get over—and real terrible that has no end. . . . A story of the death of a loved one written with great insight and emotion. Fiction.

DENTAL HEALTH

DE GROAT, DIANE, Alligator's Toothache, Crown, 1977. (P)

Alligator's predicament—a toothache and fear of the dentist—is eventually resolved through trickery and is eloquently portrayed through the three-color pen-and-ink drawings in this wordless book. Fiction.

DOSS, HELEN, All the Better to Bite With, Messner, 1976. (I)

Here is a guided tour of our teeth and mouth, introduced by a discussion of different animal teeth. Parts of the mouth and teeth, causes and prevention of tooth and gum disease, dentist office procedures, and intelligent choice of foods are all discussed in a clear text accompanied by black and white photographs and diagrams. Nonfiction.

HAMMOND, WINIFRED G., Riddle of Teeth, Coward-McCann, 1971. (I)

Most chapters of this factual book about teeth contain interesting projects for readers to try at home or in school with classmates. The author is very specific in her discussion of formation of teeth, the different kinds of teeth and how they work, the causes of caries and other dental diseases, and the fight to control and prevent the loss of teeth. Children who are preparing for othodontia can learn much from this book, and it can be used in health classes, by dentists, and for general reading about the care and protection of the teeth and mouth. Nonfiction.

KESSLER, ETHEL, Our Tooth Story; a Tale of Twenty Teeth, Dodd-Mead, 1972. (P)

Cartoonlike illustrations add to the children's story of their visits to the dentist. There is emphasis on the importance of regular checkups, the fundamentals of caring for the teeth by brushing and good diet, and the ways in which the establishment of good dental habits help protect the teeth. Nonfiction.

LESIEG, T., Tooth Book, Random House, 1981. (P)

In this beginning reader book, rhymed verses and bright, cartoon-style artwork reveal a wealth of dental facts. An excellent fun and educational book for children that conveys good feelings toward dentists and dental health. Fiction.

POMERANTZ, CHARLOTTE, Mango Tooth, Greenwillow, 1977. (P)

Posy is starting to lose her baby teeth. The first one is loosened by a mango pit, and it earns her a dime. Then go the "chicken bone tooth" and the "Turkish tootsie tooth," each providing another dime. But clever Posy nets two dimes on the fourth tooth, an "elephant tooth." Not many people can loosen a tooth on an elephant. Fiction.

RICHTER, A., and NUMEROFF, L., You Can't Put Braces On Spaces, Greenwillow, 1979. (I-U)

Eleven-year-old Neil has just started to wear braces. Neil's brother describes what Dr. Sherman did and said as he fitted Neil with braces and how his brother said they felt. Line drawings enhance this story, which presents the prospect of wearing braces as a positive event. Fiction.

ROSS, PAT, Molly and the Slow Teeth, Lee & Shepard, 1980. (P)

Molly is an unhappy second grader because while all her classmates are losing their baby teeth and getting rewards from the Tooth Fairy, she doesn't even have a loose tooth. She tries to fool the Tooth Fairy with a small white pebble, but that doesn't work. Only weeks and weeks of waiting and a hard apple finally put a gaping smile on Molly's face and her name on the class tooth chart. Fiction.

SHOWERS, PAUL, How Many Teeth? Crowell, 1962 (A Let's-read-and-find-out science book). (P)

The loss of a front tooth is common to all children and is one of childhood's great experiences. The subject is treated with respect, but the tooth loss has a light touch, with a happy, now-we-are-growing-up significance. Other facts about the teeth are informally presented. Easy-to-read with illustrations. Nonfiction.

DISEASES AND HEALTH PROBLEMS

COOER, ELANOR, Sadako and the Thousand Paper Cranes, Putnam, 1977. (I)

Sadako was 2 when the atom bomb was dropped on her hometown of Hiroshima. Now, at age 12, she has developed leukemia, and she and her supportive family must fight her disease. Fiction.

COHEN, DANIEL, Vaccination and You, Messner, 1969. (U)

The story of vaccination or immunization against disease, from the time of Edward Jenner and vaccination against smallpox, Pasteur's study of germs under microscope, and Koch's isolation of bacteria to Ehrlich's conquest of diphtheria, Salk and Sabin's efforts against polio, and Drs. Hilleman and Ender's work on a vaccine for measles. Nonfiction.

DONAHUE, PARNELL, and CAPELLAOR, HELEN, Germs Make Me Sick: a health Handbook for Kids, Knopf, 1975. (U)

Describes a wide variety of diseases and their treatment, and offers a brief discussion of germs in general. Included are diseases of the gastrointestinal tract (food poisoning, stomach sickness), the respiratory tract (colds, sore throats, sinusitis), germs on the skin (warts, acne, athlete's foot), and viral exanthems (measles, chickenpox). A separate chapter discusses "Some Diseases You Probably Won't Get," such as meningitis, rabies, and rheumatic fever. The final chapter tells about "Getting Well and Staying There." A glossary and index are appended. Nonfiction.

SAMPSON, FAY, Watch on Patterick Fell, Greenwillow, 1980. (U)

Patterick Fell is an English plant that stores nuclear waste from around the world. Teenage Roger's father is the director and his mother a distinguished coworker, and Roger has never questioned the plant's validity until the protests mount, and his younger sister joins them. When an explosion nearly levels the plant, the family rethinks its commitment. A very timely book, but some British attitudes and idioms may need explantion. Fiction.

SHARMAT, MARJORIE WEINMAN, I Want Mama, Harper & Row, 1974. (P)

Tenderly describes a young girl's concern over her mother going to the hospital. Fiction.

SILVERSTEIN, VIRGINIA B., and SILVERSTEIN, DR. ALVIN, Itch, Sniffle and Sneeze: All About Asthma, Hay Fever and Other Allergies, Four Winds, 1978. (P-I)

If any of your children sneeze every August, get those annoying itchy bumps on their skin when they eat chocolate, or have trouble breathing when they play with a puppy, this book should be passed on to them. The text succinctly tells what allergies are, how the body reacts to them, things people are allergic to, and how to cope with allergies. Nonfiction.

WINN, MARIE, The Sick Book: Questions and Answers About Hiccups and Mumps, Sneezes and Bumps, and Other Things That Go Wrong With Us, Four Winds, 1976. (P-I)

This is an informative volume about common childhood illnesses. Presented in a lively question-and-answer format, the various sections deal with colds and the flu, allergies, chickenpox, mumps, measles, skin troubles, and broken bones. Each ailment is presented so that readers will understand what happens when they are sick. A special section at the end of the book explains how our bodies work when they are healthy. Nonfiction.

DRUGS

HYDE, MARGERT O., Know About Drugs, ed. 2, McGraw-Hill, 1979. (I-U)

Along with the basic information about all drugs, the authors include facts about the use and abuse of marijuana, alcohol, coca and cocaine, cigarettes, PCP (angel dust), inert inhalants, heroin, barbiturates, methaqualone, and a wide variety of tranquilizers, amphetamines, and LSD and other hallucinogens. Nonfiction.

MARR, JOHN S., Good Drug and the Bad Drug, Evans, 1970. (I)

A city doctor has written in simple terms the course of two complete trips of drugs through the body. By means of illustrations, the good drug is shown as it travels toward the infected area in an effort to effect a cure. Having established certain basic concepts, the doctor then describes the harmful effects of a bad drug. A book that lends itself to class discussion. Nonfiction.

MOREY, WALT, Lemon Meringue Dog, Dutton. In Canada, Clarke, Irwin, 1980. (U)

Chris, age 20, is the junior member of a new Coast Guard narcotic squad that uses dogs to uncover drugs. On their first assignment on a ship, his dog Mike is curiously diverted by a surprise cache of his favorite lemon meringue pies, ruining the drug bust. Demoted, Chris buys Mike, and moonlighting as a night watchman he redeems them both by uncovering a huge and dangerous drug ring. A good action story with a low reading level. Fiction.

SHREVE, SUSAN, Nightmare of Geranium Street, Knopf, 1977. (P)

Elizabeth's family has chosen to stay on in their long-time home in a deteriorating area of Germantown, Pennsylvania. She has become the "Rex" of a club of children. When Amanda comes to live with her Aunt Tess the club—the Nightmares—become very curious about what happens in their house. Slowly it becomes evident that Tess is involved in a drug ring, as the children observe and become involved in disclosing. They never actually take drugs themselves—partly because of the strict discipline in Elizabeth's own family. An interesting and valuable picture of inner-city life from a true child's point of view. Fiction.

FAMILY

BLAINE, MARGE, Terrible Thing That Happened at Our House, Four Winds, 1975. (P-I)

Two young children dislike the changes in their family life when Mother goes back to work. Everyone has to rush around in the morning, they have to eat in the noisy, smelly school lunchroom, no one has time to listen, and there's no time for stories, games, or trips to the gas station. Things are just too topsy-turvy. Fiction.

BRANDENBERG, FRANZ, Nice New Neighbors, Greenwillow, 1977. (P)

When Mr. and Mrs. Fieldmouse and their six children move to new a home, the neighborhood children are unfriendly. The resourceful mouse children invent their own play and suddenly they are very popular. All the neighbor children beg to join in. Fiction.

BURNINGHAM, JOHN, Baby, Crowell, 1975. (P)

In a few words a young boy tells about the new baby at his home. Fiction.

BURNINGHAM, JOHN, Snow, Crowell, 1975. (P)

It snows one day, and a little boy tells of all the fun he and his mother have playing in the snow. Fiction.

HAZEN, BARBARA SHOOK, Tight Times, Viking. In Canada, Penquin Books Canada, Ltd. 1979. (P)

A youngster doesn't understand why something called "tight times" keeps him from getting a dog and causes Mommy to go to work and Daddy to lose his job. But in spite of all their problems, when the child brings home a starved kitten Mommy and Daddy say the new pet can stay. Fiction.

LIVINGSTON, CAROLE, Why Was I Adopted? Lyle Stuart, 1978. (I-U)

Presents facts of adoption in clever and appealing text and illustrations. Focuses on reasons for and ways of being adopted and how special adopted children are to parents. Concludes with questions children frequently ask. Nonfiction.

McCORD, JEAN, Turkeylegs Thompson, Atheneum. In Canada, McClelland & Stewart, 1979. (I-U)

Even pugnacious Turkeylegs (really 12-year-old Betty Ann) has a breaking point. Virtually without friends, she helps her single-parent mother care for her whiny little brother and her enchanting little sister. But buffeted by a pervert exposing himself to her, her little sister's death, and her alcoholic father's return home, she runs away to the hills she loves, but returns home to face her grief and confusion when her young friend Charlie meets her and counsels patience. A bleak, sometimes painful story, with a very believable main character. Fiction.

NAYLOR, PHYLLIS REYNOLDS, Getting Along in Your Family, Abingdon, 1976. (I-U)

Explores family life and related problems—fighting, sharing tasks, being loyal, showing love, and coping with mental disturbances, alcoholism, and divorce. Will help children understand their brothers, sisters, and parents. Nonfiction.

NOLAN, MADEENA SPRAY, My Daddy Don't Go to Work, Carolrhoda Books, 1978. (P)

A young black girl tells about her daddy who goes out every day looking for a job but just can't find a place that needs him. Although her daddy is discouraged, the little girl likes having him home to play ball with her and listen to her after school. Fiction.

PURSELL, MARGARET SANFORD, Look at Adoption, Lerner, 1977. (I-U)

Straightforward discussion of adoption, including reasons children are available and steps necessary for adoption. Nonfiction.

RAYNOR, DORKA, This Is My Father and Me, Whitman, 1973. (P-I)

Photographic essay on the relationship between father and child in many different countries. Nonfiction.

RICHARDS, ARLENE KRAMER, How to Get It Together When Your Parents Are Coming Apart, McKay, 1976. (I-U)

Through many representative stories of adolescents, this guide offers suggestions to young people for coping with divorce. Divided into three parts (marriage trouble, during the divorce, and after the divorce), the emphasis is to assuage guilt feelings on the part of the children and to provide specific addresses for finding outside help. Nonfiction.

STEIN, SARA, Adopted One: an Open Family Book for Parents and Children Together, Walker. In Canada, Beaverbooks, Ltd., 1979. (U)

Dual text for adult and child readers tells how Joshua feels about being adopted and gives parental guidance in understanding his needs for information about adoption. Black and white photographs on each page effectively express emotion. Nonfiction.

STOLZ, MARY, Go and Catch a Flying Fish, Harper & Row. In Canada, Fizhenry & Whiteside, 1979 (An Ursual Nordstrom book). (P-I)

The seemingly idyllic life of the Reddick family centers on the sea, sun, and sand of Florida's Gulf Coast. Although the three children—13-year-old Taylor and her younger brothers, aged 10 and 4—are aware that something is wrong, no one, not even her husband, Tony, is prepared for Junie's abrupt departure for "time on her own." Fiction.

TATE, ELEANORA E., Just an Overnight Guest, Dial, 1980. (I-U)

Margie is a 9-year-old black girl living with her family in a Mississippi River town. When her mother introduces Ethel, who is half white, into their warm, stable home, Margie is confused and jealous. Her father gently explains that Ethel is her cousin, her uncle Jake's child, and will be more than just an overnight guest. Some frank language makes this less suitable for younger readers. Fiction.

TAX, MEREDITH, Families, Little, Brown & Co., 1981. (P)

Positive and humorous description of different kinds of families as told by 6-year-old Angie. Includes animals (lions, dogs, chickens, ants) and people (parents, single parent, stepparents, grandparents, two women). Nonfiction.

HANDICAPS

ADAMS, BARBARA, Like It Is: Facts and Feelings About Handicaps From Kids Who Know, Walker, 1979. (I)

Six kids with handicaps tell what it's like to live in their unique worlds. The reader learns how handicapped people wish to be treated and what one can do to help. Nonfiction.

BRIGHTMAN, ALAN, Like Me, Little, Brown & Co., 1976. (P)

Rhyming text and beautiful photographs explain the concept of mental retardation for the younger reader. Nonfiction.

CHARLIP, REMY, and CHARLIP, MARY BETH, Handtalk: an ABC of Finger Spelling and Sign Language, Four Winds, 1980 (reprint of edition published by Parents' Magazine Press, 1974). (P)

All ages will enjoy learning about the ways people can talk without using their voices: finger spelling (making words letter by letter with the fingers) and signing (using the hands to convey a picture for a word or idea). Full-color pictures show children how it's done. Nonfiction.

CLIFTON, LUCILLE, My Friend Jacob, Dutton, 1980. (P)

Sam and Jacob are neighbors and the very best of friends. Though 17-year-old Jacob is mentally retarded, 8-year-old Sam learns they can love and help each other. Fiction.

DACQUINO, V.T., Kiss The Candy Days Good-bye, Delacorte, 1983.(I)

This book tells of Jimmy, who is diagnosed as having diabetes. It describes the adjustments that must be made by Jimmy, his family, and friends. Fiction.

FROEHLICH, M.W., Hide Crawford Quick, Houghton Mifflin, 1983.(I)

Twelve-year-old Gracie realizes that something is wrong when her parents' first son is born with a limb abnormality. The main plot is the eventual acceptance of this physically handicapped boy by the rest of the family. Fiction.

GRIESE, ARNOLD A., At the Mouth of the Luckiest River, Crowell, 1973. (I)

A convincing tale of Talek, an Alaskan Indian boy who becomes a leader among his people despite being crippled. Set in the 19th century. Fiction.

HERMES, PATRICIA, What If They Knew? Harcourt, 1980. (I)

Jeremy is an epileptic who learns that real friends don't care if you're different in some ways. Fiction.

JONES, RON, The Acorn People, Abingdon, 1976. (I)

Teachers may wish to read aloud some parts of this story of five severely handicapped children in a Boy Scout camp with an unprepared counselor. Older children will learn about courage through their own reading. Fiction.

KAMIEN, JANET, What If You Couldn't . . . ? A Book About Special Needs, Scribner's, 1979. (I)

An informational book about handicaps that includes "experiments" that will help children to understand the everyday problems that confront the handicapped. Nonfiction.

LASKER, JOE, He's My Brother, Whitman, 1974. (P)

Jamie is not retarded, but he is a slow learner who often becomes frustrated at school. The other children make fun of him and tease him. There are many things he can't do well, but Jamie is kind and gentle to animals, babies, and young children. He draws well and is also very good on the drums. His parents are patient and understanding. His brother and sister are good to him and make up stories to tell him they love him. Nonfiction.

LEVINE, EDNA S., Lisa and Her Soundless World, Human Science Press, 1974. (I)

Eight-year-old Lisa is deaf and attends special schools to learn to use sign language and to lip read, as well as to improve her speech. Fiction.

MILLER, EDNA, Mousekin's Close Call, Prentice-Hall, 1978. (P)

Mousekin watches some other animals protect themselves and their young by pretending to be handicapped. There's no pretending when Mousekin is caught by a weasel, but a startled one-legged sparrow comes to the rescue and proves that the handicapped are achievers too. Fiction.

PAYNE, SHERRY, A Contest, Minneapolis, Carolrhoda Books, Inc., 1982. (P)

Mike, who is in a wheelchair and has attended a special school, finds himself in a regular class. The other kids stare and are scared until the teacher devises games to show off Mike's strengths. Fiction.

PETERSEN, PALLE, Sally Can't See, Crowell, 1977 (A John Day Book). (P)

The life of a blind child and how she learns and plays is described in a brief text illustrated with color photographs. Nonfiction.

PETERSON, JEANNE WHITEHOUSE, I Have A Sister—My Sister is Deaf, Harper & Row, 1977. (P)
> Soft black-and-white drawings depict the daily life in a loving home where one child is deaf. Fiction.

PHELAN, TERRY WOLFE, The S. D. Valentine, Four Winds, 1979. (I)
> Children identify with the young people who learn how to relate to Connie, the new girl in class who must use a wheelchair. Fiction.

ROBINET, HARRIETTE GILLEM, Ride the Red Cycle, Houghton, Mifflin, 1980. (I)
> Gutsy, crippled Jerome is determined to learn to ride his tricycle, and with the help of his family, he does. Fiction.

SAVITZ, HARRIET MAY, Run, Don't Walk, Watts, 1979. (I)
> Two teenagers confined to wheelchairs take some positive actions to prevent being discriminated against because of their handicaps. Fiction.

SHAOLM, DEBRA, Special Kids Make Special Friends, Bellmore, N.Y., An Association for Children with Down Syndrome, 1984. (P)
> This simply written book, aimed at primary and beginning intermediate students, has excellent photographs. It is about children with Down Syndrome.

SIEGEL, DOROTHY SCHAINMAN, Winners: Eight Special Young People, Messner, 1978. (I-U)
> Biographical sketches of eight courageous young people, each with a different handicap. These children have not permitted their problems to curtail their activities more than is absolutely necessary. Nonfiction.

SLEPIAN, JAN, The Alfred Summer, Macmillan, 1980. (I-U)
> Lester could care less that Alfred is slightly retarded. After all, Alfred doesn't mind about Lester's cerebral palsy. Together with two other friends, they are a memorable quartet. Fiction.

SMITH, DORIS BUCHANAN, Kelly's Creek, Crowell, 1975. (I)
> Young Kelly suffers from perceptual learning problems and must find his own way to live with this handicap and achieve self-respect. Fiction.

SMITH, LUCIA B., A Special Kind of Sister, Holt, 1979. (P)
> Seven-year-old Sarah talks about her feelings for her retarded younger brother Andy. Fiction.

SULLIVAN, MARY BETH, BRIGHTMAN, ALAN J., and BLATT, JOSEPH, Feeling Free, Addison-Wesley, 1979.
> In this spin-off of the television series by the same name, handicapped children talk about their disabilities. A great aid to mainstreaming, the book is directed toward children and adults who are unprepared to interact with the handicapped. Nonfiction.

WHITE, PAUL, Janet at School, Crowell, 1978, (A John Day Book). (P)
> Janet has spina bifida and cannot move or feel her legs. As children learn about her daily life in this straightforward, caring account, they will grasp the difficulties people with this disease must overcome. Nonfiction.

WOLF, BERNARD, Don't Feel Sorry for Paul, Lippincott, 1974. (I)
> Born with his hands and feet incompletely formed, Paul is encouraged to be independent all his life. This book shows his progress. Nonfiction.

WOLF, BERNARD, Anna's Silent World, Lippincott, 1977. (P)
> Abundant black-and-white photographs show Anna at home, in school, at dancing class, and at the New York League for the Hard of Hearing. Hearing aids and the process of learning to speak are explained. Nonfiction.

MENTAL AND EMOTIONAL PROBLEMS

BONSAIL, CROSBY, Who's Afraid of the Dark? Harper & Row. In Canada, Fitzhenry & Whiteside, 1980. (P)
> A little boy tries to teach his dog Stella to be unafraid of the dark and the night noises, but the readers know it's really the boy who's scared. Fiction.

BURNINGHAM, JOHN, Friend, Crowell, 1976. (P)
> A little boy has a best friend named Arthur. The two children always play together, but sometimes they fuss and don't like each other, and Arthur goes home. Fiction.

DIXON, PAIGE, Walk My Way, Atheneum. In Canada, McClelland & Stewart, 1980. (I-U)
> Fourteen-year-old Kitty is 5 feet 11 inches tall, and clumsy. Her brutal father mistreats her, and she decides to go and live with her mother's friend who raised her. On the 50-mile trip through the woods to the coast of Maine, she meets a lost dog and an ill old man and his grandson. Through helping them, Kitty also learns how to help herself. Fiction.

GREENE, LAURA, I Am Somebody, Childrens Press. In Canada, Regensteiner, 1980. (P-I)

Story is told in the first person by a not-so-good ball player. Nathan deals with the frustration of not being chosen first, being tagged out at base, and missing an important catch. There is no miraculous ending. Nathan has a collection of feathers that he shares with a friend. He loves to play baseball, but he is better at collecting. Nonfiction.

HALL, MALCOLM, Friends of Charlie Ant Bear, Coward-McCann. In Canada, Academic, 1980. (P)

Charlie Ant Bear is jealous of his best friend Wild Bob Ding, who is liked by everyone in town because of his funny practical jokes. Gloomy Charlie buys a joke book thinking that he too can become popular. All his jokes and tricks backfire, and Charlie is feeling worse than ever, until he and Bob try one final trick that tops them all. Fiction.

HAZEN, BARBARA SHOOK, Me I See, Abingdon, 1978. (P)

Through rhymed verse and full-page illustrations, a little girl discovers the different parts of her body and how she is different from anyone else. Nonfiction.

KAVANAUGH, DORRIET, Listen to Us. The Children's Express report, edited by Dorriet Kavanaugh; produced by Children's Express and Robert Clampitt, Workman, 1978. (U)

Compilation of writings and interviews of children ages 5 to 17 on family, divorce, school, sex, handicaps, friendship, drugs, television, money, religion, discrimination, emotions, and much, much more. Readers will find that they are not alone in their growth and development, which will build increased self-confidence. Nonfiction.

LEVOY, MYRON, Alan and Naomi, Harper & Row, 1977. (I-U)

Naomi is a French Jewish girl, traumatized by Nazi brutality, who comes to live in a New York City apartment building with her mother. A neighbor boy, Alan Silverman, is asked by his parents to befriend her and help her return to reality. Though this means giving up his only sport, stickball, in which he is beginning to wear down accusing taunts of "sissy," Alan complies with his parents' wishes and establishes a special friendship with Naomi. Fiction.

THOMAS, MARLO, Free to Be . . . You and Me, McGraw-Hill, 1974. (U)

A collection of songs, poems, stories, and pictures by well-known composers, writers, and artists, with an overall theme that debunks old sexual and racial stereotypes and emphasizes the idea that anyone is free to be who they are and who they want to be. Several short stories have been added to the material on the record of the same title. Nonfiction.

NUTRITION

BERGER, MELVIN, New Food Book; Nutrition, Diet, Consumer Tips and Foods of the Future, Crowell. In Canada, Fitzhenry & Whiteside Ltd., 1978. (U)

A collection of valuable food information including nutrition, diet, consumer education, experiments designed for elementary students, food production and processing, the present food crisis and its causes and possible solutions, and up-to-date information concerning cholesterol. Nonfiction.

BORGHESE, ANITA, Down to Earth Cookbook, Revised edition, Scribner's, 1980. (U)

Introduction to natural cooking for intermediate graders. Contains explanations of terms, utensils, and ingredients, gives clear directions for all recipes, and introduces the user to unfamiliar foods. Pleasant illustrations enhance the text. Nonfiction.

COBB, VICKI, More Science Experiments You Can Eat, Lippincott, 1979. (U)

Describes food experiments that investigate spoilage, dehydration, ripening, acidity, flavorings, and extracts. In discussing additives, the author relies on the Food and Drug Administration's questionable Generally Regarded As Safe (GRAS) list. Nonfiction.

COLE, W. (compiler), Poem Stew, Lippinncott, 1981. (P-I)

Fifty-seven humorous poems about table manners, overeating and enjoying food. Fiction.

JONES, HETTIE, How to Eat Your ABC's; a Book About Vitamins, Four Winds, 1976. (I-U)

An attractive, neat format and an informal text will be appealing to many middle graders. The history of vitamin research and the roles each vitamin plays and where to get it are included. Nutrition is stressed in problem-solving menu ideas, food charts, and a few easy and yummy recipes. An important topic today in our world of junk food. This book will be of use in nutrition and food units. Nonfiction.

PERL, LILA, Eating the Vegetarian Way: Good Food From the Earth, Morrow, 1980. (U)

An in-depth discussion as to what vegetarianism is and why it has become a new trend in American eating patterns. Final chapter is devoted to recipes that would appeal to boys and girls. Nonfiction.

PINKWATER, D.M., Slaves of Spiegel: A Magic Moscow Story, Four Winds, 1982. (I-U)

Fat men from the planet Spiegel are ordered to track down the most fattening food. Includes an interplanetary cooking contest. Fiction.

U.S. DEPARTMENT OF AGRICULTURE, What's to Eat? and Other Questions Kids Ask About Food, foreword by Bob Bergland. Superintendent of Documents (U.S. Government Printing Office 001-000-04041-3), 1979.(I)

Useful for both teachers and students, this colorful book is full of facts on nutrition and includes recipes, games about food and health, and activities for consumer education. Nonfiction.

SAFETY

ELGIN, KATHLEEN, Fall Down, Break a Bone, Skin Your Knee Book, Walker, 1974. (U)

Major and minor wounds and injuries, including fractures, burns, bruises, warts, sprains, and sunburns, are discussed in text with accompanying drawings. First-aid suggestions are given. Useful for study of human body. Nonfiction.

KESSLER, LEONARD, Tale of Two Bicycles, Safety on Your Bike, Lothrop, Lee & Shepard, 1971. (P)

Humorous text and illustrations on the serious subject of bicycle safety. Freddy and Tommy both receive identical bikes for their birthdays, but from the very first, Tommy does not like his gift; he disregards all safety rules, hurts himself repeatedly, endangers others with his bad bicycle manners, and ends up demolishing his bike. Ends with safety tips for bike riders. Good addition to a primary collection. Fiction.

KESSLER, LEONARD, Who Tossed That Bat? Safety on the Ballfield and Playground, Lothrop, Lee & Shepard, 1973. (P)

Advice in verse form on safety as a participant and observer on the ballfield and playground. A delightful way for beginning readers to be reminded of sports and playground safety rules. Nonfiction.

SEXUALITY

BURN, HELEN JEAN, Getter Than the Birds, Smarter Than the Bees; No-Nonsense Answers to Honest Questions About Sex and Growing Up, Abingdon, 1969. (U)

Frank answers are given to honest questions about sex and growing up asked by adolescents. Compiled by one of the members of the Planned Parenthood Association's speaker's bureau, the book provides simple yet complete and satisfying answers to questions relating to the psychological angle of sex, the physiological differences between boys and girls, the "marriage bit," and the "no-no's." The bibliography includes selected references on aspects of sex education, films for use in sex education, and selected fiction on sexual problems. Nonfiction.

MAY, JULIAN, New Baby Comes, Creative Education, 1970. (P)

By means of illustrations and simple text, the growth of a baby is followed until its birth in a hospital and the beginning of its life as a new member of the family. Despite the low reading level, a practical book for the older child. Nonfiction.

SHEFFIELD, MARGARET, Where Do Babies Come From? Knopf, 1973. (I)

A first sex education book that has the answer to what children really want to know. All of the facts are included in the text using correct terminology. The direct illustrations are soft colored paintings. The book gracefully creates a mood of reverence for life in representing human reproduction. Adopted from a BBC award-winning program. Nonfiction.

SMOKING

MARR, JOHN S., Breath of Air and Breath of Smoke, Evans, 1971. (I-U)

The first part of the book contains a detailed description of the respiratory system with many illustrations. Then the processes of inhalation and exhalation are carefully explained again with illustrations. Without critique, the author describes the effect that smoking has on the body. Three-color illustrations are used on every page to enhance the interesting text. Nonfiction.

SONNETT, SHERRY, Smoking, Watts, 1977. (U)

The history of tobacco and smoking, how it affects people physically, and the diseases it promotes are clearly explained in this slim book. A good book for student reports and classroom units on cancer and health. Nonfiction.

APPENDIX F

SOURCES OF FREE AND LOW-COST SPONSORED INSTRUCTIONAL AIDS FOR HEALTH TEACHING

Since some organizations move, change policy, or go out of business each year, it is virtually impossible to prepare a list of sources of free and inexpensive materials that will not require revision periodically. Teachers can keep up-to-date on such changes by conferring with the librarian or by requesting that their letters of inquiry be forwarded. Teacher's manuals that accompany many health textbooks furnish the teacher with accurate and selective lists of printed materials, films and filmstrips, and their sources.

The national organizations listed with asterisks have state or regional affiliates or offices. When this is known, the teacher should first request materials or information from the nearest unit.

Abbott Laboratories
Abbott Park, D-383
North Chicago, IL 60064
(312) 937-6100

Aetna Life and Casualty Companies
Public Relations and Advertising
151 Farmington Avenue DA06
Hartford, CT 06156
(203) 273-0123

Al-Anon Family Group Headquarters*
One Park Avenue
New York, NY 10016
(212) 683-1771

Allstate
Corporate Relations Department
Allstate Plaza
Northbrook, IL 60062
(312) 291-5000

American Alliance for Health, Physical Education, Recreation, and Dance
1900 Association Drive
Reston, VA 22091
(703) 476-3400

American Automobile Association*
Traffic Safety Department
8111 Gatehouse Road
Falls Church, VA 22047
(703) 222-6000

American Cancer Society, Inc.*
90 Park Avenue
New York, NY 10016
(212) 599-8200

American Chiropractic Association*
1916 Wilson Blvd.
Arlington, VA 22201
(202) 276-8800

American Dental Association
Bureau of Health Education and Audiovisual Services
211 East Chicago Avenue
Chicago, IL 60611
(312) 440-2500

American Diabetes Association*
2 Park Avenue
New York, NY 10016
(212) 683-7444

American Dry Milk Institute, Inc.
130 North Franklin Street
Chicago, IL 60606
(312) 782-4888

American Foundation for the Blind
15 West 16th Street
New York, NY 10011
(212) 620-2000

American Institute of Baking
Communications Department
1213 Bakers Way
Manhattan, KS 66502
(913) 537-4750

American Lung Association*
1740 Broadway
New York, NY 10019
(212) 315-8700

American Medical Association*
535 North Dearborn Street
Chicago, IL 60610
(312) 645-5000

American Optometric Association
Department of Public Information
243 N. Lindbergh Blvd.
St. Louis, MO 63141
(314) 991-4100

American Osteopathic Association
212 East Ohio Street
Chicago, IL 60611
(312) 280-5800

American Podiatric Medical Association
20 Chevy Chase Circle N.W.
Washington, DC 20015
(202) 537-4900

American National Red Cross*
17th and D Streets N.W.
Washington, DC 20006
(202) 737-8300

American School Health Association
PO Box 708
Kent, OH 44240
(216) 678-1601

American Social Health Association
260 Sheridan Ave., Suite 307
Palo Alto, CA 94306
(415) 321-5134

American Veterinary Medical Association
930 North Meacham Road
Schaumburg, IL 60196
(312) 885-8070

Better Vision Institute, Inc.
230 Park Ave.
New York, NY 10169
(212) 682-1731

Channing L. Bete Co., Inc.
200 State Road
South Deerfield, MA 01373
(413) 665-7611

Consumer Information Center
Pueblo, CO 81009
(303) 323-9301

Consumer Nutrition Center
Human Nutrition Information Service
U.S. Department of Agriculture
Hyattsville, MD 20782
(301) 868-8800

Distilled Spirits Council of the United States
1250 Eye St. N.W.
Washington, DC 20005
(202) 628-3544

Environmental Protection Agency
PM 211-B
401 M St. S.W.
Washington, DC 20460
(202) 755-0707

Epilepsy Foundation of America
4351 Garden City Drive
Landover, MD 20785
(301) 459-3700

FDA/Consumer Communications (HFE-88)
5600 Fishers Lane
Rockville, MD 20857
(301) 443-3170

General Mills, Inc.
Publications & Editorial Department
9200 Wayzata Blvd.
Minneapolis, MN 55440
(612) 540-2311

The Gillette Company
Personal Care Division
Box 61
Boston, MA 02199
(617) 421-7000

The Hogg Foundation for Mental Health
University of Texas–Austin
PO Box 7998, University Station
Austin, TX 78712
(512) 471-5041

Institute of Makers of Explosives
1575 Eye St. N.W., Suite 550
Washington, DC 20005
(202) 789-0310

Kellogg Co.
235 Porter St.
Battle Creek, MI 49017
(616) 966-2000

Kemper Corporation
Long Grove, IL 60049
(312) 540-2000

Kemper Investors Life Insurance Company
120 S. LaSalle Street
Chicago, IL 60603
(312) 781-1121

Kimberly-Clark Corporation
DFW Airport Station
Box 619100
Dallas, TX 75261
(214) 830-1200

Lever Brothers Company, Inc.
Lever House
390 Park Avenue
New York, NY 10022
(212) 688-6000

March of Dimes*
1275 Mamaraneck Ave.
White Plains, NY 10605
(914) 428-7100

Mental Health Materials Center
30 E. 29th St.
New York, NY 10016
(212) 889-5760

Metropolitan Life Insurance Company
Health and Safety Education Division
One Madison Avenue
New York, NY 10010
(212) 578-2211

Muscular Dystrophy Association
810 Seventh Avenue
New York, NY 10019
(212) 586-0808

National Association for Hearing and Speech Action
(NAHSA)
10801 Rockville Pike
Rockville, MD 20852
(301) 897-8682

National Council on Alcoholism
12 West 21st Street
New York, NY 10010
(212) 206-6770

National Council on Family Relations
1910 W. Country Rd. B, Suite 147
St. Paul, MN 55113
(612) 633-6933

National Dairy Council*
6300 North River Rd.
Rosemont, IL 60018
(312) 696-1020

National Fire Protection Association
Batterymarch Park
Quincy, MA 02269
(617) 770-3000

National Health Council, Inc.
70 West 40th Street
New York, NY 10018
(212) 869-8100

National Heart, Lung, and Blood Institute
Bldg. 31; Room 5A52
National Institutes of Health
Bethesda, MD 20205
(301) 496-5161

National Institute on Drug Abuse Clearinghouse
Public Inquiries
5600 Fishers Lane
Rockville, MD 20857
(301) 443-4797

National Kidney Foundation
Two Park Ave.
New York, NY 10016
(212) 889-2210

National Institute of Mental Health
Public Inquiries
5600 Fishers Lane
Rockville, MD 20857
(301) 443-4513

National Livestock and Meat Board*
Nutritional Department
444 N. Michigan Ave.
Chicago, IL 60611
(312) 467-5520

National Mental Health Association
1021 Prince Street
Arlington, VA 22314
(703) 684-7022

National Multiple Sclerosis Society*
205 East 42nd Street
New York, NY 10017
(212) 986-3240

National Safety Council
444 N. Michigan
Chicago, IL 60611
(312) 527-4800

NIAAA National Clearinghouse for Alcohol
   Information
PO Box 2345
Rockville, MD 20852
(301) 468-2600

Office on Smoking and Health
5600 Fishers Lane
Rm 1-10
Park Building
Rockville, MD 20857
(301) 443-1575

Ortho Pharmaceuticals
RT 202
Raritan, NJ 08869
(201) 524-0400

Personal Products Company
c/o Karol Media
22 Riverview Dr.
Wayne, NJ 07470
(201) 628-9111

Pet Incorporated
Director of Home Economics
400 S. Fourth Street
St. Louis, MO 63102
(314) 621-5400

Pharmaceutical Manufacturers' Association
Department NW-601
1100 15th Street N.W.
Washington, DC 20005
(202) 835-3400

Planned Parenthood Federation of America, Inc.*
Publications Department
810 Seventh Avenue
New York, NY 10019
(212) 541-7800

President's Council on Physical Fitness and Sports
400 Sixth Street S.W.
Room 300 Donohoe Bldg.
Washington, DC 20202
(202) 755-7947

Proprietary Association
1700 Pennsylvania Ave. N.W.
Washington, DC 20006
Attention: Mary B. Alterman, Librarian
(202) 393-1700

Prudential Insurance Company of America
Public Relations and Advertising
Prudential Plaza
Box 36
Newark, NJ 07101
(201) 877-6000

Public Affairs Committee
381 Park Avenue South
New York, NY 10016
(212) 683-4331

Public Health Service
200 Independence Ave., S.W.
Washington, DC 20025
(202) 443-2403

Ralston Purina Company
Corporate Consumer Services—Public Relations
Checkerboard Square
St. Louis, MO 63164
(314) 982-1000

Rutgers Center of Alcohol Studies
Smithers Hall
New Brunswick, NJ 08903
(201) 932-2190

Schering-Plough Corporation
One Giralda Farms
Madison, NJ 07940
(201) 822-7000

Sex Information and Education Council
   of the United States
80 Fifth Ave., Suite 801
New York, NY 10011
(212) 929-2300

Smithkline & French
1500 Spring Garden St.
PO Box 7929
Philadelphia, PA 19101
(215) 751-4000

State Farm Insurance Companies
Public Relations Department
One State Farm Plaza
Bloomington, IL 61761
(309) 766-2311

Sunkist Growers, Inc.
PO Box 7888
Van Nuys, CA 91409
(213) 986-4800

Superintendent of Documents
U.S. Government Printing Office
North Capitol & H Streets N.W.
Washington, DC 20402
(202) 541-3000

The Travelers Film Library
Travelers Ins. Co.
One Tower Square
Hartford, CT 06115
(203) 277-0111

United Cerebral Palsy Association, Inc.
66 E. 34th
New York, NY 10016
(212) 481-6347

Wheat Flour Institute
600 Maryland Ave. S.W.
Suite 305 West Wing
Washington, DC 20024
(202) 484-2200

APPENDIX G

SELECTED FEDERAL HEALTH INFORMATION CLEARINGHOUSES AND INFORMATION CENTERS

AGING

National Clearinghouse on Aging
330 Independence Avenue S.W.
Washington, DC 20201
(202 245-2158
> Provides access to information and referral services that assist the older American in obtaining services. Distributes Administration on Aging publications.

ALCOHOL

National Clearinghouse for Alcohol Information (NIAAA)
PO Box 2345
Rockville, MD 20852
(301) 468-2600
> Gathers and disseminates current knowledge on alcohol-related subjects.

ARTHRITIS

Arthritis Information Clearinghouse
1700 North Moore St.
Arlington, VA 22209
(703) 558-8250

Identifies materials concerned with arthritis and related musculoskeletal diseases and serves as an information exchange for individuals and organizations involved in public, professional, and patient education. Refers personal requests from patients to the Arthritis Foundation.

BLIND AND PHYSICALLY HANDICAPPED

National Library Service for the Blind and Physically Handicapped
Library of Congress
1291 Taylor Street N.W.
Washington, DC 20542
(202) 882-5500; (800) 424-8567
> Works through local and regional libraries to provide free library service to persons unable to read or use standard printed materials because of visual or physical impairment. Provides information on blindness and physical handicaps on request. A list of participating libraries is available.

CANCER

National Cancer Institute Information Service
National Cancer Institute
Office of Cancer Communicatons
9000 Rockville Pike, Building 31, Room 10A18
Bethesda, MD 20892
(301) 496-5583

Collects information on public, patient, and professional cancer education materials and disseminates it to organizations and health care professionals.

Office of Cancer Communication
National Cancer Institute
Cancer Information Service
Bethesda, MD 20205
(301) 496-2351; (800) 638-6694

Answers requests for cancer information from patients and the general public. The National Cancer Institute sponsors a toll-free telephone number to supply cancer information to the general public.

CHILD ABUSE

Clearinghouse on Child Abuse and Neglect
  Information
PO Box 1182
Washington, DC 20013
(202) 245-2840

Collects, processes, and disseminates information on child abuse and neglect.

CONSUMER EDUCATION

Consumer Education Resource Network (CERN)
1555 Wilson Blvd., Suite 600
Rosslyn, VA 22209
(800) 336-0222

Provides reference and referral services to consumer educators, serves as a depository of information and materials, and conducts training and technical assistance programs.

CONSUMER INFORMATION

Consumer Information Center
Pueblo, CO 81009
(303) 323-9301

Distributes consumer publications on topics such as children, food and nutrition, health, exercise, and weight control. The *Consumer Information Catalog* is available free from the Center and must be used to identify publications requested.

DIABETES

National Diabetes Information Clearinghouse
Box: NDIC
Bethesda, MD 20205
(202) 842-7630

Collects and disseminates information on patient education materials and coordinates the development of materials and programs for diabetes education.

DIGESTIVE DISEASES

National Digestive Diseases Education and
  Information Clearinghouse
1555 Wilson Blvd., Suite 600
Rosslyn, VA 22209
(703) 522-0870

Provides information on digestive diseases to health professionals and consumers.

DRUG ABUSE

National Clearinghouse for Drug Abuse Information
5600 Fishers Ln., Room 10A43
Rockville, MD 20857
(301) 443-6500

Collects and disseminates information on drug abuse. Produces informational materials on drugs, drug abuse, and prevention.

ENVIRONMENTAL PROTECTION

Environmental Protection Agency (EPA)
Public Inquiries Center
PM 211-3
401 M Street S.W.
Washington, DC 20460
(202) 755-0707

Public information materials on such topics as hazardous wastes, the school asbestos project, air and water pollution, pesticides, and drinking water are available. Offers information on the agency and its programs and activities.

FAMILY PLANNING

National Clearinghouse for Family Planning
  Information
PO Box 2225
Rockville, MD 20852
(301) 881-9400

Collects family planning materials, makes referrals to other information centers, and distributes and produces materials. Primary audience is federally funded family planning clinics.

FOOD AND DRUGS

Food and Drug Administration (FDA)
Office for Consumer Communications
5600 Fishers Lane, Room 15B-32 (HFE-88)
Rockville, MD 20857
(301) 443-3170

Answers consumer inquiries for the FDA and serves as a clearinghouse for its consumer publications.

FOOD AND NUTRITION

Food and Nutrition Information Center (FNIC)
National Agricultural Library Building, Room 304
Beltsville, MD 20705
(301) 344-3719

Serves the information needs of persons interested in human nutrition, food service management, and food technology. Acquires and lends books, journal articles, and audiovisual materials dealing with these areas of concern.

GENETIC DISEASES

National Clearinghouse for Human Genetic Diseases
805 15th Street N.W., Suite 500
Washington, DC 20005
(202) 842-7617

Provides information on human genetics and genetic diseases for both patients and health care workers. Reviews existing curricular materials on genetic education.

HANDICAPPED

Clearinghouse on the Handicapped
Office for Handicapped Individuals
Washington, DC 20202
(202) 732-1244

Responds to inquiries from handicapped individuals and serves as a resource to organizations that supply information to, and about, handicapped individuals.

HEALTH INDEXES

Clearinghouse on Health Indexes
National Center for Health Statistics
Division of Analysis
3700 East-West Highway
Hyattsville, MD 20782
(301) 436-7035

Provides informational assistance in the development of health measures for health researchers, administrators, and planners.

HEALTH INFORMATION

National Health Information Clearinghouse (NHIC)
PO Box 1133
Washington, DC 20013-1133
(701) 522-2590 (in VA); (800) 336-4797

Helps the public locate health information through identification of health information resources and an inquiry and referral system. Health questions are referred to appropriate health resources that, in turn, respond directly to inquirers.

HEALTH PROMOTION AND EDUCATION

Center for Health Promotion and Education (CHPE)
1300 Clifton Road, Building 14
Atlanta, GA 30333
(404) 329-3235

Provides leadership and program direction for the prevention of disease, disability, premature death, and undesirable and unnecessary health problems through health education. Formerly called the Bureau of Health Education.

HIGH BLOOD PRESSURE

National High Blood Pressure Education Program
120/80 National Institutes of Health
Bethesda, MD 20205
(703) 558-4827

Provides information on the detection, diagnosis, and management of high blood pressure to consumers and health professionals.

HIGHWAY SAFETY

National Highway Traffic Safety Administration (NHTSA)
U.S. Department of Transportation
400 7th St. S.W.
Washington, DC 20590
(202) 426-9550; (800) 424-9393

Works to reduce highway traffic deaths and injuries. Publishes a variety of safety information brochures, conducts public information campaigns on vehicle defects and drunken driving, and maintains a toll-free hotline for consumer complaints on auto safety.

INJURIES

National Injury Information Clearinghouse
5401 Westbard Avenue, Room 615
Washington, DC 20207
(301) 492-6424

Collects and disseminates injury data and information relating to the causes and prevention of death, injury, and illness associated with consumer products. Requests of a general nature are referred to the Consumer Product Safety Commission's Communications Office.

MENTAL HEALTH

National Clearinghouse for Mental Health
   Information
Public Inquiries Section
5600 Fishers Lane, Room 15C17
Rockville, MD 20857
(301) 443-4513
   Acquires and abstracts the world's mental health literature, answers inquiries from the public, and provides computer searches for the scientific and academic communities.

PHYSICAL FITNESS

President's Council on Physical Fitness and Sports
450 Fifth St. N.W., Suite 2103
Washington, DC 20201
(202) 755-7478
   Conducts a public service advertising program and cooperates with governmental and private groups to promote the development of physical fitness leadership, facilities, and programs. Produces informational materials on exercise, school physical education programs, sports, and physical fitness for youth, adults, and the elderly.

POISON CONTROL

Division of Poison Control
Food and Drug Administration
5600 Fishers Lane
Rockville, MD 20857
(301) 443-6261
   Works with the national network of 600 poison control centers to reduce the incidence and severity of acute poisoning. Directs toxic emergency calls to a local poison control center.

PRODUCT SAFETY

U.S. Consumer Product Safety Commission (CPSC)
Washington, DC 20207
(800) 638-8326 (in the District of Columbia)
(800) 492-8363 (in Maryland)
(800) 638-8333 (in Alaska, Hawaii, the Virgin Islands, and Puerto Rico)
(301) 492-6800 (in all other states)

Evaluates the safety of products sold to the public. Provides printed materials on different aspects of consumer product safety on request. Does not answer questions from consumers on drugs, prescriptions, warranties, advertising, repairs, or maintenance.

RAPE

National Rape Information Clearinghouse
5600 Fishers Lane, Room 15-99
Rockville, MD 20857
(301) 443-1910
   Maintains a listing of rape prevention and treatment resources to help people locate services available in their community and to facilitate networking among those working in the field of sexual assault. Has little information for inquiries from the general public and prefers to refer them to local resources.

REHABILITATION

National Rehabilitation Information Center (NARIC)
4407 Eighth Street N.E.
Washington, DC 20017-2299
(202) 635-5822
   Supplies publications and audiovisual materials on rehabilitation and assists in locating information on dates, places, names, addresses, or statistics. The collection includes materials relevant to the rehabilitation of all disability groups.

SMOKING

Office on Smoking and Health
Technical Information Center
Park Building
5600 Fishers Lane, Room 116
Rockville, MD 20857
(301) 443-1575
   Offers bibliographic and reference service to researchers and others and publishes and distributes a number of titles in the field of smoking.

SUDDEN INFANT DEATH SYNDROME (SIDS)

Sudden Infant Death Syndrome Clearinghouse
1555 Wilson Blvd., Suite 600
Rosslyn, VA 22209
(703) 522-0870
   Provides information on SIDS to health professionals and consumers.

CRITERIA FOR EVALUATING THE ELEMENTARY SCHOOL HEALTH PROGRAM

CALIFORNIA STATE DEPARTMENT OF EDUCATION*

Criteria for Evaluating the Elementary School Health Program provides school personnel with a tool to use in making an evaluation of the school health program. The results of such an evaluation reveal the strengths and weaknesses of the program. Where weaknesses are revealed, the school health committee may act to bring all the available forces into action for the express purpose of securing strength in the program where weaknesses exist and for planning ways all other phases of the program may be kept strong.

The criteria are organized into four divisions: I—Administration, II—Health instruction, III—Health services, and IV—Healthful school environment. The criteria are expressed in terms of desirable practices presented in the left column. The evaluation should be made by a representative group of the faculty, including administrators, teachers, and health service personnel. The results should express judgments approved by the evaluation committee as a whole.

Provision is made for the quality of each *provision* or *practice* stated in the criteria to be judged on a four-point scale: *excellent, good, fair,* or *poor*. If the provision is not made, the practice is not followed; or if the quality is fair or poor, there is space for listing changes needed. At the top of each section, space is provided for recording recommended steps to be taken in relation to the changes needed. Care should be taken to make recommendations that will not have an adverse effect on provisions or practices already judged excellent or good.

SUGGESTED PROCEDURE FOR USING THE CRITERIA FOR EVALUATING THE ELEMENTARY SCHOOL HEALTH PROGRAM

1. Determine the membership of study group to evaluate the program.
2. Determine the need for consultant help.
3. Study thoroughly the criteria and the provisions for making the desired evaluations.

---

*Adapted from Criteria for evaluating the elementary school health program, Sacramento, Calif., 1977, California State Department of Education.
Note: Although this instrument was developed more than a decade ago, it remains one of the best models available.

4. Determine whether the program meets each criterion.
5. If the criterion is met, determine the quality of the provision or practice according to the following scale: *excellent*—near perfection; *good*—satisfactory; *fair*—slightly less than satisfactory; *poor*—unsatisfactory.
6. If the criterion is not met—that is, the provision not made or the practice not followed—indicate by a check in the appropriate column.
7. Compile a list of the changes needed and determine how the changes can best be secured.
8. Set up a priority for accomplishing the changes.
9. Develop recommendations for making the needed changes and record in appropriate space at the top of each section.
10. Submit the recommendations to the administration for action.

Criteria for evaluating the elementary school health program

Criteria	Quality of provision or practice					Changes needed
	Excellent (near perfection)	Good (satisfactory)	Fair (slightly less than satisfactory)	Poor (unsatisfactory)	Provision not made or practice not followed	
I. Administration A. The policies of the district's governing board provide for a school health program designed to help all pupils achieve the degree of health their potentialities permit through health instruction, health services, a healthful school environment—essentials of the program.	RECOMMENDED STEPS TO BE TAKEN:					
B. A written statement of the school district's point of view regarding the kind and quality of the school health program is available.	RECOMMENDED STEPS TO BE TAKEN:					
C. Responsibility for planning, developing, and administering the district's school health program is delegated by the governing board of the district to the district superintendent of schools. 1. A health committee with a membership that includes school personnel, representatives of community health services, and representatives of the other important segments of the community is assigned advisory responsibilities for the district's school health program.	RECOMMENDED STEPS TO BE TAKEN:					
D. The principal of the school has outlined the practices that are employed in operating the school health program. 1. A health council or committee with a membership that includes an administrator, teachers, health personnel, and, when possible, counselors, custodians, and school lunch personnel is assigned advisory responsibilities for the school health program.	RECOMMENDED STEPS TO BE TAKEN:					
E. Clerical help, equipment, and supplies, in keeping with the pupil population, are provided for the health services program.	RECOMMENDED STEPS TO BE TAKEN:					
F. Health personnel are adequate in number and specialization to provide needed services. 1. School nurses are available in a ratio of 1 nurse for each 1,000 to 1,400 pupils. (Distances traveled to visit homes and types of terrain should be considered in determining the desired ratio.) 2. Physicians are available for consultation and advice. 3. Dentists are available for consultation and advice.	RECOMMENDED STEPS TO BE TAKEN:					

G. The professional library and the school library are well supplied with health materials.

H. Each classroom is supplied with the materials needed for use in health instruction.
1. The classrooms for each grade are supplied with the basic textbooks in health.
2. Each classroom is supplied with health materials, in addition to adopted textbooks, that cover each phase of health.
3. The scope of the materials in each classroom is sufficient to provide for all the pupils, from the slowest to the fastest learner.

RECOMMENDED STEPS TO BE TAKEN:

I. The in-service education program for school personnel provides for health instruction to have the same emphasis as other areas of instruction.

RECOMMENDED STEPS TO BE TAKEN:

J. The in-service education program for school personnel provides for study of the school health services.

RECOMMENDED STEPS TO BE TAKEN:

II. Health instruction

A. A course of study for health, a course of study and a teacher's guide, or a combination of study and teacher's guide is provided by the school district or the office of the county superintendent of schools for use in the school.

RECOMMENDED STEPS TO BE TAKEN:

B. The course of study contains statements of the purposes of health instruction and the objectives to be sought; an outline of the contents that shows both scope and sequence; units of instruction, lists of materials and sources of materials, and recommended means and procedures for evaluating pupils' progress.
1. The scope of the content for the total program includes the following areas:
   a. Consumer health
   b. Mental-emotional health
   c. Drug use and misuse (including alcohol)
   d. Family health (including human sexuality, masculine and feminine qualities, marriage, and family planning)
   e. Oral health, vision, and hearing
   f. Nutrition
   g. Exercise, rest, and posture
   h. Diseases and disorders
   i. Environmental health hazards (including pollution, radiation hazards, accidents, and first aid)
   j. Community health resources
2. The basic program of health instruction is developed through the use of units devoted primarily to health.

Continued.

Criteria for evaluating the elementary school health program—cont'd

Criteria	Quality of provision or practice					Changes needed
	Excellent (near perfection)	Good (satisfactory)	Fair (slightly less than satisfactory)	Poor (unsatisfactory)	Provision not made or practice not followed	

II. Health instruction—cont'd

RECOMMENDED STEPS TO BE TAKEN:

3. Health instruction is enriched by making it a correlated phase of units in other subjects, such as science, social studies, and homemaking.

4. Pupils' interests and needs are used as motivation for learning.

5. Health instruction is adapted to the pupils' abilities by employing a variety of methods.

6. Instruction is enriched through the use of the up-to-date information that is made available by official and voluntary health agencies and professional associations.

7. Instruction is enriched by the use of up-to-date audiovisual materials, such as films and film strips, charts and pictures, and radio and TV programs.

III. Health services

A. A health services guide is provided by the school district or by the office of the county superintendent of schools.

RECOMMENDED STEPS TO BE TAKEN:

B. A health services committee, preferably a subcommittee of the health council or committee, has advisory responsibility for health services.

RECOMMENDED STEPS TO BE TAKEN:

C. Health services are provided in accordance with the provisions of the guide, provided, however, that the advice of the health services committee is an important consideration in decisions regarding adaptations required to meet special needs of individuals and of the school population.

RECOMMENDED STEPS TO BE TAKEN:

D. The school health services are of sufficient scope to provide school personnel the information and assistance needed to determine status of, protect, and promote the health of pupils.

RECOMMENDED STEPS TO BE TAKEN:

1. Guidance and assistance are provided in securing an appraisal of each pupil's health status.

2. School personnel, pupils, and parents are counseled regarding the results of health appraisals and ways to protect and promote one's health.

3. Procedures designed to help prevent and control disease are established.

4. First aid for the injured and emergency care for cases of sudden illness are provided.

5. School health services are coordinated with those provided by professional health agencies in the community.

		RECOMMENDED STEPS TO BE TAKEN:	

E. School health personnel encourage and guide teacher observation of pupils' health characteristics and accept referrals of pupils whose characteristics are unlike those of the well child.

F. School personnel inform and advise parents regarding medical examinations their children should have and assist in making provision for the medical examinations as necessary.
  1. Parents are advised to have medical examinations for their children before school entrance.
  2. Provision is made for pupils to have medical examinations as required by existing conditions. (Preferably this provision is made in cooperation with the local medical society.)
  3. Procedures are established for the cumulative health record to follow the pupil from grade to grade and school to school.

G. School personnel inform parents of the importance of eye examinations for children before school entrance, maintain a vision screening program, and inform and advise parents regarding eye conditions of their children that require the attention of a specialist.

H. School health personnel provide for all pupils to have group hearing tests at regular intervals, individual tests for pupils discovered with hearing difficulties; inform and advise parents regarding their children's need for examinations by ear specialists; and recommend classroom adjustments for children with hearing difficulties.

I. Health services provide for parents to be informed regarding their children's need for regular dental examinations beginning before the children's entrance to school, and for parents of children who have defective dental conditions to be informed regarding the undesirable effects of the conditions and advised regarding essential treatment.

J. Pupils' growth characteristics are observed to determine deviations in growth patterns that merit special attention.

K. Follow-up procedures are taken as necessary—begin when pupils with health difficulties are identified and conclude when the health difficulties have been corrected or their effects minimized.

L. Health counseling and guidance is provided.

M. Provisions are made for supplying teachers with health information concerning handicapped pupils and for recommending cases for whom home teaching may be necessary.

N. The health services program includes provisions for the prevention and control of communicable diseases.
  1. Parents of preschool children are advised by the school to protect their children as early as possible against communicable diseases for which immunization is available.

Continued.

Criteria for evaluating the elementary school health program—cont'd

Criteria	Quality of provision or practice					Changes needed
	Excellent (near perfection)	Good (satisfactory)	Fair (slightly less than satisfactory)	Poor (unsatisfactory)	Provision not made or practice not followed	
III. Health services—cont'd						
2. School personnel cooperate with representatives of the local health department in planning community immunization programs available to pupils.	RECOMMENDED STEPS TO BE TAKEN:					
3. The school cooperates with local health agencies in conducting a tuberculosis case-finding program for pupils and school personnel.						
O. The health services program provides emergency service for injury, sudden illness, and disasters.	RECOMMENDED STEPS TO BE TAKEN:					
1. Updated written policies and procedures for first aid and emergency care are provided to all school personnel.						
2. The policies and procedures pertaining to first aid and emergency care are approved by the local medical society or the health department.						
3. Phone numbers of parents and of physicians to call in emergencies are on file for each pupil.						
4. Parents are notified immediately in instances of serious injury or illness.						
5. Teachers are prepared to render first aid.						
6. First-aid kits are available in each classroom and in the principal's office.						
IV. Healthful school environment						
A. The school environment is protected by employing personnel whose health is good, requiring all personnel to have regular health examinations, and providing measures that encourage good health practices.	RECOMMENDED STEPS TO BE TAKEN:					
B. A wholesome emotional climate prevails and essential provisions are made for its maintenance.	RECOMMENDED STEPS TO BE TAKEN:					
1. The morale of teachers is at a high level.						
2. The following provisions are made for the maintenance of staff morale at a high level.						
a. Leaves of absence without pay are granted for specified purposes.						
b. Sabbatical leaves for study or travel are granted certificated personnel in accordance with written policies of the district.						

c. Communication is maintained between the administration and teaching personnel.

d. A teamwork approach is used in the prevention and solving of staff problems.

3. The following provisions are employed to create classroom environments that are conducive to learning.

a. The teachers adapt learning experience to each child's developmental pattern of growth and needs.

b. The daily program provides for a balance of quiet and active experiences.

c. Opportunities are provided for each child to release tension by participating in various types of esthetic and physical activities.

d. Teachers discuss required behavior standards with pupils.

e. Pupils share responsibility for securing desired classroom behavior.

f. Discipline and grading procedures are fair and consistent.

g. The teacher-pupil ratio permits the individualization of instruction to the extent required for maximal learning.

4. Pupils are given the following types of opportunities to develop as self-directing individuals:

a. To share responsibility for solving social problems in the school.

b. To assume leadership responsibility through participation in classroom and student government activities.

c. To plan and organize school activities under teacher supervision.

5. Teachers are helped by the principal and special school personnel—the school psychologist, counselors, curriculum consultants, and others—to solve problems that arise in their classes.

6. School personnel and parents are encouraged in the following ways to work cooperatively in solving the problems that are causing pupils to make less than maximum use of their abilities.

RECOMMENDED STEPS TO BE TAKEN:

C. The school food services are conducted so that each pupil has opportunity to have a wholesome and nutritionally adequate lunch in an environment that is pleasant and sanitary; and pupils are helped to learn the importance of good eating habits, eating well-balanced meals, and using good table manners.

1. A Type A lunch, a lunch that meets the nutritional standards of the Type A lunch, or both, are served daily.

2. Lunchroom and kitchen facilities are periodically inspected by sanitarians from the local health department.

RECOMMENDED STEPS TO BE TAKEN:

D. The health service unit provides the required space for each type of activity conducted in the unit and is properly equipped with built-in facilities.

Continued.

Criteria for evaluating the elementary school health program—cont'd

Criteria	Quality of provision or practice					Changes needed
	Excellent (near perfection)	Good (satisfactory)	Fair (slightly less than satisfactory)	Poor (unsatisfactory)	Provision not made or practice not followed	
IV. Healthful school environment—cont'd						
E. The school site meets the standards established for schools as set forth by state law.	RECOMMENDED STEPS TO BE TAKEN:					
1. The school is centrally located in the geographic area served.						
2. The area in which the school is located is relatively free of disturbing noises, noxious odors, and other distractions.						
3. Water drains rapidly from outdoor areas.						
F. A planned procedure is followed to detect and correct possible unsafe conditions of buildings, grounds, and equipment.	RECOMMENDED STEPS TO BE TAKEN:					
G. The buildings and play areas are designed to provide for the successful operation of the school program and are kept in good condition.	RECOMMENDED STEPS TO BE TAKEN:					
1. All doors providing exit from buildings are equipped with panic bars.						
2. Ceilings and walls of classrooms and inside corridors are constructed with sound-absorbing materials.						
3. Areas or rooms in which noise-producing activities, such as band practice and playing games, take place are located at points where noises are likely to be least disturbing to classes held in other areas.						
4. The enrollments in classes assigned to rooms are not in excess of the number of pupils for which the rooms were originally planned.						
H. Essential provisions have been made to secure in each classroom the conditions needed for eye comfort.	RECOMMENDED STEPS TO BE TAKEN:					
1. The lighting in classrooms is soft, even, properly distributed, and sufficiently bright for eye comfort.						
2. The colors of the walls, ceilings, and chalkboards are conducive to eye comfort.						

I. The classrooms and the library are heated or cooled and ventilated as required to provide good working conditions for teachers and pupils.

RECOMMENDED STEPS TO BE TAKEN:

J. Drinking fountains in the building and on the school grounds are sufficient in number, of desirable design, of proper height, conveniently located, and cleaned daily.

1. An adequate number of drinking fountains are available (one for each 75 pupils and at least one on each floor of a multistoried building).

2. The water supply is regularly inspected by health department personnel.

RECOMMENDED STEPS TO BE TAKEN:

K. The handwashing and toilet facilities are sufficient in number and kept clean.

1. The lavatories are readily accessible from classrooms and play areas.

2. Each lavatory contains at least 1 wash basin equipped with hot and cold running water for every 50 pupils using the room.

3. An adequate number of toilets for girls are available (1 for each 30 girls).

4. An adequate number of toilets and urinals are available for boys (1 toilet for each 60 boys, 1 urinal for each 30 boys).

5. A supply of liquid or powdered soap is available near each wash basin.

6. The supply of toilet paper and hand towels is replenished each day at specified intervals.

RECOMMENDED STEPS TO BE TAKEN:

L. Fire prevention equipment is conveniently located and inspected at regular intervals.

1. All school personnel know the location of fire signal switches in the school and of fire alarm boxes near the school.

2. Fire extinguishers are of a type approved by the local fire department and are inspected at regular intervals by fire officials.

RECOMMENDED STEPS TO BE TAKEN:

M. The procedures to be followed in the case of various types of disasters are known by all school personnel and pupils.

1. Written procedures to be followed in times of disaster are displayed in prominent places throughout the school.

2. School personnel and pupils have practices and know the procedure to be followed in case of a fire, an earthquake, or other disaster.

3. Fire drills are held monthly.

4. Drills for disasters other than those that might be caused by fire are held at specified intervals throughout the school year.

RECOMMENDED STEPS TO BE TAKEN:

GENERAL CRITERIA FOR EVALUATING HEALTH INSTRUCTIONAL MATERIALS AND COMPARATIVE TEXT ANALYSIS

GENERAL CRITERIA FOR EVALUATING HEALTH INSTRUCTIONAL MATERIALS*

The following criteria are to help you evaluate health instructional materials. Indicate your judgment by circling the appropriate number. Each item must be rated. A separate evaluating sheet is necessary for each set of materials considered for recommendation.

NOTE: Comments that would add to this evaluation would be appreciated. Please use last page.

EVALUATED BY _____ DATE _____

COMMITTEE _____ SCHOOL _____

Data for materials evaluated:

Author _____
Title _____
Publisher or producer _____
Copyright date _____ Type of material _____
Grade level of material being evaluated _____
Is this material part of a series?   Yes ☐ Series grade level _____
                                       No ☐
Title of series _____
Cost per item _____

*Modified from: Handbook I: Guidelines for the development of instructional materials selection policies, Olympia, Wash., State Office of Public Education.

SUMMARY OF EVALUATION

	High				Low	M*	NA†
I. Text format	5	4	3	2	1	0	0
II. Audiovisual format considerations	5	4	3	2	1	0	0
III. Organization and overall content	5	4	3	2	1	0	0
IV. Bias content	5	4	3	2	1	0	0
V. Teacher's guide	5	4	3	2	1	0	0
VI. Additional support materials	5	4	3	2	1	0	0
VII. Purchase priority	5	4	3	2	1		

I. TEXT FORMAT	High				Low	M	NA
1. General appearance	5	4	3	2	1	0	0
2. Size and color practical for classroom use	5	4	3	2	1	0	0
3. Binding: durability and flexibility	5	4	3	2	1	0	0
4. Quality of paper	5	4	3	2	1	0	0
5. Readability of type	5	4	3	2	1	0	0
6. Appeal of page layouts	5	4	3	2	1	0	0
7. Usefulness of chapter headings	5	4	3	2	1	0	0
8. Appropriateness of illustrations	5	4	3	2	1	0	0
9. Usefulness of references, index, bibilography, appendix	5	4	3	2	1	0	0
10. Consistency of format	5	4	3	2	1	0	0

II. AUDIOVISUAL FORMAT AND CONSIDERATIONS	High				Low	M	NA
1. Sound quality	5	4	3	2	1	0	0
2. Picture quality	5	4	3	2	1	0	0
3. Emotional impact	5	4	3	2	1	0	0
4. Other qualities: vitality, style, imagination	5	4	3	2	1	0	0
5. Authoritative and well-researched, free of propaganda	5	4	3	2	1	0	0
6. Length suitable to audience and content	5	4	3	2	1	0	0
7. Durability	5	4	3	2	1	0	0
8. Usefulness in more than one subject area: write areas here _____	5	4	3	2	1	0	0

_____
_____

III. ORGANIZATION AND OVERALL CONTENT: COVERAGE OF HEALTH AREAS (How comprehensive is the coverage?)	High				Low	M	NA
1. Anatomy and physiology	5	4	3	2	1	0	0
2. Community health (e.g., noise, chemical, water pollution control; community resources)	5	4	3	2	1	0	0
3. Consumer health (e.g., evaluating health products, use of medicines, components of health examinations, health care delivery system)	5	4	3	2	1	0	0

*Missing; material should have had item but does not.
†Not applicable.

Continued.

SUMMARY OF EVALUATION—cont'd

Organization and overall content—cont'd	High				Low	M	NA
4. Disease prevention (e.g., lifestyle and disease; emotional illness; cancer; cardiovascular disorders; immunizations; diseases of interest to ethnic groups; oral health)	5	4	3	2	1	0	0
5. Adult lifestyle (e.g., changing roles; decisions about sex, marriage, and family; careers)	5	4	3	2	1	0	0
6. Fitness (e.g., benefits of fitness, fitness regimen, grooming and self-concept, fatigue, balanced diets, obesity, ethnic foods)	5	4	3	2	1	0	0
7. Growth and development (e.g., reproduction process, prenatal concerns, tools of inheritance, birth defects, genetic counseling, effects of drugs and nutrition on developing embryo and fetus)	5	4	3	2	1	0	0
8. Mental health (e.g., coping skills, stress, human needs and emotions, self-concept, mental illness, psychological growth and development, stereotyping)	5	4	3	2	1	0	0
9. Safety and first aid	5	4	3	2	1	0	0
10. Smoking, drugs, and alcohol (psychoactive drugs, medical use prescription and over-the-counter drugs)	5	4	3	2	1	0	0
11. Nutrition (e.g., basic necessities; balance; metabolism; changing needs; facts, fads, and fallacies; preparation)	5	4	3	2	1	0	0

IV. BIAS CONTENT	High				Low	M	NA
1. Presents more than one viewpoint of controversial issues	5	4	3	2	1	0	0
2. Presents accurate facts when generalizations are made	5	4	3	2	1	0	0
3. Includes all socioeconomic levels and settings and all ethnic groups	5	4	3	2	1	0	0
4. Gives balanced treatment of the past and present	5	4	3	2	1	0	0
5. Promotes the diverse character of our nation by:	5	4	3	2	1	0	0
(a) Presenting the positive nature of cultural differences	5	4	3	2	1	0	0
(b) Using languages and models that treat all human beings with respect, dignity, and seriousness	5	4	3	2	1	0	0
(c) Including characters that help students identify positively with their heritage and culture	5	4	3	2	1	0	0

SUMMARY OF EVALUATION—cont'd

	High				Low	M	NA
(d) Portraying families realistically (one parent, two parents, several generations)	5	4	3	2	1	0	0
(e) Portraying the handicapped realistically	5	4	3	2	1	0	0
6. Includes minorities and women by:	5	4	3	2	1	0	0
(a) Presenting their roles positively but realistically	5	4	3	2	1	0	0
(b) Having their contributions, inventions, or discoveries appear alongside those of white men	5	4	3	2	1	0	0
(c) Depicting them in a variety of occupations and at all levels in a profession	5	4	3	2	1	0	0
(d) Having their work included in materials	5	4	3	2	1	0	0
(e) Presenting information from their perspective	5	4	3	2	1	0	0
(f) Having appropriate illustrations	5	4	3	2	1	0	0

V. TEACHER'S GUIDE FOR TEXTS OR AUDIOVISUAL MATERIALS

	High				Low	M	NA
1. Easy to use	5	4	3	2	1	0	0
2. Answers provided	5	4	3	2	1	0	0
3. Background information	5	4	3	2	1	0	0
4. Teaching strategies	5	4	3	2	1	0	0
5. Ideas for motivation, follow-up, extension	5	4	3	2	1	0	0
6. Guidelines for evaluation	5	4	3	2	1	0	0
7. Inclusion of script	5	4	3	2	1	0	0
8. Bibliography	5	4	3	2	1	0	0

VI. ADDITIONAL SUPPORT MATERIALS THAT ACCOMPANY TEXT

Please list the materials (e.g., workbooks, tests) and use separate form for each one listed

_____

_____

_____

USE THIS SPACE FOR COMMENTS:

COMPARATIVE TEXT ANALYSIS

The following form, entitled "Comparative Text Analysis," is included as an aid for those who may have the opportunity to review numerous texts in the process of selecting one for local adoption. It can also be used to build a case for replacing old health textbooks. Although the format is designed for facilitating comparison of texts, the items are appropriate for evaluating a single text.

Using the following rating scale, evaluate the material in each area identified.

High	. . . .	Low	Missing	Not Applicable
4	3 2	1	0	NA

Fill in *title*, *publisher*, and *copyright date* for each text.

A. *TECHNICAL QUALITY*
   1. General appearance
   2. Readability of type
   3. Quality of paper and binding
   4. Appropriateness of illustrations
   5. Format and general organization
B. *EFFECTIVENESS OF MATERIAL*
   1. Adapts to individual needs and interests
   2. Has appropriate sequential development
   3. Provides varied teaching and learning strategies
   4. Provides for measuring student achievement
   5. Provides management system for tracking student progress
   6. Provides clearly organized teacher edition
C. *CONTENT*
   1. Consistent with district, program, and course goals
   2. Reflects respect for personal worth
   3. Aids in building positive attitudes and understandings
   4. Depicts cultural diversity
   5. Deals effectively with issues and problems
   6. Offers accurate and realistic treatment of subject
   7. Incorporates balanced viewpoints
   8. Makes provision for distinguishing between fact and opinion
   9. Stimulates critical thinking
D. *CRITERIA FOR SEX BIAS*
   1. Material divides qualities such as leadership, imagination, intelligence, and courage approximately evenly between male and female characters.
   2. Females and males are equally represented as central characters in story and illustrative materials.
   3. Both men and women are shown performing similar work in related fields.
   4. Males and females are shown working together.
   5. People are referred to by their own names and roles as often as they are referred to as someone's spouse, parent, or sibling.
   6. Stereotyping language such as "women chatting"/"men discussing" is avoided.

Fill in *title, publisher,* and *copyright date* for each text.

7. Biographical or historical materials include a variety of male and female contributions to society.
8. Both males and females are given credit for discoveries and contributions to social, artistic, and scientific fields.
9. Groups that may include both males and females are referred to in "neutral" language such as people, mail carriers, fire fighters, or legislators.

E. *CRITERIA FOR RACIAL/ETHNIC BIAS*
   1. Materials contain racial/ethnic balance in main characters and in illustrations.
   2. Oversimplifications and generalizations about racial groups are avoided in illustrations and in text material.
   3. Minority characters are shown in a variety of lifestyles in active, decision-making, and leadership roles.
   4. The vocabulary of racism is avoided.
   5. Minority characters are given credit for discoveries and contributions to social, artistic, and scientific fields.

Using the following rating scale, evaluate the material in each area identified.

High . . . . *Low*	*Missing*	*Not Applicable*
4 3 2 1	0	NA

SUMMARY INFORMATION

Fill in *title, publisher,* and *copyright date* for each text.

List total points for each area by Publisher and Title.
A. TECHNICAL QUALITY
B. EFFECTIVENESS OF MATERIAL
C. CONTENT
D. SEX BIAS
E. RACIAL/ETHNIC BIAS

Grand total scores

Additional rationale for selection of these materials: _____

_____

_____

SIGNS AND SYMPTOMS OF HEALTH DEFECTS AND ILLNESSES

Point of observation	Physical signs	Behavior	Complaints
General appearance and behavior	Excessive thinness; excessive overweight; very small or very large in body build for age; pallor; weary expression; poor posture; dark circles under or puffiness of eyes; unusual gait or limp; uncleanliness; lethargic and unresponsive; facial tic	Acts tired or apathetic; is easily irritated; makes frequent trips to toilet; has persistent-nervous habits, such as muscular twitching or biting of nails or lips; is subject to spasms (fits), fainting spells, or frequent nosebleeds; gets short of breath after mild exertion and climbing stairs; lacks appetite; vomits frequently; has frequent accidents	Feels tired; does not want to play; has aches or pains; feels sick to stomach; feels dizzy
Hair and scalp	Stringy, lusterless hair; small bald spots; crusty sores on scalp; nits in hair	Scratches head frequently	Head itches
Ears	Discharge from ears; cotton in ear; tired, strained expression long before day is over; watchful, sometimes bewildered expression	Is persistently inattentive; asks to have questions repeated; habitually fails to respond when questioned; mispronounces common words; cocks one ear toward speaker; fails to follow directions	Has earache; has buzzing or ringing in ears; ears feel stuffy; hears noises in head
Eyes	Inflamed or watery eyes; frequent styes; red-rimmed, encrusted, swollen lids; crossed eye; recurring styes; sensitivity to light	Holds book too close to, or too far from, eyes; squints at book or blackboard; persistently rubs or blinks eyes; reads poorly; attempts to brush away blur; tilts head to one side; tends to reverse words or syllables; tends to lose place on page; shuts or covers one eye; unable to see distant things clearly	Headaches; dizziness; nausea; eyes ache, itch, smart, or feel scratchy; cannot see well (blurred or double vision); sensitivity to light
Mouth and teeth	Cavities in teeth; excessive stains; tartar at necks of teeth; malocclusion (uneven bite); irregular teeth; bleeding or inflamed gums; swollen jaw; sores in mouth; cracking of lips at corners of mouth	Acts depressed or resentful if many missing teeth or severe malocclusion subjects him or her to teasing or adverse comments from other children; this behavior is especially likely to occur in adolescence	Has toothache; mouth or gums feel sore

Point of observation	Physical signs	Behavior	Complaints
Nose and throat (upper respiratory tract)	Frequent or long-continued colds; persistent nasal discharge; persistent mouth breathing; enlarged glands in neck	Is often absent from school because of a cold; constantly clears throat or has frequent coughing or sneezing spells; is always sniffling or blowing nose; breathes persistently through mouth	Throat feels sore or scratchy; has difficulty in swallowing; nose feels stuffy or sore
Skin	Rashes or inflamed skin areas; scales and crusts; persistent sores, pimples, and blackheads on face; boils; hives; persistent warts; accidental injuries, such as cuts, scratches, bruises, burns, blisters; dry, red, rough skin	Is always scratching; is subject to skin irritations (hives, eczema, puzzling rashes, etc), which suggest sensitivity to one or more substances (allergic manifestations); is easily bruised	Skin itches or burns; is concerned about pimples, blackheads, and other skin conditions that affect personal appearance

Condition	Signs and symptoms	
Allergy	Stuffy and runny nose; sneezing; persistent cough; swollen eyelids; rash; itching; watery and burning eyes; paleness; mouth breathing	Tired and listless, recurrent headaches, recurrent gastrointestinal cramps, vomiting, diarrhea
Cancer	Leukemia; tires easily; irritable, pale (anemic), recurrent and serious infections, prolonged bleeding from injuries	Brain tumors; irritability, fatigability, decreased appetite and activity, intermittent headache
Child abuse	Bruises, untreated sores, burns, skin injuries; wears long-sleeved shirts or blouses to hide bruises, etc.	Hungry for affection, difficulty relating to others, displays behavioral extremes—timid/fearless, passive/aggressive; undiagnosed learning problems
Child neglect	No one to look after child, inadequate home management; need for health services—dental care, eyeglasses, immunizations	Malnutrition—underweight, fatigue, lack of muscle tone; no breakfast, food, or lunch money
Contagious diseases of childhood	Chill or chilliness; fever (flushed face, lassitude, malaise); sore or scratchy throat; red, watery eyes; watery nasal discharge	Tight, dry cough; sneezing; headache, earache, or aching in back or legs; nausea or vomiting
Diabetes	Constant urination, abnormal thirst, unusual hunger	Rapid loss of weight, irritability, obvious weakness and fatigue, nausea and vomiting
Diabetic insulin reaction*	Excessive hunger, perspiration, pallor, headache, dizziness, nervousness—trembling, confusion, crying	Irritability, drowsiness, fatigue, blurred vision, poor coordination, abdominal pain or nausea
Drug misuse and abuse	Physical: possible odor on breath and clothes; mouth and nose irritations; red, watery eyes; fingers with burns from smoking; poor appetite or weight loss; distraction of time and sense of perception; needle marks and scars on body; appearance of intoxication; dryness of mouth and nose	Behavior: changes in attendance, discipline and academic performance; display of unusual degrees of activity and excitement; display of unusual inactivity—moodiness, depression; deterioration of physical appearance and concern for health habits; unpredictable outbreaks of temper and flare-ups
Epilepsy	Dazed look, loss of consciousness	Tremors of any or all groups of muscles, odd gestures or movements (e.g., chewing or lip-smacking), occasional loss of muscle control (involuntary urination)
Heart problems	Pale, blue lips; short of breath on rest or exertion; undersized, deformed chest	Rapid pulse at rest, clubbed fingers, easily fatigued, undernourished, fainting after exertion or excitement

*Give sugar immediately in form of sugar, fruit juice, carbonated beverages, or candy.

Continued.

Condition	Signs and symptoms	
Hyperkinesis	Extreme overactivity, inattentiveness, impulsiveness, emotional explosiveness, short attention span, failure to progress in school at expected rate	Restless, oscillating mood swings, fidgeting, difficulty in sitting still, clumsiness, aggressive behavior, low frustration level
Lead poisoning	Fatigue, lethargy, stomach pains, constipation, vomiting, anemia, irritability	Temper tantrums, severe headaches, unsteady walking, insomnia, convulsions, loss of coordination, poor appetite or paleness; may be no symptoms
Nutrition	General appearance: fatigue slouch or posture; round shoulders or flabby muscles; excessively thin with spindly legs; lack of or finicky appetite; fails to gain weight steadily; excessively fat or poor distribution of fat; strained and worried look; listless and inactive or high-strung and overactive; easily fatigued and possibly irritable and difficult to manage Hair: dry, coarse, brittle, lacking luster, dull	Eyes: tiny red line (engorged capillaries) extending around or across the cornea and inward toward pupil; dark circles under eyes; inflammation and crusting of lids Teeth and gums: decayed teeth; swollen, bleeding, or spongy gums; or abnormal color Tongue: beefy red and magenta Mouth: scarring, fissuring, or sores on angles of lips Skin: small nodules (like gooseflesh) or scaly and rough Chest, knees, legs and feet: pigeon-breasted, knock-kneed, bow-legged, flatfooted—abnormal bone growth
Posture	Head tilted to side when reading or listening Head tilted forward when sitting, standing or walking Feet pointed inward or outward; stands with weight on inner ankles (pronated); drage or scuffles feet	Shoulders not level: one higher, lower, or forward Round shoulders with protruding shoulder blades One hip higher or more prominent Knees pointed inward (knock-kneed), outward or hyperextended (bowlegs)
Rheumatic fever	Failure to gain weight, or loss in weight; pallor; irritability	Poor appetite, repeated colds and sore throats, unexplained nosebleeds, muscle or joint pains
Sexually transmitted diseases	Syphilis: Within 10 to 90 days—small sore (chancre) at site where germs entered body tissue 6 weeks to 6 months—rash on palms or soles of feet; falling hair; ugly sores on body, in mouth, under arms, between legs or toes Herpes simplex: Blisters on genitalia, sometimes on buttocks and thighs	Gonorrhea: Within 3 to 8 days in males—burning sensation on urination, pus from urethra; in females—no pain, male signs may not appear until serious damage to bodily organs occurs Nongonococcal urethritis (NGU): pain on urination
Sickle cell anemia	Pain in arms and legs, swelling in joints, loss of appetite	Weakness, pain in abdomen, jaundice
Social-emotional maladjustment	Overtimidity: withdrawing, crying easily Overaggressiveness: bullying, quarreling, boisterousness; cruel behavior Excessive daydreaming: persistent inattentiveness Extreme sensitiveness to criticism: cries easily, temper tantrums Difficulty in reading or reciting Failure to advance in school at normal rate despite good physical health and adequate intellectual capacity Stuttering or other forms of speech difficulty	Excess boasting or showing off Poor sportsmanship Undue restlessness: hyperactivity, habit tics, stammering, nail biting Frequent accidents or near accidents Poor coordination Abnormal sex behavior Unhappy and depressed Gradual deterioration or marked sudden drop in educational achievement Lack of interest or motivation Withdrawal, shyness, inferiority feelings

Condition	Signs and symptoms	
	Lying, stealing, cheating, truancy	Intense ambition, especially if inconsistent with potential
	Resistance to authority: constant complaints of unfairness, "picked on," may engage in vandalism	Inconsistent bladder or bowel control
		Constantly seeking attention or popularity
"Strep" sore throat	Fever, difficulty in swallowing, swollen neck glands	
Suicidal melancholia	Sudden shift in quality of work; excess use of drugs and alcohol; changes in early behavior and learning patterns; extreme fatigue; boredom; decreased appetite; inability to concentrate; truancy; gives away prized possessions	Open signs of mental illness—delusions, hallucinations; distress signals—"Notice me; I need help; you'll be sorry when I'm dead"
Tuberculosis	Persistent cough, blood in sputum, nervousness, lack of energy, easy fatigability, fever	Loss of weight, chest pain, rapid pulse, night sweats or afternoon fever, pallor, feeling of tiredness

GOOD HEALTH CHARACTERISTICS OF CHILDREN

Physical	Social-emotional	Work habits
Endurance: completes a task without undue fatigue	Enthusiastic	Attentive
Enjoys vigorous play	Objective interests: friends, hobbies, games, work, people	Carries a task through to completion
Alert, buoyant, pleasant	Curious: interested in a variety of things	Ability to concentrate
Looks refreshed in morning	Enters into activities	Persistent in work
Assumes good posture	Happy, cheerful, agreeable, friendly	Works independently
Posture expresses buoyancy, alertness, success, happiness	Refrains from quarreling	Orderly in work habits
Prompt, efficient muscular coordination	Confident: expects success, meets failure	Shows originality and initiative
Poise: freedom from unnecessary activity	Shares group responsibility	Creative
Muscles firm	Protects others' property	Takes responsibility
Hair: natural luster	Appreciation and understanding for others	Prompt in meeting appointments
Clear skin, clear bright eyes, clean, neat in appearance, inoffensive breath, wholesome appetite	Does things for the group, not for self alone	Responds quickly and cheerfully to directions
	Shows courage in meeting difficulties	Shares group responsibility
	Cooperative with peers	Cooperative with peers
	Adapts to new situations	
	Exercises emotional control	

Growth and Development Characteristics

Physical development	Characteristics	Health education implications
	3 to 5 years of age	
Growth continues at moderately rapid rate	Needs vigorous outdoor activity	Rest and sleep; adequate amounts needed; provide rest periods
Permanent body build evident	Becoming more independent; doing things for self; needs freedom	Dental health: emphasis on food selection and care of teeth
Head and upper body reach adult proportions	Needs to learn to get along with others, to share, to take turns	Emotional health: needs attention, freedom, and learning to share and get along; provide restraints with love and care
Legs and arms lengthening	Temper tantrums less likely; may begin to call names, "I don't like you"; much quarreling, hitting, fighting	
Bone growth proceeding and cartilage almost completely replaced by bone		Nutrition: emphasis on adequate diet and amounts of food; needs protein, minerals, and vitamins
Girls ahead of boys in skeletal development; usually lighter and shorter than boys	Learns through play; crayons, blocks, large pencils	Sex education: answer questions with simple understandings
Height and weight gradually increasing	Language development increases; understands words; can give simple reasons and explanations; can absorb much information; asks questions	Safety: provide concern for school and playground accident prevention
Primary teeth usually developed		
Heart rate, respiration, and blood pressure usually stable	Can play longer without fatigue	Exercise: allow for vigorous play involving large muscle activities; small muscle coordination not developed
Large muscle weight increasing; boys with more muscle tissue than girls; girls more fatty tissue	Begins to identify own sex; asks why mothers and fathers are different	
Brain at 90% of adult weight	Responds when treated as individual	
	More self-reliant; can wash and dress self; attention hard to hold	
	5 to 7 years of age	
Growth is relatively slow: at age 7 may be 2 to 3 inches and 3 to 6 pounds yearly	On entering school may be a resumption of earlier tensional behavior; thumbsucking, nail biting, toilet lapses	Mental health:
		Wants to get along with peers
Large muscles better developed than small ones; improving by age 7	Eager to learn, exuberant, restless; exaggerates, overactive, and susceptible to fatigue; dawdling may occur	Praise, warmth, and patience with independence and encouraging support from adults
Some postural defects may have been established by age of 6		Some responsibilities without pressure of being required to make decisions or meet rigid standards
Hand-eye coordination is incomplete; 90% are right-handed; small muscle control difficult, especially of fingers and hands	Criticism difficult; thrives on encouragement	Help make adjustments in playground; withdrawn child needs encouragement to find place in group
Eyeballs are still increasing in size; tendency toward farsightedness	Attention span short but increasing; interested in activity, not results; learns best through active participation	
Heart is in a period of rapid growth		Provide sense of accomplishment for each child; engage in real tasks; needs freedom
Permanent teeth begin to appear;	Has difficulty making decisions	

Continued.

479

Physical development	Characteristics	Health education implications
	5 to 7 years of age—cont'd	
baby teeth begin to be lost Susceptible to respiratory infections; childhood diseases (measles, mumps, chickenpox, etc.), rheumatic fever Lungs relatively small Tires easily Teeth: 6-year molars appearing and loss of primary teeth	Self-assertive; aggressive; wants to be first; becoming self-dependent; can take care of own toilet needs and dressing; likes to climb and jump; by 7 is apt to be talkative and prone to exaggeration; competition developing Interest of boys and girls diverging, less play together; gets along best in small groups Able to assume some responsibility concerning right and wrong and simple tasks; acts grown up at times Bright eyes, color in face, great vitality Enjoys rhythms, active play, fairy tales, comics, TV, myths, dramatic play and stories Moods fluctuate; quick resistance to bathing	Provide active participation in learning with concrete objects Exercise and safety: active, boisterous games for large muscles; stress safety Vision care: protect eyes Sleep and rest: need 11 or more hours of sleep and possibly daytime naps Dental health: emphasis on tooth care Disease control: development of personal hygiene; cover coughs, sneezes, fingers away from mouth, washing hands, and others
	8 to 10 years of age	

Growth still slow and steady; some children reach plateau preceding growth of preadolescence; differences in individual bone ossification may vary as much as 5 to 6 years; girls' growth spurts at about 10 years
Small muscles developing; manipulative skill increasing
Poor posture may develop; presence may indicate attention; chronic infection, fatigue, orthopedic difficulties, emotional maladjustment, etc.
Hand-eye coordination improved; hands ready for crafts
Eyes ready for both nearsightedness and farsightedness; nearsightedness may develop during eighth year
Incisors and lower bicuspids appear; often a period of dental neglect; orthodontia may be necessary
Internal changes in glands and body structure taking place; wide range in beginning of sexual maturity; period of rapid growth comes earlier for girls, it lasts longer in boys:
Boys: beginning puberty cycle 10 to 13 years; ends 14 to 18½ years
Girls: appearance of menstruation 10 to 16 years; average 12 years
Lungs and digestive and circulatory systems still developing
	Wants to do well but loses interest if discouraged or pressured; sensitive to criticism
	Gangs strong and of one sex only, of short duration and changing membership; response to structured groups and activities
	Allegiance to peers instead of adult in case of conflict; wants a "best friend"
	Capable of prolonged interest; often makes plans and goes ahead on his or her own; increased attention span; realism replacing fantasy
	Enjoys conforming to rules of game, testing his or her skill against perfection; can be fairly responsible and dependable
	Gaining self-control; conscience becoming strong; awareness of self-energy
	Fairly good eater; may neglect vegetables
	Decisive, responsible, dependable, reasonable, strong sense of right and wrong; much arguing over fairness of games
	Is untidy, deliberately throws over table manners, handwashing, hair combing; protests parents' choice of new clothes; general coolness toward all adults
	Is prone to accidents
	Health usually good; has much energy
	Fond of sports and games, collections, comics, adventure stories
		Mental health:
		  Self-concept; values
		  Needs friends and group membership
		  Training in skills without pressure
		  Wise guidance and channeling of interests rather than domination or overcritical standards
		  Praise, encouragement; warmth from adults
		  Help gain self-confidence by excelling in one thing
		  Definite responsibility; reasonable explanations; no talking down
		Exercise:
		  Activities involving use of whole body; sports and games
		  Posture development in need of attention
		Sleep and rest: 10 to 12 hours sleep
		Nutrition: balanced intake of foods
		Dental health: care of teeth reemphasis
		Disease control: handwashing, hair washing, food washing, etc.
		Safety: accident prevention
		Sex education: growth and developmental changes

Physical development	Characteristics	Health education implications
	11 to 13 years of age	
A "resting period" followed by a period of rapid growth in height, then weight; usually starts somewhere between 9 and 13 years; girls usually taller and heavier at 11 years than boys	Wide range of individual differences and maturity level	Mental health:
	Gangs or groups important; prestige is more important than adult approval; gang interest is changing to interest in one or two best friends (girls more than boys)	Self-image; success experiences
Rapid muscular growth; uneven growth of different parts of body; awkwardness prevalent; posture may be slovenly	Loves parents but does not show it, cool toward adults	Warm affection, approval, no nagging or condemnation
		Increase opportunities for independence
Secondary sex characteristics beginning to develop; may cause embarrassment; in girls hip and breast development; in boys voice changes	Strong sense of responsibility about matters thought to be important	Relations with others
	Girls mature earlier than boys; girls are taller, heavier	Sense of belonging and peer group relations
		Values development
Heart developing; blood pressure may fall; more rest is needed	Strong interest in sex, much teasing and antagonism between boy and girl groups; sex consciousness may cause self-consciousness and shyness	Individual health and emotional counseling
Permanent dentition of 28 teeth is completed by 13 to 14 years		Nutrition: adequate diet importance
Resistance to infection may be low	Child approaching adolescence often becomes hypercritical, changeable, rebellious, uncooperative; exhibits extremes of conduct from independence to childish dependence; may rebel against rules	Rest and sleep: 9 to 11 hours of sleep
		Exercise: sports and games, both individual and team
	Interest in activities to earn money	Dental health: care of teeth
	Reading differences in ability and tastes apparent	Safety: accident prevention and first aid
	Ravenous but finicky appetite may develop	Disease control: acne especially
	May be overanxious about own health and normalcy	Sex education:
	Competition is keen; development of coordination and skills through games	Physical and social changes
		Boy-girl relations
	Awkwardness and laziness common because of rapid and uneven growth; may need rest	Sexually transmitted diseases
		Reproduction

INDEX